CRC SERIES IN MEDICINAL CHEMISTRY

Series Editor-in-Chief

Matthew Verderame
Professor of Medicinal Chemistry
Head, Department of Chemical and
Physical Sciences
Albany College of Pharmacy
Albany, New York

Handbook of Chemotherapeutic Agents (Volumes I and II)

Handbook of CNS Agents and Local Anesthetics

Handbook of Autonomic Drugs and Autacoids

Handbook of Cardiovascular and Anti-Inflammatory Agents

CRC
Handbook of Hormones, Vitamins, and Radiopaques

Editor

Matthew Verderame, Ph.D.

Professor of Medicinal Chemistry
Head, Department of Chemical and Physical Sciences
Albany College of Pharmacy
Albany, New York

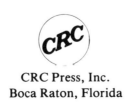

CRC Press, Inc.
Boca Raton, Florida

Library of Congress Cataloging-in-Publication Data
Main entry under title:

Handbook of hormones, vitamins, and radiopaques.

  Includes bibliographies and index.
  1. Hormones—Handbooks, manuals, etc.   2. Vitamins—
Handbooks, manuals, etc.   3. Contrast media—Handbooks,
manuals, etc.   I. Verderame, Matthew.   [DNLM:
1. Contrast Media.   2. Hormones.   3. Vitamins.
WK 102 H236]
QP571.H34   1986   615'.36   85-19500
ISBN 0-8493-3291-5

DEDICATION

To my typist and companion and the mother of our four children — Fran.

PREFACE

Handbook of Hormones, Vitamins, and Radiopaques is a companion to five other handbooks in this pharmaceutically related set published by CRC Press. The titles of the other five follow: **Handbook of Chemotherapeutic Agents** (Volumes I and II); **Handbook of CNS Agents and Local Anesthetics; Handbook of Autonomic Agonists and Antagonists and Autacoids;** and **Handbook of Cardiovascular and Anti-Inflammatory Agents**.

The six handbook represent a systematic collection of selective chemical and pharmacological reference data on drugs drawn from the major categories of therapeutically important agents. For the principal classes of drugs, or for individual drugs which do not belong to a particular class, the following topics are addressed: *Mechanism of Action, Structure-Activity Relationships, Pharmacokinetics, Uses and Dosage, Toxicity* (including *Drug Interactions*), and *Physical-Chemical and Other Data*. Drug metabolism data are heavily emphasized in the pharmacokinetics sections. The term "toxicity" is used broadly to also include side effects. Generally included in the physical chemical and other data sections is such information on the drug as the chemical name, formula, melting point, pKa value(s), solubility and stability data, physical description, salt forms, and any other property deemed worthy of inclusion.

Other topics generally considered include historical aspects leading to or associated with the development of the class of drugs, possible causes of the condition or disease state for which the drugs are used, life cycles of organisms against which the chemotherapeutic agents are used, testing methods employed in the screening of potentially useful compounds, and review articles covering the fields. Chemical syntheses are not emphasized. However, this topic received significant attention in a few chapters. Figures are used appropriately to illustrate a point or concept, especially in the mechanism of action sections.

In this series of reviews, emphasis is placed on the most useful drugs associated with each physiological class or disease entity. The monograph format is used extensively, not only to donote the most useful members, but also to provide a close examination of these agents. Comparative pharmacological or therapeutic data on the principal drugs within the classes provide additional, practical information.

Monographs of drugs with useful multiple functions are appropriately placed in more than one chapter and cross referenced. Though necessitating some repetition of data, these monographs generally complement each other and maintain a continuity of thought and application.

Newer and/or experimental drugs have also been included to round out the coverage and to present current knowledge and possible future trends.

This set of reference books should have appeal and utility for the practioners and students of medicinal chemistry, pharmacology, pharmacy and medicine. It should also be useful to researchers in the pharmaceutical industry and in other allied health professions.

A special debt of gratitude is extended to the many contributors who labored long and diligently to prepare their manuscripts for publication. Also, for their counsel and cooperation, the dedicated assistance of the Advisory Board is acknowledged with sincere appreciation.

The editorial assistance of the CRC staff and, in particular, the coordinating efforts of Ms. Amy Skallerup must not go unmentioned.

Finally, it is our hope that the reader will find these first edition handbooks interesting, useful, and valuable. Comments for improvement will be gratefully received.

Matthew Verderame, Ph.D.
Albany, New York
Editor

THE EDITOR

Matthew Verderame, Ph.D., is Professor of Medicinal Chemistry and Head of the Department of Physical Sciences at the Albany College of Pharmacy, Union University. Dr. Verderame received his undergraduate education at the University of Connecticut, where he received an M.S. degree in Pharmacy in 1952 and the Ph.D. degree in 1955 in Pharmaceutical Chemistry. In 1954, he joined the faculty at the Albany College of Pharmacy as an Assist Professor and moved through the ranks to his present position. Dr. Verderame's education was enhanced by his attendance of NSF-sponsored institutes at the University of North Carolina in 1962, Michigan State University in 1964, Duke University in 1969, and State University of New York in Albany in 1974. From 1955 through 1968, Dr. Verderame received consecutive year-long research grants from the Sterling-Winthrop Research Institute. In 1968 and again in 1973, he was cited for his contributions to teaching by receiving the Lederle Award. Courses which he regularly teaches include Medicinal Chemistry, Qualitative Organic Analysis, and Drug Analysis. The principal areas of synthetic research of Dr. Verderame include the preparation of various derivatives of cystein, methionine, and piperazine as possible anti-infective agents. He also synthesized organo tin compounds and ether derivatives of cyclic hydrocarbons as possible anti-infective agents. He has authored several publications. Dr. Verderame is a member of the American Chemical Society, Rho Chi, Sigma Xi, Phi Sigma, Rho Pi Phi, the American Association for the Advancement of Sciences, the New York Academy of Sciences, and the American Association of University Professors.

CONTRIBUTORS

Thomas T. Andersen, Ph.D.
Assistant Professor
Department of Biochemistry
Albany Medical College of Union
 University
Albany, New York

Robert W. Brueggemeier
Assistant Professor of Medicinal
 Chemistry and Pharmacognosy
College of Pharmacy
Ohio State University
Columbus, Ohio

James A. Dias, Ph.D.
Assistant Professor
Department of Biochemistry
Albany Medical College of Union
 University
Albany, New York

D. Ellis, Ph.D.
Senior Biochemist
Smith Kline and French Research, Ltd.
Welwyn, England

John C. Emmett
Head, Medicinal Chemistry II
Smith Kline and French Research, Ltd.
Welwyn, England

Richard A. Ferrari, Ph.D.
Group Leader in Pharmacology
Department of Pharmacology
Sterling-Winthrop Research Institute
Rensselaer, New York

Paul W. Fletcher, Ph.D.
Assistant Professor
Department of Biochemistry
Albany Medical College of Union
 University
Albany, New York

Edmund J. Hengesh, Ph.D.
Professor of
 Pharmaceutical Chemistry
School of Pharmacy
Ferris State College
Big Rapids, Michigan

M. Margaret King, Ph.D.
Assistant Member
Biomembrane Research Program
Oklahoma Medical Research Foundation
and
Associate Professor in Research
 Biochemistry
Department of Biochemistry and
 Molecular Biology
Health Sciences Center
Oklahoma City, Oklahoma

Paul D. Lesson
Section Leader
Merck Sharp & Dohone Research Labs
Neuroscience Research Centre
Harlow, England

Robert A Mararian, Ph.D.
Professor of Medicinal Chemistry
College of Pharmacy
Univeristy of Oklahoma
Health Sciences Center
Oklahoma City, Oklahoma

J. Thomas Pento, Ph.D.
Professor of
 Pharmacodynamics and Toxicology
College of Pharmacy
University of Oklahoma
Health Sciences Center
and
Adjunct Professor of Pharmacology
School of Medicine
Health Science Center
Oklahoma City, Oklahoma

Leo E. Reichert, Jr., Ph.D.
Professor and Chairman
Department of Biochemistry
Albany Medical College of Union
 University
Albany, New York

Patrick M. Sluss, Ph.D.
Assistant Professor
Department of Biochemistry
Albany Medical College of Union
 University
Albany, New York

David D. Shaw, Ph.D.
Clinical Project Director
Sterling-Winthrop Research Institute
Rensselaer, New York

Anthony H. Underwood
Head of Pharmacological Biochemistry
Smith, Kline and French Research, Ltd.
Welwyn, England

TABLE OF CONTENTS

ANDROGENS, ANABOLICS, AND ANTIANDROGENS

Robert W. Brueggemeier

INTRODUCTION AND HISTORICAL PERSPECTIVE

The class of steroid hormones which is responsible for the primary and secondary sex characteristics of the male are called androgens. The hormone testosterone (1) is the predominant circulating androgen and is produced mainly

testosterone (1)

by the testes. This steroid and other endogenous androgens not only affect the development and maturation of the male genitalia and sex glands but also influence other tissues such as kidney, liver, and brain. In addition, androgens exert general growth-promoting properties on various skeletal muscles; these general responses are referred to as anabolic effects. This report will discuss the endogenous androgens, synthetic analogs, various anabolic agents, and the antiandrogens, with a focus on those synthetic preparations currently available. More extensive presentations of the topic of androgens and anabolic agents have appeared in several recently published books.[1-7]

The role of the testes in the development and maintenance of the male sex characteristics and the dramatic physiological effects of castration have been recognized for many years. The elucidation of the molecules responsible for these actions has only occurred in the last 50 years. In 1931, the first androgen was isolated in a very small amount from human urine and was named androsterone (2) by the chemist Butenandt.[8,9] Dehydroepiandrosterone (3) was the second androgenic molecule isolated from human urine in 1934. Because of the central role of the testes in male physiology, research efforts concentrated on isolation of the active testicular component, and in 1935 the hormone testosterone was isolated in crystalline form from testicular extracts by Laqueur et al.[10] The structure and chemical synthesis was quickly confirmed.[11,12]

androsterone (2)   dehydroepiandrosterone (3)

Until 1968, testosterone was thought to be the active form of the endogenous androgens in man. At that time two independent research laboratories demonstrated that the testosterone molecule was converted in target tissues such as prostate and seminal vesicles to 5α-dihydrotestosterone (DHT, 4).[13,14] A soluble receptor protein was later demonstrated to bind specifically to DHT and was necessary for the hormone's actions in the target tissues.

5α-dihydrotestosterone (**4**)

The androgens also exert an anabolic effect, with this increased retention of nitrogen in the body and increased protein synthesis first being demonstrated in 1935 in animals[15] and in 1938 in humans.[16] The majority of chemical, biological, and clinical efforts associated with the androgens have focused on the general anabolic effects of these steroids.

TESTOSTERONE

Physiological Roles

The hormone testosterone affects many organs in the body. Its most dramatic effects are observed on the primary and secondary sex characteristics of the male. These actions are first manifested in the developing male fetus when the embryonic testis begins to secrete testosterone. Differentiation of the Wolffian ducts into the vas deferens, seminal vesicles, and epididymis occurs under this early influence of testosterone, as does the initiation of the development of external genitalia and the prostate.[17] Testosterone also influences the steroid metabolic patterns of the liver in the developing male fetus.[18]

At puberty further development of the sex organs (prostate, penis, seminal vesicles, and vas deferens) is again evident and under the control of androgens. Additionally, the testes now begin to produce mature spermatozoa. Other effects of testosterone, particularly on the secondary sex characteristics, are observed. Hair growth on the face, arms, legs, and chest is stimulated. The larynx develops and a deepening of the voice occurs. The male's skin at puberty thickens and the sebaceous glands proliferate. General body growth is initiated, including increased muscle mass and protein synthesis, a loss of subcutaneous fat, and increased skeletal maturation and mineralization. these latter effects reflect the anabolic actions of testosterone. Finally, testosterone influences the sexual behavior, mood, and aggressiveness of the male from the time of puberty.

Biosynthesis

The major site of the biosynthesis of androgens is the testis, but various androgens can also be synthesized and secreted by other endocrine organs such as the adrenal gland and the ovary. Testosterone is the principal circulating androgen and is secreted by the Leydig cell of the testis. The steroid dehydroepiandrosterone, secreted by the adrenal gland and the ovarian androgen androstenedione (**5**) can be readily converted to testosterone in peripheral tissues and increase circulating levels of testosterone.

androstenedione (**5**)

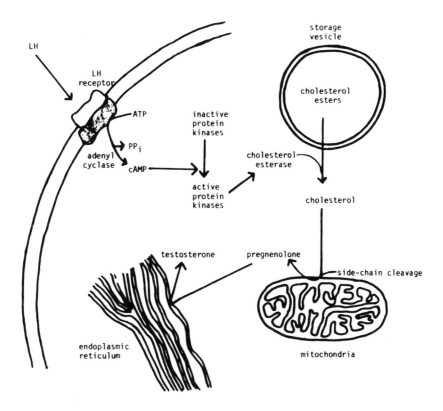

FIGURE 1. Cellular events of steroidogenesis. (From Counsell, R. E. and Brueggemeier, R.W., *Burger's Medicinal Chemistry, Part II,* 4th ed., Wolff, M. E., Ed., John Wiley & Sons, New York, 1979, 873. With permission.)

The biosynthesis of testosterone in the testis is under the regulation of the gonadotropin luteinizing hormone (LH), which is also referred to as interstitial cell-stimulating hormone (ICSH). The other pituitary gonadotropin, follicle stimulating hormone (FSH), acts on the germinal epithelium and is important for sperm development. The secretion of these pituitary hormones is, in turn, regulated by circulating testosterone levels in a negative feedback mechanism. This feedback mechanism in the male is not as well understood as that for the gonadotropins in the female. Recent research suggests that the regulation of gonadotropin release in the male is related to the presence of aromatizable androgens such as testosterone in the circulation.[19]

The biochemical events of steroidogenesis in the Leydig cell are analogous to those that occur in other steroid-producing endocrine tissues[20,21] and are summarized in Figure 1. LH initiates the events by binding to a membrane-bound receptor on the outer surface of the Leydig cell. This hormone-receptor interaction activates adenylate cyclase located on the inside of the cell membrane, which in turn converts ATP to cAMP. The intracellular concentration of cAMP is increased and results in an activation of certain protein kinases. This cascade mechanism results in the conversion of an inactive cholesterol esterase to the active form. Consequently, cholesterol esters are converted to free cholesterol. The cholesterol is then translocated to the mitochondria and converted by a mixed-function oxidase to pregnenolone. Finally pregnenolone is converted to testosterone by several enzymatic transformations.

The rate-limiting step of the biosynthesis of the steroid hormones is the conversion of cholesterol to pregnenolone the enzymatic reaction referred to as the cholesterol side-chain cleavage reaction. This transformation requires molecular oxygen and NADPH and is cat-

cholesterol (6)

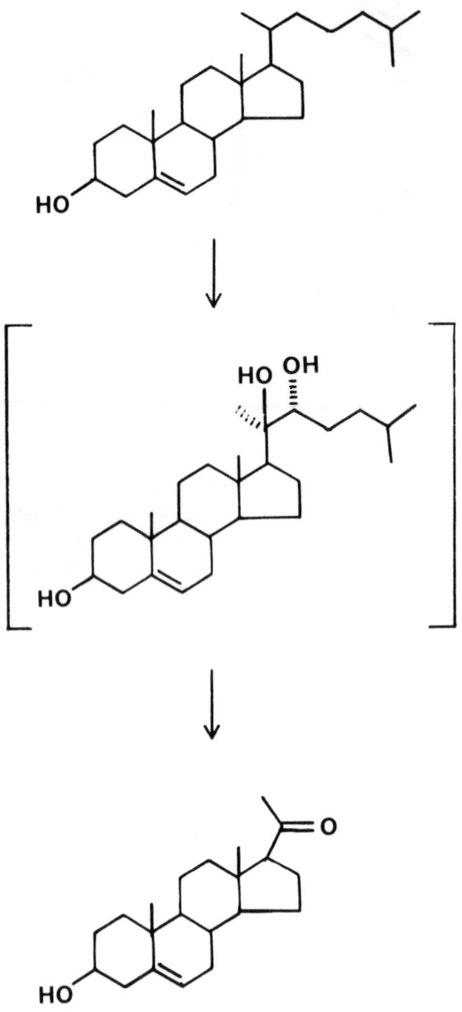

20R, 22R-diol (7)

pregnenolone (8)

FIGURE 2.   Cholesterol side chain cleavage reaction.

alyzed by a cytochrome P450 enzyme complex. The proposed mechanism for this conversion is oxidation at C-20 and C-22 to yield the intermediate 20R,22R-diol (Figure 2). A third oxidation results in the cleavage of the bond between C-20 and C-22 to produce pregnenolone. A series of enzymatic conversions follow in the smooth endoplasmic reticulum of the cell leading to the formation of testosterone from pregnenolone. Two interconverting pathways have been described for this biosynthesis, the ''4-ene'' and the ''5-ene'' pathways. The ''5-ene'' pathway, with the intermediate dehydroepiandrosterone, is the preferred route of the biosynthesis and thus the more important one.[22] The critical enzymes in these conversions are 17α-hydroxylase, C_{17}-C_{20}-lyase, the 3β-hydroxysteroid dehydrogenase and $\Delta^{4,5}$-isomerase complex, and 17β-hydroxysteroid dehydrogenase; the biosynthetic scheme is shown in Figure 3.

Metabolism

For decades, the primary function of metabolism was thought to be the inactivation of testosterone and the mechanism for the excretion of the steroid in the urine. However, the identification of metabolites of testosterone formed in the peripheral tissues and the potent and sometimes different biological activities of these products emphasized the importance

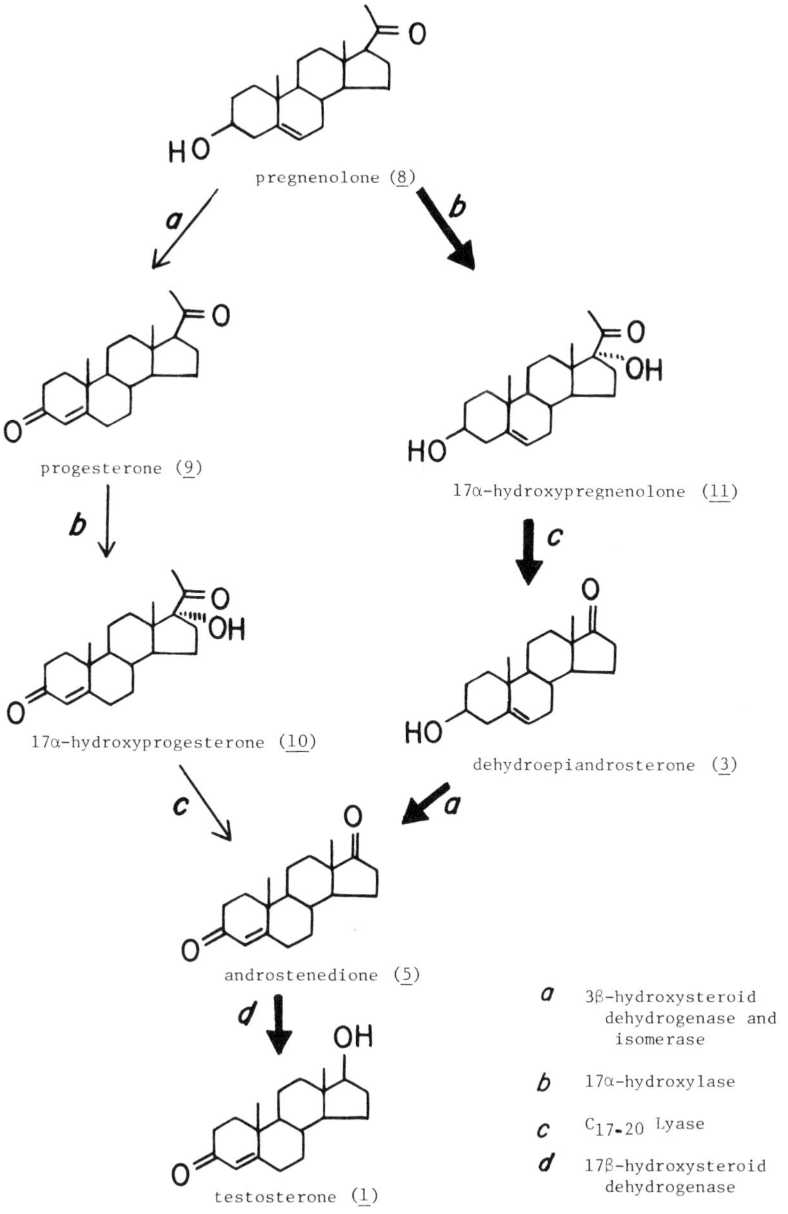

FIGURE 3. Enzymatic conversion of pregnenolone to testosterone.

of the metabolic transformations of androgens in endocrinology. Two active metabolites of testosterone have received considerable attention — the reductive metabolite dihydrotestosterone and the oxidative metabolite estradiol. The biological importance of these steroids will be discussed in greater detail in the following section on mechanism of action of testosterone.

The general pathways for in vivo and in vitro testosterone metabolism have been extensively reviewed.[23-27] The principal liver metabolites in man arise from the actions of 3α-, 3β-, and 17α-hydroxysteroid dehydrogenases and 5α and 5β-reductases, providing the numerous compounds shown in Figure 4. Testosterone metabolism has also been examined in prostatic tissues and similar transformation patterns are observed. The primary metabolites

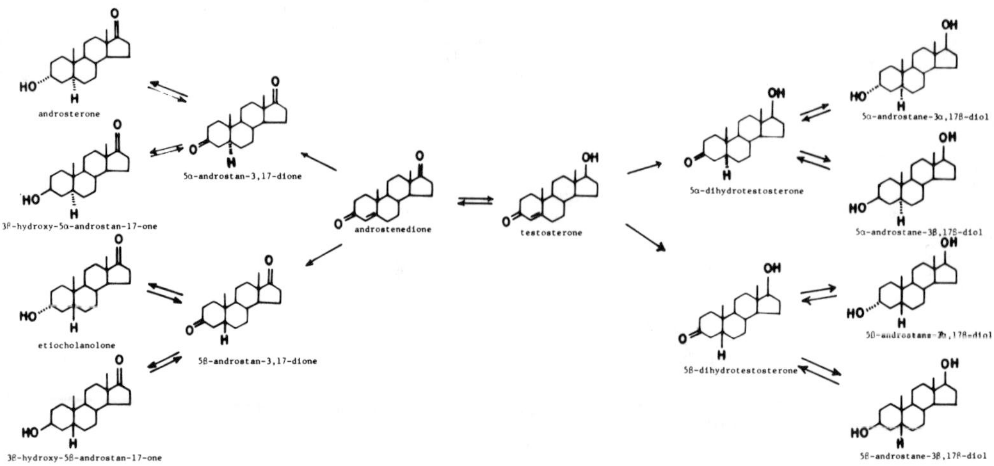

FIGURE 4.   Reductive metabolites of testosterone.

present in the urine are androsterone **2** and etiocholanolone **13,** both excreted as glucuronide and sulfate conjugates.

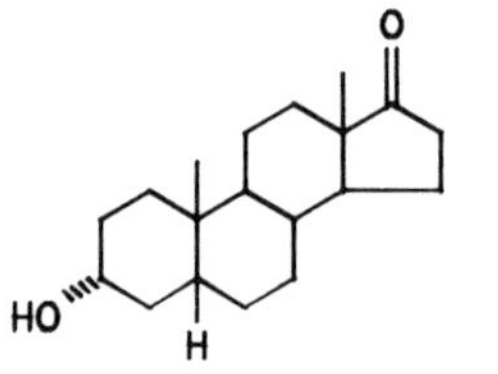

etiocholanolone (**13**)

   The conversion of testosterone to 5α-dihydrotestosterone by 5α-reductase in androgen target tissues serves as a major step in the mechanism of action of the hormone. This enzyme is present in both the microsomal fraction and the nuclear membrane of the cell.[28] The irreversible enzymatic reaction requires NADPH as the cofactor, which provides the hydrogen for carbon-5.[29] The 5α-reductase from rat ventral prostrate tissues exhibits a broad range of substrate specificity for various C_{19} and C_{21} steroids;[26] this is also observed in inhibition studies.[30] In addition, testosterone and DHT both influence the levels of 5α-reductase in target cells.[31] The full extent of the regulation of this important ezyme in androgen-sensitive tissues remains to be elucidated.

   The conversion of testosterone and androstenedione to estrogens is another metabolic transformation that leads to an active hormone. The enzymatic activity has been termed aromatase and was first identified by Ryan[32] in the microsomal fraction from human placental tissue. This cytochrome P450 enzyme complex requires 3 mol of NADPH and 3 mol of molecular oxygen to convert 1 mol of androgen to estrogen. The currently proposed mechanism for aromatization is shown in Figure 5 and involves the formation of 19-hydroxyandrostenedione **14** and 19-*gem*-diol **15** from the first two oxidations. The third oxidation has been proposed to involve the oxidation of the carbon at the 3 position, giving 2β-hydroxy-19-oxoandrostenedione **16**.[32] Substrate specificity studies have aided in examining the structural requirements of the active site,[34-36] as have various inhibitor studies. 4-Hydroxyandrostenedione[37-39] and several 7α-substituted androstenedione derivatives[40,41] are among the most potent inhibitors of aromatase.

   Examinations of the metabolic transformations of androgens in the brain have been ex-

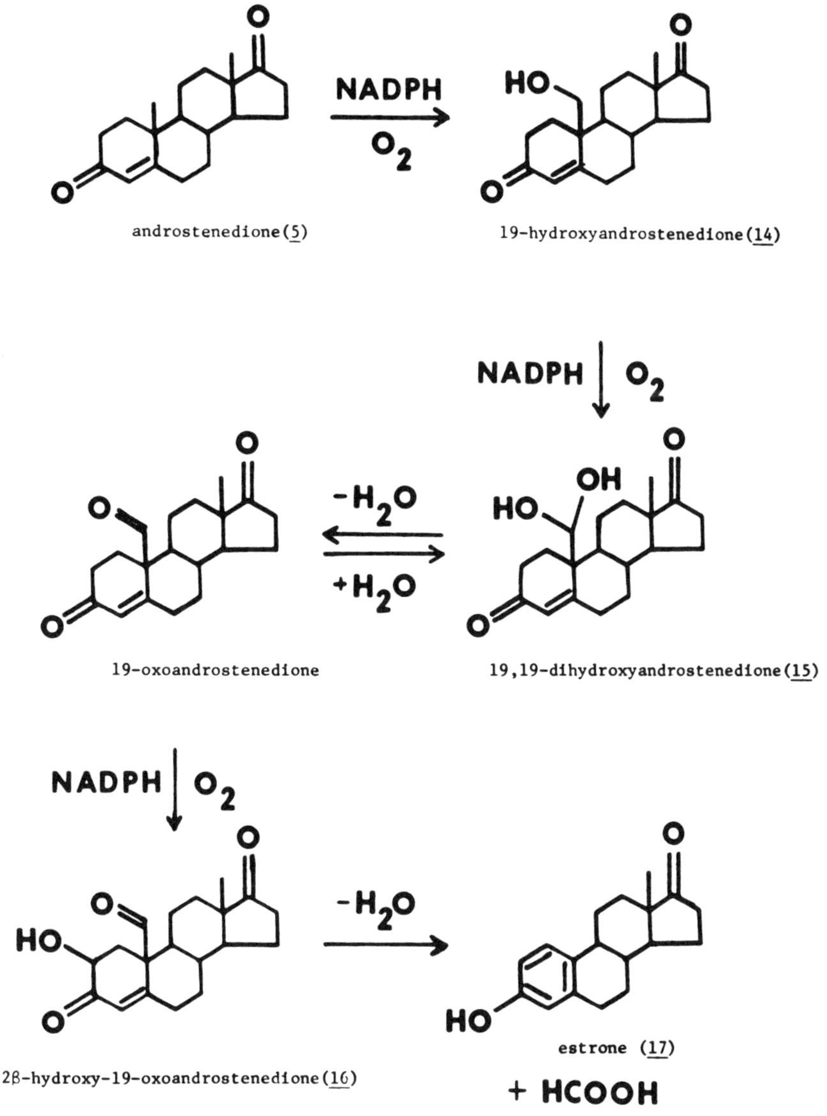

FIGURE 5.   Aromatization.

tensive in the past 2 decades. Testosterone can be converted to DHT, androstenedione, 5α-androstane-3,17-dione, and 5α-androstane-3β,17β-diol in brain tissues.[41–46] These reduced androgens can influence the release of hypothalamic and pituitary hormones.[47] Aromatase activity is also present in neuroendocrine tissues and the conversion of androgens to estrogens in these tissues may explain some of the CNS actions on regulation of gonadotropin release and on sexual behavior.[48] Further research efforts on both 5α-reductase and aromatase activities in neuroendocrine tissues will provide additional information and probe the significance of these metabolic pathways in endocrinology.

Mechanism of Action

Considerable evidence has been gathered over the past 2 decades on the mechanism by which androgens exert their effects on certain biological tissues. The androgens act through regulation of protein synthesis in target cells via the formation of a steroid-receptor complex.

A Mechanism of Action of Testosterone

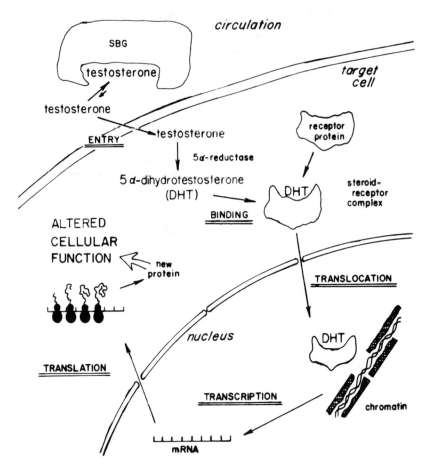

FIGURE 6.   Mechanism of action of testosterone in prostatic tissue. (From Counsell, R.E. and Brueggemeier, R. W., *Burger's Medicinal Chemistry,* Part II, 4th Ed., Wolff, M. E., Ed., John Wiley & Sons, New York, 1979, 873. With permission.)

Extensive reviews on the mechanism of androgen action and the similar mechanisms of the other steroid hormones have appeared.[49-54]

The current concept of the mechanism of action of testosterone in target cells evolved from studies employing rat ventral prostate (Figure 6). Testosterone was found to be rapidly converted to DHT in target tissues, and furthermore DHT was the androgen selectively retained.[55,56] Thus, the proposed mechanism of action of testosterone begins by the conversion of testosterone to DHT by 5α-reductase. Present in the cytosol of prostate cells are proteins that bind DHT with extremely high affinity and specificity.[57] Following the formation of this DHT-receptor complex, a conformational change or activation occurs, triggering the translocation of the steroid-receptor complex into the nucleus of the cell. The nuclear steroid-receptor complex then interacts with the chromatin present in the target cell and results in the increased production of messenger RNA (mRNA).[58-60] The exact events that occur in the nucleus of the cell are not fully understood. Finally, the elevated levels of mRNA lead to an increase in protein synthesis and subsequent stimulation of cell growth and differentiation.

The mechanism of action of androgens in other tissues also involves the formation and translocation of a steroid-receptor complex. Androgen receptors have been identified in other tissues such as seminal vesicles,[61,62] testis,[63,64] epididymis,[63,65] kidney,[66] brain,[67–69] liver,[70] and androgen-sensitive tumors.[71,72] However, DHT is not the only functioning form of androgen in other androgen-sensitive tissues. DHT is rapidly biosynthesized in tissues like prostate but it is not readily formed in certain other tissues such as kidney. The dog prostate specifically binds 5α-androstane 3α,17α-diol with a cytosolic receptor protein,[73] thus, also demonstrating the species variation as well as a different functioning androgen. Less research emphasis focused on the mechanism of anabolic action of the androgens. Testosterone has greater activity than DHT in the androgen-mediated growth of muscle both in vivo and in tissue culture.[74–76] Cytosolic receptor proteins specific for testosterone have also been identified in muscle tissues.[77–83] Thus, the involvement of specific receptor proteins, their translocation into the nucleus, and the resulting increase in protein synthesis are the common mechanisms of action of the androgens in a variety of target tissues.

SYNTHETIC ANDROGENS

Clinical Uses and Bioassays

The primary use of synthetic androgens is the treatment of disorders of testicular function and of cases with decreased testosterone production. Several types of clinical conditions result from testicular dysfunction. Information on the biochemistry and mechanism of action of testosterone that has accumulated over the past 20 years has greatly aided in the elucidation of the underlying pathophysiology of these diseases. Two recent reviews describe in greater detail the mechanisms involved in disorders of testicular function and androgen resistance.[84,85]

Hypogonadism arises from the inability of the testis to secrete androgens and can be caused by various conditions. These hypogonadal diseases can, in many cases, result in disturbances in sexual differentiation and function and/or sterility. Primary hypogonadism is the result of a basic disorder in the testes, while secondary hypogonadism results from the failure of pituitary and/or hypothalamic release of gonadotropins and thus, diminished stimulation of the testis. Usually primary hypogonadism is not recognized in early childhood (with the exception of cryptorchidism) until the expected time of puberty. This testosterone deficiency is corrected by androgen treatment for several months, at which time the testes are evaluated for possible development. Long-term therapy is necessary if complete testicular failure is present. Patients with Klinefelter's syndrome, a disease in which a genetic male has an extra X chromosome, have low testosterone levels and can also be treated by androgen replacement.

Male pseudohermaphroditism include disorders in which genetically normal men do not undergo normal male development. One type, testicular feminization, is observed in patients which have normal male XY chromosomes, but the male genitalia and accessory sex glands do not develop. Rather, the patients have female external genitalia. These patients are unresponsive to androgens and have defective androgen receptors.[86–88] Another type of male pseudohermaphroditism results from a deficiency of the enzyme 5α-reductase.[89,90] Since DHT is necessary for early differentiation and development, the patients again develop female genitalia; later, some masculinization can occur at the time of puberty due to elevated testosterone levels in the blood. A third disorder is Reifenstein syndrome, an incomplete pseudohermaphroditism. In these patients, the androgen levels are normal, 5α-reductase is present, and elevated LH levels are found. Partially deficient androgen receptors are present in these patients.[86,88] In most cases of male pseudohermaphroditism androgen replacement has little or no effect and thus, steroid treatment is not recommended.

Deficiencies of circulating gonodotropins lead to secondary hypogonadism. This condition can be caused by disorders of the pituitary and/or hypothalamus resulting in diminished secretions of neurohormones. The lack of stimulation of the seminiferous tubules and the Leydig cells due to the low levels of these neurohormones decreases androgen production.

Drugs such as the neuroleptic phenothiazines and the stimulant marihuana can also interfere with release of gonadotropins. The use of androgens in secondary hypogonadism is symptomatic.

Synthetic androgens have also been used in women for the treatment of endometriosis, abnormal uterine bleeding, and menopausal symptoms. However, their utility is severely limited by the virilizing side effects of those agents. Two weak androgens, calusterone and 1-dehydrotestolactone, are used clinically in the treatment of mammary carcinoma in women. The mode of action of these drugs in the treatment of breast cancer is unknown, and is not simply related to their androgenicity.[91] More recent evidence on the ability of these compounds to inhibit estrogen biosynthesis catalyzed by aromatase suggests that they effectively lower estrogen levels in vivo.[92]

Bioassays for determining androgenic properties examined the ability of the synthesized steroid to either increase the weight of accessory sex glands like the prostate and seminal vesicles in rats or increase in the growth of the comb of the capon rooster.[93] In vitro evaluation of the relative affinity of potential androgens for the androgen receptor has also become important in assessing biological activity.[94,95]

Structure-Activity Relationships

The natural hormone testosterone is ineffective as an androgen when given orally and has a short duration of action when administered parenterally because of rapid hepatic metabolism. Synthetic androgens were prepared to provide orally active compounds or medicinal agents which would have a prolonged action. In addition, synthetic efforts focused on the separation of androgenic effects of the hormone from the anabolic properties. This section will deal with those agents which retain the androgenic effects, while those with anabolic activity will be discussed in a later section.

Examination of the biological activity of testosterone and its precursors and metabolites provides information of the biologically important regions of the molecule. These steroids with a 3-ketone have greater activity than the reduced 3-hydroxyl metabolites. On the other hand, the 17β-hydroxy steroids have greater androgenic properties than the 17-ketone analogs. Reduction of the 4,5-double bond to 5α-DHT, as discussed earlier, enhances the affinity of the C_{19} molecule, whereas 5β-reduced metabolites are inactive androgens. Thus, the A/B trans ring juncture and the 3-keto functionality are necessary for androgenicity, with a 17β-hydroxyl moiety enhancing the biological activities of C_{19} steroids.

Early modifications of the testosterone molecule were designed to increase the oral activity of the agents. Alkylation of the 17α-position produced the compound 17α-methyltestosterone (**18**) and conferred oral activity on the compounds. However, increasing the length of the alkyl chain led only to a decrease in activity.[96] Preparation of the 17β-esters of testosterone was found to greatly prolong the duration of androgenic effects. This modification enhances the lipid solubility of the steroid and, after injection, permits a local depot effect. The propionate, enanthate, and cypionate esters of testosterone are available (**19, 20, 21**).

17α-methyltestosterone (**18**)

esters of testosterone

Other synthetic compounds which retain androgenic activity include the 1-dehydro isomer of DHT (**22**),[97] and several halogenated analogs. 4-Chlorotestosterone (**23**) has androgenic activity and has been tested

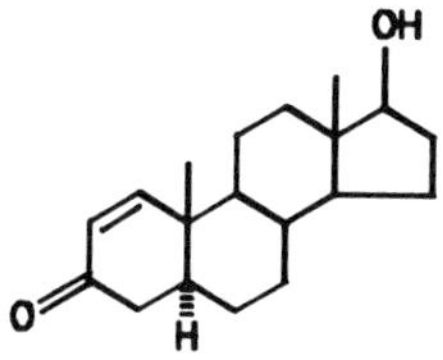

DHT (**22**)

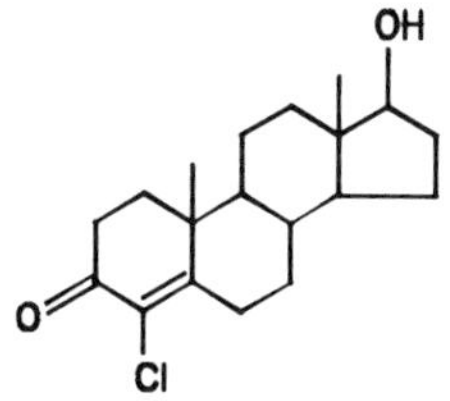

4-chlorotestosterone (**23**)

clinically for its efficacy.[98] The introduction of a 9α-fluoro and 11β-hydroxy substitutents (analogous to synthetic glucocorticoids) gives the compound halotestin (**24**), which is an orally active androgen.

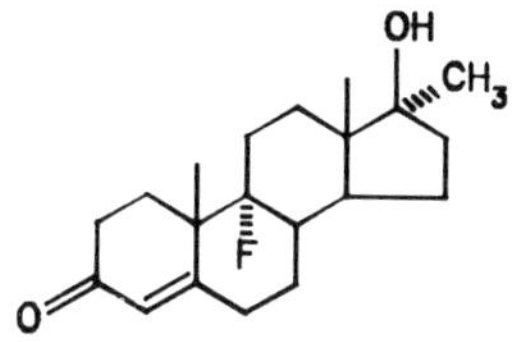

halotestin (**24**)

Several synthetic steroids having weak androgenic activity are being utilized in patients. Calusterone (**25**) and 1-dehydrotestolactone (Teslac, **26**) are agents used in the treatment of advanced metastatic breast cancer.[99–101]

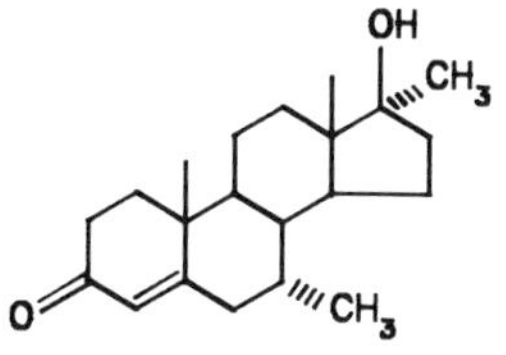

calusterone (**25**)

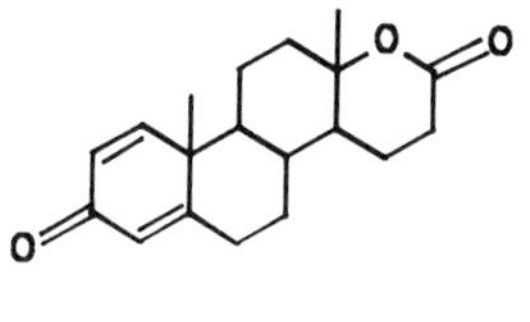

Teslac (**26**)

The introduction of a fused isoxazole ring at positions 2 and 3 of the steroid nucleus of a 17α-ethinyl testosterone produced the compound marketed under the tradename of Danazol (**27**).[102] This agent exhibits only weak androgenic activity but selectively inhibits the release of gonadotropins from the

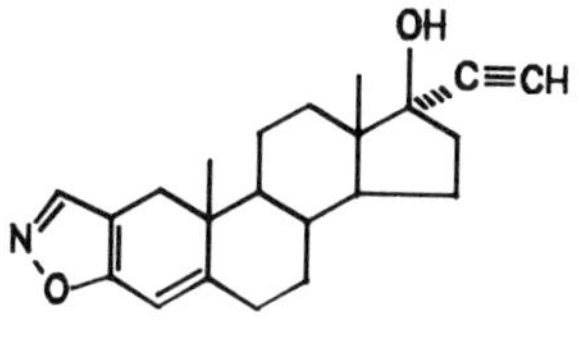

Danazol (**27**)

pituitary. The regulation of reproduction with this agent is promising. Finally, similar modifications of the testosterone nucleus have resulted in agents with increased anabolic activity, which will be discussed in a later section.

Pharmacokinetics

Numerous factors are involved in the absorption, distribution, and metabolism of the synthetic androgens and the physicochemical properties of these steroids greatly influence the pharmacokinetic parameters. The lipid solubility of a synthetic steroid is an important factor in its intestinal absorption. The acetate ester of testosterone demonstrated enhanced absorption from the gastrointestinal tract over both testosterone and 17α-methyltestosterone.[103] Injected solutions of testosterone in oil result in the rapid absorption of the hormone from the injection site; however, rapid metabolism greatly decreases the biological effects of the injected testosterone. The esters of testosterone are much more nonpolar and, when injected intramuscularly, are absorbed more slowly. As a result, the commercial preparations of testosterone propionate are administered every 2 or 3 days. Increasing the size of the ester functionality enables the testosterone esters such as the ethanate or cypionate to be given in a depot injection lasting 2 to 4 weeks.

Once absorbed, the steroids are transported in the circulation primarily in a protein-bound complex. Testosterone and other androgens are reversibly associated with certain plasma proteins and the unbound fraction can be absorbed into target cells to exert its action. A plasma protein termed sex steroid binding globulin (SBG) or testosterone-estradiol binding globulin (TEBG) has a very high affinity for the endogenous steroid.[104,105] This plasma protein functions not only to transport testosterone or estradiol in the bloodstream but also to serve as a storage reservoir for the hormone and to protect testosterone from metabolic inactivation. SBG contains high affinity, low capacity binding sites with a dissociation constant of approximately $1 \times 10^{-9} M$.[106] The structure-binding relationships of the natural and synthetic androgens to SBG have been extensively investigated.[107-114] A 17α-hydroxyl group is essential for binding and the presence of a 17α-substituent such as the 17α-methyl moiety decreases its affinity. The 5α-reduced androgens bind with the highest affinity. A much smaller quantity of the androgen is bound to other plasma proteins, principally albumin and corticosteroid-binding globulin or transcortin (CBG).

The metabolism of the synthetic androgens is similar to that of testosterone. The introduction of the 17α-methyl group greatly retards the metabolism, thus providing oral activity. Reduction of the 4-en-3-one system in synthetic androgens to give the various α- and β-isomers occurs in vivo.[115-117] Finally, aromatization of the A ring can also occur.[34,35,118]

Toxicities

The use of androgens in women and children can often result in virilizing or masculinizing side effects. In boys an acceleration of the sexual maturation is seen, while in girls and women growth of facial hair and deepening of the voice can be observed.[119,120] These effects are reversible when medication is stopped; however, prolonged treatment can produce effects that are irreversible. Inhibition of gonadotropin secretion by the pituitary can also occur in patients receiving androgens.

Both males and females experience salt and water retention resulting in edema. This edema can be treated by either maintaining a low-salt diet or by using diuretic agents. Liver problems are also encountered with some of the synthetic androgens. Clinical jaundice and cholestasis can develop after the use of the 17α-alkylated products.[121-124] Various clinical laboratory tests for hepatic function such as bilirubin concentrations, sulfobromophthalein retention, and glutamate transaminase and alkaline phosphatase activities are affected by these androgen analogs.

Table 1 is a compilation of the names, structures, chemical data, biological activity, and dosage forms of the synthetic androgens.

Table 1
ANDROGENS

Structure and chemical name	Generic name	Trade Names	Chemical data	Biological data		Dosage forms
				Relative androgenicity	Relative androgen receptor affinity	
17β-hydroxyandrost-4-en-3-one	Testosterone	Android-T Malestrone Oreton	mol wt = 288.41 mp = 155°C λ_{max} = 240 nm	1.0	1.0	Aqueous suspension (25, 50, and 100 mg/mℓ)
	Testosterone acetate	Primotest Virosterone Aceto-sterandryl	E = 15,800 mol wt = 330.44 mp = 140—141°C	—	—	Pellets (75 mg)
R = CH₃ R = CH₂CH₃	Testosterone propionate	Aceto-testoviron Perandrone A Oreton Perandren Sterandryl Testoviron	mol wt = 344.48 mp = 118—122°C	—	—	Tablets (10 mg) Oily solution (25, 50, and 100 mg/mℓ)

Table 1
ANDROGENS (continued)

Structure and chemical name	Generic name	Trade Names	Chemical data	Biological data		Dosage forms
				Relative androgenicity	Relative androgen receptor affinity	
$R = CH_2(CH_2)_4CH_3$	Testosterone enanthate	Androtardyl Delatestryl Testoenant	mol wt = 400.48 mp = 36—37.5°C	—	—	Oily solution (100 and 200 mg/mℓ)
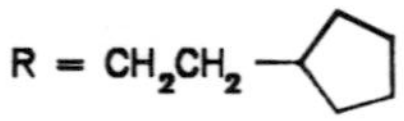 $R = CH_2CH_2-$	Testosterone cypionate	Depo-testosterone	mol wt = 412.59 mp = 101—102°C	—	—	Oily solution (50, 100, or 200 mg/mℓ)
Dihydrotestosterone and esters	Dihydrotestosterone Androstanolone Stanolone	Anaboleen Anabolex Apeton Protona	mol wt = 290.43 mp = 181°C	2.0	1.4	
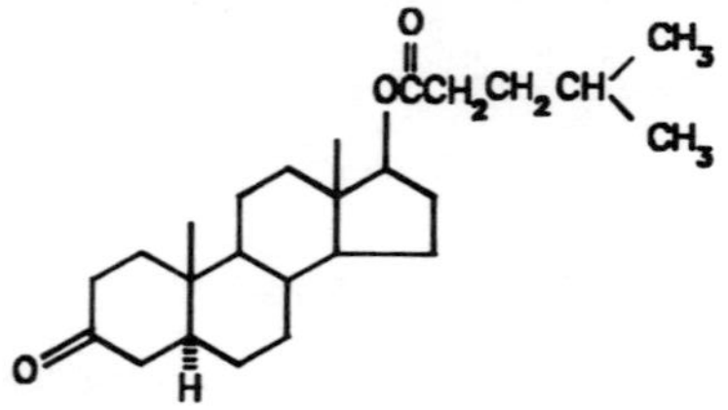 17β-hydroxy-5α-androstan-3-one	Dihydrotestosterone valerianate	Apeton Depot	mol wt = 388.4	—		

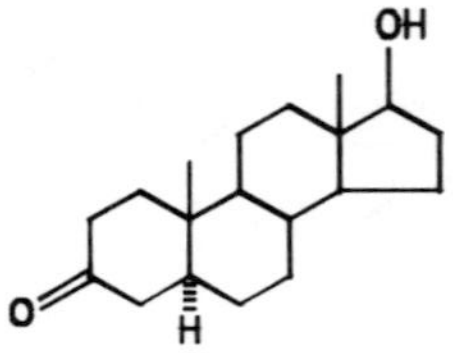

Testosterone derivatives

Chemical name	Generic name	Trade/other names	Physical data			Dosage forms
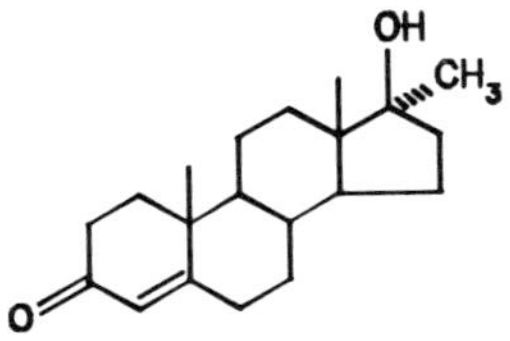 17β-hydroxy-17α-methylandrost-4-en-3-one	Methyltestosterone	Anertan, Android, Metandren	mol wt = 302.44, mp = 161—166°C	3.0	1.5	Tablets (5, 10, and 25 mg) Capsules (10 mg)
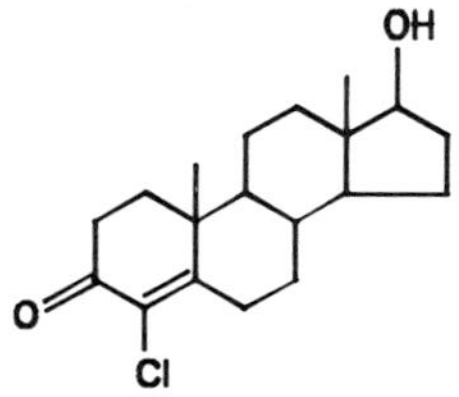 4-chloro-17β-hydroxyandrost-4-en-3-one	Chlorotestosterone, Clostebol	Oreton Methyl, Testoviron, Steranabol	mol wt = 322.89, mp = 188—190°C, λ$_{max}$ = 256 nm, E = 13,500	0.4		
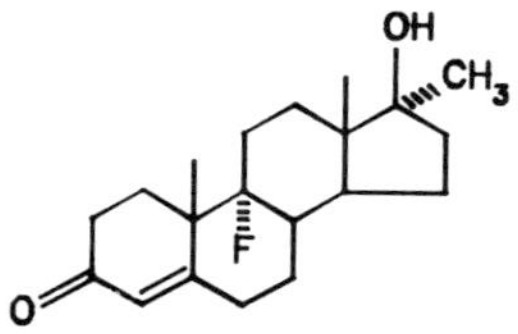 9α-fluoro-11β,17β-dihydroxy-17α-methylandrost-4-en-3-one	Fluoroxymesterone	Androfluorene, Fluotestin, Halotestin, Oratestin, Ultandren	mol wt = 366.45, mp = 270°C (dec), λ$_{max}$ = 240 nm, E = 16,700	11.0		Tablets (2, 5, and 10 mg)

Table 1 (continued)
ANDROGENS

Structure and chemical name	Generic name	Trade Names	Chemical data	Biological data		Dosage forms
				Relative androgenicity	Relative androgen receptor affinity	
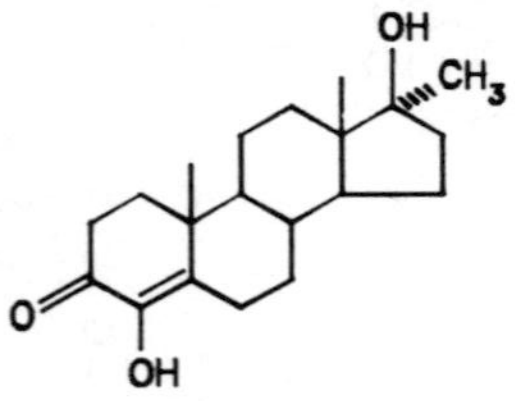 4,17β-dihydroxy-17α-methyl-androst-4-en-3-one	Oxymesterone	Oranabol Sanaboral Theranabol	mol wt = 318.44 mp = 169—171°C λ_{max} = 278 nm	1.5		
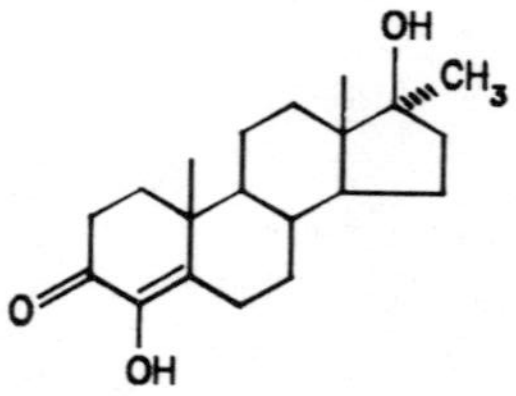 7α,17α-dimethyl-17β-hydroxyandrost-4-en-3-one	Bolasterone	Myagen	mol wt = 316.49 mp = 163—165°C	0.6	0.3	

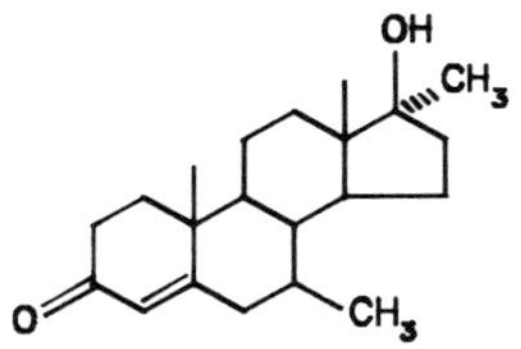

7β,17α-dimethyl-17β-hydroxyandrost-4-en-3-one

Miscellaneous Androgens

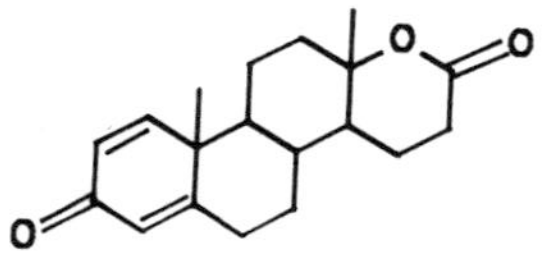

17α-oxo-D-homo-androsta-1,4-diene-3,17-dione

17α-ethinylandrost-4-eno-[2,3-d]-isoxazol-17β-ol

Name	Trade name	Properties		Dosage forms
Calusterone	Methosarb	mol wt = 316.49, mp = 127—129°C, λmax = 243 nm	0.1	Tablets (50 mg)
			<0.1	
Δ^1—Testololactone 1-Dehydrotestololo-lactone	Teslac	mol wt = 300.38, mp = 218—219°C, λmax = 242 nm		Tablets (50 and 500 mg) Aqueous suspension (100 mg/ml)
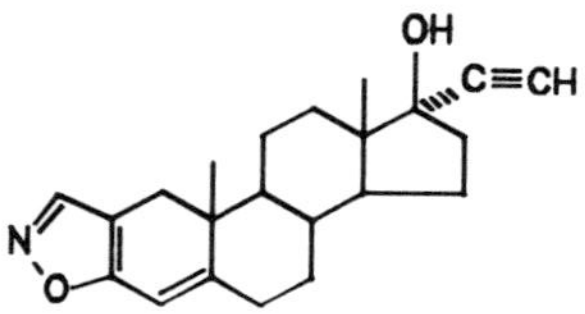 Danazol	Danocrine Danol	mol wt = 337.47, mp = 224.4—226.8°C, λmax = 286, E = 11,300		Capsules (200 mg)

ANABOLIC AGENTS

Clinical Uses and Bioassays

Many synthetic analogs of testosterone were prepared in order to separate the anabolic activity of the C_{19} steroids from their androgenic activity. Although the goal of a pure synthetic anabolic which retains no androgenic activity has not been accomplished, numerous preparations are now available on the market which have high anabolic/androgenic ratios.

The primary criterion for assessing anabolic activity of a compound is the demonstration of a marked retention of nitrogen. This nitrogen-retaining effect is the result of an increase of protein synthesis and a decrease in protein catabolism in the body.[125] Thus, the urinary nitrogen excretion, particularly urea excretion, is greatly diminished. The castrated male rat serves as the most sensitive animal model for nitrogen retention, although other animals have been utilized.[126-128] Another bioassay for anabolic activity involves examination of the increase in mass of the levator ani muscle of the rat upon administration of an anabolic agent.[129,130] This measure of myotrophic effect correlates well with the nitrogen retention bioassay and the two are usually performed in the determination of anabolic activity.[131]

Anabolic steroids exert other effects on the body as well. Skeletal mineralization and bone maturation are enhanced by androgens and anabolics.[132] These agents will decrease calcium excretion by the kidney and result in increased deposition of both calcium and phosphorus in bone. Androgenic and anabolic agents also can influence red blood cell formation. Two mechanisms of action of this erythropoiesis involving increased erythropoietin production and enhanced responsiveness of the tissue have been described.[133]

These various biological activities of the anabolics have prompted the use of these agents in treatment protocols, with varying success. Clinical trials have demonstrated the effectiveness of the anabolic steroids in inducing muscle growth and development in some diseases.[134] Anabolic steroids are effective in the symptomatic treatment of various malnourished states due to their ability to increase protein synthesis and decrease protein catabolism. Treatment of diseases such as malabsorption, anorexia nervosa, emaciation, and malnutrition as a result of psychoses includes dietary supplements, appetite stimulants, and anabolics.[134-139] Improved postoperative recovery with adjunctive use of anabolic agents has been demonstrated in numerous clinical studies.[134,140-144] However, their usefulness in other diseases such as muscular dystrophies and atrophies and in geriatics has not been observed.

In addition, the myotrophic effects have also led to the use and the abuse of these agents by athletes.[145] Conflicting reports on the effectiveness of anabolics to increase strength and power in healthy males have resulted from clinical trials. Several groups reported no significant differences between groups of male college-age students receiving anabolics and weight training and those groups receiving placebo plus the weight training in double blind studies.[146-149] Other reports cited some improvement in strength and power, but they utilized small numbers of subjects or were only single blind studies.[150-153] Even though clinical studies do not indicate the efficacy of anabolics for healthy males, an alarming percentage of amateur and professional athletes utilize anabolic steroids[154] which are readily available "on the street". The use of these steroids for increasing strength and power is banned in international sports.

Anabolic steroids also have the ability to lower serum lipid levels in vivo.[134,155-157] The most widely studied agent is oxandrolone, which dramatically lowers serum triglycerides and, to a lesser extent, cholesterol levels at pharmacological doses.[158-160] The proposed mechanism of this hypolipidemic effect includes both an inhibition of triglyceride synthesis[161] and an increased clearance of the triglycerides.[162] The androgenic side effects of the anabolics and the lack of superiority over conventional hypolipidemic agents have curtailed its use for treatment of these conditions.

The stimulation of erythropoiesis by anabolics has resulted in the use of these agents for the treatment of various anemias.[133,163] Anemias arising from deficiencies of the bone marrow are particularly responsive to pharmacological doses of anabolic agents. Treatment of aplastic anemia with anabolics and corticosteroids has been proven effective.[163-166] Secondary anemias resulting from inflammation, renal disease, or neoplasia are also responsive to anabolic steroid administration.[133,167-170] Finally, synthetic anabolics have been prescribed for women with osteoporosis[132] and for children with delayed growth.[161] These applications have produced limited success; however, the virilizing side effects severely limit their usefulness, particularly in children.

Structure-Activity Relationships

The first compound to be tested which enhanced anabolic actions while minimizing androgenic effects was the testosterone analog in which the methyl group at C-19 was replaced with a hydrogen atom. This compound, 19-nortestosterone (nandrolone, **28**), has approximately equal anabolic activity but only 0.1 the androgenic activity of testosterone.[130,172,173] These reports prompted the preparation of other 19-nortestosterone analogs, including the 17α-methyl (**29**) and 17α-ethyl (**30**) analogs which have been used clinically.[174]

nandrolone R=H (**28**)
normethandrone R=CH₃ (**29**)
norethandrone R=CH₂CH₃ (**30**)

Introduction of another double bond at carbons 1 and 2 of the testosterone molecule also resulted in anabolic agents.[175] Methandrostenolone (**31**) exhibits two times the oral anabolic activity of 17α-methyltestosterone with fewer

methandrostenolone (**31**)

androgenic effects.[176-179] Additionally, introduction of double bonds in rings B and/or C led to agents with enhanced anabolic activities. An anabolic/androgenic ratio of 5/1 was observed in the unsaturated steroid ethyldienolone (**32**).[180] A triene analog, methyltrienolone (**33**), exhibited a surprising 300-fold anabolic effect as compared with methyltestosterone following oral administration in castrated rats.[181] However, in humans the biological effects did not correlate, and the compound only demonstrated weak activity[182-184] and produced severe hepatic dysfunction at very low doses.[184] Because of its high affinity for the androgen receptor, ³H-methyltrienolone is used as the radioligand in receptor binding studies.[185]

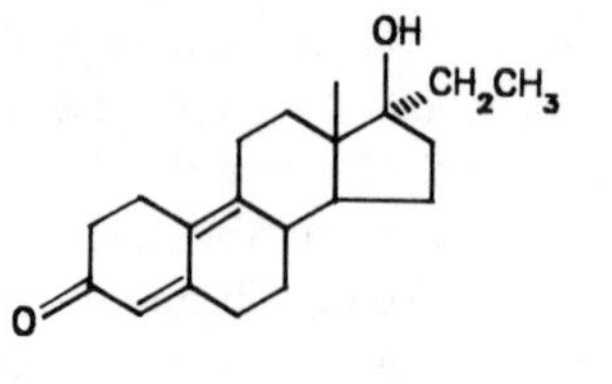

ethyldienolone (**32**) 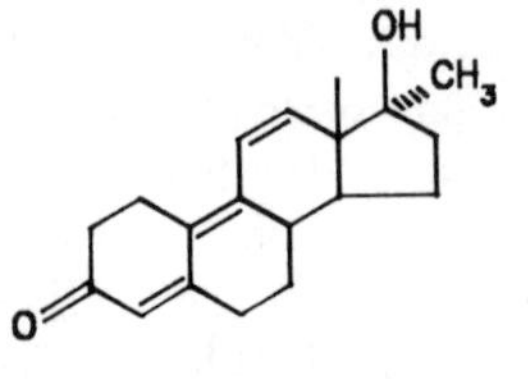   methyltrienolone (**33**)

Substitutions of alkyl moieties on the steroid nucleus in place of certain hydrogen atoms have resulted in useful anabolics. 2α-Methyl-5α-androstan-17β-ol-3-one (drostanolone, **34**) demonstrates anabolic activity in both animals and humans.[186,187] The 2,2-dimethyl and the 2-methylene analogs had little anabolic or androgenic activity.[186,188,189] Interestingly, the most widely studied anabolic steroid has been 2-hydroxymethylene-17α-methyl-5α-andros-tan-17β-ol-3-one (oxymetholone, **35**), with three times the anabolic activity and 0.5 times the androgenic activity of

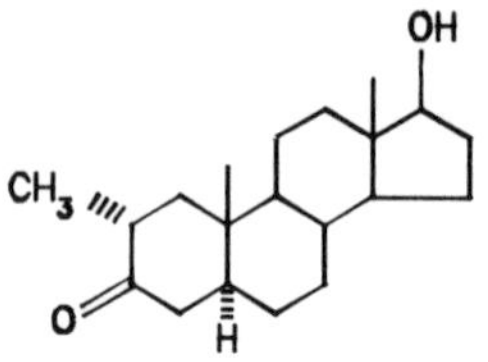

drostanolone (**34**) 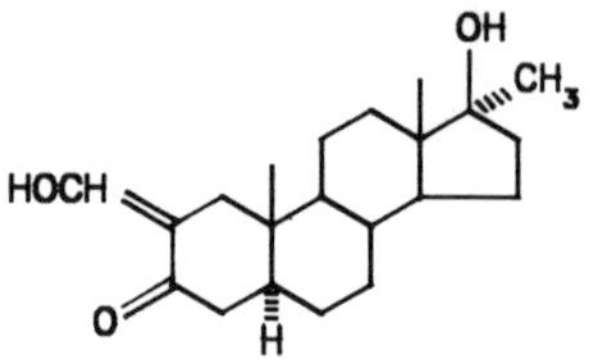   oxymetholone (**35**)

methyltestosterone.[187,190-192] A 1-methyl-1-ene derivative, methenolone (**36**), is a potent anabolic (5 times testosterone) with weak androgenic activity (only 0.1 times testoster-one).[193-195] In contrast, the 1α-methyl dihydro analog (mesterolone, **37**) and the 1-dehydro analog **22** are both androgenic.[97,196,197] These studies and those of androgenic analogs suggest and exquisite sensitivity of the androgen and anabolic receptors and the differences of the structural requirements for binding to the receptor. A detailed analysis of the

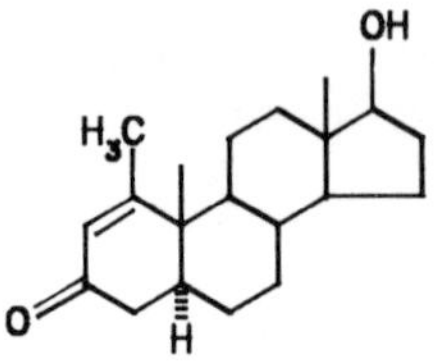

methenolone (**36**) 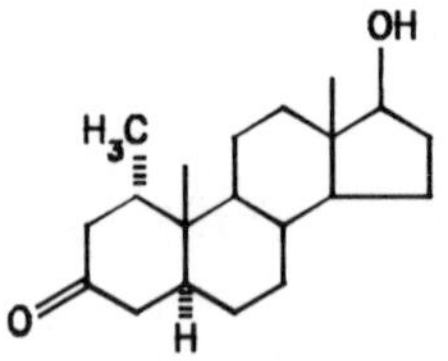   mesterolone (**37**)

structure-activity relationships for these anabolic steroids will require future binding studies with the anabolic receptor(s). A final alkylated anabolic agent is $7\alpha,17\alpha$-dimethyltestoster-one, bolasterone (**38**), which demonstrates 6.6 times the myotrophic effect of methyltes-tosterone.[198,199] Its 7β-epimer, calusterone (**25**), was mentioned earlier and has very little anabolic and androgenic activity, enabling it to be used as a nonvirilizing agent for the treatment of advanced breast cancer.

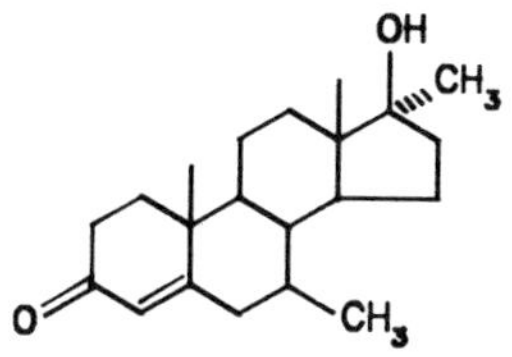

bolasterone (**38**)

A number of bioisosteric analogs of testosterone have been synthesized and evaluated for biological activity. A potent anabolic agent produced by these studies is oxandrolone (**39**), having 3 times the anabolic effects of methyltestosterone and only 0.24 times the androgenic activity in animal studies.[200,201] In humans, oxandrolone demonstrates an even greater enhancement of anabolic activity and is a very effective myotrophic agent without androgenic side effects at low doses.[202,203]

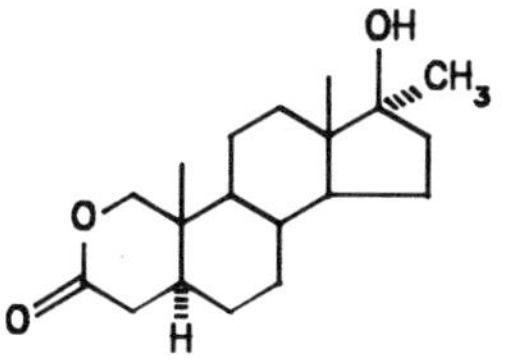

oxandrolone (**39**)

The 2-thia and 2-aza analogs of testosterone demonstrated no significant biological activities in bioassays.[7]

In an attempt to decrease androgenic activity, the 3-deoxy steroid 17α-methyl-5α-androstan-17β-ol (**40**) was prepared.[204] Unfortunately,

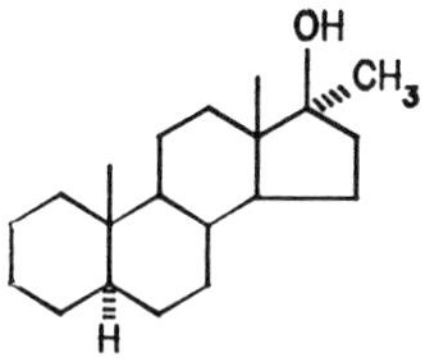

17α-methyl-5α-androstan-17β-ol (**40**)

this compound retained androgenic activity in animals and in humans.[205] Nonetheless, it led to the preparation of unsaturated analogs ethylestrenol (**41**) and 17α-methyl-5α-androst-2-en-17β-ol (**42**) which demonstrated enhanced anabolic effects and diminished androgenicity.[204,206-210] On the

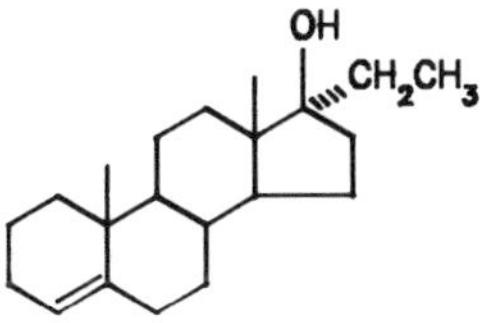

ethylestrenol (**41**)

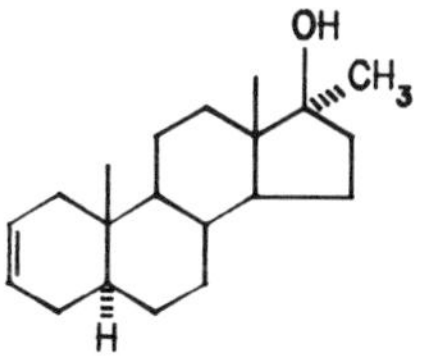

17α-methyl-5α-androst-2-en-17β-ol (**42**)

other hand, the sulfur, selenium, and telerium bioisosteres of this 3-deoxy series (**43, 44, 45**) have exhibited good androgenic activity.[211-215]

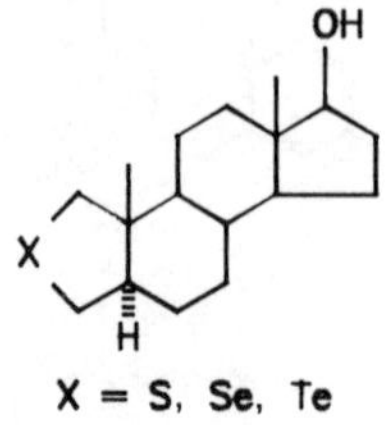

(**43,44,45**) X = S, Se, Te

The final modifications of the androstane molecule that have yielded clinically useful anabolic agents are the introductions of heterocyclic rings fused to the A ring. The simple 2α,3α-cyclopropyl analog **46** and the 2α,3α-epithiol derivative **47** were found to be active anabolic agents.[216,217] Another fused-ring derivative is stanazolol (**48**), containing a pyrazole ring at carbons 2 and 3 of the steroid system. It is effective clinically at a dose of 6 mg/day with no androgenic side effects.[218-221] The isoxazole isostere androisoxazole (**49**) also exhibits anabolic activity with an anabolic/androgenic ratio of 40.[222] Interestingly, its 17α-ethinyl derivative is danazol (**27**) which has minimal androgenic activity but is a potent inhibitor of gonadotropin release.[102]

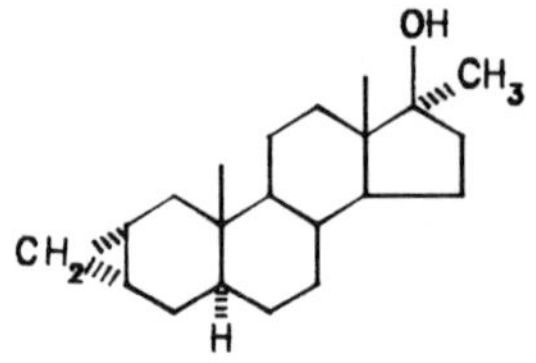

2α,3α-cyclopropyl analog (**46**)

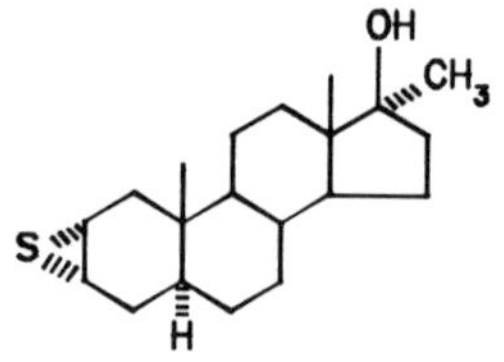

2α,3α-epithiol derivative (**47**)

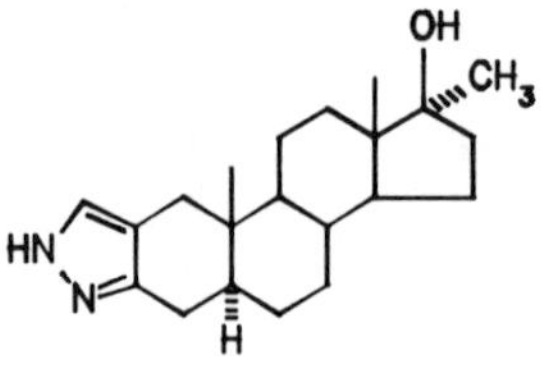

stanazolol (**48**)

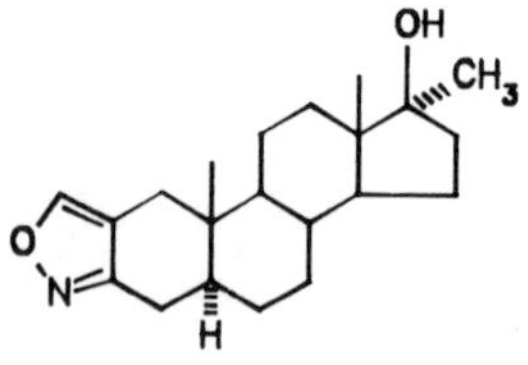

androisoxazole (**49**)

Pharmacokinetics

The absorption, distribution, and metabolism of the various anabolic steroids are quite similar to those pharmacokinetic properties of the endogenous and synthetic androgens discussed earlier in the chapter.[7,223] Again, lipid solubility is critical for the absorption of these agents following oral or parenteral administration. The 17α-methyl group retards the metabolism of the compounds and provides orally active agents. Other anabolics such as methenolone are orally active without a 17α-substituent, indicating that these steroids are poor substrates for 17α-hydroxysteroid dehydrogenase.[194,195] Reduction of the 4-en-3-one system in synthetic anabolics to give the various α-and β-isomers occurs in vivo.[115] The 3-deoxy agent 17α-methyl-5α-androstan-17α-ol was shown to be extensively converted to the 3-keto derivative by liver homogenate preparations.[224] The metabolic fates of stanzolol and danazol have been reported,[225,226] with the major metabolites being heterocycle-ring opened derivatives and their deaminated products. Finally, both the unchanged anabolics and their metabolites are primarily excreted in the urine as the glucuronide or sulfate conjugates.

Toxicities

The major side effect of the anabolic steroids is the residual androgenic activity of the molecules. The virilizing actions are undesirable in adult males as well as in females and children. In addition, many anabolic steroids can suppress the release of gonadotropins from the anterior pituitary and lead to lower levels of circulating hormones and potential reproductive problems. Headaches, acne, and elevated blood pressure are common in individuals taking anabolics. The salt and water retention induced by these agents can produce edema.

The most serious toxicity resulting from the use of anabolic steroids is subsequent liver damage. Liver damage including jaundice and cholestasis can occur after use of the 17α-alkylated C_{19} steroids.[121-124] Also, individuals who have received anabolic agents over an extended period have developed hepatic adenocarcinomas.[227-230] Such clinical reports serve to underscore the inherent risks associated with anabolic steroid use in amateur athletes for no demonstrable benefits.

Table 2 is a compilation of the names, structures, chemical data, biological activity, and dosage forms of the synthetic androgens.

ANTIANDROGENS

Clinical Uses and Bioassays

A majority of the recent research efforts in the area of androgens and anabolic agents have concentrated on the preparation and biological activities of the antiandrogens. An antiandrogen is defined as a substance which antagonizes the actions of testosterone and, when administered with an androgen, blocks or diminishes the effectiveness of the androgen at various androgen-sensitive tissues. Such compounds are of interest in both a biochemical and a physiological sense for examining the various actions of the androgens in the cell. In addition, antiandrogens have therapeutic potential in the treatment of acne, virilization in women, hyperplasia and neoplasia of the prostate, baldness, and for male contraception.

Antiandrogens may act to block the action of testosterone at several possible sites. First, such compounds could interfere with the entrance of the androgen into the target cell. A second site of action of an antiandrogen may be to block the conversion of the steroid such as testosterone to its more active metabolite dihydrotestosterone. Third, competition for the high affinity binding sites on the androgen receptor molecule may account for antiandrogenic effects. Finally, certain agents can act in the pituitary to lower gonadotropin secretion and thus, diminish the production of testosterone by the testis. The substances described in this section act through at least one of these mechanisms. Several reviews on the antiandrogens have recently appeared.[231-233]

Initial clinical studies demonstrate the potential therapeutic benefits of the antiandrogens. The agent cyproterone acetate (**50**) has produced quite satisfactory results in the treatment of acne, seborrhea, and hirsutism.[234-240] Therapeutic effectiveness of this agent in the treatment of prostatic carcinoma has been reported.[241-245]

Structure-Activity Relationships

Several steroidal and nonsteroidal compounds with demonstrated antiandrogenic activity have been utilized clinically.[232] The first compounds used as antiandrogens were the estrogens and progestins.[246] Steroidal estrogens and diethylstilbesterol are used in the treatment of prostatic carcinoma[247-250] and exert their action via a suppression of the release of pituitary gonadotropins. Progestational compounds have also been utilized for antiandrogenic actions

Table 2
ANABOLICS

Structure and chemical name	Generic name	Trade names	Chemical data	Anabolic activity — Nitrogen retention	Anabolic activity — Myotrophic	Dosage form
Testosterone 17β-hydroxyandrost-4-en-3-one	Testosterone	Android-T Malestrone Oreton Primotest Virosterone	mol wt = 288.41 mp = 155°C λ_{max} = 240 nm E = 15,800	1.0	1.0	Aqueous suspension (25, 50, and 100 mg/mℓ) Pellets (75mg)
19-Nortestosterone derivatives 17β-hydroxyestr-4-en-3-one	19-Nortestosterone nandrolone	Nerobolil Nortestonate	mol wt = 274.39 mp = 112°C λ_{max} = 241 nm E = 17,000	0.8	1.0	
	Nandrolone phenpropionate	Durabol Durabolin Nandrolin	mol wt = 406.54 mp = 95—96°C	—	2.2	Oily solution (25 and 50 mg/mℓ)

	Name	Trade names	Properties			
R=CH₂(CH₂)₇CH₃	Nandrolone decanoate	Deca-Durabol Deca-Durabolin Abolon	mol wt = 428.63 mp = 32—35°C	—	3.2	Oily solution (50 and 100 mg/mℓ)
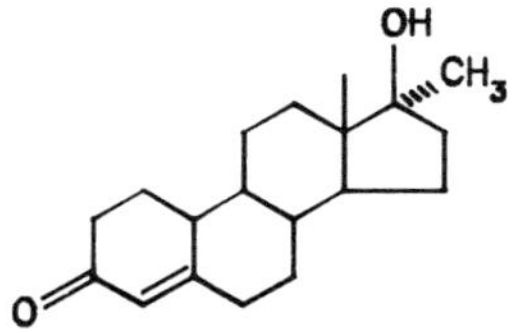 17β-hydroxy-17α-methylestra-4-en-3-one	Normethandrone	Methalutin Orgasteron	mol wt = 288.41 mp = 156—158°C λ_{max} = 240 nm E = 16,500	4.0	4.5	
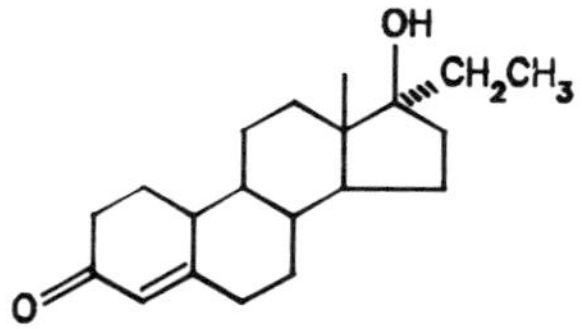 17α-ethyl-17β-hydroxyestra-4-en-3-one	Norethandrolone	Nilevar Solevar	mol wt = 302.44 mp = 140—141°C λ_{max} = 240 nm E = 16,500	3.9	4.0	
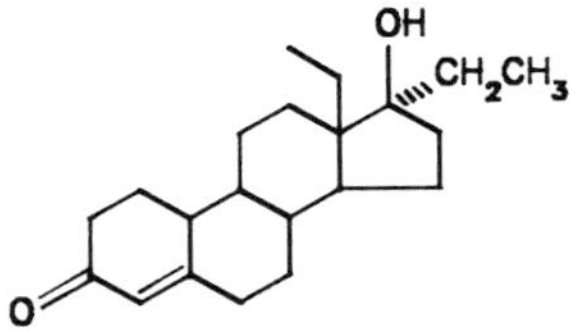 13β,17α-diethyl-17β-hydroxygon-4-en-3-one	Norbolethone	Genabol	mol wt = 326.47 mp = 144—145°C λ_{max} = 241 nm E = 16,500	3.4	—	

Table 2 (continued)
ANABOLICS

Structure and chemical name	Generic name	Trade names	Chemical data	Anabolic activity		Dosage form
				Nitrogen retention	Myotrophic	
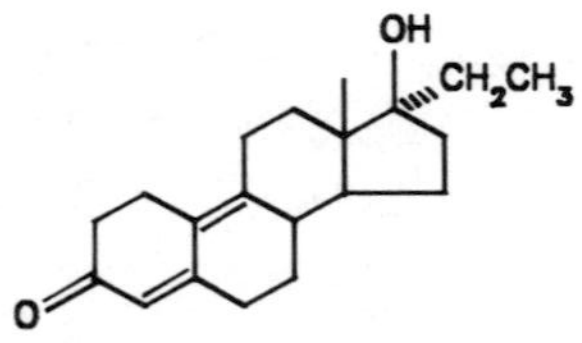 17α-ethyl-17β-hydroxyestra-4,9,11-trien-3-one	Ethyldienolone		mol wt 300.40	—	—	
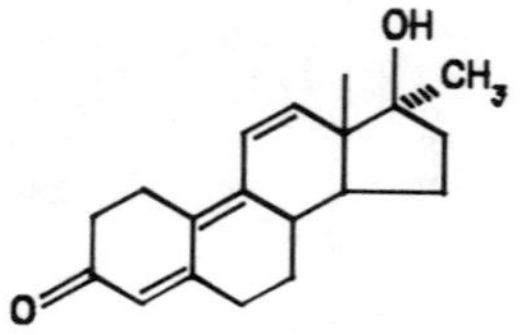 17α-methyl-17β-hydroxyestra-4,9,11-trien-3-one	Methyltrienolone	R 1881	mol wt = 284.38 mp = 170°C	—	—	
Androstane derivatives						
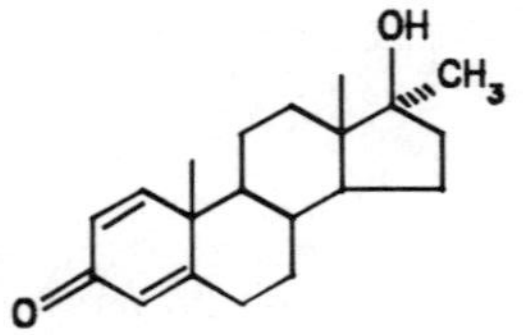	Methandrostenolone Methandienone 1-Dehydromethyl-testosterone	Danabol Dianabol Nabolin Nerobil	mol wt = 300.42 mp = 163—164°C λ_{max} = 245 nm E = 15,600	0.6	1.4	Tablet (5 mg)

Structure / IUPAC name	Common name	Brand name	Properties			
17β-hydroxy-17α-methylandrosta-1,4-dien-3-one	Drostanolone 2α-Methylandrostanolone	Drolban Masterone	mol wt = 304.48 mp = 149—153°C	—	1.3	
17β-hydroxy-2α-methyl-5α-androstan-3-one	Drostanolone propionate	Mastizol	mol wt = 360.52 mp = 126—130°C	—	1.5	Oily solution (50 mg/mℓ)
17β-hydroxy-17α-methyl-5α-androstan-3-one	Mestanolone Methylandrostanolone	Androstalone Ermalon	mol wt = 304.46 mp = 192—193°C	0.8	0.8	

Table 2 (continued)
ANABOLICS

Structure and chemical name	Generic name	Trade names	Chemical data	Anabolic activity		Dosage form
				Nitrogen retention	Myotrophic	
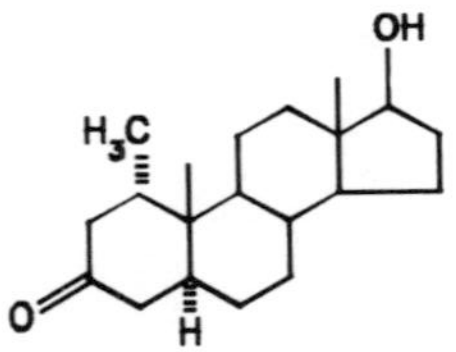 17β-hydroxy-1α-methyl-5α-androstan-3-one	Mesterolone	Androviron Mestoran Mestoranum	mol wt = 304.46 mp = 203.5—205°C	—	—	
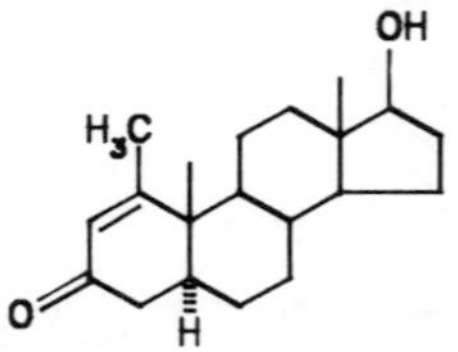 17β-hydroxy-1-methyl-5α-androst-1-en-3-one	Methenolone	Nibol Primobolan	mol wt = 302.44 mp = 149.5—152°C	—	5.0	
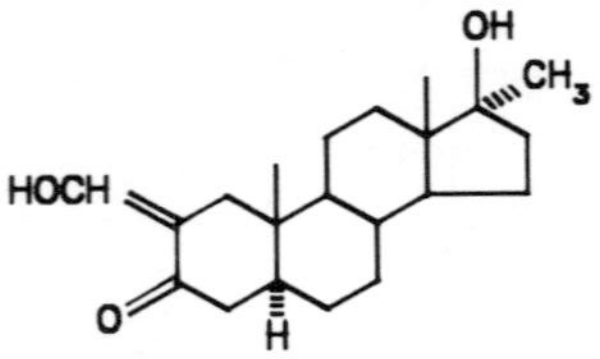	Oxymetholone	Adroyd Anadrol Anadroyd Anapolon Anasterone Nastenon Protanabol Synasteron	mol wt = 332.47 mp = 178—180°C λ_{max} = 285 nm E = 10,000	2.75	2.8	Tablets (5, 10, and 50 mg)

17β-hydroxy-2-hydroxymethylene-17α-methyl-5α-androstan-3-one

3-Deoxyandrostane derivatives

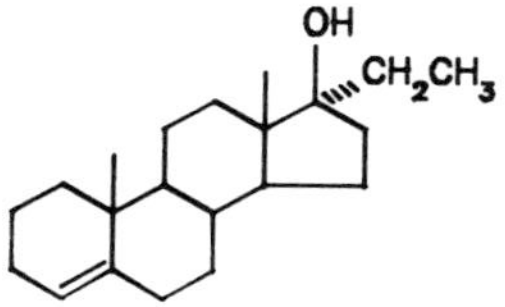

17α-ethylandrost-4-en-17β-ol

Ethylestrenol	Duraboral-O Maxibolin Orabolin Orgaboral Orabolin Orgabolin	mol wt = 288.46 mp = 76—78°C	1.7	2.0	Elixir (2 mg/5 mℓ) Tablets (2 mg)
Oxandrolone	Anavar Provita	mol wt = 306.43 mp = 235—238°C	3.0	3.0	Tablets (2.5 mg)
		mol wt = 320.54 mp = 173—174°C	11.0	—	

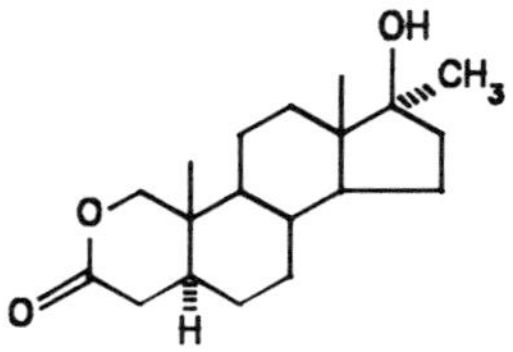

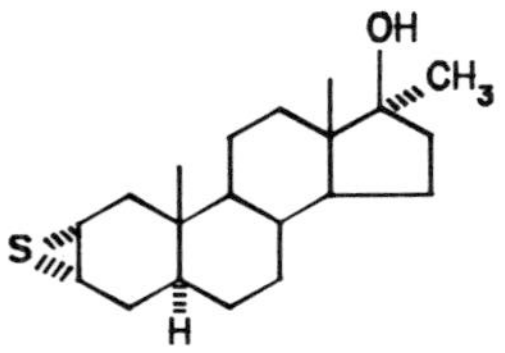

Heterocyclic anabolics

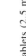

17β-hydroxy-17α-methyl-2-oxa-5α-androstan-3-one

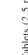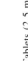

2,3α-epithio-17α-methyl-5α-androstan-17β-ol

Table 2 (continued)
ANABOLICS

Structure and chemical name	Generic name	Trade names	Chemical data	Anabolic activity		Dosage form
				Nitrogen retention	Myotrophic	
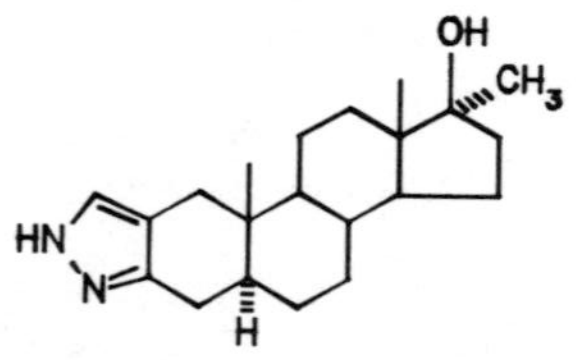 17α-methyl-5α-androstano-[3,2-c]-pyrazol-17β-ol	Stanazolol	Stanozol Winstrol Tevabolin	mol wt = 328.48 mp = 229.8—242°C λ_{max} = 223 E = 4740	10.0	7.5	Tablets (2 mg)
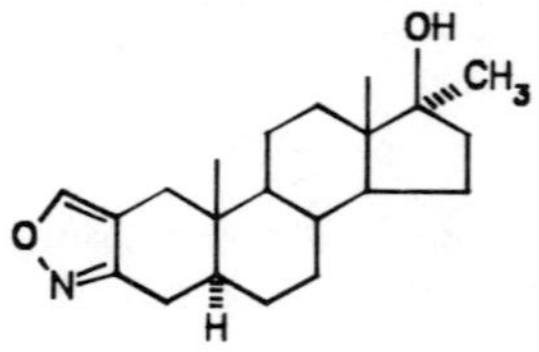 17α-methyl-5α-androstano-[3,2-c]-isoxazol-17β-ol	Androisoxazole	Androxan Neo-Ponden	mol wt = 329.47 mp = 169—170°C λ_{max} = 226 nm E = 5130	1.5	1.7	

with limited success.[251] The inherent hormonal activities of these compounds and the development of more selective antiandrogens have limited the clinical applications of estrogens and progestins as antiandrogens.

A modified progestin which is a potent antiandrogen and has minimal progestational activity is the agent cyproterone acetate (50). This compound

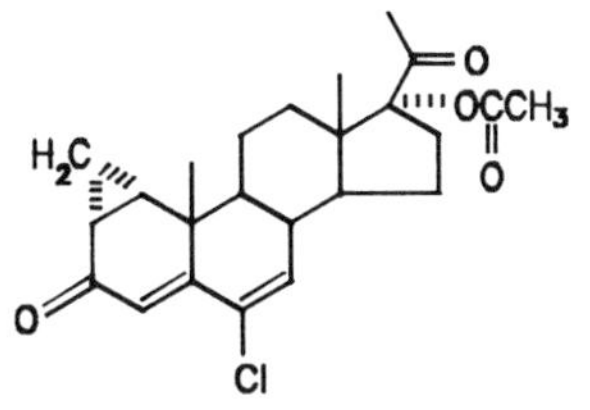

cyproterone acetate (50)

was originally prepared in search of orally active progestins, but was quickly recognized for its ability to suppress gonadotropin release.[252-259] It was later demonstrated that this compound also bound with high affinity to the androgen receptor and thus, competed with DHT for the binding site.[260-263] Cyproterone acetate has received the most clinical attention in antiandrogen therapy.[234-245] Other pregnane compounds that exhibit antiandrogenic actions are medrogesterone[264] (51), A-norprogesterone[265] (52), and gestonorone capronate[266] (53).

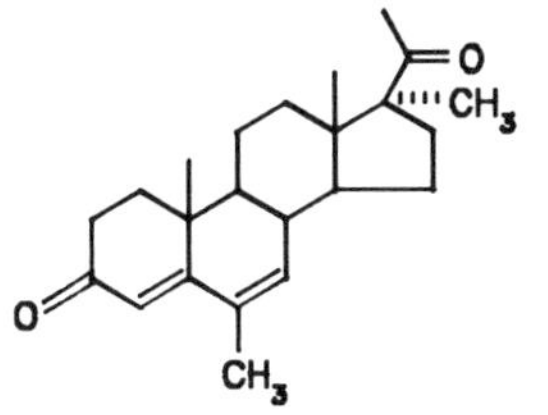

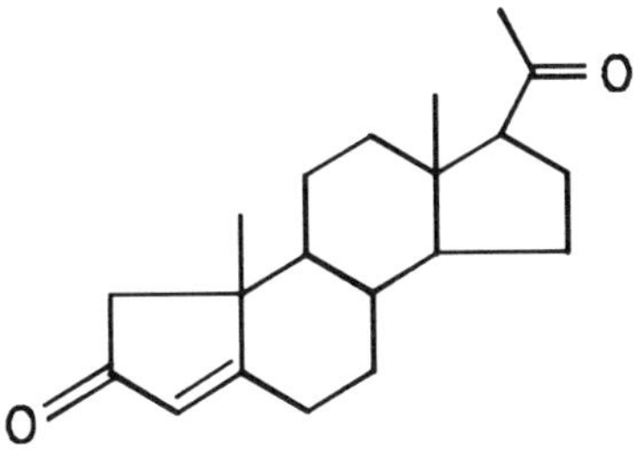

A-norprogesterone (52)

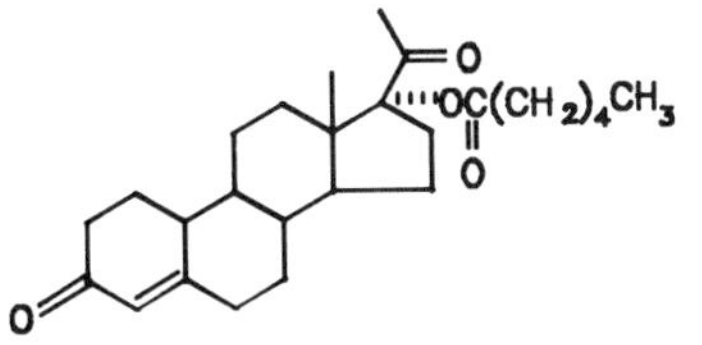

gestonorone capronate (53)

Medrogesterone exerts its antiandrogenic effects by inhibiting 5α-reductase and thus preventing the formation of DHT,[267,268] while gestonorone capronate interferes with the uptake process in target cells.[266]

Several androstane derivatives demonstrate antiandrogenic properties. 17α-Methyl-B-nor-testosterone (54) was prepared and tested in 1964 for

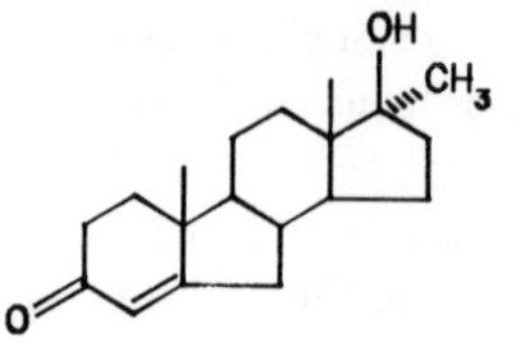

17α-methyl-β-nortestosterone **(54)**

antihormonal activity.[269] Within the next decade, several other androstane analogs were prepared and found to possess antiandrogenic activity, including BOMT[270,271] **(55)**, R 2956[272] **(56)**, SC 9420[273,274] **(57)**, and TSAA291[275,276] **(58)**.

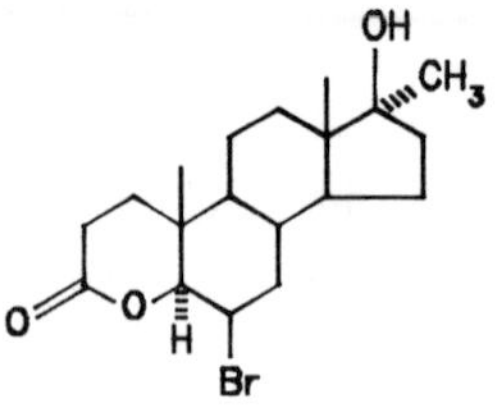

BOMT **(55)**

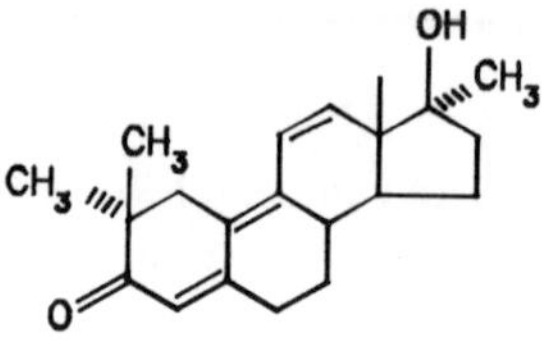

R 2956 **(56)**

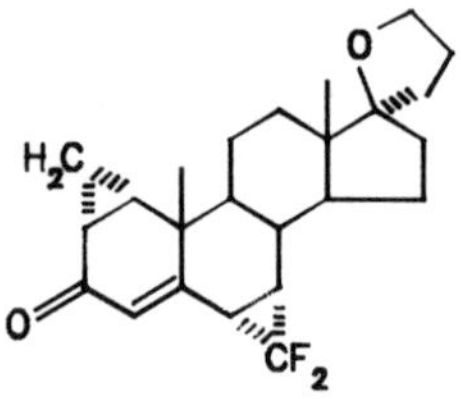

SC 9420 **(57)**

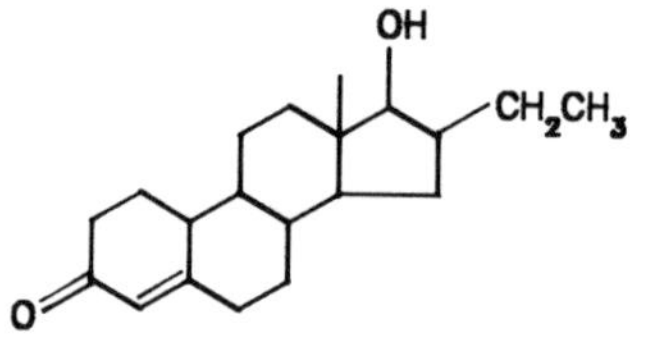

TSAA291 **(58)**

As expected, the mechanism of antiandrogenic action of these synthetic steroids is the competition with androgens for the binding sites on the receptor molecule.[277-281] Recently, numerous A- and B-ring modified steroids were examined for antiandrogenic activity and the ability to bind to the androgen receptor,[282,283] demonstrating that the structural requirements of receptor binding site can accommodate some degree of flexibility in the A and/or B rings of antiandrogenic molecules.

The absolute requirement of a steroidal compound for interaction with the androgen receptor was invalidated when the potent nonsteroidal antiandrogen flutamide **(59)** was introduced.[284,285] Subsequent receptor studies[281,286,287] demonstrated that this compound competed with DHT for the binding sites. The side-chain of flutamide allows sufficient flexibility for the molecule to assume a structure similar to an androgen. In addition, an hydroxylated metabolite **(60)** has been identified and is a more powerful antiandrogen in vivo and has a higher affinity for the receptor than the parent compound.[281,288]

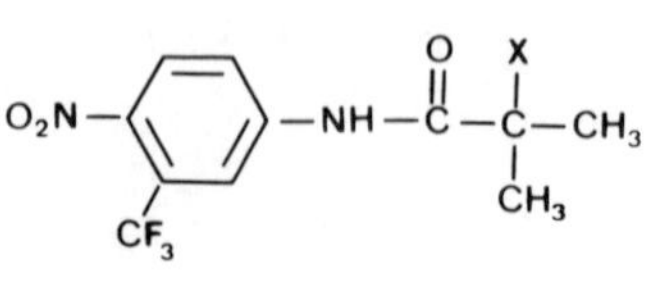

flutamide X = H **(59)**
metabolite X = OH **(60)**

DIMP[289] (**61**), R 23908[246] (**62**), and RO5-2537[290] (**63**) are other nonsteroidal antiandrogens and have recently been shown to interact with the androgen receptor to varying degrees.[281]

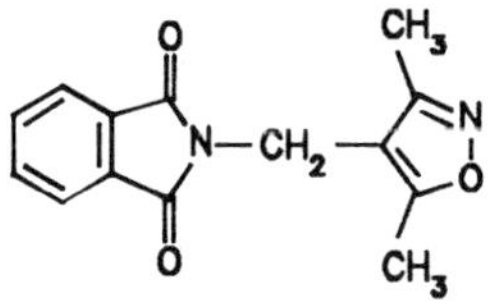

DIMP (**61**) 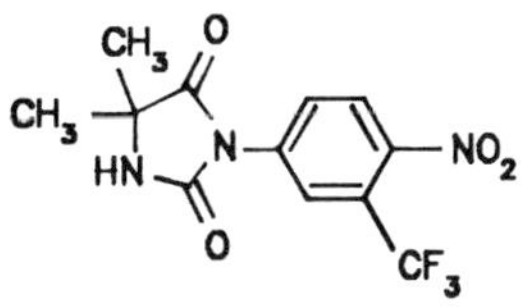   R 23908 (**62**)

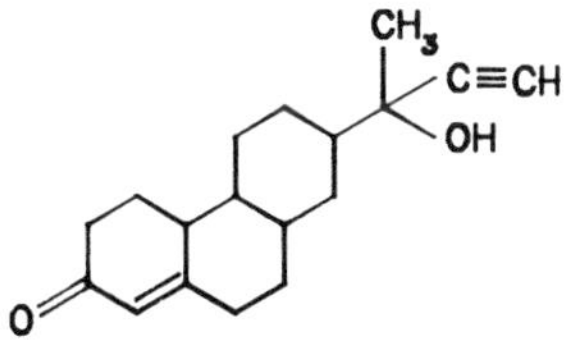

RO5-2537 (**63**)

Pharmacokinetics

The steroidal antiandrogens exhibit similar pharmacokinetic properties to the androgens and anabolic agents. The lipophilicity of the compounds influences the androgens and anabolic agents. The lipophilicity of the compounds influences absorption both orally and from injection sites.[291-295] Reductions of the 3-ketone and 4,5 double bond are common routes of metabolism.[291] An unusual metabolite of cyproterone acetate, 15α-hydroxycyproterone acetate, was isolated and identified in both animals and man.[296] The nonsteroidal antiandrogen flutamide is rapidly absorbed and extensively metabolized in vivo.[297,298] As described earlier, the hydroxy metabolite **60** of flutamide is a more potent antiandrogen.[281,288] Finally, the antiandrogens are primarily excreted as the glucuronide and sulfate conjugates in the urine.

Toxicities

Side effects ot these agents have been identified from various clinical trials. Testicular atrophy and decreased spermatogenesis have been observed during treatment with cyptorterone acetate.[299,300] Antiandrogens can also impair libido and result in impotency.[301] Certain antiandrogens such as cyproterone acetate and medrogesterone also exhibit inherent progestational activity, suppress corticotropin release, and have some androgenic effects.[302-304] On the other hand, no hormonal activities were observed for the nonsteroidal flutamide.[298]

Table 3 is a compilation of the names, structures, chemical data, biological activity, and dosage forms of the antiandrogens.

SUMMARY

The steroid testosterone is the major circulating sex hormone of the male and serves as the prototype for this class of medicinal agents, the androgens and the anabolics. The endogenous androgens are biosynthesized from cholesterol in various tissues in the body; the majority of the circulating androgens are made in the testes under the stimulation of the gonadotropin LH. A critical aspect of testosterone and its biochemistry is that this steroid is converted in various cells to other active steroidal agents. The reduction of testosterone to dihydrotestosterone is necessary for some of the androgenic actions of testosterone in androgen target tissues such as the prostate. On the other hand, oxidation of testosterone

Table 3
ANTIANDROGENS

Generic name	Trade name	Chemical data	Relative antiandrogenic activity	Dosage forms
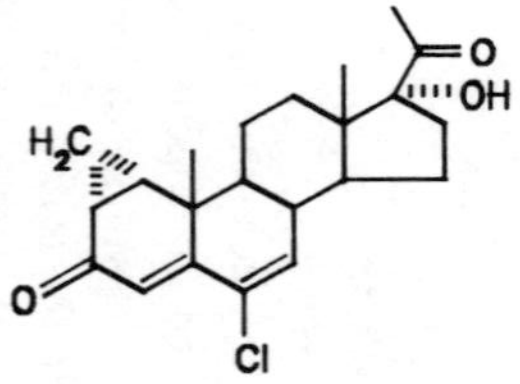 Cyproterone		mol wt = 287.39 mp = 237.5—240°C		
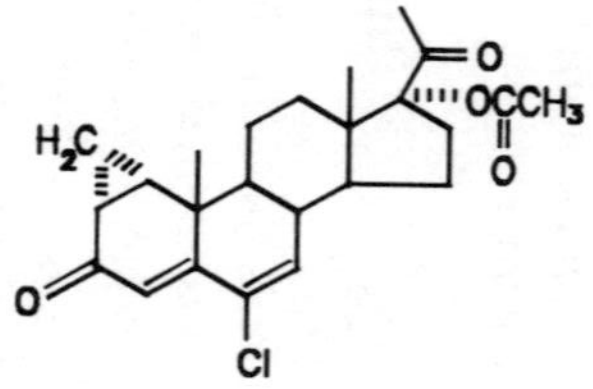 Cyproterone acetate	Androcur	mol wt = 329.04 mp = 200—201°C λ_{max} = 281 E = 17,280	1.0	Tablet (50 mg)

Structure and chemical name

Progestin derivatives

6-chloro-17α-hydroxy-1α,2α-meth-ylenepregna-4,6-diene-3,20-dione

17α-acetoxy-6-chloro-1α,2α-methy-lenepregna-4,6-diene-3,20-dione

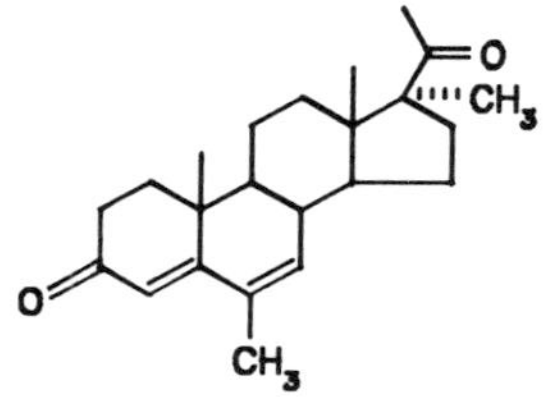

Medrogesterone
Colpro
Colprone
Prothil

mol wt = 324.40
mp = 144—146°C
λ_{max} = 288 nm
E = 25,000

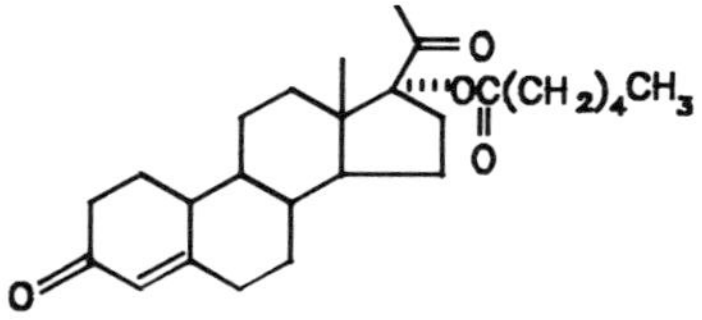

6,17α-diemethylpregna-4,6-diene-3,20-dione

Gestonorone
Caproate
Depostat

mol wt = 414.59
mp = 123—124°C
λ_{max} = 239
E = 17,500

17α-hydroxy-19-norpregn-4-ene-3,20-dione hexanoate
Androstane derivatives

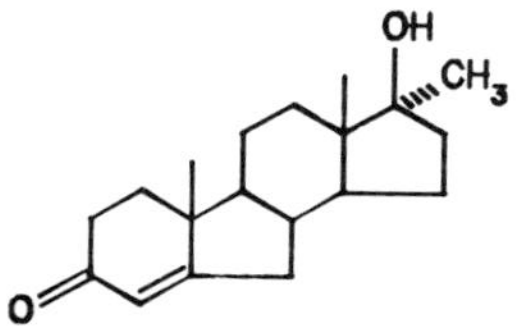

17β-hydroxy-17α-methyl-B-norandrost-4-en-3-one

Table 3 (continued)
ANTIANDROGENS

Generic name	Trade name	Chemical data	Relative antiandrogenic activity	Dosage forms
BOMT		mol wt = 385.35 mp = 163—164°C	0.8	
R 2956				
SC 9420		mol wt = 402 mp = 183—185°C λ_{max} = 243 E = 11,600		

Structure and chemical name

6β-bromo-17β-hydroxy-17α-methyl-4-oxa-5α-androstan-3-one

17β-hydroxy-2α,2β,17α-trimethyl-estra-4,9,11-trien-3-one

Structure	Name	Data	Value
6α,7α-difluoromethylene-4′,5′-di-hydro-1α,2α-methylene-17(R)-spiro-[androst-4-ene-17,2′(3′H)-furan]-3-one	TSAA291	mol wt = 302 mp = 152—153°C	
16β-ethyl-17β-hydroxyestr-4-en-3-one	Nonsteroidal antiandrogens		
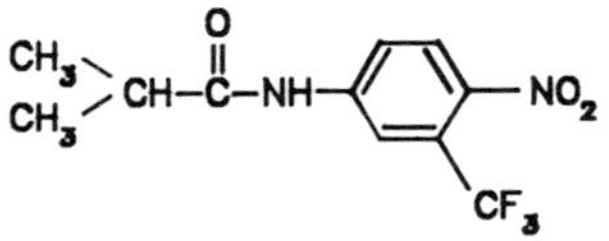 2-methyl-N-[4-nitro-3-(trifluoromethyl)phenyl]propanamide	Flutamide	mol wt = 276.22 mp = 111.5—112.5°C	0.63
N-(3,5-dimethyl-4-isoxazolylmethyl)phthalimide	DIMP		0.78

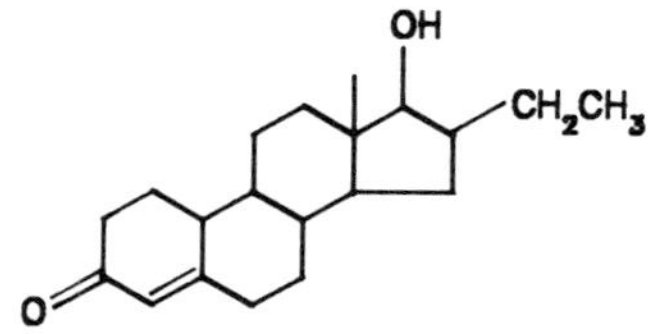

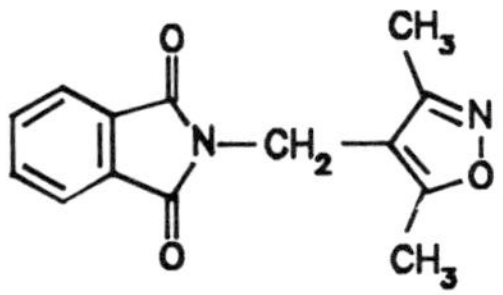

Table 3 (continued)
ANTIANDROGENS

Generic name	Trade name	Chemical data	Relative antiandrogenic activity	Dosage forms
R 23908			1.1	
RO 5-2537				

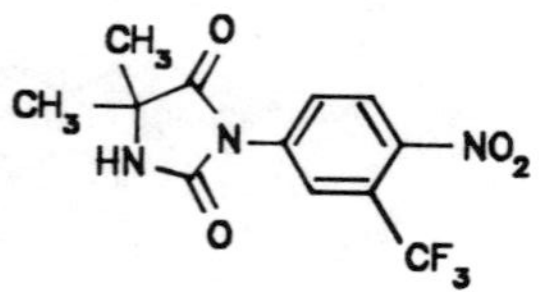

Structure and chemical name

5,5-dimethyl-3-(4¹-nitro-3¹-trifluoro-methyl)phenyl)-2,4-imidazolidinedione

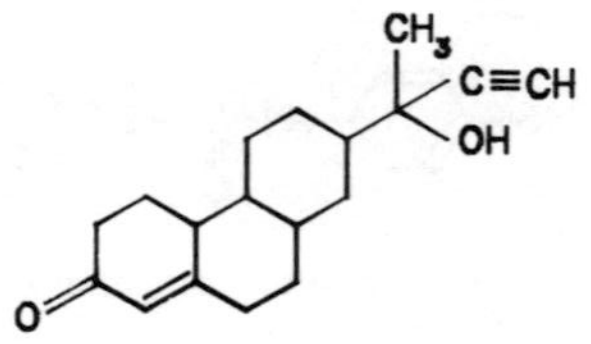

[2-((1-ethinyl-1-hydroxyethyl)]-7-oxo-1,2,3,4,4α,4β,5,6,7,9,10,10α-dodecahydrophenanthrene

by the enyzme aromatase to yield the estrogens is crucial for certain CNS actions. Investigation of these enzymatic conversions of circulating testosterone continue to be a fruitful area of biochemical research on the roles of the steroid hormones in the body. Additionally, the elucidation of the mechanism of action of the androgens in various target tissues receives on-going emphasis. Many androgenic actions of testosterone are due to the binding of dihydrotestosterone to its cytosolic receptor, followed by translocation into the nucleus and stimulation of the synthesis of new mRNA. Other actions of testosterone, particularly the anabolic actions, appeared to be mediated through a specific receptor for testosterone itself. Many of the intricate biochemical events that occur during the action of the androgens in their target cells remain for further clarification. Nevertheless, receptor studies of new agents are an important biological tool in the evaluation of the compunds for later, in-depth pharmacological testing.

The synthetic androgens and anabolics were prepared to impart oral activity to the androgen molecule, to separate the androgenic effects of testosterone from its anabolic effects and to improve upon its biological activities. These research efforts have provided several effective drug preparations for the treatment of various androgen-deficient diseases, for the therapy of diseases characterized by muscle wasting and protein catabolism, for postoperative adjuvant therapy, and for the treatment of certain hormone-dependent cancers. The synthetic anabolics have also resulted in the abuse of these agents in athletics. Finally, the most recent area of research is the development of the antiandrogens, both steroidal and nonsteroidal agents. Such compounds have therapeutic potential in the treatment of acne, virilization in women, hyperplasia and neoplasia of the prostate, baldness, and for male contraception. Thus, the numerous biological effects of the male sex hormone testosterone and the varied chemical modifications of the androstane molecule have resulted in the development of effective medicinal agents for the treatment of androgen-related diseases.

REFERENCES

1. **Vida, J. A.**, *Androgens and Anabolic Agents: Chemistry and Pharmacology,* Academic Press, New York, 1969.
2. **Eik-Nes, K. B.**, *The Androgens of the Testes,* Marcel Dekker, New York, 1970.
3. **Munson, P. L., Diczfalusy, E., Glover, J., and Olsen, R. E., Eds.,** *Vitamins and Hormones,* Vol. 33, Academic Press, New York, 1975.
4. **Kochakian, C. D.**, *Anabolic-Androgenic Steroids,* Springer-Verlag, Basel, 1976.
5. **Martini, L. and Motta, M., Eds.,** *Androgens and Antiandrogens,* Raven Press, New York, 1977.
6. **Singhal, R. L. and Thomas, J. A.,** *Advances in Sex Hormone Research,* Vol. 2, University Park Press, Baltimore, 1976.
7. **Counsell, R. E. and Brueggemeier, R. W.,** The male sex hormones and analogs, in *Burger's Medicinal Chemistry, Part II,* 4th ed., Wolff, M. E., Ed., John Wiley & Sons, New York, 1979, 873.
8. **Butenandt, A.,** Über die Chemische untersuchung der Sexualhormon, *Angew. Chem.,* 44, 905, 1931.
9. **Butenandt, A. and Tscherning, K.,** Über Androsteron, ein Krystallisiertes männliches Sexualhormon; Isolierung und Reindarstellung aus Männerharn, *Z. Physiol. Chem.,* 229, 167, 1934.
10. **David, K., Dingemanse, E., Freud, J., and Laqueur, E.,** Über krystallinisches männliches Hormon aus Hoden (Testosteron), wirksamer als aus Harn oder aus Cholestrin bereites Androsteron, *Z. Physiol. Chem.,* 233, 281, 1935.
11. **Butendant, A. and Hanisch, G.,** Über die umwandlung des dehydroAndrosterons in Δ^4-Androsten-ol-(17)-on-(3) (testosteron); ein Wegzur darstellung des Testosterons aus Chloestrin, *Chem. Ber.,* 68, 1859, 1935.
12. **Ruzicka, L.,** The testicular hormones, *J. Am. Chem. Soc.,* 57, 2011, 1935.
13. **Bruchovsky, N. and Wilson, J. D.,** The intracellular binding of testosterone and 5α-androstan-17β-ol-3-one by rat prostate, *J. Biol. Chem.,* 243, 5953, 1968.
14. **Anderson, K. M. and Liao, S.,** Selective retention of dihydrotestosterone by prostatic nuclei, *Nature (London),* 219, 277, 1968.

15. **Kochakian, C. D. and Murlin, J. D.,** Effect of male hormone on the protein and energy metabolism of castrate dogs, *J. Nutr.,* 10, 437, 1935.

16. **Kenyon, A. T., Sandiford, I., Bryan, A. H., Knowlton, K., and Koch, F. C.,** Effect of testosterone propionate on nitrogen, electrolyte, water and energy metabolism in eunuchoidism, *Endocrinology,* 23, 135, 1938.

17. **Villee, D. B.,** *Human Endrocrinology, A Developmental Approach,* W. B. Saunders, Philadelphia, 1975.

18. **Gustafsson, S. and Lundquist, A.,** Specificity of neonatal, androgen-induced imprinting of hepatic steroid metabolism in rats, *Science,* 191, 203, 1976.

19. **Naftolin, F., Ryan, K. J., Davies, I. J., Reddy, V. V., Flores, F., Petro, Z., White, R. J., Takaoka, Y., and Wolin, L.,** The formation of estrogens by central neuroendocrine tissues, *Rec. Progr. Horm. Res.,* 31, 295, 1975.

20. **Catt, K. J. and Dufau, M. L.,** Basic concepts of the mechanism of action of peptide hormones, *Biol. Reprod.,* 14, 1, 1976.

21. **Schluster, D., Burstein, S., and Cooke, B. A.,** *Molecular Endocrinology of Steroid Hormones,* John Wiley & Sons, New York, 1976, 230.

22. **Eik-Nes, K. B.,** Biosynthesis and secretion of testicular steroids, in *Handbook of Physiology,* Section 7, Vol. 5, Greep, R. O. and Astwood, E. B., Eds., American Physiological Society, Washington, D.C., 1974, 95.

23. **Dorfman, R. I. and Ungar, F.,** *Metabolism of Steroid Hormones,* Academic Press, New York, 1965.

24. **Ofner, P.,** Effects and metabolism of hormones in normal and neoplastic prostate tissue, in *Vitamins and Hormones,* Vol. 26, Harris, R. S., Wool, I. G., and Lorraine, J. A., Eds., Academic Press, New York, 1968, 237.

25. **Hartiala, K.,** Metabolism of hormones, drugs and other substances by the gut, *Physiol. Rev.,* 53, 496, 1973.

26. **Wilson, J. D.,** Metabolism of testicular androgens, in *Handbook of Physiology,* Section 7, Vol. 5, Greep, R. O. and Astwood, E. B., Eds., American Physiological Society, Washington, D. C., 1974, 491.

27. **Givens, J. R.,** Normal and abnormal androgen metabolism, *Clin. Obstet. Gynecol.,* 21, 115, 1978.

28. **Bruchovsky, N. and Wilson, J. D.,** The conversion of testosterone to 5α-androstan-17β-ol-3-one by rat prostate *in vivo* and *in vitro, J. Biol. Chem.,* 243, 2012, 1968.

29. **Wilton, D. C. and Ringold, H. J.,** Mechanism of enzymatic reduction of Δ^4 3-ketosteroids by rat liver enzymes, in *Third International Congress of Endocrinology, Mexico, 1968,* Excerpta Medica, Amsterdam, 1968, 105.

30. **Skinner, R. W. S., Pozderac, R. V., Counsell, R. E., and Weinhold, P. A.,** The inhibitive effects of steroid analogues in the binding of tritiated 5α-dihydrotestosterone to receptor proteins from rat prostate tissues, *Steroids,* 25, 189, 1975.

31. **Moore, R. J. and Wilson, J. D.,** The effect of androgenic hormones on the reduced nicotinamide adenine dinucleotide phosphate: Δ^4-3-ketosteroid 5α-oxidoreductase of rat ventral prostate, *Endocrinology,* 93, 581, 1973.

32. **Ryan, K. J.,** Biological aromatization of steroids, *J. Biol. Chem.,* 234, 268, 1959.

33. **Goto, J. and Fishman, J.,** Participation of a nonenzymatic transformation in the biosynthesis of estrogens from androgens, *Science,* 195, 80, 1977.

34. **Ryan, K. J.,** Estrogen formation by the human placenta: studies on the mechanism of steroid aromatization by mammalian tissues, *Acta Endocrinol. (Copenhagen), Suppl.,* 51, 350, 1960.

35. **Ryan, K. J.,** Biogenesis of estrogens, in *Proceedings of the Fifth International Congress on Biochemistry,* Popjak, G., Ed., Macmillan, New York, 1963, 381.

36. **Gual, C., Morato, T., Hayano, M., and Dorfman, R. I.,** Biosynthesis of estrogens, *Endocrinology,* 71, 920, 1962.

37. **Brodie, A. M. H., Schwarzel, W. C., Shaikh, A. A., and Brodie, H. J.,** The effect of an aromatase inhibitor, 4-hydroxy-androstene-3,17-dione, on estrogen-dependent processes in reproduction and breast cancer, *Endocrinology,* 100, 1684, 1977.

38. **Brodie, A. M. H., Wu, J. T., Marsh, D. A., and Brodie, H. J.,** Aromatase. II. Studies on the antifertility effect of 4-acetoxy-4-androstene-3,17-dione, *Biol. Reprod.,* 18, 365, 1978.

39. **Brodie, A. M. H., Marsh, D., and Brodie, H. J.,** Aromatase Inhibitors. IV. Regression of hormone-dependent, mammary tumors in the rat with 4-acetoxy-4-androstene-3,17-dione, *J. Steroid Biochem.,* 10, 432, 1979.

40. **Brueggemeier, R. W., Floyd, E. E., and Counsell, R. E.,** Synthesis and biochemical evaluation of inhibitors of estrogen biosynthesis, *J. Med. Chem.,* 21, 1007, 1978.

41. **Brueggemeier, R. W., Snider, C. E., and Counsell, R. E.,** Substituted C_{19} analogs as inhibitors of estrogen biosynthesis, *Cancer Res.,* 42, 3334s, 1982.

42. **Jaffe, R. B.,** Testosterone metabolism in target tissues. Hypothalamic and pituitary tissues of the adult rat and human fetus, and the immature rat epiphysis, *Steroids,* 14, 483, 1969.

43. **Sholiton, L. J. and Werk, E. E.,** The less polar metabolites produced by incubation of testosterone-4-14C with rat and bovine brain, *Acta Endocrinol. (Copenhagen),* 61, 641, 1969.

44. **Sholiton, L. J., Hall, I. J., and Werk, E. E.,** The iso-polar metabolites produced by incubation of [4-14C] testosterone with rat and bovine brain, *Acta Endocrinol. (Copenhagen),* 63, 512, 1970.

45. **Stern, J. J. and Murphy, M.,** The effects of cyproterone acetate on the spontaneous activity and seminal vesicle weight of male rats, *J. Endocrinol.,* 50, 441, 1971.

46. **Massa, R., Stupnika, E., Kniewald, Z., and Martini, L.,** The transformation of testosterone into dehydrotestosterone by the brain and the anterior pituitary, *J. Steroid Biochem.,* 3, 385, 1972.

47. **Martini, L.,** Androgen reduction by neuroendocrine tissues: physiological significance, in *Subcellular Mechanisms in Reproductive Neuroendocrinology,* Naftolin, F., Ryan, K. J., and Davies, I. J., Eds., Elsevier, Amsterdam, 1976, 327.

48. **Naftolin, F., Ryan, K. J., and Davies, I. J.,** Androgen aromatization by neuroendocrine tissues, in *Subcellular Mechanisms in Reproductive Neuroendocrinology,* Naftolin, F., Ryan, K. J., and Davies, I. J., Eds., Elsevier, Amsterdam, 1976, 347.

49. **O'Malley, B. W. and Means, A. R.,** *Receptors for Reproductive Hormones,* Plenum Press, New York, 1974.

50. **King, R. J. B. and Mainwaring, W. P.,** *Steroid-Cell Interactions,* University Park Press, Baltimore, 1974.

51. **Liao, S.,** Cellular receptors and mechanisms of action of steroid hormones, *Int. Rev. Cytol.,* 41, 87, 1975.

52. **Williams-Ashman, H. G. and Reddi, A. H.,** Androgenic regulation of tissue growth and function, in *Biochemical Actions of Hormones,* Vol. 2, Litwack, G., Ed., Academic Press, New York, 1972, 257.

53. **Chan, L. and O'Malley, O. W.,** Mechanisms of action of the sex steroids, *N. Engl. J. Med.,* 294, p. 1322, 1372, 1430, 1976.

54. **Mainwaring, W. I. P.,** *The Mechanism of Action of Androgens,* Springer-Verlag, Basel, 1977.

55. **Bruchovsky, N. and Wilson, J. D.,** The conversion of testosterone to 5-alpha-androstan-17-beta-ol-3-one by rat prostate *in vivo* and *in vitro, J. Biol. Chem.,* 243, 2012, 1968.

56. **Mainwaring, W. I.,** The binding of (1,2-3H) testosterone within nuclei of the rat prostate, *J. Endocrinol.,* 44, 323, 1969.

57. **Fang, S. and Liao, S.,** Androgen receptors. Steroid- and tissue-specific retention of a 17-beta-hydroxy-5-alpha-androstan-3-one protein complex by the cell nuclei of ventral prostate, *J. Biol. Chem.,* 246, 16, 1971.

58. **Mainwaring, W. I. and Peterken, B. M.,** A reconstituted cell-free system for the specific transfer of steroid-receptor complexes into nuclear chromatin isolated from the rat ventral prostate gland, *Biochem. J.,* 125, 285, 1971.

59. **Tymoczko, J. L. and Liao, S.,** Retention of an androgen-protein complex by nuclear chromatin aggregates: heat-labile factors, *Biochem. Biophys. Acta,* 252, 607, 1971.

60. **Mainwaring, W. I., Wilce, P. A., and Smith, A. E.,** Studies on the form and synthesis of messenger ribonucleic acid in the rat ventral prostate gland, including its tissue-specific stimulation by androgens, *Biochem. J.,* 137, 513, 1974.

61. **Tvter, K. J. and Unhjem, O.,** Selective uptake of androgen by rat seminal vesicle, *Endrocrinology,* 84, 963, 1969.

62. **Stern, J. M. and Eisenfeld, A. J.,** Androgen accumulation and binding to macromolecules in seminal vesicles: inhibition cyproterone, *Science,* 166, 233, 1969.

63. **Mainwaring, W. I. and Mangan, F. R.,** A study of the androgen receptors in a variety of androgen-sensitive tissues, *J. Endocrinol.,* 59, 121, 1973.

64. **Hansson, V., McLean, W. S., and Smith, A. A.,** Androgen receptors in rat testis, *Steroids,* 23, 823, 1974.

65. **Tindall, D. J., French, F. S., and Nayfeh, S. N.,** Androgen uptake and binding in rat epididymal nuclei, *in vivo, Biochem. Biophys. Res. Commun.,* 49, 1391, 1972.

66. **Ritzin, E. M., Nayfeh, S. N., French, S. F., and Aronin, A.,** Deficient nuclear uptake of testosterone in the androgen-insensitive (Stanley-Gumbreck) pseudo-hermaphrodite male rat, *Endocrinology,* 91, 116, 1972.

67. **Jovan, P., Samperez, S., and Thieulant, M. L.,** Testosterone receptors in purified nuclei of rat anterior hypophysis, *J. Steroid Bicohem.,* 4, 65, 1973.

68. **Sar, M. and Stumpf, W. E.,** Autoradiographic localization of radioactivity in the rat brain after the injection of 1,2-³H-testosterone, *Endocrinology,* 92, 251, 1973.

69. **Cardinali, D. P., Nagle, C. A., and Rosner, J. M.,** Metabolic fate of androgens in the pineal organ: uptake binding to cytoplasmic proteins and conversion of testosterone into 5-alpha-reduced metabolites, *Endocrinology,* 95, 179, 1974.

70. **Roy, A. K., Milin, B. S., and McMinn, D. M.,** Androgen receptor in rat liver: hormonal and developmental regulation of the cytoplasmic receptor and its correlation with the androgen-dependent synthesis of alpha 2 u-globulin, *Biochem. Biophys. Acta,* 354, 213, 1974.

71. **Bruchovsky, N. and Meakin, J. W.,** The metabolism and binding of testosterone in androgen-dependent and autonomous transplantable mouse mammary tumors, *Cancer Res.,* 33, 1689, 1973.

72. **Bruchovsky, N., Sutherland, D. J., Meakin, J. W., and Minesita, T.,** Androgen receptors: relationship to growth response and to intracellular androgen transport in nine variant lines of the Shionogi mouse mammary carcinoma, *Biochem. Biophys. Acta,* 381, 61, 1975.

73. **Evans, C. R. and Pierrepoint, C. G.,** Demonstration of a specific cytosol receptor in the normal and hyperplastic canine prostate for 5 alpha-androstane-3 alpha, 17 alpha-diol, *J. Endocrinol.,* 64, 539, 1975.

74. **Gloyna, R. E. and Wilson, J. D.,** A comparative study of the conversion of testosterone to 17-beta-hydroxy-5-alpha-androstan-3-one (Dihydrotestosterone) by prostate and epididymis, *J. Clin. Endocrinol.,* 29, 970, 1969.

75. **Hansson, V., Tveter, K. J., Unhjem, O., and Djoseland, O.,** Studies on the interaction between androgens and macromolecules in male accessory sex organs of rat and man, *J. Steroid Biochem.,* 3, 427, 1972.

76. **Giannopoulos, G.,** Binding of testosterone to uterine components of the immature rat, *J. Biol. Chem.,* 248, 1004, 1973.

77. **Powers, M. L. and Florini, J. R.,** A direct effect of testosterone on muscle cells in tissue culture, *Endocrinology,* 97, 1043, 1975.

78. **Jung, I. and Baulieu, E. E.,** Testosterone cytosol "receptor" in the rat levator ani muscle, *Nature (London) New Biol.,* 237, 24, 1972.

79. **Michel, G. and Baulieu, E. E.,** Récepteur cytosoluble des androgénes dans un muscle strié squelettique, *C. R. Acad. Sci. Ser. D Paris,* 279, 421, 1974.

80. **Krieg, M.,** Characterization of the androgen receptor in the skeletal muscle of the rat, *Steroids,* 28, 261, 1976.

81. **Krieg, M. and Voigl, K. D.,** Biochemical substrate of androgenic actions at a cellular level in prostate, bulbocavernosus/levator ani and in skeletal muscle, *Acta Endocrinol. (Copenhagen) Suppl.,* 214, 43, 1977.

82. **Snochowski, M., Dahlberg, E., and Gustafsson, J. A.,** Characterization and quantification of the androgen and glucocorticoid receptors in rat skeletal muscle cytosol, *Eur. J. Biochem.,* 111, 603, 1980.

83. **Snochowski, M., Soartok, T., Dahlberg, E., Eriksson, E., and Gustafsson, J. A.,** Androgen and glucocorticoid receptors in human skeletal muscle cytosol, *J. Steroid Biochem.,* 14, 765, 1981.

84. **Odell, W. D. and Swerdloff, R. S.,** Abnormalities of gonadal function in men, *Clin. Endocrinol.,* 8, 149, 1978.

85. **Griffin, J. E. and Wilson, J. D.,** The syndromes of androgen resistance, *N. Engl. J. Med.,* 302, 198, 1980.

86. **Griffin, J. E., Punyashthiti, K., and Wilson, J. D.,** Dihydrotestosterone binding by cultured human fibroblasts: comparison of cells from control subjects and from patients with hereditary male pseudohermaphroditism due to androgen resistance, *J. Clin. Invest.,* 57, 1342, 1976.

87. **Kaufman, M., Straisfeld, C., and Pinsky, L.,** Male pseudohermaphroditism presumably due to target organ unresponsiveness to androgens: deficient 5α-dihydrotestosterone binding to cultured skin fibroblasts, *J. Clin. Invest.,* 58, 345, 1976.

88. **Griffin, J. E.,** Testicular feminization associated with a thermolabile androgen receptor in cultured human fibroblasts, *J. Clin. Invest.,* 64, 1624, 1979.

89. **Walsh, P. C., Madden, J. D., Harrod, M. J., Goldstein, J. L., MacDonald, P. C., and Wilson, J.D.,** Familial incomplete male pseudohermaphroditism, type 2: decreased dihydrotestosterone formation in pseudovaginal perineoscrotal hypospadias, *N. Engl. J. Med.,* 291, 944, 1974.

90. **Imperato-McGinley, J., Guerrero, L., Gautier, T., and Peterson, R. E.,** Steroid 5α-reductase deficiency in man: an inherited form of male pseudohermaphroditism, *Science,* 186, 1213, 1974.

91. **Segaloff, A.,** Hormones and breast cancer, *Rec. Progr. Horm. Res.,* 22, 351, 1966.

92. **Siiteri, P. K. and Thompson, E. A.,** Studies on human placental aromatase, *J. Steroid Biochem.,* 6, 317, 1975.

93. **Dorfman, R. I.,** Biosassay, in *Methods in Hormone Research,* Vol. 2, Dorfman, A., Ed., Academic Press, New York, 1962, 275.

94. **Liao, S., Liang, T., Fang, S., Casteneda, E., and Shao, T.,** Steroid structure and androgenic activity. Specificities involved in the receptor binding and nuclear retention of various androgens, *J. Biol. Chem.,* 248, 6154, 1973.

95. **Skinner, R. W. S., Pozderac, R. V., and Counsell, R. E.,** The inhibitive effects of steroid analogues in the binding of tritiated 5alpha-dihydrotestosterone to receptor proteins from rat prostate tissue, *Steroids,* 25, 189, 1975.

96. **Drill, V. A. and Riegel, B.,** Structural and hormonal activity of some new steroids, *Rec. Progr. Horm. Res.,* 14, 29, 1958.

97. **Counsell, R. E., Klimstra, P. D., and Colton, F. B.,** Anabolic agents. Derivatives of 5alpha-androst-1-ene, *J. Org. Chem.,* 27, 248, 1962.

98. **Sola, G. and Baldratti, G.,** Myotrophic (anabolic) activity of 4-substituted testosterone analogs, *Proc. Soc. Exp. Biol. Med.,* 9, 22, 1957.

99. **Rosso, R., Porcile, G., and Brema, F.,** Antitumor activity of calusterone in advanced breast cancer, *Cancer Chemother. Rep.,* 59, 890, 1975.

100. **Goldenberg, I. S., Waters, M. N., Ravdin, R. V., Ansfield, F. J., and Segaloff, A.,** Androgenic therapy for advanced breast cancer in women, *JAMA,* 223, 1267, 1973.

101. **Gordan, G. S., Wessler, S. W., and Avioli, L. V.,** Calusterone in the therapy for advanced breast cancer, *JAMA,* 219, 483, 1972.

102. **Potts, G. O.,** Pharmacology of Danazol, *J. Int. Med. Res.,* 5(Suppl. 3), 1, 1977.

103. **Schedl, H. P. and Clifton, J. A.,** Small intestinal absorption of steroids, *Gastroenterology,* 41, 491, 1961.

104. **Pearlman, W. H. and Crépy, O.,** Steroid-protein interaction with particular reference to testosterone binding by human serum, *J. Biol. Chem.,* 242, 182, 1967.

105. **Guériguian, J. and Pearlman, W. H.,** Separation of testosterone-binding protein of human pregnancy serum form CBG, *Fed. Proc. Fed. Am. Soc. Exp. Biol.,* 26, 757, 1967.

106. **Mercier-Bodard, C., Alfsen, C., and Baulieu, E. E.,** Sex steroid binding plasma protein (SBP), *Acta Endocrinol. Copenhagen,* 147, 204, 1970.

107. **Murphy, B. E. P.,** Binding of testosterone and estradiol in plasma, *Can. J. Biochem.,* 46, 299, 1968.

108. **Steeno, O., Heyns, W., Van Baelen, H., and De Moor, P.,** Testosterone binding in human plasma, *Ann. Endocrinol. (Paris),* 29, 141, 1968.

109. **De Moor, P., Steeno, O., Heyns, W., and Van Baelen, H.,** The steroid binding beta-globulin in plasma: pathophysiological data, *Ann. Endocrinol. (Paris),* 30, 233, 1969.

110. **Horton, R., Kato, T., and Sherins, R.,** A rapid method for the estimation of testosterone in male plasma, *Steroids,* 10, 245, 1967.

111. **Vermeulen, A. and Verdonck, L.,** Studies on the binding of testosterone to human plasma, *Steroids,* 11, 609, 1968.

112. **Kato, T. and Horton, R.,** Studies of testosterone binding globulin, *J. Clin. Endocrinol. Metab.,* 28, 1160, 1968.

113. **Mercier-Bodard, C. and Baulieu, E. E.,** Récentes études des protéines plasmatiques liant la testostérone, *Ann. Endocrinol. (Paris),* 29, 159, 1968.

114. **Murphy, B. E. P.,** Further studies of the specificity of the sex hormone-binding globulin of human plasma, *Steroids,* 16, 791, 1970.

115. **Segaloff, A., Gabbard, R. B., Carriere, B. T., and Rongone, E. L.,** The metabolism of 4-14C-17-alpha-methyltestosterone, *Steroids,* 1(Suppl.), 149, 1965.

116. **Engel, L. L., Alexander, J., and Wheeler, M.,** Urinary metabolites of administered 19-nortestosterone, *J. Biol. Chem.,* 231, 159, 1958.

117. **Bruchovsky, N. and Wilson, J. D.,** The conversion of testosterone to 5-alpha-androstan-17-beta-ol-3-one by rat prostate *in vivo* and *in vitro, J. Biol. Chem.,* 243, 2012, 1968.

118. **Gual, C., Morato, T., Hayano, M., Gut, M., and Dorfman, R. I.,** Biosynthesis of estrogens, *Endocrinology,* 71, 920, 1962.

119. **Plantier, H. A.,** Precocious pubescence-iatrogenic, *New Engl. J. Med.,* 270, 141, 1964.

120. **Hortling, H., Malmio, K., and Husi-Brummer, L.,** Norandrostenolone phenylpropionate and norandrostenolone decanoate in the treatment of metastasizing mammary carcinoma, *Acta Endocrinol. (Copenhagen) Suppl.,* 39, 132, 1961.

121. **De Lorimier, A. A., Gordan, G. S., Lowe, R. C., and Carbone, J. V.,** Methyl-testosterone, related steroids, and liver function, *Arch. Intern. Med.,* 116, 289, 1965.

122. **Arias, I. M.,** Effects of anabolic steroids in liver function, in *Influence of Growth Hormone, Anabolic Steroids and Nutrition in Health and Disease,* Gross, F., Ed., Springer-Verlag, Basel, 1962, 434.

123. **Frasier, S. D.,** Androgens and athletes, *Am. J. Dis. Child.,* 125, 479, 1973.

124. **Westaby, D., Ogle, S. J., Paradinas, F. J., Randell, J. B., and Murray-Lyon, I. M.,** Liver damage from long-term methyl testosterone, *Lancet,* 2, 261, 1977.

125. **Landau, R. L.,** The metabolic effects of anabolic steroids in man, in *Androgenic-Anabolic Steroids,* Kochakian, C. D., Ed., Springer-Verlag, Basel, 1976, 45.

126. **Stafford, R. O., Bowman, B. J., and Olson, K. I.,** Influence of 19-nortestosterone cyclopentylpropionate on urinary nitrogen of castrate male rat, *Proc. Soc. Exp. Biol. Med.,* 86, 322, 1954.

127. **Henderson, E. and Weinberg, M.,** Endocrine review; methylandrostenediol, *J. Clin. Endocrinol.,* 11, 641, 1951.

128. **Stucki, J. C., Forbes, A. D., Northam, J. I., and Clark, J. J.,** An assay for anabolic steroids employing metabolic balance in the monkey: the anabolic activity of fluoroxymesterone and its 11-keto analogue, *Endocrinology,* 66, 585, 1960.

129. **Eisenberg, E. and Gordan, G. S.,** Levator ani muscle of rat as index of myotrophic activity of steroidal hormones, *J. Pharmacol. Exp. Ther.,* 99, 38, 1950.

130. **Hershberger, L. G., Shipley, E. G., and Meyer, R. K.,** Myotrophic activity of 19-nortestosterone and other steroids determined by modified levator ani muscle method, *Proc. Soc. Exp. Biol. Med.,* 83, 175, 1953.

44   *CRC Handbook of Hormones, Vitamins, and Radiopaques*

131. **Edgren, R. A.,** A comparative study of the anabolic and androgenic effects of various steroids, *Acta Endocrinol. (Copenhagen),* 44(Suppl. 87), 1, 1963.
132. **Spencer, H., Friedland, J. A., and Lewin, I.,** Effect of androgens on bone, calcium, and phosphorus metabolism, in *Anabolic-Androgenic Steroids,* Kochakian, C. D., Ed., Springer-Verlag, Basel, 1976, 419.
133. **Gurney, C. W.,** The hematologic effects of androgens, in *Anabolic-Androgenic Steroids,* Kochakian, C. D., Ed., Springer-Verlag, Basel, 1976, 483.
134. **Kopera, H.,** Miscellaneous uses of anabolic steroids, in *Anabolic-Androgenic Steroids,* Kocha Kian, C. D., Ed., Springer-Verlag, Basel, 1976, 535.
135. **Huseman, C. and Johanson, A.,** Growth hormone deficiency in anorexia nervosa, *J. Pediatr.,* 87, 946, 1975.
136. **Tec, L.,** Anorexia nervosa — follow-up on a special method of treatment, *Am. J. Psychiatry,* 127, 1702, 1971.
137. **Sansoy, P. M., Naylor, R. A., and Shields, L. M.,** Anabolic action and side effect of oxandrolone in 34 mental patients, *Geriatrics,* 26, 139, 1971.
138. **Morrison, B. O.,** Use of analeptic, antidepressant and anabolic drugs in treatment of the aged, *J. Mich. St. Med. Soc.,* 60, 723, 1961.
139. **Kolodny, A. L.,** Methandrostenolone (Dianabol) in the clinical management of weight deficit, *Med. Tms. (N.Y.),* 91, 9, 1963.
140. **Buchner, H.,** Zur Frage der hormonalen Beeinflussung des posttraumatischen Eriveizverlustes, *Wien. Med. Wschr.,* 111, 576, 1961.
141. **Konrad, R. M., Ammedick, U., Hupfauer, W., and Ringler, W.,** Der Effekt anaboler Steroide auf die Stickstoffbilanz bei Patienten nach Lungenoperationen, *Chirung,* 38, 168, 1967.
142. **Ammedick, U., Konrad, R. M., and Gotzen, E.,** Über die Wirksamkeit anaboler Steroide in der postoperativen Phase, *Med. Ernahr.,* 9, 121, 1968.
143. **Tweedle, D. E. F., Walton, C., and Johnston, I. D. A.,** The effect of a long-acting anabolic steroid on nitrogen balance during the anabolic phase of recovery from abdominal surgery, *Br. J. Surg.,* 59, 300, 1972.
144. **Renzi, A. A. and Chart, J. J.,** Interaction of methandrostenolone and adrenocortical hormones, *Proc. Soc. Exp. Biol. Med.,* 110, 259, 1962.
145. **Ryan, A. J.,** Athletics, in *Anabolic-Androgenic Steroids,* Kochakian, C. D., Ed., Springer-Verlag, Basel, 1976, 516.
146. **Casner, S., Early, R., and Carlson, B. R.,** Anabolic steroid effects on body composition in normal young men, *J. Sports Med. Phys. Fit.,* 11, 98, 1971.
147. **Fahey, T. D. and Brown, C. H.,** The effects of an anabolic steroid on the strength, body composition and endurance of college males when accompanied by a weight training program, *Med. Sci. Sports,* 5, 272, 1973.
148. **Golding, L. A., Freydinger, J. E., and Fishel, S. S.,** Weight, size and strength — unchanged by steroids, *Phys. Sports Med.,* 2, 39, 1974.
149. **Strömme, S. B., Meen, H. D., and Aakvaag, A.,** Effects of an androgenic-anabolic steroid on strength development and plasma testosterone levels in normal males, *Med. Sci. Sports,* 6, 203, 1974.
150. **Ariel, G. and Saville, W.,** Effect of anabolic steroids on reflex components, *J. Appl. Physiol.,* 32, 795, 1972.
151. **Ariel, G.,** The effect of anabolic steroid upon skeletal muscle contractile force, *J. Sports Med. Phys. Fit.,* 13, 187, 1973.
152. **Johnson, L. C., Fisher, G., Silvester, L. J., and Hofheins, C. C.,** Anabolic steroid: effects on strength, body weight, O_2 uptake and spermatogenesis in mature males, *Med. Sci. Sports,* 4, 43, 1972.
153. **Steinbach, M.,** Über den Einfluβ Anaboler Wirkstoffe auf Korpergewicht, Muskelkraft und Muskeltraining, *Sportarzt Sportmedizin,* 11, 485, 1968.
154. **Wade, N.,** Anabolic steroids: doctors denounce them, but athletes aren't listeneing, *Science,* 176, 1399, 1972.
155. **Howard, R. P. and Furman, R. H.,** Metabolic and serum lipid effects of methylandrostane and methylandrostene pyrazoles, *J. Clin. Endocrinol.,* 22, 43, 1962.
156. **Dingman, J. F. and Jenkins, W. H.,** Dihydrotestosterone-hypocholesterolemic androgenic hormone, *Metabolism,* 11, 273, 1962.
157. **Weisenfeld, S., Akgun, S., and Newhouse, S.,** Effect of anabolic drugs on response of blood sugar and free fatty acids to glucagon, *Diabetes,* 12, 375, 1963.
158. **Glueck, C. J.,** Progestins, anabolic androgens, estrogens: effects on triglycerides and lipases, *Clin. Res.,* 17, 475, 1971.
159. **Glueck, C. J.,** Effects of oxandrolone on plasma triglycerides and postheparin lipolytic activity in patients with types III, IV, and V familial hyperlipoproteinemia, *Metabolism,* 20, 691, 1971.
160. **Doyle, A. E., Pinkus, N. B., and Green, J.,** The use of oxandrolone in hyperlipidaemia, *Med. J. Aust.,* 1, 127, 1974.

161. **Sachs, B. A. and Wolfman, L.,** Effect of oxandrolone on plasma lipids and lipoproteins of patients with disorders of lipid metabolism, *Metabolism,* 17, 400, 1968.

162. **Glueck, C. J., Ford, S., Steiner, P., and Fallat, R.,** Triglyceride removal efficiency and lipoprotein lipases-effects of oxandrolone, *Metabolism,* 22, 807, 1973.

163. **Shahidi, N. T.,** Androgens and erythropoiesis, *New Engl. J. Med.,* 289, 72, 1973.

164. **Killander, A., Lundmark, K., and Sjolin, S.,** Idiopathic aplastic anemia in children: results of androgen treatment, *Acta Paediatr. Scand.,* 58, 10, 1969.

165. **Branda, R. F., Amsden, T. W., and Jacob, H. S.,** Randomized study of nandrolone therapy for refractory anemia, (abstract), *Clin. Res.,* 22, 607A, 1974.

166. **Hughes, D. W.,** Aplastic anaemia in childhood: a reappraisal. II. Idiopathic and acquired aplastic anaemia, *Med. J. Aust.,* 2, 361, 1973.

167. **Hendler, E. D., Goffinet, J. A., Ross, S., Longnecker, R. E., and Bakovic, V.,** Controlled study of androgen therapy in anemia of patients on maintenance hemodialysis, *New Engl. J. Med.,* 291, 1046, 1974.

168. **Blumberg, A. and Keller, H.,** Erythropoiesis in anephric patients, *Schweiz. Med. Wschr.,* 101, 1887, 1971.

169. **Fried, W., Jonasson, O., Lang, G., and Schwartz, F.,** The hematologic effect of androgen in uremic patients, *Ann. Intern. Med.,* 79, 823, 1973.

170. **Keyssner, J., Hauswaldt, C., Uhl, N., and Hunstein, W.,** Testosteronbehandlung renaler Anämie, *Schweiz. Med. Wschr.,* 104, 1938, 1974.

171. **Daniel, W. A. and Bennett, D. L.,** The use of anabolic-androgenic steroids in childhood and adolescence, in, *Anabolic-Androgenic Steroids,* Kochakian, C. D., Ed., Springer-Verlag, Basel, 1976, 441.

172. **Saunders, F. J. and Drill, V. A.,** The myotrophic and androgenic effects of 17-ethyl-19-nortestosterone and related compounds, *Endocrinology,* 58, 567, 1956.

173. **Barnes, L. E., Stafford, R. O., Guild, M. E., Thole, L. C., and Olson, K. J.,** Comparison of myotrophic and androgenic activities of testosterone propionate with 19-nortestosterone and its esters, *Endocrinology,* 55, 77, 1954.

174. **Colton, F. B., Nysted, L. N., Reigel, B., and Raymond, A. L.,** 17-akyl-19-nortestosterones, *J. Am. Chem. Soc.,* 79, 1123, 1957.

175. **Sala, G., Baldratti, G., Ronchi, R., Clini, V., and Bertazzoli, C.,** Attivitá-anabolica di una serie di nuovi derivati del testosterone, *Sperimentale,* 106, 490, 1956.

176. **Gordan, G. S.,** Experimental basis for anabolic therapy, *Arch. Intern. Med.,* 100, 744, 1957.

177. **Arnold, A., Potts, G. O., and Beyler, A. L.,** Evaluation of the protein anabolic properties of certain orally active anabolic agents based on nitrogen balance studies in rats, *Endocrinology,* 72, 408, 1963.

178. **Desaulles, P. A.,** Anabolic hormones from the experimental point of view, *Helv. Med. Acta,* 27, 479, 1960.

179. **Dorfman, R. I. and Kincl, F. A.,** Relative potency of various steroids in an anabolic-androgenic assay using the castrated rat, *Endocrinology,* 72, 259, 1963.

180. **Edgren, R. A., Peterson, D. L., Jones, R. C., Nagra, C. L., Smith, H., and Hughes, G. A.,** Biological effects of synthetic gonanes, *Rec. Progr. Hormone Res.,* 22, 305, 1966.

181. **Tremololieres, J. and Pequignot, E.,** Anabolisme protéique produit chez l'homme par un nouveau steroide: la méthyltriénolone, *Presse Med.,* 73, 2655, 1965.

182. **Kruskemper, H. L. and Noell, G.,** Liver toxicity of a new anabolic agent: methyltrienolone, *Steroids,* 8, 13, 1966.

183. **Kruskemper, H. L., Morgner, K. D., and Noell, G.,** Klinische Pharmakologie von Tirenolonen, einer Gruppe neuartiger anabol wirksamer Oestrun — Derivate, *Arzneim. Forsch.,* 17, 449, 1967.

184. **Halden, A., Walter, R. M., and Gordan, G. S.,** Antitumor efficacy and toxicity of methyltrienolone (NSC-92858) in advanced breast cancer, *Cancer Chemother. Rep.,* 54, 453, 1970.

185. **Bonne, C. and Raynaud, J. P.,** Assay of androgen binding sites by exchange with methyltrienolone (R 1881), *Steroids,* 27, 497, 1976.

186. **Abe, O., Herraneu, H., and Dorfman, R. I.,** Influence of 2α-methyl-17β-hydroxy-5α-androstan-3-one on incorporation of glycine-2-C[14] into proteins of a rat mammary fibroadenoma. A possible bioassay method, *Proc. Soc. Exp. Biol. Med.,* 111, 706, 1962.

187. **Berkowitz, D.,** The treatment of postgastrectomy weight loss with two new anabolic agents, *Clin. Res.,* 8, 199, 1960.

188. **Counsell, R. E. and Klimstra, P. D.,** Anabolic Agents. 2-Methylene-5α-androstane derivatives, *J. Med. Chem.,* 6, 736, 1963.

189. **Dorfman, R. I. and Dorfman, A. S.,** The assay of subcutaneously injected androgens in the castrated rat, *Acta Endocrinol. (Copenhagen),* 42, 245, 1963.

190. **Sola, G.,** Clinical evaluation of the anabolic effect of 4-hydroxy-17α-methyltestosterone, *Helv. Med. Acta,* 27, 519, 1960.

191. **Meyerson, R. M.,** Clinical and metabolic studies on a new anabolic steroid, oxymetholone, *Am. J. Med. Sci.,* 241, 732, 1961.

192. **Glas, W. W. and Lansing, E. H.,** Oxymetholone as an anabolic agent in geriatric patients, *J. Am. Geriatr. Soc.,* 10, 509, 1962.
193. **Suchowsky, G. K. and Junkmann, K.,** Anabolic steroids and their side-effects, *Acta Endocrinol. (Copenhagen),* 39, 68, 1962.
194. **Pelc, B.,** Steroid derivatives. XXVIII. Preparation of 1-methyl-5α-androstane derivatives, *Collect. Czech. Commun.,* 29, 3089, 1964.
195. **Weller, O.,** Comparative studies on the metabolic effect of testosterone and 1-methyl-delta-androstenolone in cases with primary hypogonadism, *Endokrinology,* 42, 34, 1962.
196. **Neumann, F., Wiechert, R., Kramer, M., and Raspé, G.,** Tierexperimentelle Untersuchungen mit einem neuen Androgen, Mesterolon (1α-Methyl-5α-androstan-17β-ol-3-on), *Arzneim. Forsch.,* 16, 455, 1966.
197. **Weller, O.,** Die androgene Wirkung von 1α-Methyl-5α-androstan-17β-ol-3-on im Vergleich zum 17α-Methyl-Δ4-androsten-17β-ol-3-on, *Arzneim. Forsch.,* 16, 465, 1966.
198. **Arnold, A., Potts, G. O., and Beyler, A. L.,** The ratio of anabolic to androgenic activity of 7:17-dimethyltestosterone, oxymesterone, mestanolone and fluoxymesterone, *J. Endocrinol.,* 28, 87, 1963.
199. **Korst, D. R., Bowers, C. Y., Flokstra, J. H., and McMahon, F. G.,** Clinical evaluation of a new anabolic agent 7α, 17α-dimethyltestosterone (bolasterone), *Clin. Pharmacol. Ther.,* 4, 734, 1963.
200. **Pappo, R. and Jung, C. J.,** 2-oxasteroids: a new class of biologically active compounds, *Tetrahedron Lett.,* 365, 1962.
201. **Lennon, H. D. and Saunders. F. J.,** Anabolic activity of 2-oxa-17α-methyl-dihydrotestosterone (oxandrolone) in castrated rats, *Steroids,* 4, 689, 1964.
202. **Fox, M., Minot, A. S., and Liddle, G. W.,** Oxandrolone: a potent anabolic steroid of novel chemical configuration, *J. Clin. Endocrinol. Metab.,* 22, 921, 1962.
203. **Ray, C. G., Kirschvink, J. F., Waxman, S. H., and Kelley, V. C.,** Studies of anabolic steroids. III. The effect of oxandrolone on height and skeletal maturation in mongoloid children, *Am. J. Dis. Child.,* 110, 618, 1965.
204. **Nutting, E. F., Klimstra, P. D., and Counsell, R. E.,** Anabolic-androgenic activity of A-ring modified androstane derivatives. I. A comparison of parenteral activity, *Acta Endocrinol. (Copenhagen),* 53, 627, 1966.
205. **Nutting, E. F., Klimstra, P. D., and Counsell, R. E.,** Anabolic-androgenic activity of A-ring modified androstane derivatives. II. A comparison of oral activity, *Acta Endocrinol. (Copenhagen),* 53, 635, 1966.
206. **Overbeek, G. A., Delver, A., and deVisser, J.,** Pharmacological comparisons of anabolic steroids (ethylestrenol, nandrolone esters), *Acta Endocrinol. (Copenhagen), Suppl.,* 63, 7, 1961.
207. **Kalliomaki, A., Pirila, A. M., and Ruikka, I.,** A therapeutic trial with ethyl-estrenol in geriatric patients, *Acta Endocrinol. (Copenhagen),* 63, 124, 1962.
208. **Kopera, H.,** Clinical experiences with anabolic steroids in some special indications, in *Hormonal Steroids, Biochemistry, Pharmacology, and Therapeutics,* Vol. 2, Martini, L. and Pecile, A., Eds., Academic Press, New York, 1965, 195.
209. **Walser, A. and Schoenenberger, G.,** Metabolic research on ethylestrenol, *Schweiz Med. Wschr.,* 92, 897, 1962.
210. **Edwards, J. A. and Bowers, A.,** Δ² — hormone analogs, *Chem. Ind. (London),* 1961, 1962.
211. **Wolff, M. E. and Zanati, G.,** Thia steroids. I. 2-thia-A-nor-5-alpha-androstan-17-beta-ol, an active androgen, *J. Med. Chem.,* 12, 629, 1969.
212. **Wolff, M. E., Zanati, G., Shanmagasundarum, G., Grupte, S., and Aadahl, G.,** Thia steroids. 3. Derivative of 2-thia-a-nor-5-alpha-androstan-17-beta-ol as probes of steroid-receptor interactions, *J. Med. Chem.,* 13, 531, 1970.
213. **Wolff, M. E. and Zanati, G.,** Preparation and androgenic activity of novel heterocyclic steroids, *Experientia,* 26, 1115, 1970.
214. **Zanati, G., Gaare, G., and Wolff, M. E.,** Heterocyclic steroids. V. Sulfur, selenium, and tellurium 5-alpha-androstane derivatives and their 7-alpha-methylated congeners, *J. Med. Chem.,* 17, 561, 1974.
215. **Skinner, R. W. S., Pozderac, R. V., Counsell, R. E., Hsu, C. F., and Weinhold, P. A.,** Androgen receptor protein binding properties and tissue distribution of 2-selena-a-nor-5-alpha-androstan-17-beta-ol in the rat, *Steroids,* 30, 15, 1977.
216. **Wolff, M. E., Ho, W., and Kwok, R.,** The steroid-receptor complex. Some considerations based on sp-2-hybridized systems, *J. Med. Chem.,* 7, 577, 1964.
217. **Klimstra, P. D., Nutting, E. F., and Counsell, R. E.,** Anabolic agents. 2,3-epithioandrostane derivatives, *J. Med. Chem.,* 9, 693, 1966.
218. **Potts, G. O., Arnold, A., and Beyler, A. L.,** Comparative nitrogen retaining and androgenic activities of certain orally active steroids, *Int. Congr. Hormonal Steroids,* Milan, May 14, 1962, 211.
219. **Potts, G. O., Beyler, A. L., and Burnham, D. F.,** Myotrophic and androgenic activities of androstanazole. A new heterocyclic steroid, *Proc. Soc. Exp. Biol. Med.,* 103, 383, 1960.
220. **Burnett, P. C.,** A steroidal pyrazole as an anabolic agent in the treatment of geriatric mental patients, *J. Am. Geriatr. Soc.,* 11, 979, 1963.

221. **Mullin, W. G. and diPillo, F.**, Influence of stanozolol on hemoglobin levels, *N.Y. St. J. Med.*, 63, 2795, 1963.

222. **Manson, A. J., Stonner, F. W., Neumann, H. C., Christiansen, R. G., Clarke, R. L., Ackerman, H. J., Page, D. F., Dean, J. W., Phillips, D. K., Potts, G. O., Arnold, A., Beyler, A. L., and Clinton, R. O.**, Steroidal heterocycles. VII. Androstano-[2,3-d]isoxazoles and related compounds, *J. Med. Chem.*, 6, 1, 1963.

223. **Kochakian, C. D. and Arimasa, N.**, The metabolism *in vitro* of anabolic-androgenic steroids by mammalian tissues, in *Anabolic-Androgenic Steroids*, Kochakian, C. D., Ed., Springer-Verlag, Basel, 1976, 287.

224. **Wolff, M. E. and Kasuya, Y.**, C-3-oxygenation of 17α-methyl-5α-androstan-17β-ol by rabbit liver homogenate, *J. Med. Chem.*, 15, 87, 1972.

225. **Rosi, D., Neumann, H. C., Christiansen, R. G., Schane, H. P., and Potts, G. O.**, Isolation, synthesis, and biological activity of five metabolites of danazol, *J. Med. Chem.*, 20, 349, 1977.

226. **Davison, C., Banks, W., and Fritz, A.**, The absorption, distribution and metabolic fate of danazol in rats, monkeys and human volunteers, *Arch. Int. Pharmacodyn. Ther.*, 221, 294, 1976.

227. **Bernstein, M. S., Hunter, R. L., and Yachnin, S.**, Hepatoma and peliosis hepatitis in Fanconi's anemia, *N. Engl. J. Med.*, 284, 1135, 1971.

228. **Henderson, J. T., Richmond, J., and Sumerling, M. D.**, Androgenic-anabolic steroid therapy and hepatocellular carinoma, *Lancet*, 1, 934, 1973.

229. **Johnson, F. L., Feagler, J. R., Lerner, K. G., Majerus, P. W., Siegel, M., Hartman, J. R., and Thomas, E. D.**, Association of androgenic-anabolic steroid therapy with development of hepatocellular carcinoma, *Lancet*, 2, 1273, 1971.

230. **Ishak, K. G.**, Hepatic neoplasms associated with contraceptive and anabolic steroids, in *Carcinogenic Hormones*, Lingeman, C. H., Ed., Springer-Verlag, Basel, 1979, 73.

231. **Steinbeck, H. and Neumann, F.**, Androgen antagonists: chemistry and influence on neural-gonadal function, in *Reproductive Endocrinology*, Vokaer, R. and DeBock, G., Eds., Pergamon Press, Oxford, 1975, 135.

232. **Martini, L. and Motta, M., Eds.**, *Androgens and Antiandrogens*, Raven Press, New York, 1977.

233. **Raynaud, J. P.**, The mechanism of action of anti-hormones, in *Advances in Pharmacology and Therapeutics*, Vol. 1, Jacob, J., Ed., Pergamon Press, Oxford, 1979, 259.

234. **Hammerstein, J., Meckies, J., Leo-Rossberg, I., Moltz, L., and Zielke, F.**, Use of cyproterone acetate (CPA) in the treatment of acne, hirsutism, and virilism, *J. Steroid Biochem.*, 6, 827, 1975.

235. **Burton, J. L., Laschet, U., and Shuster, S.**, Reduction of serum excretion in man by the antiandrogen cyproterone acetate, *Br. J. Dermatol.*, 89, 487, 1973.

236. **Hammerstein, J. and Cupceancu, B.**, Behandlung des hirsutismus mit cyproteronacetat, *Dtsh. Med. Wochenschr.*, 94, 829, 1969.

237. **Ismail, A. A., Davidson, D. W., Souka, A. R., Barnes, E. W., Irvine, W. J., Kilimnik, H., and Vanderbeeken, Y.**, The evaluation of the role of androgens in hirsutism and the use of a new anti-androgen "cyproterone acetate" for therapy, *J. Clin. Endocrinol. Metab.*, 39, 81, 1974.

238. **Cittadini, E. and Barreca, P.**, Use of antiandrogens in gynecology, in *Androgens and Antiandrogens*, Martini, L. and Motta, M., Eds., Raven Press, New York, 1977, 309.

239. **Mahesh, V. B.**, Excessive androgen secretion and use of antiandrogens in endocrine therapy, in *Androgens and Antiandrogens*, Martini, L. and Motta, M., Eds., Raven Press, New York, 1977, 321.

240. **Ebling, F. J.**, Antiandrogens in dermatology, in *Androgens and Antiandrogens*, Martini, L. and Motta, M., Eds., Raven Press, New York, 1977, 341.

241. **Geller, J., Fruchtman, B., Newman, H., Roberts, T., and Sylva, R.**, Effect of progestational agents on carcinoma of the prostate, *Cancer Chemother. Rep.*, 51, 441, 1967.

242. **Bracci, U. and DiSilverio, F.**, Il cancro della prostata: nostri attuali orientamenti terapeutici, *Progr. Med.*, 29, 779, 1973.

243. **Bracci, U.**, Interet de la cyprotereone a dans les metastases du carcinoma de la prostate, *J. Urol. Nephrol.*, 79, 405, 1973.

244. **DiSilverio, F. and Gagliardi, V.**, Il cancro della prostata: orientamenti terapeutici nell forme estrogeno resistenti, *Boll. Soc. Urol.*, 5, 198, 1968.

245. **Bracci, U. and diSilverio, F.**, Role of cyproterone acetate in urology, in *Androgens and Antiandrogens*, Martini, L. and Motta, M., Eds., Raven Press, New York, 1977, 333.

246. **Raynaud, J. P., Azadian-Boulanger, G., Bonne, C., Perronnet, J., and Sakis, E.**, Present trends in antiandrogen research, in *Androgens and Antiandrogens*, Martini, L. and Motta, M., Eds., Raven Press, New York, 1977, 281.

247. **Huggins, C. and Hodges, C. V.**, Studies on prostatic cancer; effect of castration, of estrogen and of androgen injection on serum phosphatases in metastatic carcinoma of prostate, *Cancer Res.*, 1, 293, 1941.

248. **Huggins, C., Stevens, R. E., Jr., and Hodges, C. V.**, Studies on prostatic cancer; effects of castration on advanced carcinoma of prostate gland, *Arch. Surg.*, 43, 209, 1941.

249. **Sutherland-Rawlings, E. A. P.,** Thrombosis and carcinoma of the prostrate, *Br. Med. J.,* 111, 643, 1970.
250. **Dodds, E. C.,** Synthetic oestrogens in cancer, *Biochem. J.,* 39, i, 1945.
251. **Geller, J., Fruchtman, B., Meyer, C. and Newman, H.,** Effect of progestational agents on gonadal and adrenal cortical function in patients with benign prostatic hypertrophy and carcinoma of the prostate, *J. Clin. Endocrinol. Metab.,* 27, 556, 1967.
252. **Neumann, F.,** Methods for evaluating antisexual hormones, in *Methods in Drug Evaluation,* Mantegazza, P. and Piccinini, F., North-Holland, Amsterdam, 1966, 548.
253. **Mietkiewski, K., Malendowicz, L., and Lukaszyk, A.,** Cytological and cytochemical comparative study on the effect of cyproterone (anti-androgen) and gonadectomy on the gonadotrophic cells of the hypophysis in male rats, *Acta Endocrinol. (Cophenhagen),* 61, 293, 1969.
254. **Neri, R. O.,** Antiandrogens, *Adv. Sex. Hormone Res.,* 2, 233, 1976.
255. **Neumann, F.,** Pharmacology and potential use of cyproterone acetate, *Hormone Metab. Res.,* 9, 1, 1977.
256. **Fixson, U.,** Preliminary report on a new orally active gestagen (SH 714), *Geburtsh. Frauenheilk,* 23, 371, 1963.
257. **Junkmann, K. and Neumann, F.,** Zum Wirkungsmechanismus von an Feten antimaskulin Wirksamen Gestagenen, *Acta Endocrinol. (Copenhagen) Suppl. 90,* 139, 1964.
258. **Neumann, F., Gräf, K. J., Hasan, S. H., Schenck, B., and Steinbeck, H.,** Central actions of antiandrogens, in *Androgens and Antiandrogens,* Martini, L. and Motta, M., Eds., Raven Press, New York, 1977, 163.
259. **Neumann, F., Berswodt-Wallace, R. von, Elger, W., Steinbeck, H., Hahn, J., and Kramer, M.,** Aspects of androgen-dependent events as studied by anti-androgens, *Rec. Progr. Hormone Res.,* 26, 337, 1970.
260. **Fang, S., Anderson, K. M., and Liao, S.,** Receptor proteins for androgens. On the role of specific proteins in selective retention of 17-beta-hydroxy-5-alpha-androstan-3-one by rat ventral prostate *in vivo* and *in vitro, J. Biol. Chem.,* 244, 6584, 1969.
261. **Fang, S. and Liao, S.,** Antagonistic action of antiandrogens on the formation of a specific dihydrotestosterone-receptor protein complex in rat prostate, *Mol. Pharmacol.,* 5, 420, 1969.
262. **Stern, J. and Eisenfeld, A. J.,** Distribution and metabolism of ^{3}H-testosterone in castrated male rats; effects of cyproterone, progesterone, and unlabeled testosterone, *Endocrinology,* 88, 1117, 1971.
263. **Mangan, F. R. and Mainwaring, W. I. P.,** An explanation of the antiandrogenic properties of 6α-bromo-17β-hydroxy-17β-methyl-4-oxa-5α-androstan-3-one, *Steroids,* 20, 331, 1972.
264. **Jagarinec, N. and Givner, M. L.,** Measurement of a progestational and antiandrogenic compound by a competitive protein binding assay, *Steroids,* 23, 561, 1974.
265. **Lerner, L. J., Bianchi, A., and Borman, A.,** A-norprogesterone, an androgen antagonist, *Proc. Soc. Exp. Biol. Med.,* 103, 172, 1960.
266. **Orestano, F., Altwein, J. E., Knapstein, P., and Bandhauer, K.,** Mode of action of progesterone, gestonorone capronate (Deprostat) and cyproterone acetate (Androcur) on the metabolism of testosterone in human prostatic adenoma: *in vitro* and *in vivo* investigations, *J. Steroid Biochem.,* 6, 845, 1975.
267. **Mainwaring, W. I. P.,** Modes of action of antiandrogens: a survey, in *Androgens and Antiandrogens,* Martini, L. and Motta, M., Eds., Raven Press, New York, 1977, 151.
268. **Tan, S. Y., Antonipillai, I., and Murphy, B. E. P.,** Inhibition of testosterone metabolism in the human prostate, *J. Clin. Endocrinol. Metab.,* 39, 936, 1974.
269. **Saunders, H. L., Holden, K., and Kerwin, J. F.,** The anti-androgenic activity of 17α-methyl-B-nortestosterone (SKF 7690), *Steroids,* 3, 687, 1964.
270. **Boris, A. and Uskokovic, M.,** A new antiandrogen, 6α-bromo-17β-hydroxy-17α-methyl-4-oxa-5α-androstan-3-one, *Experientia,* 26, 9, 1970.
271. **Boris, A., DeMartino, L., and Trmal, T.,** Some endocrine studies of a new antiandrogen, 6α-bromo-17β-hydroxy-17α-methyl-4-oxa-5α-androstan-3-one (BOMT), *Endocrinology,* 88, 1086, 1971.
272. **Baulieu, E. E. and Jung, I.,** A prostatic cytosol receptor, *Biochem. Biophys. Res. Commun.,* 38, 599, 1970.
273. **Rasmusson, G. H., Chen, A., Reynolds, G. F., Patanelli, D. J., Patchett, A. A., and Arth, G. E.,** Antiandrogens. 2′,3′α-tetrahydrofuran-2′-spiro-17-(1,2α-methylene-4-androsten-3-ones), *J. Med. Chem.,* 15, 1165, 1972.
274. **Brooks, J. R., Busch, F. D., Patanelli, D. J., and Steelman, S. L.,** A study of the effects of a new antiandrogen on the hyperplastic dog prostate, *Proc. Soc. Exp. Biol. Med.,* 143, 647, 1973.
275. **Hiraga, K., Tsunehiko, A., and Takuichi, M.,** Synthesis and steric hinderances in 13β-isopropylgonanes, *Chem. Pharm. Bull. (Tokyo),* 13, 1294, 1965.
276. **Goto, G., Yoshiska, K., Hiraga, K., Masouka, M., Nakayama, R., and Miki, T.,** Synthesis and antiandrogenic activity of 16β-substituted 17β-hydroxysteroids, *Chem. Pharm. Bull. (Tokyo),* 26, 1718, 1978.
277. **Mangan, F. R. and Mainwaring, W. I. P.,** An explanation of the antiandrogenic properties of 6α-bromo-17β-hydroxy-17α-methyl-4-oxa-5α-androstane-2-one, *Steroids,* 20, 331, 1972.

278. **Azadian-Boulanger, G., Bonne, C., Sechi, J., and Raynaud, J. P.,** Antiandrogenic activity of R2956 (17β-hydroxy-2,2,17α-trimethylestra-4,9,11-trien-3-one). I. Endocrinological profile, *J. Pharmacol. (Paris),* 5, 509, 1974.

279. **Bonne, C. and Raynaud, J. P.,** Mode of spironolactone antiandrogenic action: inhibition of androstanolone binding to rat prostate androgen receptor, *Mol. Cell Endocrinol.,* 2, 59, 1974.

280. **Corvol, P., Michaud, A., Menard, J., Freifeld, M., and Mahoudean, J.,** Antiandrogen effect of spirolactones: mechanism of action, *Endocrinology,* 97, 52, 1975.

281. **Wakeling, A. E., Furr, B. J. A., Glen, A. T., and Hughes, L. R.,** Receptor binding and biological activity of steroidal and nonsteroidal antiandrogens, *J. Steroid Biochem.,* 15, 355, 1981.

282. **Starka, L., Sulcova, J., Broulik, P. D., Joska, J., Fajkos, J., and Doskocil, M.,** Screening for antiandrogenic activity of some 4,5-cyclo-A-nor-3,5-secoandrostanes, *J. Steroid Biochem.,* 8, 939, 1977.

283. **Starka, L., Hanapl, R., Bicikova, M., Cerny, V., Fajkos, J., Kosal, A., Kocovsky, P., Kohout, L., and Velgova, H.,** Steroids with modified ring A or B: screening for potential antiandrogenic and synandrogenic activity, *J. Steroid Biochem.,* 13, 455, 1980.

284. **Neri, R., Florance, K., Koziol, P., and van Cleave, S.,** A biological profile of a nonsteroidal antiandrogen SCH 13521 (4′-nitro-3′trifluoromethylisobutyranilide), *Endocrinol.,* 91, 427, 1972.

285. **Neri, R. O. and Monahan, M.,** Effects of a novel nonsteroidal antiandrogen on canine prostatic hyperplasia, *Invest. Urol.,* 10, 123, 1972.

286. **Peets, E. A., Henson, M. F., and Neri, R.,** On the mechanism of the antiandrogenic action of flutamide (α-α-α-trifluoro-2-methyl-4′-nitro-m-propionotoluidide) in the rat, *Endocrinology,* 94, 532, 1974.

287. **Liao, S., Howell, D. K., and Chuag, T.,** Action of a nonsteroidal antiandrogen, flutamide, on the receptor binding and nuclear retention of 5α-dihydrotestosterone in rat ventral prostate, *Endocrinology,* 94, 1205, 1974.

288. **Neri, R. and Perts, E. A.,** Biological aspects of antiandrogens, *J. Steroid Biochem.,* 6, 815, 1975.

289. **Boris, A., Scott, J. W., DeMartino, L., and Cox, D. C.,** Endocrine profile of a nonsteroidal antiandrogen N-(3,5-dimethyl-4-isoxazolylmethyl) phthalimide (DIMP), *Acta Endocrinol. (Copenhagen),* 72, 604, 1973.

290. **Boris, A.,** Endocrine studies of a nonsteroid anti-androgen and progestin, *Endocrinology,* 76, 1062, 1965.

291. **Tanayama, S., Yoshida, K., Kondo, T., and Kanai, Y.,** Disposition and metabolism of 16β-ethyl-17β-hydroxy-4-estren-3-one (TSAA-291), a new antiandrogen in rats, *Steroids,* 33, 65, 1979.

292. **Speck, U., Wendt, H., Schulze, P. E., and Jentsch, D.,** Bio-availability and pharmacokinetics of cyproterone acetate — ^{14}C and ethinyl oestradiol-[^3H] after oral administration as a coated tablet (SH B 209 AB), *Contraception,* 14, 151, 1976.

293. **Hümpel, M., Wendt, H., Schulze, P. E., Dogs, G., Weiss, C., and Speck, U.,** Bioavailability and pharmacokinetics of cyproterone acetate after oral administration of 2.0 mg cyproterone acetate in combination with 50 μg ethinyl oestradiol to 6 young women, *Contraception,* 15, 579, 1977.

294. **Hümpel, M., Dogs, H., Wendt, H., and Speck, U.,** Plasmaspiegel und Pharmakokinetik von Cyproteronacetate nach oraler Applikation als 50-mg-Tablette bei 5 Männein, *Arzneim. Forsch.,* 28, 319, 1978.

295. **Frölich, M., Vader, H. L., Walma, S. T., and De Rooy, H. A. M.,** Cyproterone acetate in blood of hirsute women during long-term treatment. The absorption and elimination after oral application, *J. Steroid Biochem.,* 13, 1097, 1980.

296. **Bhargava, A. S., Seeger, A., and Günzel, P.,** Isolation and identification of 15β-hydroxy cyproterone acetate as a new metabolite of cyproterone acetate in dog, monkey and man, *Steroids,* 30, 407, 1977.

297. **Katchen, B. and Buxbaum, S.,** Disposition of a new, nonsteroid, antiandrogen, alpha, alpha, alpha-trifluoro-2methyl-4′-nitro-m-propion (Flutamide), in men following a single oral 200 mg dose, *J. Clin. Endocrinol. Metab.,* 41, 373, 1975.

298. **Neri, R. O.,** Studies on the biology and mechanism of action of nonsteroidal antiandrogens, in *Androgens and Antiandrogens,* Martini, L. and Motta, M., Raven Press, New York, 1977, 179.

299. **Neumann, F. and Von Berswordt-Wallrabe, R.,** Effects of the androgen antagonist cyproterone acetate on the testicular structure, spermatogenesis and accessory sexual glands of testosterone-treated adult hypophysectomized rats, *J. Endocrinol.,* 35, 363, 1966.

300. **Hammerstein, J.,** Male contraception, in *Androgens and Antiandrogens,* Martini, L. and Motta, M., Eds., Raven Press, New York, 1977, 327.

301. **Horn, H. J.,** Role of antiandrogens in psychiatry, in *Androgens and Antiandrogens,* Martini, L. and Motta, M., Eds., Raven Press, New York, 1977, 351.

302. **Neumann, F. and Junkmann, K.,** A new method for determination of virilizing properties of steroids on the fetus, *Endocrinology,* 73, 33, 1963.

303. **Neri, R. O., Monahan, M. D., Meyer, J. G., Alfonso, B. A., and Tabachnick, I. I. A.,** Biological studies on an anti-androgen, *Eur. J. Pharmacol.,* 1, 438, 1967.

304. **Lerner, L. J.,** Androgen antagonists, *Pharmacol. Ther. B,* 1, 217, 1975.

FEMALE SEX HORMONES, ANTIESTROGENS, AND ANTIOVULATORY AGENTS

Robert A. Magarian, J. Thomas Pento, and M. Margaret King

FEMALE SEX HORMONES

ESTROGENS

Introduction

The female reproductive steroids, 17β-estradiol and progesterone, are produced and secreted primarily by the ovary; although, small amounts of these hormones are produced by the adrenal medulla. In 1900 Knauer[1] established that a hormonal substance from the ovary controlled female reproductive function. Later Doisy and co-workers[2,3] isolated the reproductive steroids from the urine of pregnant women.

The ovaries produce two types of active steroid hormones whose actions are interrelated in the regulation of the process of sexual development and reproduction in the female. The first group is referred to as the estrogens and includes 17β-estradiol, estrone, and estriol. The second type of ovarian hormone is progesterone. The developing ovarian follicles secrete estrogens during the first half of the female menstrual cycle in response to the action of the follicle stimulating hormone (FSH) from the anterior pituitary. At approximately day 14 of the cycle the mature follicle ruptures and ovulation occurs under the influence of luteinizing hormone (LH) which is also secreted by the anterior pituitary. Following ovulation the ruptured follicle is transformed into a corpus luteum, within the ovary, which secretes both estrogens and progesterone. Toward the end of the cycle the corpus luteum begins to degenerate due to the loss of gonadotropin (LH and FSH) stimulation. Thus, the secretion of estrogen and progesterone decreases which leads to sluffing of the uterine endometrium, menstrual bleeding, and the onset of another menstral cycle.

The secretion of estrogens and progesterone from the ovaries is stimulated (+) by FSH and LH from the anterior pituitary and gonadotropin-releasing hormone (GnRH) from the hypothalamus as outlined in Figure 1. The elevated levels of estrogen and progesterone in the circulation, which vary with the phase of the menstrual cycle, inhibit (−) the secretion of GnRH, FSH, and LH by means of a negative feedback loop. FSH and LH also exert a negative feedback loop on the secretion of GnRH from the hypothalamus. Since the hypothalamus is part of the cerebral cortex, the regulation of GnRH, FSH, LH, and the ovarian hormones are also influenced by psychological and emotional factors via the central nervous system.

Mechanism of Action

Steroidal and nonsteroidal estrogens are known to produce typical estrogenic actions in estrogen-responsive tissues (e.g., breast, female reproductive tract, pituitary, and hypothalamus) by reaction with specific estrogen receptors which are located in the cell cytoplasm and nucleus. A schematic outline of the major events known to be involved in an estrogenic response is presented in Figure 2. Estrogens in the circulation cross the cell membrane by passive diffusion and bind to the cytoplasmic estrogen receptor (R_c) with very high affinity (Kd = approximately $10^{-10}\,M$). The original estrogen-receptor complex (E-R_c) is converted to a different species (E-$R_c{}'$) which is translocated into the nucleus of the cell. Within the nucleus the nuclear estrogen-receptor complex (E-R_n) promptly affects the expression of genetic material and stimulates RNA, DNA, and protein synthesis, which in turn produces

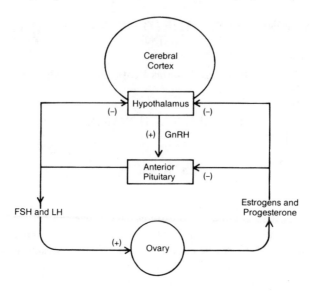

FIGURE 1.   Outline of the central mechanism for the secretion of the ovarian hormones; (+)-secretory stimulation, (−) secretory suppression.

CELL IN AN ESTROGEN-DEPENDENT TISSUE

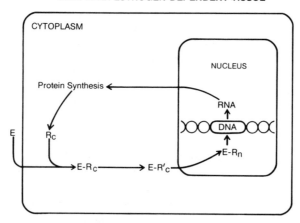

FIGURE 2.   Schematic outline of the estrogenic mechanism of action.

the ultimate expression of estrogenic activity in estrogen-dependent target tissue. The estrogenic action within the nucleus also causes the regeneration of existing cytoplasmic receptors or the synthesis of new receptors.

Estrogen actions in general are characterized by the changes which take place during puberty in the female. These actions include growth and maturity of the female reproductive tract (i.e., vagina, uterus, and fallopian tubes), growth and development of breast tissue, general anabolic effects on body growth, and development of the feminine body contour, growth of pubic hair, regional pigmentation, and psychological and emotional effects which are associated with sexual drive, and feminine behavior.

Estrogen and progestin actions also include stimulation of the growth and maturation of the uterine endometrium observed during the normal adult menstrual cycle and the characterisitc utero-placental and breast development observed during pregnancy and lactation.

Pharmacokinetics

Most estrogens used therapeutically are well absorbed through the skin, mucous membranes, gastrointestinal tract, and parenteral sites of injection. Absorption from the parenteral sites may be delayed due to esterification of the estrogen in the oil-based parenteral preparations.

Natural estrogens are absorbed readily by the oral route; however, they are promptly metabolized to less active products. Thus, the oral route of administration for natural estrogens is not very effective. Synthetic estrogens such as ethinyl estradiol and diethylstilbestrol are more slowly metabolized by the liver, and for this reason have a longer duration of action and are much more effective than natural estrogens when administered by the oral route.

The liver is the major site of estrogen metabolism. It is here that 17β-estradiol is metabolized to estrone and estriol which are the major products of estrogen metabolism. Quantitatively, hydroxylation at positions 2 and 16 appears to be the most prominent metabolic transformation. The specific enzymatic systems involved in estrogen metabolism (usually microsomal) utilize NADPH and O_2. However, interconversion of estradiol and estrone also occurs in other tissues including the placenta.[4]

Catechol-O-methyltransferase catalyzes the O-methylation of specific hydroxylated estrogen metabolites (especially 2-hydroxy compounds) by S-adenosylmethionine. These methoxy metabolites and their conjugates are excreted in the urine.

Estrogens and estrogen metabolites are excreted primarily as conjugates of glucuronic and sulfuric acids. The major estrogen conjugates are the C-3 glucuronides of estrone and 2-hydroxyestrone, also estrone sulfate esterified at the C-3 position. Sulfation at C-17 and formation of the 3,17-disulfate of estradiol has been reported. The estrogen conjugates produce estrogenic activity by the oral route of administration which indicates that the conjugated estrogens are less susceptible to hepatic degradation than the parent estrogens.[4,5]

Both the conjugated and nonconjugated estrogens are bound (50 to 75%) to specific and nonspecific plasma proteins. The conjugated estrogens are ionized and water soluble, and thus, urinary excretion is favored. However, a small amount of the circulating estrogens and estrogen metabolites are excreted in the bile and appear in the feces, or are reabsorbed from the intestine and returned to the circulation.

In normal adult premenopausal women the blood levels of the active estrogens (estradiol, estrone, estriol) vary considerably during the menstrual cycle. Estrogen blood levels are the lowest during the first 5 to 6 days of the cycle and range from 50 to 150 pg/mℓ. This is followed by a gradual rise in estrogen levels to a mid-cycle peak of 150 to 600 pg/mℓ followed by a gradual decline in estrogen levels.[5-7] Following menopause and ovarian atrophy estrogen blood levels remain very low.[8]

Uses

The discovery that certain nonsteroidal compounds, especially stilbene derivatives, were able to produce all of the physiological effects of naturally occurring estrogens, even when given by the oral route, proved to be of great therapeutic importance. Some of these include diethylstilbestrol, hexestrol, and ethinyl estradiol. Ethinyl estradiol, given orally is 50 times more effective than water-soluble estrogenic preparations or 30 times that of estradiol benzoate injected intramuscularly.

Estrogens are used as substitution therapy following ovariectomy, natural menopause, X-ray or radium therapy, and for general menopausal symptoms. Evidence is not convincing that therapy can prevent arteriosclerotic cardiovascular disease although they have been used effectively to retard the progression of postmenopausal osteoporosis. Menstrual irregularities such as amenorrhea may be treated with the estrogens. Used cyclically, they are useful for the treatment of secondary amenorrhea. In young women, the estrogens are used for treatment of failure of steroidogenesis (hypogonadism). Local application is useful in the treatment of cervicitis, vulvovaginitis, kraurosis vulvae, and atrophic or senile vaginitis. Estrogens are effective for only short periods of time in the treatment of endometriosis. Treatment of moderate to severe vasomotor symptoms prior to menstruation is a common use of estrogens, including headache, tension, breast engorgement, and nipple tenderness. They are also of value in decreasing electrolyte imbalance premenstrually.

Less commonly the estrogens are used as hypocholesterolemic drugs since they decrease plasma cholesterol. Additionally, they have been used to treat *acne vulgaris* and hirsutism. As anticancer therapy the estrogens are effective in the inhibition of prostatic cancer in men and breast carcinoma, as well as carcinoma in other areas of the reproductive tract in women, especially when they are 4 years or more postmenopausal. They are used occasionally in the treatment of postpartum breast engorgement, although the benefits must be carefully weighed against an associated increased risk of peripheral thromboembolism especially in the use of high dosages.

In order to minimize possible adverse effects, estrogens are generally administered at the lowest effective dosage level for the shortest possible time interval. Patients who have been on a high-dose or long-term protocol of estrogen therapy, should be discontinued or reduced in dose level gradually.

Administration should be cyclic and for short-term use only for premenstrual vasomotor symptoms, and menopausal atrophic vaginitis or kraurosis vulvae. Dosages are usually 3 weeks on and 1 week off with attempts being made to decrease or discontinue medication every 3 to 6 months. Cyclic administration for longer periods of time is useful in the treatment of postmenopausal symptoms, ovariectomy, primary amenorrhea, osteoporosis, and female hypogonadism.

When given for postpartum breast engorgement, estrogen treatment is only for a few days.

Estrogens are administered chronically primarily for the treatment of carcinoma. Specifically chronic estrogen therapy is used for treatment of inoperable and metastatic breast cancer in postmenopausal women and inoperable prostatic cancer in men. Progestin therapy is often used concommitantly with chronic estrogen therapy for a period of 10 days each month. This procedure mimics physiological hormone cycle and induces a cyclical uterine bleeding. Studies have indicated that combined estrogen-progestin therapy may decrease the high risk of endometrial carcinoma known to occur as a result of chronic estrogen therapy.

Precautions

Estrogens should be used with caution in patients who are known to suffer from epilepsy, cardiac insufficiency, or cerebrovascular disease, asthma, migraine headaches, mental depression, renal dysfunction, benign cystic breast disease, diabetes mellitus, hepatic disorders, gall bladder disease, endometriosis, hypertension, jaundice, or uterine abnormalities such as fibroids and tumor-associated hypercalcemia or other metabolic bone diseases.

Estrogens have an effect on epiphyseal closure and thus should be used carefully in young patients with incomplete bone growth.

Many of the estrogen products contain tartrazine and may cause allergic reactions, including bronchial asthma in susceptible persons. This response is seen more commonly in persons who also have aspirin sensitivity.

Evidence suggests that estrogens increase the risk of endometrial, breast, cervical, vaginal, and liver cancer. Extra caution should be exercised in prescribing estrogens to women with breast nodules, fibrocystic disease, or a family history of breast cancer. In women taking oral contraceptives, hepatocellular carcinoma has been reported, as have benign hepatic adenomas.

Severe hypercalcemia may occur as a result of estrogen therapy, and is especially common in patients with breast cancer and bone metastases.

Hypertension occurs frequently in women undergoing estrogen therapy, especially for menopause. Monitoring of blood pressure should be common with estrogen therapy.

Increased sun sensitivity may occur during estrogen therapy. Patients should be warned about possible increases in photosensitivity and cautioned to avoid prolonged UV light or sun exposure.

Diabetics should be given estrogens cautiously, and carefully observed during therapy, since a decrease in glucose tolerance is common as a result of estrogen treatment.

Estrogens increase the risk of both cervical and uterine carcinoma, thus warranting frequent periodic examinations. In men taking large doses for prostatic cancer, hypercalcemia may occur.

In mature women, chronic estrogen use may cause spotting or break-through vaginal bleeding. After discontinuation of estrogen therapy, withdrawal bleeding usually occurs.

Carbohydrate tolerance may deteriorate during estrogen treatment with a resultant decrease in glucose tolerance. Diabetes mellitus may be exacerbated. In persons already having a type 4 hyperlipidemia, serum triglycerides may rise resulting in a dangerous hyperlipidemic state. The composition of bile is altered due to estrogen therapy and after long-term therapy, an increased incidence of gall stones has been reported. Porphyria may be provoked, although this occurs only rarely. Several reports have been made of an increased incidence of carcinoma of the endometrium exclusively involving menopausal women treated with estrogens.[9,12]

Carcinoma can be expected to occur more frequently in the estrogen-stimulated than in the inactive endometrium.[13,14] Induced endometrial carcinoma is unknown in childhood or adolescence. Because estrogens do increase the risk of both cervical and uterine carcinoma, periodic examinations are advisable.

Contraindications

Estrogens should not be used during pregnancy since many studies suggest a high degree of correlation between their use and congenital malformations. This is especially true in the use of diethylstilbestrol (DES). Daughters of mothers having taken DES during pregnancy have been reported to develop reproductive tract abnormalities, as well as cancer of the vagina and/or cervix as they reach sexual maturity. No effective purpose for the use of estrogens during pregnancy has been shown, and the adverse effects on the fetus are well documented.[15-18]

Estrogens should not be used in abnormal undiagnosed genital bleeding or in cases of a history of hypersensitivity to estrogens. Their use should be avoided in any of the thromboembolic and thrombophlebitic disorders, thrombophlebitis and thrombosis especially if these disorders are associated with a previous estrogen use.

Use of estrogens by nursing mothers is not recommended since they are excreted in the breast milk and inhibit lactation. It is difficult to predict the potential adverse effects to the nursing infant.

Patients with known or suspected breast cancer, or other suspected estrogen-dependent neoplasias, should not be subjected to estrogen therapy. The only exception is in patients being treated specifically for metastatic breast carcinoma.

Estrogens alter hepatic function and therefore should not be used in patients with a history of cholestatic hepatitis, previous jaundice with pregnancy, or as a reaction to other medications. The composition of the bile is altered, and an increase in the incidence of gall stones after long-term use has been reported. Gall bladder disease shows a two- to threefold increase in women undergoing postmenopausal estrogen therapy.

Estrogens are believed to increase the incidence of breast cancer in premenopausal women. Nodular masses of various sizes which regress spontaneously have been observed in the breast parenchyma during high-dosage estrogen therapy being given to arrest growth in girls with tall stature. Similar nodules are occasionally seen in girls undergoing spontaneous puberty. There is no indication that carcinoma of the breast arises during estrogen therapy.

Toxicity

Nausea and vomiting, "hot flashes", and anorexia are among the most frequent side effects of estrogen therapy. During estrogen therapy there is quite frequently an increased retention of water although, less frequently, estrogens may actually decrease salt and water accumulation. Breast tenderness is often caused by estrogen therapy and is likely due, at least in part, to the retention of electrolytes and water. Additionally, estrogens may cause breast engorgement and tenderness by promoting the proliferation of the secretory acini and ducts. The additional accumulation of water disappears within a few days of stopping the estrogens. Concommitant to this fluid and electrolyte retention is commonly an elevation of blood pressure during estrogen treatment occurring in as many as 15 to 40% of women.[19,20] This condition has been attributed, at least in part, to known changes in the concentration of blood proteins. Thyroxine and glucocorticoid binding proteins are increased which may alter endocrine relationships. Aldosterone secretion is known to be increased, accounting for the sodium retention as well as the abnormal incidence of hypertension seen in estrogen users. In adolescent girls receiving estrogen therapy for excessive height (estrogens are known inducers of epiphyseal closure)[21,22] systolic blood pressures commonly rise to 135 mmHg. Therapy is not usually stopped for this reason, however.

Thromboembolic complications during treatment with ovulatory inhibitors are well known, with the risk of complications being almost as high as in pregnancy. In adolescents, these complications are extremely rare although as high as 25% complain of calf-muscle cramps. No indication of any disorder of limb perfusion has, however, been found. Estrogens are known to effect changes in the concentration of some of the blood clotting factors, and much evidence indicates a resulting increase in thrombophlebitis and thromboembolism in both the superficial and deep veins.[23] Pulmonary and cerebral embolism mesenteric vascular occlusion and coronary thrombosis occur more rarely. Statistically, women over 35 years of age and having blood type O are most susceptible to these latter anomolies.

Migraine headache is another very common complication of estrogen therapy, especially in older women. Induced migraine is more rare in adolescents. High doses of estrogens often cause dizziness. Headache is also more frequent at high doses but does occur even with low doses. Nausea and dizziness are more frequently seen with ethinyl estradiol therapy than with treatment with the conjugated estrogens. Malaise, irritability, and depression are frequent problems with high estrogen doses, but occur only occasionally with small dosages.

Estrogens may induce changes in the skin such as rash, itching, yellowing, increasing pigmentation, some loss of scalp hair, and spider angiomas. Some patients express allergic reactions such as simple rashes, erythema nodosum, erythema multiforme, and cholestatic jaundice. In women, chronic use of estrogens may cause changes in vaginal bleeding, spotting, prolonged bleeding, breakthrough bleeding, or complete cessation of bleeding, lumps in breasts, mental depression, and thick, curd-like vaginal discharge (vaginal candidiasis). General and less frequent side effects include shortness of breath, slurred speech, loss of coordination, sudden vision changes, diarrhea, irritability, increased photosensitivity, stomach, side, chest, or groin pains, and yellowing of the eyes. An effect on libido is common, usually decreasing in males and increasing in females. Nausea, vomiting, and anorexia are frequent side effects of estrogen therapy. In both men and women venous thrombosis is common.

During oral contraceptive treatment, occasional rises in alkaline phosphatase, the transaminases, and aminopeptidases are seen. The values usually return to normal following cessation of therapy. The possible increase of both benign and malignant hepatoma in young women treated with oral contraceptives must be a consideration in their use.

Long-term use of ovulatory inhibitors results in amenorrhea for up to 6 months or even longer in 1% of women. In adolescent girls treated with high doses of estrogens for excessive growth in height, and over long periods before menarche, there is almost always a prolonged amenorrhea lasting up to 1.5 years.

Drug Interactions

Antidepressants — Simultaneous use of high doses of estrogens may result in a potentiation of tricyclic antidepressant side effects and reduce the effectiveness of the antidepressant.

Rifampin and other inducers of hepatic enzymes — Simultaneous use of estrogens and rifampin may result in significantly reduced estrogenic effects due to an acceleration of estrogen metabolism.

Oral anticoagulants — Estrogens may reduce the anticoagulant effective dose when given concurrently. If simultaneous usage of estrogens and anticoagulants is required, an increased dosage of anticoagulants may be necessary.

Other drug interactions with estrogens — may occur with carbeamazepin, phenobarbital, phenytoin, or primidone.

Structure-Activity Relationship*

The steroidal estrogen, 17β-estradiol, is the most potent of the three natural estrogens (Table 1), and is the major secretory product of the ovary. It is readily oxidized in the body to estrone, which subsequently is reduced to estriol. These transformations take place in the liver where estradiol is rapidly metabolized, making it ineffective by the oral route. Estrone has one third the activity of estradiol, while estriol has one sixtieth the activity. By the oral route, estriol is more active than estradiol, and estrone is the least active.

The three estrogens have in common an unsaturated A ring and a phenolic hydroxyl group at the C-3 position. Modification of 17β-estradiol through epimerization of the C-17-OH group to the α-configuration, or the removal of either or both of the C-3- and C-17-OH groups results in a less active estrogen.[24] Unsaturation in the B ring will also produce a weaker estrogen.

Chemical modifications of the natural estrogens make them effective orally, because of the protection from liver inactivation provided by the substituent groups. For example, the introduction of 17α-ethinyl group in estradiol yields a highly potent semisynthetic estrogen, ethinyl estradiol (Table 1), possessing oral activity. The ethinyl group is thought to slow the oxidation step of the 17-OH to the keto group. This estrogen and its derivatives are widely used and are incorporated with progestins (q.v.) for regulation of the menstrual cycle and as antifertility agents. Ester derivatives (benzoate and cypionate) of the natural and synthetic estrogens have an increased duration of action and are hydrolyzed in vivo to the free estrogens.

Recently, more attention has been given to the importance of the steroid molecule in estradiol. Earlier workers[25,26] considered the steroid skeleton as a spacer to hold the C-3-OH and the C-17-OH groups at the appropriate distance apart. However, it has been reported[3] that the steroid skeleton now contributes more to binding than the two hydrogen bonding groups. This contribution is made through hydrophobic binding and π-complex formation with the aromatic ring. These two effects have been found to be important for the binding of the steroid skeleton to the receptor, but hydrophobic binding is now considered to be the more important factor.[27,28]

The nonsteroidal estrogens (Table 2) are potent compounds that are also effective by mouth. One of the first agents prepared,[29] and still the most potent is DES. In most studies it is as potent as estradiol and is highly active orally. Its duration of action is longer suggesting a slower rate of degradation in the body. Officially, DES is known as the *trans*-isomer* (E), which can exist in a quasi-steroidal configuration resembling the natural hormone, estradiol. The *cis*-isomer** (Z) is much less active (1/10) and this difference in activity is attributed to the shortened interatomic distance between the terminal hydroxyl groups.

---

* See also individual preparations for other discussions.

** See monograph on DES.

Table 1
NATURAL ESTROGENS USED IN THERAPY

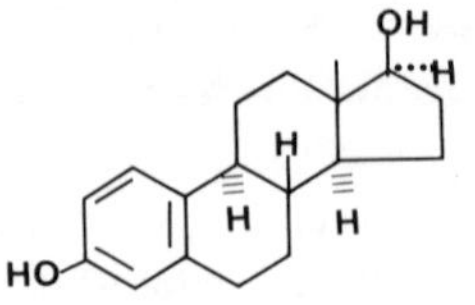

ESTRADIOL

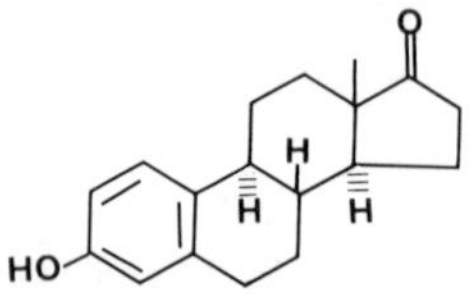

ESTRONE

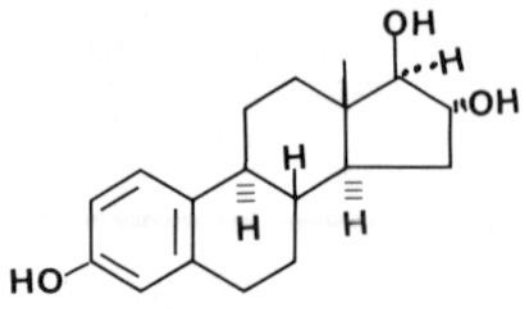

ESTRIOL

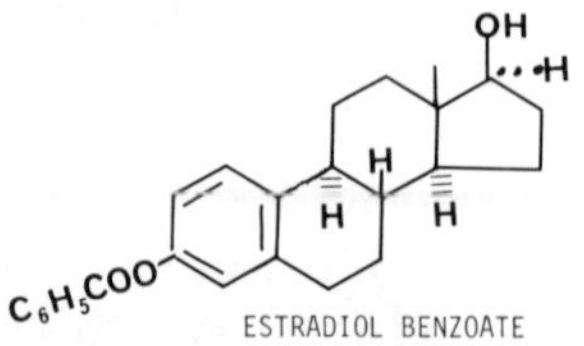

ESTRADIOL BENZOATE

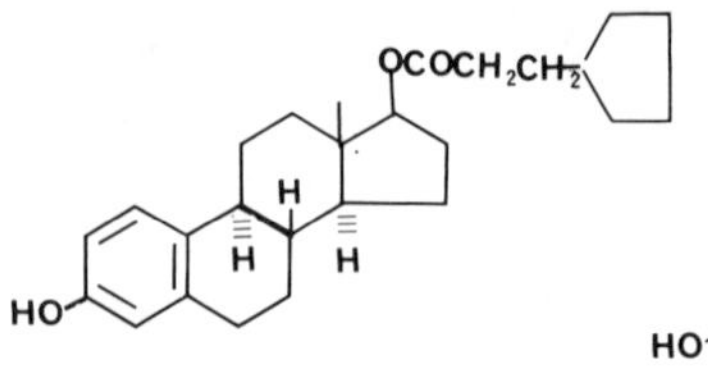

ESTRADIOL CYPIONATE

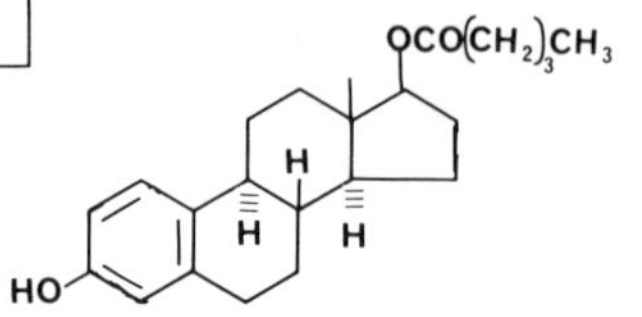

ESTRADIOL VALERATE

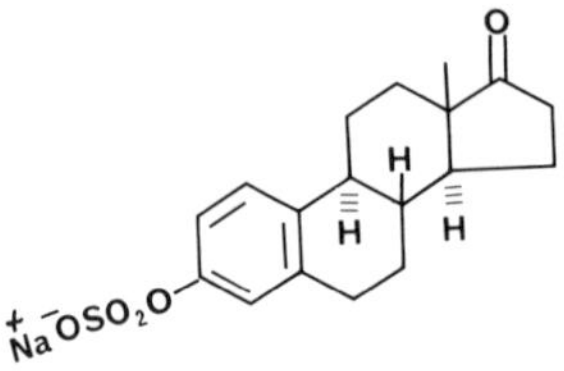

SODIUM ESTRONE
SULFATE

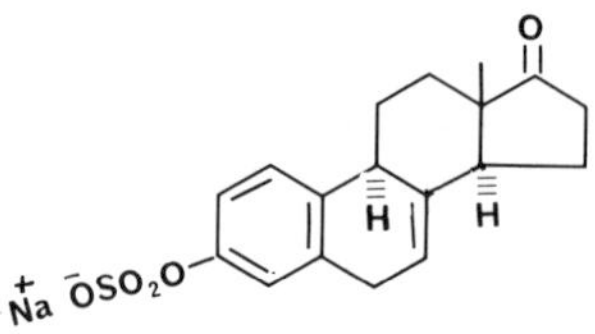

SODIUM EQUILIN
SULFATE

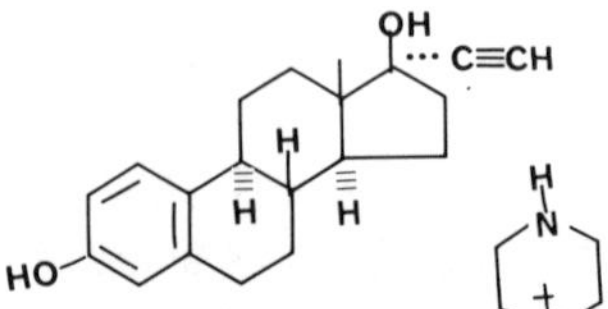

ETHINYL ESTRADIOL

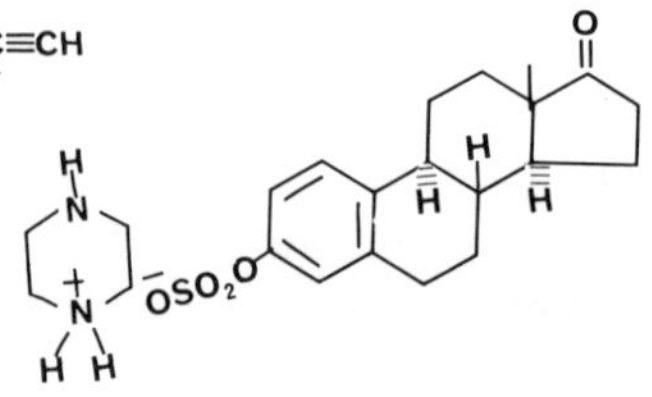

ESTROPIATE

Both DES and estradiol conform to Schueler's[25,30] hypothesis that the activity of steroids and nonsteroids is due to a similar interatomic distance ("critical distance") between terminal hydrogen bonding groups such as, the phenolic hydroxyl groups in DES and the C-3 and C-17 hydroxyl groups in estradiol. Other steroidal and nonsteroidal estrogens also conform to this hypothesis. X-ray crystallography has revealed that this distance in DES and estradiol is 12.1 Å and 10.9 Å respectively.[31] Fullerton[31] suggests that since hydrated estradiol, like DES, has a critical distance of 12.1 Å, this interatomic distance might be essential for receptor binding, and more than likely involves water molecules, since X-ray crystallographic analysis has shown water molecules bonded to the C-17-OH group in estradiol.

Since DES was reported in 1938 by Dodds et al.[29] many analogs and structural changes have been made.[32-35]

Hexestrol (Table 2) is the *meso* form of 2,4-*bis(p*-hydroxyphenyl)-*n*-hexane. This dihydro

Table 2
SYNTHETIC ESTROGENS USED IN THERAPY

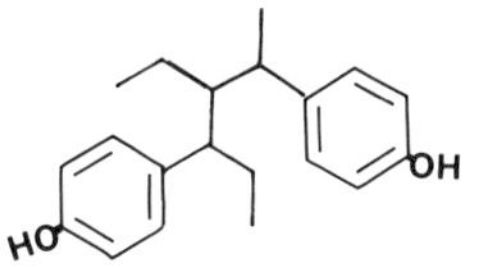

BENZESTROL

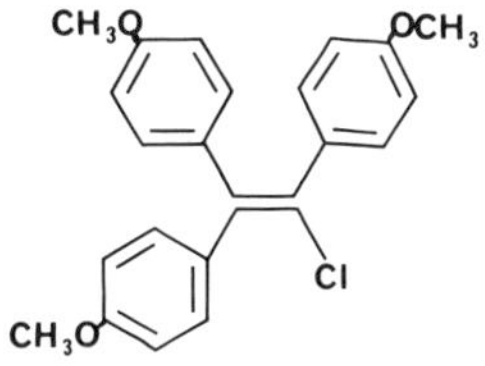

CHLOROTRIANISENE

DIETHYLSTILBESTROL

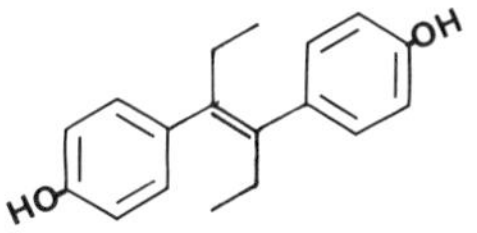

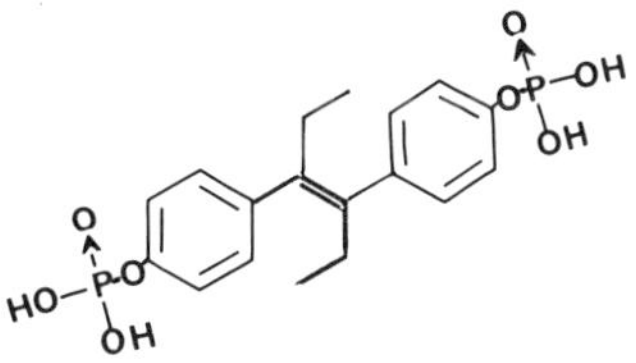

DIETHYLSTILBESTROL DIPHOSPHATE

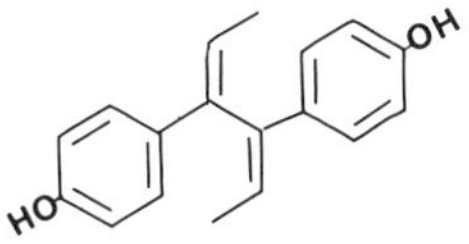

DIENESTROL

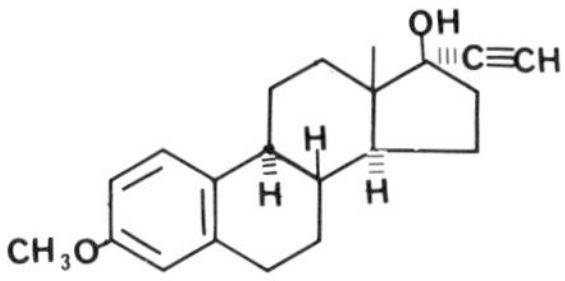

MESTRANOL

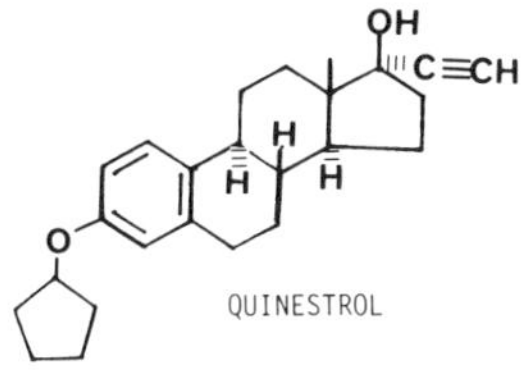

QUINESTROL

analog of DES is less active than DES, but more active than the dl-stereoisomers. Many derivatives of hexestrol have been studied by Katzenellenbogen and co-workers.[36]

Physical-Chemical and Other Data

Included are the following classes of estrogens.

1. Natural estrogens (structures are shown in Table 1)
   Estradiol
   Estrone
   Estradiol benzoate
   Estradiol cypionate
   Estradiol valerate
   Conjugated estrogens
   Esterified estrogens
   Estropipate
   Ethinyl estradiol
2. Synthetic estrogens (structures are shown in Table 2)
   Benzestrol
   Chlorotrianisene
   Diethylstilbestrol

Diethylstilbestrol diphosphate
Dienestrol
Mestranol
Quinestrol

NATURAL ESTROGENS

ESTRADIOL

Estradiol is a white crystalline, odorless solid which is stable in air, but is hygroscopic; mp 173 to 179°C (80% alcohol*); $C_{18}H_{24}O_2$; mol wt 272.39. It is insoluble in water; freely soluble in alcohol; soluble in acetone and other organic solvents; and slightly soluble in vegetable oil.

It is the most potent naturally occurring estrogen; formed by the ovary, placenta and testes; isolated from follicular fluid of sow ovaries and from the urine of pregnant mare.[37] Estradiol is prepared from other steroids, but is usually prepared through the reduction of the 17-keto group of estrone (q.v.)[38,39] The preparation is found also in several U.S. patents: 2,096,744, 2,225,419, and 2,361,847 (1938, 1941, 1944 to Schering).

The esters of estradiol are usually used in place of estradiol since they are not destroyed as readily. Estradiol can be used, however, to supplement parenteral treatment with the ester derivatives. The oral route is ineffective and not recommended since most of the hormone is destroyed by the liver. The plasma halflife for parenteral estradiol is about 1 hr.

Chemical names and synonyms — (1) Estra-1,3,5(10)-triene-3,17-diol,(17β)-; (2) estra-1,3,5(10)-triene-3,17β-diol; 17β-estradiol; dihydrotheelin; CAS-50-28-2.

Uses — Also see introduction. Estradiol is used for estrogen replacement (female hypogonadism; ovariectomy; primary ovarian failure; moderate to severe vasomotor symptoms; atrophic vaginitis or kraurosis vulvae associated with menopause; and as an antineoplastic) in inoperable and progressing prostatic carcinoma.

Administration and dosage — Replacement therapy, usual oral adult dose: 1 mg daily for 21 days, the dosage being repeated cyclically following 7 days of no mediciation; i.m. (oil or sterile suspension), usual adult dose: 0.5 mg to 1.5 mg 2 to 3 times a week for 3 weeks, the dosage being repeated cyclically following 1 week of no medication.

Postpartum breast engorgement — Intramuscular, usual adult dose: 1.5 to 2.2 mg daily. *Note:* the use of estrogens for the prevention of postpartum breast engorgement is no longer recommended due to the increased possibility of clot formation at the larger doses required for effectiveness. Also, the efficacy of this usage is questionable, since in many cases the breasts fill up to some degree in spite of treatment.

Dosage forms and strengths usually available — Tablets: 0.2, 0.5, 1, and 2 mg; sterile suspension: 0.5 and 1 mg/mℓ; 2.2, 2.5, 4.4, and 11 mg/10 mℓ; 5.5 mg/25 mg; injection (in oil): 0.1, 0.2, and 0.5 mg/mℓ; 1 mg/mℓ.

Proprietaries — Estrace (Mead Johnson)

ESTRONE

Estrone is a white crystalline solid in the dl form, stable in air; mp 251 to 254°C (acetone). The d-form is the natural form and exists as a white crystalline solid; mp 254.5 to 256°C (acetone); $C_{18}H_{22}O_2$; mol wt 270.37. It is slightly soluble in water at room temperature; soluble in some organic solvents, slightly soluble in ether and vegetable oils. One gram of

* Recrystallization solvent.

the hormone is soluble in 250 mℓ of ethanol, 50 mℓ of acetone, and 110 mℓ of chloroform, all at 15°C.

Estrone is a 17-keto metabolite of 17β estradiol (q.v.) which is considerably less potent than the latter. It was isolated in 1929 as the first sex hormone by Doisy et al.[2,3] and by Butenandt.[40] It is found in urine of pregnant women and mares, in human placenta, in follicular fluid of many animals, and in urine of bulls and stallions. The synthesis,[41,42] stereochemistry,[43] and estrone synthesis[44-46] are well documented in the literature.

Chemical names and synonyms — (1) Estra-1,3,5(10)-trien-17-one, 3-hydroxy-; (2) 3-hydroxyestra-1,3,5(10)-trien-17-one; theelin; folliculin; follicular hormone; CAS-53-16-7.

Uses — See estradiol.

Administration and dosage — Estrogenic supplement (i.m.) usual adult dose: give 0.1 to 2 mg/week, administer as a single dose or in divided doses; antineoplastic-prostatic carcinoma (inoperable and progressing), i.m., usual adult dose: administer 2 to 4 mg, 2 or 3 times a week. A response to therapy usually occurs within 3 months of the initial therapy. If no response is observed, the hormone should be continued until the disease is again progressive. Sterile estrone and estrone potassium sulfate suspension — estrogen supplement — i.m., usual adult dose: administer 0.05 to 1 mℓ/week in a single or divided doses; abnormal uterine bleeding due to hormonal imbalance: from 2 to 5 mg for several days; inoperable progressing prostatic cancer: 2.0 to 4.0 mg, 2 or 3 times a week. Response should be seen in 3 months; inoperable progressing breast cancer: administered chronically, 5 mg, 3 or more times per week.

Dosage forms and strengths usually available — Sterile aqueous estrone suspension and estrone in oil are available in injectable forms of 1 mg/mℓ (1-mℓ vials); 2 mg/mℓ(10- and 30-mℓ vials); 5 mg/mℓ (1.5, 10, and 30 mℓ vials) to be administered intramuscularly only. Sterile estrone and estrone potassium sulfate suspension; 2 mg of estrone and 1 mg of estrone potassium sulfate per mℓ (available in 10-mg vials).

Proprietaries — Bestrone (Bluco); Estro-Med (Medics); Estrusol (SMP): Kestrone-5 (Hyrex); Theelin Aqueous (Parke-Davis). A component in: Di-Met (Organon), Spanestrin-P (Salvage), Estrofol (Tutag), Estrojet-2 (Mayrand), Estraqua (Kay Pharm), Gravigen Aqueous (Bluco); Foygen Aqueous (Foy).

ESTRADIOL BENZOATE

Estradiol benzoate is a white crystalline solid, odorless and stable; mp 191 to 196°C (alcohol); $C_{25}H_{28}O_3$; mol wt 376.50. It is soluble in alcohol, acetone, chloroform, and dioxane; slightly soluble in ether and vegetable oils; very low solubility in water.

This hormone can be prepared by the benzoylation of the 3-hydroxyl group of estradiol (q.v.). This ester acts as a pro-drug, releasing β-estradiol over several days at the site of injection; thus, these low levels of estrogen are more effective than higher doses of rapidly destroyed estradiol when used alone.

Chemical names and synonyms — (1) Estra-1,3,5(10)-triene-3,17-diol, (17β)-, 3-benzoate; (2) estradiol 3-benzoate; β-estradiol benzoate; CAS-50-50-0.

Uses — See estradiol.

Administration and Dosage — Intramuscular initially: 1.0 to 1.66 mg 2 or 3 times weekly for 2 or 3 weeks, then gradually decreased to the lowest effective maintenance dose, usually 0.33 to 1.0 mg 2 times per week.

Dosage forms and strengths usually available — Injection (in oil): 10 and 33.3 mg/10 mℓ.

ESTRADIOL CYPIONATE

Estradiol cypionate is a white crystalline solid, mp 151 to 152°C (benzene-ether); $C_{26}H_{36}O_3$;

mol wt 396.57. It is soluble in ether, methanol, benzene, chloroform, peanut oil, corn oil, and sesame oil, but insoluble in water.

This ester has a more prolonged action than the benzoate and valerate esters. Its effect lasts from 1 to 2 months. Cottonseed oil is usually the vehicle in the cypionate injectable form.

It is obtained by treating estradiol 3,17β-diclopentane propionate with potassium carbonate (U.S. patent 2,611,773 to Upjohn). Estradiol 3,17β-dicyclopentane propionate is prepared by treating estradiol with cyclopentanepropionyl chloride in pyridine (OTT, U.S. patent same as above).

Chemical names and synonyms — (1) Estra-1,3,5(10)-triene-3,17-diol, (17β)-,17-cyclopentanepropanoate; (2) estradiol 17-cyclopentanepropionate; CAS-313-06-4.

Use — See estradiol and its benzoate and valerate esters.

Administration and dosage — Estrogen supplement, female hypogonadism: i.m., 1.5 to 2.0 mg administered at monthly intervals; menopausal symptoms, i.m. at 1.0 to 5.0 mg administered at 3- to 4-week intervals.

Dosage forms and strengths usually available - Injection (in oil): 1, 2, and 5 mg/mℓ (vials of 5 and 10 mℓ).

Proprietaries — Depo-Estradiol Cypionate (Upjohn); Depestro (Kay Pharm); dep-Gynogen (O'Neal); Depogen (Hyrex); Dura-Estrin (Hauck); E-Ionate P.A. (Tutag); Estra-C (North Amercian); Estra-D (Seatrace); Estro-Cyp (Keene); Estroject-L.A. (Maryland); Spendepiol (Spencer-Mead).

ESTRADIOL VALERATE

This estrogen is white cyrstalline solid, mp 144 to 145°C; $C_{23}H_{32}O_3$; mol wt 356.50. It is almost insoluble in water and fairly soluble in oils.

Estradiol valerate is slowly absorbed from an oil suspension providing 2 to 3 weeks of estrogenic effect from a single i.m. injection. Sesame and castor oils are usually used as a vehicle.

This ester is prepared similarly to the esterification process described in estradiol cypionate, except for the acid chloride used: U.S. patents 2,205,627 and 2,233,025.

Chemical names and synonyms — (1) Estra-1,3,5(10)-triene-3,17-diol (17β)-,17-pentanoate; (2) estradiol 17-valerate; CAS-979-32-8.

Use, administration and dosage — For treatment of moderate to severe vasomotor symptoms; atrophic vaginitis or kraurosis vulvae associated with menopause, i.m.: 10 to 20 mg once per month; for the treatment of prostatic carcinoma, i.m.: 30 mg or more, once per week or every two weeks.

Dosage forms and strengths usually available — Available in 10, 20, and 40 mg/mℓ (vials of 5 and 10 mℓ).

Proprietaries — Delestrogen (Squibb); Dioval (Keene); Duragen (Hauck); Estate (Savage); Estradiol L.A. (North American); Estraval-P.A. (Tutag); Gynogen L.A. (O'Neal); Repestrogen (Spencer-M); Valergen (Hyrex).

CONJUGATED ESTROGENS

Conjugated estrogens are amorphous preparations containing water-soluble conjugated forms of mixed estrogens: 50 to 65% of the sodium salt of the sulfate ester of estrone (sodium estrone sulfate, Table 1) and 20 to 35% of the sodium salt of the sulfate ester of equilin (sodium equilin sulfate, Table 1) isolated from pregnant mares' urine. The total estrogenic potency of the preparation is expressed in terms of an equivalent quantity of sodium estrone sulfate.

The preparation can be found in U.S. patents 2,565,115 (1951 to Squibb) and 2,720,483 (1955 to Olin Mathieson). The conjugated estrogens are orally active and are specifically used for declining ovarian function symptoms.

Use, administration, and dosage — Estrogenic supplement; menopausal symptoms, ovariectomy, primary ovarian failure, and to retard progression of osteoporosis. Usual oral adult dose: 0.625 to 1.25 mg, 1 to 3 times per day for 21 days with no medication for 7 days; menopausal patients with atrophic vaginitis or kraurosis vulvae may require an upward range from 0.3 mg/day for relief of symptoms, and may be used in conjuction with vaginal dosage forms; female hypogonadism, usual oral adult dose: 0.625 to 1.25 mg, 1 to 3 times per day for 20 days with no medication for the next 10 days. Dosage is repeated cyclically until vaginal bleeding occurs. If bleeding occurs before the 10-day period is completed, an oral progestin (q.v.) is sometimes combined with the estrogen on days 16 through 20.

Antineoplastic-breast carcinoma (inoperable and progressing in selected men and post-menopausal women), usual oral adult dose: 10 mg, 3 times per day for at least 3 months; prostatic carcinoma (inoperable and progressing), usual oral adult dose: 1.25 to 2.5 mg, 3 times per day. Phosphatase determinations and symptomatic improvement can monitor the effectiveness of therapy.

Prevention of postpartum breast engorgement (not recommended, see estradiol) — usual oral adult dose: 3.75 mg every 4 hr for 5 doses, or 1.25 mg every 4 hr for 5 days. Conguated estrogens for injection — usual adult dose for abnormal uterine bleeding (hormonal imbalance) — i.m. or i.v.: 25 mg repeated in 6 to 12 hr if needed. For a more rapid response, i.v. administration is preferred, but should be administered slowly to prevent a flushing reaction.

Dosage forms and strengths usually available — Tablets: 0.3, 0.625, 1.25, and 2.5 mg. Injection: 25 mg; vaginal cream: each gram contains 0.625 mg.

Proprietaries — Evestrone (Delta Drug); Premarin (Ayerst); Sodestrin-H (Tutag); Premarin Vaginal Cream (Ayerst). A component in the following: Milprem (Wallace); PMB-400 (Ayerst).

ESTERIFIED ESTROGENS

Esterified estrogens are amorphous preparations (white or dull yellow powder) containing water-soluble esterified estrogens: not less than 75% and not more than 85% of sodium estrone sulfate and not less than 6% and not more than 15% sodium equilin sulfate in such proportions that the total of both esterified estrogens is not less than 90%, calculated on the basis of the total esterified estrogens content.

Use — See conjugated estrogens.

Administration and dosage — Given cyclically (3 weeks on and 1 week off) for short term use only; moderate to severe vasomotor symptoms associated with menopause, usual oral adult dose: 1.25 mg, dosage may be increased to 2.5 or 3.75 mg/day if a satisfactory response is not obtained in 3 or 4 days; atrophic vaginitis and kraurosis vulvae, usual oral adult dose: a range of 0.3 to 1.25 mg/day; ovariectomy and primary ovarian failure, usual oral adult dose: a 20-day estrogen-progestin cyclic regimen of 2.5 to 7.5 mg/ day in divided doses for 20 days will produce the hormone pattern of the ovary, so bleeding is from a progestational endometrium. During the last 5 days of estrogen therapy, an oral progestin is given. If bleeding occurs before this regimen is concluded, therapy is discontinued and resumed on the 5th day of bleeding; female hypogonadism, usual oral adult dose: 2.5 to 7.5 mg/day are administered to bring about sexual and somatic maturation, cyclic in divided doses for 20 days followed by a 10-day rest period. If bleeding does not occur by the end of this period, the same dosage schedule is repeated. If bleeding occurs before the end of the 10-day period, a 20-day estrogen-progestin cyclic regimen is begun as in primary ovarian failure; given chronically, prostatic carcinoma (inoperable and progressing), usual oral adult dose: 1.25 to 2.5 mg 3 times/day for several weeks. Effectiveness of therapy can be monitored by phosphatase determinations and symptomatic response. Half of the initial dosage is usually satisfactory for the maintenance dose; breast cancer (inoperable and progressing), usual oral adult dose in postmenopausal women and selected men: 10 mg, 3 times daily for at least 3 months.

Dosage forms and strengths usually available — Tablets: 0.3, 0.625, 1.25, and 2.5 mg.

Proprietaries — Amnestrogen (Squibb); Estratab (Reid-Provident); Menest (Beecham Labs).

ESTROPIPATE

Estropipate, formerly known as piperazine estrone sulfate, is a white crystalline powder (U.S. patent 3,525,738), which may have a slight odor; begins to melt at 190°C but solidifies and finally melts at 245°C with decomposition; $C_{18}H_{22}O_5S \cdot C_4H_{10}N_2$; mol wt 436.56. It has the following solubility: 1 g dissolves in over 2000 mℓ of water, alcohol, chloroform, and ether.

Crystalline estrone is solubilized as the sulfate (U.S. patent 2,917,522 to Parke-Davis) and stabilized with piperazine (1:1) acting as a buffer preventing the precipitation of the free 3-sulfate ester in acidic pharmaceutical preparations.

Chemical names and synonyms — (1) Estra-1,3,5(10)-trien-17-one, 3-(sulfooxy)-, compound with piperazine (1:1); (2) estrone hydrogen sulfate compound with piperazine (1:1); CAS-7280-37-7; CAS-481-97-0 (estrone hydrogen sulfate).

Uses — See estrone.

Administration and dosage — Estrogen supplement for female hypogonadism, ovariectomy, or primary ovarian failure, usual oral adult dose: the equivalent of 1.25 to 2.5 mg of estrone sulfate per day for 21 days, the dosage being repeated cyclically following 8 to 10 days of no medication, if withdrawal bleeding does not occur by the 10th day. The duration of therapy to produce withdrawal bleeding will vary according to the responsiveness of the endometrium. If satisfactory withdrawal bleeding does not occur, an oral progestin may be given in addition to estrogen during the 3rd week of the cycle; menopausal symptoms, usual oral adult dose: the equivalent of 0.625 to 5 mg of estrone sulfate per day for 21 days, the dosage being repeated cyclically following 7 days of no medication; intravaginal application, usual adult dose: 2 to 4 g/day for 3 weeks omitting application the 4th week. Vaginal application of estrogens has been used usually in the treatment of atrophic vaginitis or kraurosis vulvae associated with menopause or after ovariectomy.

Dosage forms and strengths usually available — Tablets: 0.625 mg (equivalent to 0.75 mg of estropipate); 1.25 mg (equivalent to 1.5 mg of estropipate); 2.5 mg (equivalent to 3 mg of estropipate); 5 mg (equivalent to 6 mg of estropipate); vaginal cream: 1.5 mg/g.

Proprietaries: — Ogen (Abbott).

ETHINYL ESTRADIOL

Ethinyl estradiol exists as white, fine needles; mp 141 to 146°C (methanol-water), dehydrates after melting and after further heating, melts at 182 to 184°C; $C_{20}H_{24}O_2$; mol wt 296.41. It is almost insoluble in water; soluble in ethanol (1:6), ether (1:4), acetone (1:5), dioxone (1:4), chloroform (1:20), and soluble in vegetable oils. The preparation of this hormone is from estrone[47] and other methods can be found in many patents: German patent 702,063; British patent 516,444; U.S. patents 2,243,887, 2,251,939, 2,265,976, and 2,267,257.

The 17α-ethinyl group bestows a great advantage upon estradiol over other estrogens by delaying the decomposition of the estradiol molecule during oral absorption, making it a potent oral estrogen. Consequently this preparation is effective at low doses. Ethinyl estradiol is 15 to 20 times more active orally, but equal to estradiol in potency by injection. This estrogen is a component with progestin in oral contraceptive preparations (q.v.).

Chemical names and synonyms — (1) 19-Norpregna-1,3,5(10)-trien-20-yne-3,17-diol, (17α)-; (2) 19-Nor-17α-pregna-1,3,5(10)-trien-20-yne-3,17-diol; ethynyl-estradiol; CAS-57-63-6.

Use, administration, and dosage — Given cyclically for short-term use only. Menopausal symptoms, usual oral adult dose: 0.02 or 0.05 mg once per day (or can be effective at 0.02 mg every other day) given for 21 days, the dosage being repeated cyclically following 7 days of no medication; female hypogonadism, usual oral adult dose: 0.05 mg per day for 2 weeks, followed by a progestin (q.v.) during the successive 2 weeks of a theoretical menstrual cycle, the dose being repeated cyclically. Given chronically for palliation, anti-neoplastic; breast carcinoma (inoperable and progressing in appropriately selected postmenopausal women, usual oral adult dose: 1 mg, 3 times per day; prostatic carcinoma (inoperable and progressing), usual oral adult dose: 0.15 to 2 mg daily.

Dosage forms and strengths usually available — Tablets: 0.02, 0.05, and 0.5 mg.

Proprietaries — Estinyl (Schering-Plough); Feminone (Upjohn).

Antiovulatory (oral contraceptive) preparations containing ethinyl estradiol include ethynodiol diacetate and ethinyl estradiol tablets; norethindrone and ethinyl estradiol tablets; norethindrone acetate and ethinyl estradiol tablets; nogestrel and ethinyl estradiol tablets.

SYNTHETIC ESTROGENS

BENZESTROL

Benzestrol, a white crystalline powder, melts at 162 to 166°C; $C_{20}H_{26}O_2$; mol wt 298.41. It is insoluble in water but soluble in acetone, ether, ethanol, methanol, and vegetable oil. It is only slightly soluble in chloroform, benzene, petroleum ether, and dilute ethanol.

This synthetic estrogen was prepared by Stuart et al.[48] It resembles diethylstilbestrol (q.v.) when drawn in a similar spatial arrangement. This is possible since the two adjacent ethyl groups avoid an eclipsed conformation; thus, keeping the phenolic groups *trans* to each other.

Chemical names and synonyms — (1) Phenol-4,4′-(1,2-diethyl-3-methyl-1,3-propane-diyl)*bis*-; (2) 4,4′-1(diethyl-3-methyltrimethylene)diphenol; CAS-85-95-0.

Use, administration, and dosage — Use and contraindications are the same as with other estrogens, but have lower untoward responses; usual oral adult dose: 0.5 to 5 mg daily.

Dosage forms and usual strengths available — Tablets: 1, 2, and 5 mg.

CHLOROTRIANISENE

Chlorotrianisene is a stable, odorless, white crystalline solid. It melts at 114 to 116°C (methanol); $C_{23}H_{21}ClO_3$; mol wt 380.86. It is insoluble in water, soluble in alcohol, ether, acetone, chloroform, benzene, carbon tetrachloride, and vegetable oils. It is prepared by reacting tri-*p*-anisylethylene or tri-*p*-anisylethanol with chlorine in carbon tetrachloride (British patent 561,508, 1944 to I.C.I.); can be synthesized from *p*-(*p*-anisoyl)anisole (U.S. patent 2,430,891, 1947 to Merrell).

Chlorotrianisene is a long acting synthetic estrogen which acts as a prodrug. It is more active orally than by injection, suggesting that the liver is converting it into a more active form. By injection, the estrogen is slowly released from lipid tissues, giving it a long duration of action, which makes cyclic therapy difficult.

Chemical names and synonyms — (1) Benzene,1,1′,1″-(1-chloro-1-ethenyl-2-ylidene)-tris[4-methoxy]-; (2) chlorotris(*p*-methoxyphenyl)ethylene; (3) tri-*p*-anisylchloroethylene; CAS-569-57-3.

Use, administration, and dosage — Menopausal symptoms, usual oral adult dose: 12 to 25 mg daily given cyclically for 30 to 60 days; female hypogonadism, usual oral adult dose: 12 to 25 mg daily for 21 days following 6 to 7 days of no medication. On oral progestin may be given the last 5 days of therapy. The cycle can be repeated after the 5th day of induced uterine bleeding; prostatic carcinoma, usual oral adult dose: 12 to 25 mg daily; postpartum breast engorgement (not recommended — see note on estradiol); usual oral adult dose: 12 mg, 4 times per day for 7 days or 50 mg every 6 hr for 6 doses. A 72-mg capsule can be administered twice daily for 2 days. The first dose is given 8 hr after delivery.

Dosage forms and strengths usually available — Capsules: 12, 25, and 72 mg (for postpartum breast engorgement see above).

Proprietaries — TACE (Merrell-National).

DIETHYLSTILBESTROL (DES)

Diethylstilbestrol is a white, odorless crystalline powder; mp 169 to 172°C (benzene); $C_{18}H_{20}O_2$; mol wt 268.34. It is insoluble in water; soluble in alcohol, ether, and chloroform. This stilbene derivative like the other derivatives is light sensitive.

Diethylstilbestrol is a potent synthetic, nonsteroidal estrogen, which is always the *trans*-isomer (E)*. The *cis*-isomer (Z)* is almost inactive in biological activity, and is unstable, reverting to the *trans*-isomer.[49] DES was first prepared by Dodds and co-workers[29] (see introduction).

DES can be prepared from various starting materials, e.g., desoxyanisoin, anisoin, and anisole. The shortest and most convenient route starts with anethole hydrobromide.[50] There are also comprehensive reviews[32,51] on the synthesis of this synthetic estrogen.

DES is capable of producing all of the pharmacological and therapeutic effects of natural estrogens. It may be taken orally in the form of enteric-released tablets or vaginally in the form of suppositories. This agent in large doses (25 mg twice per day for 5 days starting within 72 hr of insemination) can be used as a postcoital contraceptive in emergencies.

Chemical names and synonyms — (1) Phenol,4,4′-(1,2-diethyl-1,2-ethenediyl)*bis*-, (E);(2) α,α-diethyl-(E)-4,4′-stilbenediol; stilbestrol; stilboestrol; DES; CAS-56-53-1.

Use, administration, and dosage — Estrogen supplement, menopausal symptoms,** ovariectomy, primary ovarian failure, or female hypogonadism; usual oral adult dose: 0.2 to 0.5 mg per day for 21 days, following 7 days of no medication; breast carcinoma (inoperable and progressing) in selected men and postmenopausal women); usual oral adult dose: 15 mg daily; prostatic carcinoma (inoperable and progressing), usual oral adult dose: 1 mg to 3 mg initially and increased as needed, but reduced to 1 mg as soon as possible

---

*   In determining configuration for some trisubstituted and tetrasubstituted ethylenes, the two atoms or groups on each doubly-bonded carbon are arranged in their CAHN-INGOLD-PRELOG sequence. Then the group of higher priority on the one carbon and the group of higher priority on the other carbon are looked at to determine whether they are on the same side of the molecule or on opposite sides. The letter Z (zusammen, together) is used to denote on the same side, and the letter *E* (entgegen, opposite) means on opposite sides.

**   Patients with atrophic vaginitis may require up to 2 mg daily for relief of symptoms. Vaginal suppositories used concomitantly with the oral form may provide faster relief; usual adult dose of vaginal suppositories: 0.1 to 0.5 mg once or twice daily for 10 to 14 days.

since higher doses (5 mg for prolonged periods) may increase the risk of cardiovascular embolism.

Dosage forms and strengths usually available — Tablets: 0.1, 0.25, 0.5, 1, and 5 mg; tablets (enteric-coated): 0.1, 0.25, 0.5, 1, and 5 mg vaginal suppositories: 0.1 and 0.5 mg.

Proprietaries — Diethylstilbestrol (Lilly).

DIETHYLSTILBESTROL DIPHOSPHATE

This is a white crystalline powder from dilute hydrochloric acid; mp 204 to 206°C (dec); $C_{18}H_{22}O_8P_2$; mol wt 428.32. It is surprisingly soluble in water and stable solutions are maintained at a pH of 10; U.S. patents 2,828,244 (1958 to Miles Labs). The disodium salt $(C_{18}H_{20}Na_2O_8P_2)$ is a white crystalline, water soluble solid; mp 230°C (begins melting at 190°C). Its aqueous solutions are reported to have a pH of 4.8, 5.0, and 6.5.

This ester is prepared by treating DES with phosphorus oxychloride in pyridine; U.S. patents 2,234,311 and 2,802,854; sodium salts, U.S. patent 2,971,975.

Diethylstilbestrol diphosphate is used only for prostatic carcinoma since it is reputed to be more effective and to have fewer side effects than other estrogens. Although its mode of action is not known, it is speculated that DES diphosphate is hydrolyzed in the cancer cell by acid phosphatase, a rich component in the cancer cell, yielding DES.

Chemical names and synonyms — (1) Phenol, 4,4'-(1,2-diethyl-1,2-ethenediyl)-*bis*-, *bis*(dihydrogen phosphate), (E)-; (2) α,α'-diethyl-(E)-4,4'-stilbenediol *bis*(dihydrogen phosphate); Fosfestrol; CAS-522-40-7.

Use, administration, and dosage — Prostatic carcinoma (inoperable and progressing usual oral adult dose: 50 mg 3 times daily. The dosage is increased gradually to 200 mg or more, 3 times per day. If relief is not obtained with high oral dosages, i.v. administration should be tried; i.v. infusion, usual adult dose: the first day, 0.5 g dissolved in 300 mℓ of saline or 5% dextrose to be given slowly 20 to 30 drops per min intravenously during the first 10 to 15 min and then the rate of flow adjusted so the entire amount is given in 1 hr. This procedure should be followed for at least 5 days increasing the dosage to 1 g each day. After the 5 day treatment, a maintenance dose of 0.25 to 0.5 g can be administered in the same manner, once or twice a week, or maintenance may be reached using tablets.

Dosage forms and strengths usually available —Tablets: 50 mg; ampuls: 5-mℓ ampuls containing 0.25 g of DES phosphate as a solution of its sodium salt. The solution must be diluted before i.v. infusion.

Proprietaries — Stilphostrol (Dome).

DIENESTROL

This estrogen forms white needles from dilute alcohol, mp 227 to 228°C; sublimes at 130°C (1 mmHg); mp 231 to 234°C; $C_{18}H_{18}O_2$; mol wt 266.34. It is insoluble in water and vegetables oils, but soluble in alcohol, acetone, methanol, ether, and chloroform.

Dienestrol was prepared by Dodds et al.[52] and Hobday and Short.[53] U.S. patents 2,464,203 and 2,465,505. The (E) (E) configuration is described by Koch[54] and Lane.[55]

Chemical names and synonyms — (1) Phenol, 4,4'-(1,2-diethylidene-1,2-ethanediyl) *bis*-, (E,E)-; (2) 4,4'-diethylideneethylene)diphenol; CAS-84-17-3.

Use, administration, and dosage — Dienestrol is a potent estrogen which is restricted to vaginal use only in the treatment of atrophic vaginitis and kraurosis vulvae; usual adult dose: intravaginal, 6 g of cream containing 0.6 mg of dienestrol, once or twice daily for 1 or 2 weeks, the dose being reduced to one half, 3 to 6 g/day or every other day for an additional 2 weeks. If maintenance dose is needed, 3 to 6 g of cream are applied 1 to 3 times per week; suppositories usual adult dose: 0.7 to 1.4 mg once or twice daily for 1 to

2 weeks, the dose being reduced to 0.7 mg daily or every 2nd day, for an additional 1 or 2 weeks.

Dosage forms and strengths usually available — Intravaginal cream: 0.01% (0.1 mg/g); vaginal suppositories: 0.7 mg.

MESTRANOL

Mestranol is a white crystalline solid, mp 150 to 151°C (methanol or acetone); $C_{21}H_{26}O_2$; mol wt 310.44. It is insoluble in water; slightly soluble in alcohol, somewhat soluble in ether, and soluble in chloroform.

This hormone is prepared from estrone;[56] U.S. patent 2,666,769 (1954 to Searle).

Mestranol is not used alone even though it is an effective estrogen. Its discovery as a contaminant in the preparation of the progestin, norethynodrel, led to its incorporation into oral contraceptives with other progestins.

Chemical names and synonyms — (1) 19-Norpregna-1,3,5(10)-trien-20-yn-17-ol, 3-methoxy-, (17α)-; (2) 3-methoxy-19-nor-17α-pregna-1,3,5(10)-trien-20-yn-17-ol; CAS-72-33-3.

Use, administration and dosage — See antiovulatory agents (oral contraceptives).

Dosage forms and strengths available — See antiovulatory agents (oral contraceptives).

Preparations containing mestranol — Ethynodiol diacetate and mestranol tablets; norethindrone and mestranol tablets; norethynodrel and mestranol tablets.

QUINESTROL

This is a white crystalline, odorless solid; mp 107 to 108°C; $C_{25}H_{32}O_2$; mol wt 364.51. It is insoluble in water, but soluble in alcohol, chloroform, and ether.

This preparation of quinestrol is described by Ercoli and Gardi[57] and in U.S. patents 3,159,543 and 3,231,567. It is a potent orally effective synthetic estrogen, the 3-cyclopentylether of ethinyl estradiol.

Chemical names and synonyms — (1) 19-Norpregna-1,3,5(10)-trien-20-yn-17-ol,3-(cyclopentyloxy)-, (17α)-; (2) 3-(cyclopentyloxy)-19-nor-17α-pregna-1,3,5,(10)-trien-20-yn-17ol; CAS-152-43-2.

Use, administration, and dosage: (see ethinyl estradiol) — Estrogen supplement; menopausal symptoms, ovariectomy, female hypogonadism, primary ovarian failure — usual oral adult dose: intially, 100 μg (0.1 mg) daily for 7 days, followed by 1 week of no medication, after which a maintenance dose of 100 μg (0.1 mg) once a week is given. The weekly maintenance dose may be increased to 200 μg (0.2 mg) if needed.

Dosage forms and strengths usually available — Tablets: 100 μg (0.1 mg).

Proprietaries — Estrovis (Warner-Lambert)

PROGESTATIONAL AGENTS (PROGESTINS OR PROGESTOGENS)

Introduction
See estrogens.

Mechanism of Action
Progesterone and synthetic progestins act at a specific cytoplasmic receptor in target tissue to produce progestin activity by a mechanism which is similar to that outlined in Figure 2 for the estrogens. The progestin-receptor complex is translocated to the cell nucleus where protein synthesis is initiated, and results in the ultimate expression of a progestin response.[58]

Progestins cause the maturation of the uterine endometrium into a secretory state but only following an estrogen-stimulated growth phase. This progestational action transforms the uterine endometrium into an environment where implantation of the fertilized ovum and placental development can take place. In the myometrium, progestins antagonize the estrogen-induced contractile response. The cervical glands are stimulated by progestins to produce a thick, viscid mucopolysaccharide secretion in place of the estrogen-induced watery secretion which occurs during the first half of the menstrual cycle. In the vagina progestin activity causes cellular folding of the desquamated cells and increases the number of polymorphonuclear neutrophils. During pregnancy progestins acting with estrogens cause the maturation of the mammary glands for lactation.

Pharmacokinetics

The progestins are readily absorbed across the gastrointestinal tract and from parenteral sites of injection. However, as with the natural estrogens, the use of the oral route with progesterone, the natural endogenous progestin is limited due to rapid hepatic metabolism and possible transformation in the intestinal mucosa during the absorption. Most of the synthetic progestins are resistant to metabolism and thus, are very effective by the oral route.[59] Once absorbed, the progestins are bound to plasma proteins and a small amount is stored in adipose tissue.

The major metabolite of progesterone is $3\alpha,20\alpha$-dihydroxy-5β-pregnane (pregnanediol), a reduction product formed primarily by the liver, where it is conjugated with either glucuronic acid or sulfate to form the chief urinary metabolites of progesterone. Progesterone is also hydroxylated at the C-6 position. In addition, the C-20 ketone group of progesterone is reduced extrahepatically to form 20α and β hydroxy isomers.

The major urinary metabolite of progesterone is the glucuronide of pregnane-3,20-diol. The halflife of endogenous progesterone is very short, or approximately 2 to 3 min. Synthetic progestins have a much longer halflife in the body. Most of an oral dose of progestin is excreted in the urine and a small amount of appears in the feces via biliary excretion or as unabsorbed material.

As with estrogens, the blood level of progesterone varies considerably during the menstrual cycle in adult premenopausal women. Progesterone levels are the lowest during the first half of the menstrual cycle and range from 0 to 2 ng/mℓ. The level of progesterone rises rapidly following ovulation at mid-cycle and reaches a peak of 10 to 25 ng/mℓ on day 18 to 22 of the cycle and decreases rapidly toward the end of the cycle.[4,5] In postmenopausal women progesterone blood levels remain very low.[8]

Uses

Progestins are used primarily in conjunction with estrogens in the treatment of secondary amenorrhea, dysfunctional uterine bleeding and endometriosis.

Additionally, they decrease uterine motility as a contraceptive function. They are used to decrease premenstrual tension, although like the estrogens, they may also cause salt and water retention, worsening the tension phenomenon. Progestins are used cyclically for the treatment of infertility in cases where the uterus is not receptive to implantation. They inhibit spontaneous uterine contractions and may induce secretory changes in the endometrium.

Progestins may be combined with the estrogens also in the treatment of female sexual infantilism to bring about maturation and development of the genitalia. Conversely, progestins alone are used for the treatment of mastodynia to decrease breast size.

In very large doses, the progestins may be used as an antineoplastic agent for the treatment of endometrial carcinoma.

The progestins may be given cyclically for treatment of infertility especially in cases where the uterus is not receptive to implantation. Here their function is to sustain the secretory endometrium during the second half of the menstrual cycle. They are used cyclically in combination with the estrogens as contraceptive agents and for the treatment of secondary amenorrhea and dysfunctional uterine bleeding. Dosing is on a 20, 21, or 28 day cycle where day 1 of the cycle is the first day menstrual bleeding begins. Periodic administration of progestins consisting of 6 to 10 days is normally used for treatment of amenorrhea and abnormal uterine bleeding due to hormonal imbalance in the absence of pathological causes.

Very large doses of 1 or more grams 1 or more times per week (1 to 7 g/week) for periods up to 12 weeks may be used for progestins in the treatment of advanced uterine carcinoma.

Precautions

Progestins may display some anabolic or androgenic activity, and thus, should not be used during pregnancy due to the possibility of masculinization of the female fetus. Use during the first 4 months of pregnancy is not recommended due to the potential risk of birth defects in the developing fetus. They should not be used in lactating mothers since they are secreted in the milk, and effects on the nursing infant have not been determined.

Ophthalmologic effects have been noted during the use of progestins including papilledema and retinal vascular lesions leading to partial or complete loss of vision. Medication should be discontinued immediately following any change in vision or in cases of migraine.

Patients with a history of thrombophlebitic or cerebrovascular disorders, retinal thrombosis, and pulmonary embolism should be observed carefully. Caution should be observed with the use of progestins in persons with hypertension or fluid retention problems such as asthmatics, epileptics, or persons with cardiac or renal dysfunction due to its influence on sodium and water retention.

Persons with a history of depression should be observed carefully for a recurrence or worsening of the condition as a result of progestin therapy. Photosensitivity may occur as a result of progestin therapy and thus, patients should be cautioned against prolonged exposure to ultraviolet or sunlight. Persons with thyroid disease, hepatic dysfunction, and diabetes should be medicated with caution (see estrogens for further precautions).

Contraindications

The use of progestins is not recommended during the first trimester of pregnancy. Birth defects, especially heart and limb defects have been reported to occur in the children of pregnant women treated with the progestins. There is little evidence that the use of progestins is even an effective treatment modality during pregnancy. The progestins are contraindicated in persons with thromboembolic and thrombophlebitic disorders as well as cerebral apoplexy, impaired liver function, undiagnosed vaginal bleeding, or missed abortion. They are not recommended for persons with either known or suspected breast or genital carcinomas.

Toxicity

Breakthrough bleeding, spotting, changes in menstrual flow, and amenorrhea have been observed in women undergoing progestin therapy. Edema and hypertension due to a transient increase in sodium and chloride retention is not uncommon. Increases or decreases in body weight have been reported. Nausea, vomiting, diarrhea, headache, fatigue, hirsutism, urticaria, ulcerative stomatitis, pruritus vulvae, and a tendency toward vaginal candidal infections and galactorrhea have also been reported. Cholestatic jaundice, allergic rash, acne, melasma and chloasma, breast tenderness and secretion, alopecia, and mental depression may result from progestin therapy. Some progestins have both estrogenic and androgenic actions (see side effects of estrogens), and may increase the cutaneous pigmenting effect of estrogens. Isolated instances of coughing, dyspnea, chest constriction, and other allergic-type reactions have been reported. Local reactions at the site of injection may occur in some patients. Most progestins have a thermogenic effect and exert some effect on tissue retention of water within the intercellular spaces.

Table 3
PROGESTINS USED IN THERAPY

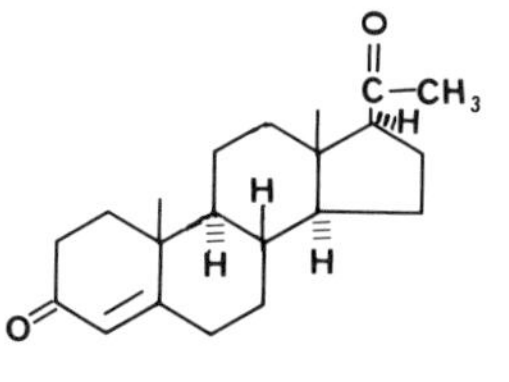

PROGESTERONE

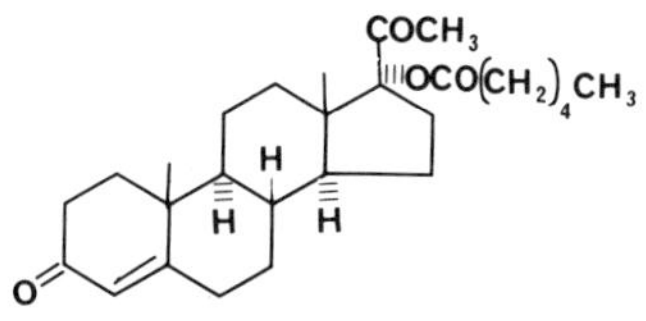

HYDROXYPROGESTERONE CAPROATE

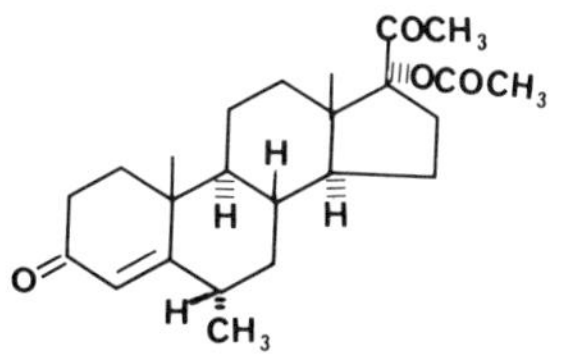

MEDROXYPROGESTERONE ACETATE

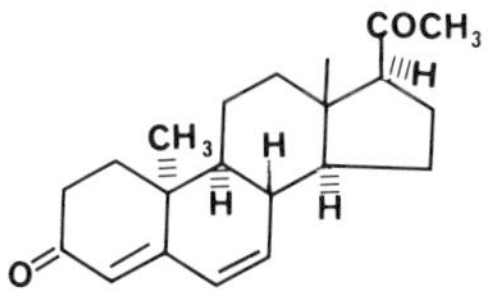

DYDROGESTERONE

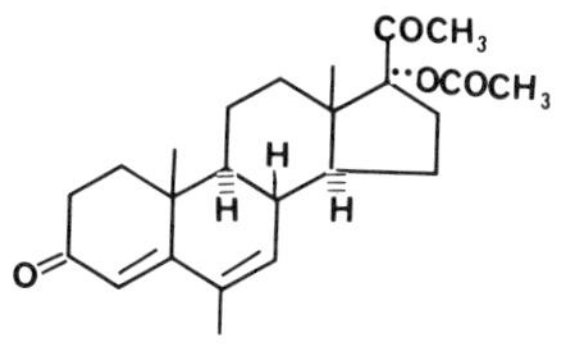

MEGESTROL ACETATE

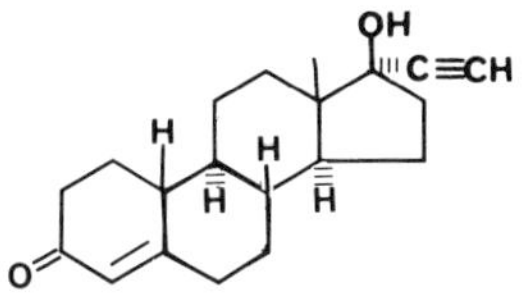

NORETHINDRONE

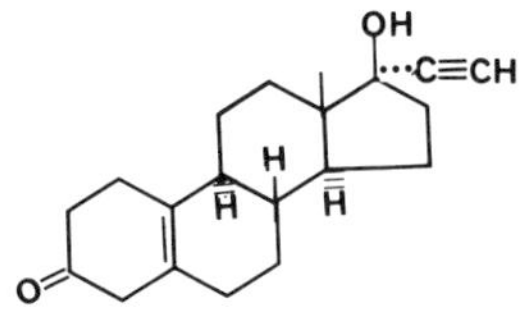

NORETHYNODREL

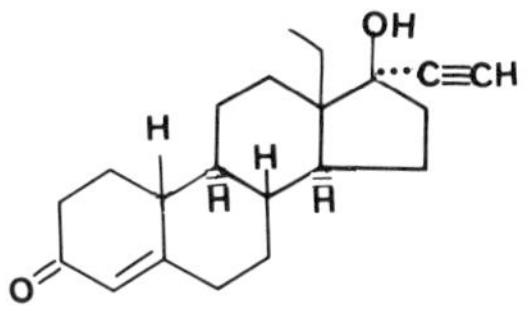

NORGESTREL

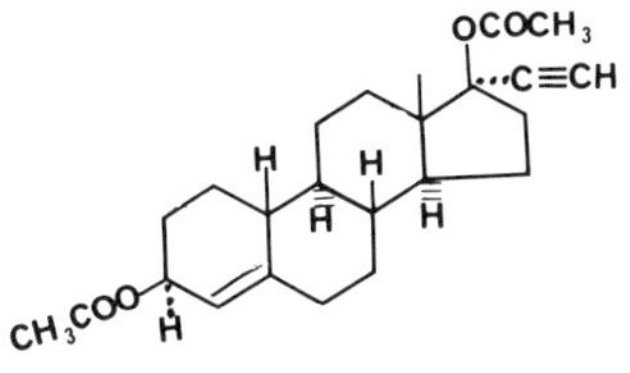

ETHYNODIOL DIACETATE

Structure-Activity Relationships

In 1937, 17α-ethinyltestosterone, ethisterone, was found to have some weak oral pro-gestational activity but was greater than natural progesterone. This surprising observation was not utilized by researchers in the design of new progestational agents until almost 10 years later. Researchers once again turned their attention to the structure of testosterone for additional clues, which ultimately led to the discovery of 19-nor steroids, i.e., steroids lacking the 19-angular methyl group. Two derivatives of 19-nortestosterone, norethindrone, and norethynodrel (Table 3), were found to be orally effective. The former is a potent oral progestin in man and only has mild androgenic properties. Isomerization of its Δ^4 bond to $\Delta^{5,10}$ gave norethynodrel. These two substances were prepared independently and in different laboratories,[60,61] and became the progestational components of the first contraceptives. Re-duction of the 3-keto group of norethindrone provides ethynodiol, a potent progestin in man which is used as the diacetate. The 18-homolog of norethindrone is norgestrel, found to be 100 times as progestational as norethindrone based on the endometrial changes in immature rabbits (Clauberg test).

17α-Hydroxyprogesterone has little or no progestational activity; however, esterification of the 17α-hydroxy group to form the acetate ester gave a substance that possessed high activity both by injection and orally, and which had a prolonged duration of action.[62,63] The caproate ester is inactive orally, but is a long-acting injectable progestin.[64] Other interesting acetoxyprogesterone derivatives are medroxyprogesterone acetate and megestrol acetate. Both are many times more potent than progesterone and each is quite effective by the oral route of administration, but megestrol acetate is more effective orally, suggesting that oral absorption may be improved by C_6-C_7 unsaturation in the B-ring.

Physical-Chemical and Other Data

Included are the following progestational agents (see Table 3).

- Dydrogesterone
- Ethynodiol diacetate
- Hydroxyprogesterone caproate
- Medroxyprogesterone acetate
- Norethindrone
- Norethindrone acetate
- Norethynodrel
- Norgestrel
- Progesterone
- Megestrol acetate

DYDROGESTERONE

Dydrogesterone is a white to light yellow, odorless, crystalline solid; mp 169 to 170°C (acetone-hexane); $C_{21}H_{28}O_2$; mol wt 312.45. It is soluble in chloroform and alcohol, but insoluble in water and ether.

Its preparations are described by Westerhof and Reerink[65] and Rappoldt and Westerhof[66] and in U.S. patent 3,198,792.

It is a good progestin, but lacks antiovulatory activity and is not as effective as other progestins in treating some menstrual disorders.

Chemical names and synonyms — (1) Pregna-4,6-diene-3,20-dione, (9β,10α)-; (2) 9β,10α-pregna-4,6-diene-3,20-dione; CAS-152-62-5.

Use, administration, and dosage — Primary or secondary amenorrhea, usual oral adult dose: 5 to 10 mg once or twice daily usually on days 15 through 25 of the menstrual cycle; functional uterine bleeding, usual oral adult dose: 5 to 10 mg once or twice daily for 5 to 10 days, the dosage is reduced to 10 mg/day from days 21 through 25 of the menstrual cycle, and repeated cyclically as needed.

Note: Usually 30 mg/day is the usual upper limit.

Dosage forms and strengths usually available — Tablets: 5 and 10 mg.

ETHYNODIOL DIACETATE

Ethynodiol diacetate is a white, odorless, crystalline solid; mp 126 to 127°C (methanol-water); $C_{24}H_{32}O_4$; mol wt 384.51. It is insoluble in water; soluble in alcohol and ether, but much more soluble in chloroform.

Several methods for the preparation of this progestin have been reported.[67] Ethynodiol diacetate is one of the most potent orally effective contraceptive substances. It is several times stronger a progestational substance than norethindrone and norethynodrel and also displays some estrogenic characteristics.[68,69]

Chemical names and synonyms — (1) 19-Norpreg-4-en-20-yne-3,17-diol, diacetate, (3β, 17α)-; (2) 19-nor-17α-pregn-4-en-20-yne-3β,17-diol diacetate; CAS-297-76-7.

Use, administration, and dosage — See ethynodiol diacetate, ethinyl estradiol tablets, ethynodiol diacetate, and mestranol tablets in the Antiovulatory Agents section.

HYDROXYPROGESTERONE CAPROATE

Hydroxyprogesterone caproate is a white crystalline solid, sometimes with an odor; mp 119 to 121°C (needles from isopropyl ether or methanol); $C_{27}H_{40}O_4$; mol wt 428.59. It is insoluble in water, slightly soluble in ether, and has solubility in sesame oil which is more than likely due to the ester function. Its preparation is described in U.S. patent 2,753,360 awarded to Schering AG, in 1956.

This hexanoate ester is a long acting progestin (see SAR), having a duration of action from 1 to 2 weeks. It is many times more potent than progesterone and its onset of action is slower. The long duration of action may be due to the 17-ester function causing steric hindrance to the enzymatic reduction of the 20-keto group.

Chemical names and synonyms — (1) Pregn-4-ene-3,20-dione, 17-[(1-oxohexyl)oxy]-; (2) 17-hydroxypregn-4-ene-3,20-dione hexanoate; CAS-630-56-8.

Use, administration, and dosage — Primary and secondary amenorrhea; abnormal uterine bleeding due to hormonal imbalance, i.m.; usual dose: 375 mg, repeated every 4 weeks for 4 cycles; production of secretory endometrium and desquamation: 375 mg every 4 weeks; uterine adenocarcinoma in advanced stage; 1 g once per day to 1 or more times each week (1 to 7 g/week) until relapse occurs or, if no desirable results are obtained, until a total of 12 weeks of therapy; to test for endogenous estrogen production: 250 mg. Bleeding 7 to 14 days after injection indicates endogenous estrogen. A second injection may be given 4 weeks after the first.

Dosage forms and strengths usually available — Injection: 125 mg/mℓ (10-mℓ vials) and 250 mg per mℓ (5-mℓ vials).

Proprietaries — Delalutin (Squibb); Deprolutin-250 (Seatrace); Duralutin (Hauck); Hydrosterone (Spencer-Mead); Hylutin (Hyrex); Hyprogest 250 (Keene); Hyproval P.A. (Tutag); Pro-Depo (North American).

MEDROXYPROGESTERONE ACETATE

This drug is a white cyrstalline powder; mp 207 to 209°C (methanol); $C_{24}H_{34}O_4$; mol wt 386.53. It is insoluble in water, soluble in acetone and chloroform, somewhat soluble in alcohol and methanol, and slightly soluble in ether. Medroxyprogesterone acetate has been synthesized by methods reported by Babcock et al.[70] and Ringold et al.[71] This substance is a very potent orally active progestin and because of the marked enhancement in biological activity of various steroids through the introduction of the 6α-methyl group, much effort has been devoted to improving the synthesis of these substances.[72] The 6α-methyl group is thought to slow the rate of reduction on the 4-ene-3-one system in ring A. Similarly, the 17α-acetate group also slows the reduction of the 20-keto group as explained for the hexanoate ester above, thereby prolonging its duration of action.

Chemical names and synonyms — (1) Pregn-4-ene-3,20-dione, 17-(acetyloxy)-6-methyl-,(6α)-; (2) 17-hydroxy-6α-methylpregn-4-ene-3,20-dione acetate; CAS-71-58-9.

Use, administration and dosage — Secondary amenorrhea, usual oral adult dose: 5 to

10 mg daily for 5 to 10 days, usually during the latter half of the menstrual cycle; functional uterine bleeding, usual oral adult dose: 5 to 10 mg daily for 5 to 10 days, beginning on days 16 or 21 of the menstrual cycle; contraceptive (sterile suspension), i.m.: 150 mg, repeated every 3 months; endometrial or renal carcinoma: initially, 400 mg to 1 g, repeated once a week, maintenance dose: 400 mg or as needed. *Note:* The parenteral form is used in the U.S. only as an investigational contraceptive.

Dosage forms and strengths usually available — Tablets: 2.5 and 10 mg; sterile suspension: 100 and 400 mg/mℓ.

Proprietaries — Provera (Upjohn); Amen (Carnick); Curretab (Reid-Provident).

NORETHINDRONE

Norethindrone is a white cyrstalline powder; mp 203 to 204°C (ethyl acetate); $C_{20}H_{26}O_2$; mol wt 298.41. It is insoluble in water; soluble in chloroform; and slightly soluble in ether and alcohol.

Its preparation is from 19-nor-4-androstene-3,17-dione;[61] and as described in U.S. patents 2,744,122 and 2,849,462.

Chemical names and synonyms — (1) 19-Norpregn-4-en-20-yn-3-one, 17-hydroxy-, (17α)-; (2) 17-hydroxy-19-nor-17α-pregn-4-en-20-yn-3-one; CAS-68-22-4; 19-norethisterone.

Use administration, and dosage — Amenorrhea; abnormal uterine bleeding due to hormonal imbalance, usual oral adult dose: 5 to 20 mg/day on days 5 to 25 of the menstrual cycle; endometriosis, usual oral adult dose: initially, 10 mg daily for 2 weeks, the daily dosage then being increased by 5 mg at 2-week intervals to a total of 30 mg daily, continued for 6 to 9 months, or until breakthrough bleeding, at which time therapy is temporarily discontinued; oral contraception, usual oral adult dose: 0.35 mg (350 μg) daily.

Dosage forms and strengths usually available — Tablets: 0.35 mg (350 μg) and 5 mg. See also norethindrone and mestranol tablets.

Proprietaries — Micronor (Ortho); Nor-Q.D. (Syntex); Norlutin (Parke Davis). Combined with an estrogen in the following preparations: Brevicon (Syntex); Modicon (Ortho); Norinyl (Syntex); Noriday (Syntex); Neocon (Ortho); Ovcon (Mead Johnson).

NORETHINDRONE ACETATE

The acetate is a white, crystalline powder; mp 161 to 162°C (methylene chloride-hexane); $C_{22}H_{28}O_3$; mol wt 340.46. It is insoluble in water; soluble in chloroform and dioxane, and slightly soluble in alcohol and ether.

Norethindrone acetate is the acetylated derivative of norethindrone. Its uses are similar to those of norethindrone, but its potency is twice that of the nonester.

Chemical names and synonyms — (1) 19-Norpregn-4-en-20-yn-3-one, 17(acetyloxy)-, (17α)-; (2) 17-hydroxy-19-nor-17α-pregn-4-en-20-yn-3-one acetate; CAS-51-98-9.

Use, administration, and dosage — Amenorrhea or functional uterine bleeding, usual oral adult dose: 2.5 to 10 mg daily on days 5 through 25 of the menstrual cycle; endometriosis, usual oral adult dose: initially, 5 mg daily for 2 weeks, then the daily dose is increased by 2.5 mg at 2-week intervals to a total of 15 mg/day, continued for 6 to 9 months unless discontinued temporarily for breakthrough bleeding.

Dosage forms and strengths usually available — Tablets: 5 mg.

Proprietaries — Norlutate (Parke-Davis). Combined with an estrogen in the following preparations: Norlestrin (Parke-Davis); Zorane (Lederle). See norethindrone acetate and ethinyl estradiol tablets.

NORETHYNODREL

Norethynodrel is a white, odorless, crystalline solid; mp 169 to 170°C (aqueous methanol); $C_{20}H_{26}O_2$; mol wt 298.41. It is soluble in chloroform, somewhat soluble in alcohol and ether, and only slightly soluble in water.

The preparation of this progestin is found in U.S. patents 2,691,028 and 2,725,389. This hormone is the $\Delta^{5,10}$ isomer of norethindrone. Isomerization in the body to norethindrone is not thought to occur too readily. The Δ^4 isomer is much more active however, which would suggest that isomerication is not a fast process as might be expected. Both are orally active and possess androgenic side effects, which can be attributed to the 17-OH group, a feature in testosterone.

Chemical names and synonyms — (1) 19-Norpregn-5(10)-en-20-yn-3-one, 17-hydroxy-, (17α)-; (2) 17-hydroxy-19-nor-17α-pregn-5(10)-en-20-yn-3-one; CAS-68-23-5.

Use, administration, and dosage — See the antiovulatory preparation, norethynodrel, and mestranol tablets.

NORGESTREL

Norgestrel is a white crystalline solid; mp 203 to 206°C (methanol or ethyl acetate), or 205 to 207°C; $C_{21}H_{28}O_2$; mol wt 312.44. It is insoluble in water, somewhat soluble in alcohol, and soluble in chloroform; (−) form, crystals from methanol-chloroform, mp 239 to 241°C; (+) form, mp 238 to 242°C.

The preparation of the racemate was reported by Hughes et al.[73] and Smith et al.[74] and in a British patent 1,041,280. Structurally, this progestin is related to norethindrone and norethynodrel, bearing an ethyl group in place of the C_{13}-methyl. It is used only in oral contraceptive preparations (q.v.), even though it is much more potent as a progestational agent than is norethindrone.

Chemical names and synonyms — (1) 18,19-Dinorpregn-4-en-20-yn-3-one, 13-ethyl-17-hydroxy-, (17α)-(±)-; (2) (±)-13-ethyl-17-hydroxy-18,19-dinor-17α-pregn-4-en-20-yn-3-one; CAS-6533-00-2.

Use, administration, and dosage — Only used in oral contraceptives, usual oral adult dose: 75μg (0.075 mg) daily.

Dosage forms and strengths usually available — Tablets: 75 μg (0.075 mg).

Proprietaries — Ovrette (Wyeth); Microlut (Schering A.G., W. Berlin). Combined with an estrogen in the preparation Ovral (Wyeth); see norgestrel and ethinyl estradiol.

PROGESTERONE

Progesterone is a white crystalline powder, existing in two crystalline forms; mp 127 to 131°C and mp 121°C; $C_{21}H_{30}O_2$; mol wt 314.47. It is insoluble in water, soluble in alcohol and acetone, and sparingly soluble in vegetable oils.

Progesterone, an active principle from the corpus luteum, secreted during the latter half of the menstrual cycle, and during pregnancy by the placenta exerts an antiovulatory effect when administered during days 5 to 25 of the normal cycle. It is not orally effective and hence is administered intramuscularly. It is isolated from the corpus luteum of pregnant sows.[75,76] The structure was elucidated by Butenandt et al.[77] and the synthesis of the dl-form was reported by Johnson et al.[78] Preparations from other steroids are described in a review by Strain[79] and in U.S. patents 2,379.832, 2,232.438, and 2,314.185.

Chemical names and synonyms — (1) Pregn-4-ene-3,20-dione; (2) progesterone; CAS-57-83-0.

Use, administration, and dosage — intramuscularly; amenorrhea, usual adult dose: 5

to 10 mg/day for 6 to 8 consecutive days before expected menstruation; functional uterine bleeding, usual adult dose: 50 to 100 mg for one dose only, or 5 to 10 mg once daily for 6 days. Bleeding may cease within 6 days. When estrogen is given, progesterone is administered after 2 weeks of estrogen therapy. Injections are stopped if menstrual flow begins during treatment.

Dosage forms and strengths usually available — Injection (oil): 25 mg/mℓ (10-mℓ vials); 50 mg/mℓ (10-mℓ vials), and 100 mg/mℓ (10-vials); sterile suspension: 25, 50, and 100 mg/mℓ (all in 10 mℓ vials).

Proprietaries — Femotrone (Bluco); Progelan (Lannett); Progestaject-50 (Maryland); Profac-O (Kay Pharmacal). Component in the following preparations: Syngesterone (Pfizer) and Syngestrets (Pfizer).

MEGESTROL ACETATE

Megestrol acetate is a white crystalline solid; mp 214 to 216°C (methanol); $C_{24}H_{32}O_4$; mol wt 384.50. It is insoluble in water, soluble in chloroform, and slightly soluble in alcohol and ether.

The preparation of this progestin is described by Ringold and co-workers[71] and in several U.S. patents, 2,891,079, 3,356,573, and 3,400,137. Biological[80] and metabolic[81] studies were conducted by Chang and Cooper respectively.

Chemical names and synonyms — (1) Pregna-4,6-diene-3,20-dione, 17-(acetyloxy)-6-methyl-; (2) 17-hydroxy-6-methylpregna-4,6-diene-3,20-dione acetate; CAS-595-33-5.

Use — Megesterol acetate is a potent antiovulatory agent and has neither estrogenic nor androgenic effects, but is indicated only as an antineoplastic agent and not indicated for other uses.

Administration and dosage — Endometrial carcinoma, usual oral adult dose: 40 to 80 mg four times per day; mammary carcinoma, usual oral adult dose: 40 mg four times per day.

Dosage forms and strengths usually available — Tablets: 20 and 40 mg.

Proprietaries — Megace (Mead Johnson).

ANTIESTROGENS

Introduction

In a general sense, any compound which reduces the biological activity of an estrogen may be considered an antiestrogen. Thus, androgens and progestins which alter estrogenic activity could be considered partial antiestrogens. However, with the development of specific competitive estrogen antagonists the term antiestrogen now applies mainly to agents with relatively specific competitive antiestrogenic effects. The first competitive antiestrogen was discovered in 1956 when Segal and Thompson[82] found that the weakly estrogenic compound chlorotrianisene (Table 2) was capable of inhibiting the pituitary enlargement caused by estradiol. Subsequently a number of weakly estrogenic compounds which competitively inhibit the response to potent estrogens, such 17β-estradiol (Table 1) and diethylstilbestrol (Table 2), have been developed. Thus, these agents act as partial estrogen agonists. Some of the antiestrogenic agents appear to exert a different degree of estrogenic/antiestrogenic effect on various target tissue. For example, clomiphene (Table 4), which is used as a female fertility agent, produces a greater antiestrogenic action in the hypothalamus and pituitary than in peripheral tissue such as the uterus and breast. Therefore, clomiphene is used to stimulate the secretion of the gonadotropins (LH and FSH) from the anterior pituitary in infertile women. Conversely, tamoxifen (Table 4), which is used in the treatment of breast cancer, produces a greater peripheral than central antiestrogenic action. The obvious draw-

Table 4
DIHYDRONAPHTHALENE AND TRIARYLETHYLENE ANALOGS

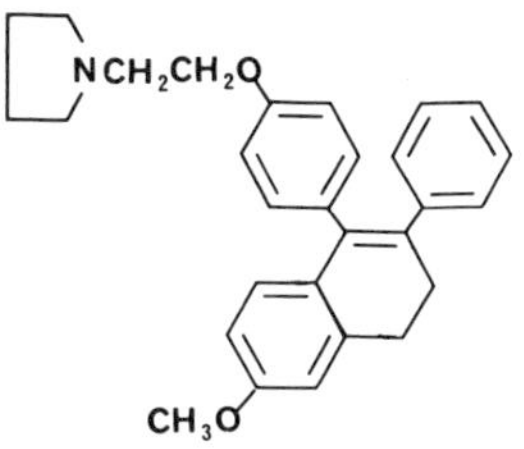

NAFOXIDINE

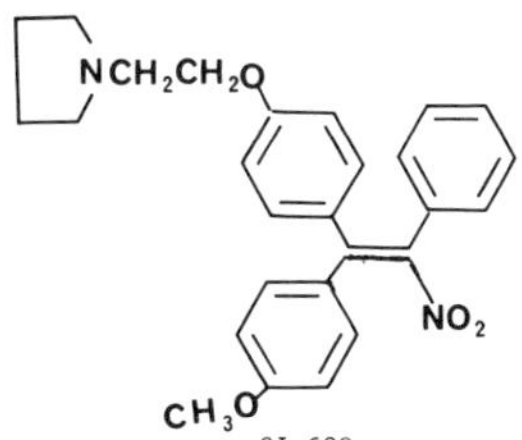

CI-628

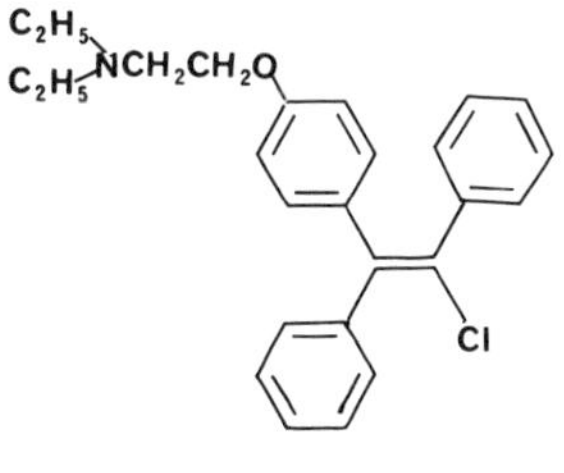

ENCLOMIPHENE

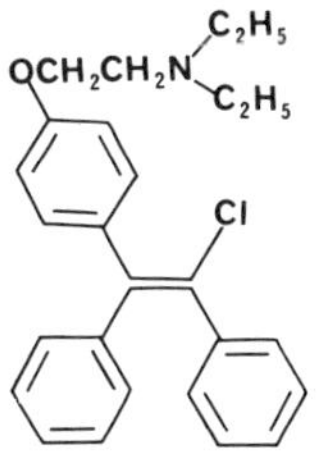

ZUCLOMIPHENE

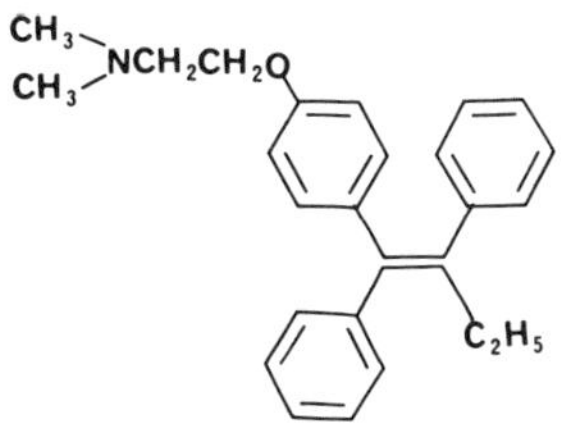

TAMOXIFEN
(I.C.I. 46,474)

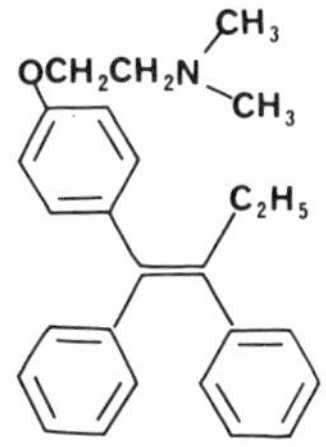

(I.C.I. 47,699)

back to the use of pharmacological doses of a partial estrogen agonist in the treatment of a estrogen-dependent tumor has led to the search for compounds which are completely antiestrogenic and devoid of estrogen agonist activity.

Mechanism of Action

With reference to the basic model of estrogen action within estrogen-dependent tissue (illustrated in Figure 2) it is theoretically possible that antiestrogens could disrupt the sub-cellular scheme of estrogenic activity at one or a number of specific stages as outlined in Figure 3. Since most antiestrogens display a relatively low affinity for the cytoplasmic estrogen receptor (R_c) in vitro[83,84] it has been suggested that premature dissociation or competitive antagonism for active estrogens to the R_c may be responsible for antiestrogenic effects. However, it is known that the triphenylethylene antiestrogens, such as clomiphene and tamoxifen, are translocated into the nucleus and produce an initial estrogenic response.[85] In addition, antiestrogens such as monohydroxytamoxifen have a relatively high affinity for the estrogen receptor.[86]

Clark and associates[87] have demonstrated that natural estrogens cause nuclear retention of the estrogen receptor for relatively short periods of time (4 to 6 hr for estradiol) while nonsteroidal antiestrogens cause the retention of the nuclear receptor (R_n) for several weeks since these compounds are slowly cleared from the body. Thus, the triphenylethylene antiestrogens cause accumulation and long term retention of R_n; however, nuclear retention is not accompanied by replenishment of R_c.[88,89] Therefore, the target tissue becomes insensitive

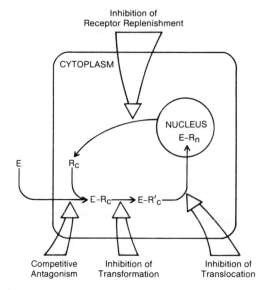

FIGURE 3. Potential mechanism of antiestrogens in estrogen-dependent tissue.[70]

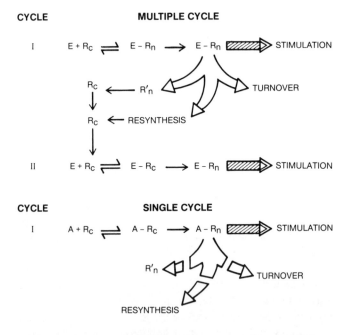

FIGURE 4. Proposed antiestrogen (A) mechanism of action. (From Liisberg, S., Godtfredson, O., and Vangedal, S., *Tetrahedron*, 9, 149, 1960. With permission.)

to subsequent cycles of estrogenic stimulation as illustrated in Figure 4. Thus, it appears that the nonsteroidal antiestrogen-receptor complex reacts with nuclear genetic material in an anomalous manner which initiates a selflimiting response.[87] Since tamoxifen and other triphenylethylene antiestrogens are known to be partial estrogen agonists, it would seem to be therapeutically beneficial to employ antiestrogens without estrogen agonist activity.[90] Recently, nonsteroidal antiestrogens which produce little or no estrogen agonist activity have been reported.[91-93]

Pharmacokinetics

The antiestrogens are well absorbed by the oral route. Maximal concentrations of tamoxifen found in the circulation occur at 4 to 7 hr following oral administration. In general, nonsteroidal antiestrogens have a longer halflife in the body than estrogenic steroids. The decline in plasma concentrations of tamoxifen is biphasic; however, the terminal halflife is greater than 1 week. Approximately 95% of a single dose of clomiphene is excreted in 5 days. Hydroxylation and conjugation are the major metabolic pathways for tamoxifen which occur primarily in the liver. The major metabolites of tamoxifen are 4-hydroxytamoxifen and 3,4-dihydroxytamoxifen. In addition, N-desmethyltamoxifen has been identified as a minor metabolite. It has been shown that both metabolites exhibit a stronger apparent binding affinity than tamoxifen for the estrogen receptor. However, 4-hydroxytamoxifen is a more potent antiestrogen and 3,4-dihydroxytamoxifen a less potent antiestrogen than the parent compound. Thus, it has been suggested that most of the in vivo antiestrogenic activity of tamoxifen is due to its hydroxylated metabolites.[94] Following biliary excretion and enterohepatic recirculation, tamoxifen, clomiphene, and their metabolites are excreted primarily in the feces.

Uses

See Introduction.

Precautions

Caution should be exercised in the use of tamoxifen in patients with leukopenia or thrombocytopenia. The occurrence of these two problems has been reported during the use of tamoxifen, but it has not been clearly shown that these effects are due to tamoxifen therapy. Transient decreases in platelet counts have been reported in patients undergoing tamoxifen therapy for breast cancer, returning to normal levels even with continuing treatment. Hemorrhagic tendencies have not been reported, however. Occasional complete blood counts, including platelets, may be warranted.

Since tamoxifen may be an oncogenic agent in experimental animals, this must be considered as a possibility in humans. Teratogenic properties have been reported in rabbits and rats, manifested as skeletal abnormalities. At dose levels somewhat higher than that used in humans, tamoxifen has been reported to affect reproductive functions in rats. That tamoxifen is safe to use in pregnancy has not been established.

Caution should be exercised in the prescription of clomiphene to patients with abnormal vaginal bleeding of undetermined origin, fibroid tumors of the uterus, impaired hepatic function, mental depression, or thrombophlebitis (see specific estrogen precautions).

Patients with a sensitivity to pituitary gonadotropins may have an exaggerated response to clomiphene.

Clomiphene is teratogenic in animals and has resulted in fetal death and congenital malformations. Even though a direct cause-and effect relationship has not been established, caution should be used in prescribing clomiphene.

Contraindications

Clomiphene therapy is not recommended in patients with ovarian cysts, since further enlargement may occur. Patients with impaired liver function or neoplastic lesions should be given clomiphene with caution. It is not recommended for use during pregnancy.

Toxicity

The most commonly reported adverse reactions to tamoxifen therapy include hot flashes, nausea, and vomiting. Less frequently vaginal bleeding, vaginal discharge, menstrual irregularities, and skin rashes have been reported.

Increased bone and tumor pain as well as local disease flare-ups possibly requiring analgesics, have been reported and are sometimes associated with a good antitumor response. Sudden increase in size of pre-existing lesions in soft tissues may occur, often associated with a marked erythema both within and surrounding the lesions. Occasionally the development of new lesions has been reported. These reactions in bone and involved tissue usually subside rapidly. Occasionally hypercalcemia, depression, dizziness, headache, peripheral edema, anorexia, and pruritis vulvae have been reported to occur. Rarely patients have been reported to develop retinal abnormalities.

In humans, overdosage has not been reported. LD_{50} studies performed in animals, and utilizing very high dosages resulted in respiratory difficulties and convulsions at the highest test dosages. Treatment for overdosage is not known, but must be symptomatic.

At recommended dosage levels, side effects resulting from clomiphene therapy are rare with both the incidence and severity being dependent upon dose level and duration of treatment.

Multiple pregnancies are increased to eight times normal with clomiphene. Major side effects include cystic enlargement of the ovaries, cyclic ovarian pain, breast enlargement, nausea, and hot flashes. Less frequently, blurred vision and scintillating scotoma may occur. All side effects are reversible upon cessation of therapy, except multiple pregnancy.

Structure-Activity Relationships

Two compounds currently available as antiestrogens for clinical use are clomiphene and tamoxifen. Nafoxidine, another antiestrogen is not available as yet (Table 4).

In its crude form, clomiphene is a mixture of the *cis* (zuclomiphene) and the *trans* (enclomiphene) geometric isomers,[95] but it was found later that only the *trans* isomers of triphenylethylenes were antiestrogenic.[96] Clomiphene was found to be an antiestrogen with antifertility properties in laboratory animals,[97,98] but clinical tests showed that it stimulated ovulation in humans[99] and is now available as a fertility agent.

Of all the compounds that have been tested for antiestrogenic and antifertility effects in laboratory animals, four have surfaced as being the most important in endocrinologic research and are listed in Table 4. They are nafoxidine,[100,101] CI-628,[102] clomiphene,[103] and tamoxifen.[104,105]

Once it was discovered that advanced breast cancer responded to endocrine ablation, much attention was directed to the use of antiestrogens as a substitute for surgery. In the laboratory, tamoxifen[106,107] inhibited the initiation, and nafoxidine,[108] enclomiphene,[109] CI-628,[110] and tamoxifen[111] inhibited the growth of hormone-dependent rat mammary carcinomas. In clinical tests nafoxidine,[112] clomiphene (mixed isomers),[113] and tamoxifen[114,115] have been shown to be effective in bringing about tumor regression in nearly 30% of advanced breast cancer patients.

Tamoxifen, as represented in Table 4 (I.C.I. 46,474), has become the antiestrogen of choice in the treatment of advanced breast cancer, because of its low incidence of side effects. It is a partial estrogen with antiestrogenic properties in the immature rat uterus, and its isomer (I.C.I. 47,699) is a full estrogen.[96,104]

The importance of the aminoethoxy side chain occupying a certain position in space for effective antiestrogenic activity has been demonstrated among a group of nafoxidine derivatives by Lednicer et al.[116] Abbott et al.[117] have shown that the substitution of two methyl groups *ortho* to the ether oxygen attached to the phenyl ring restricts the position of the side chain in space and hence, reduces the ability of tamoxifen to compete with $[^3H]$-17β-estradiol for the estrogen receptors in vitro.

Physical-Chemical and Other Data

The following sections discuss clomiphene citrate and tamoxifen citrate.

CLOMIPHENE CITRATE

Clomiphene citrate is a white, odorless powder; mp 116.5 to 118°C; $C_{26}H_{28}ClNO \cdot C_6H_8O_7$; mol wt 598.09. It is insoluble in ether, slightly soluble in water and chloroform, and sparingly soluble in alcohol.

Its preparation is described in a U.S. patent, 2,914,563 and the stereochemistry of the geometric isomers is reported by Ernst and coworkers.[118] Clomiphene citrate is a mixture of both (Z) and (E) isomers.

Chemical names and synonyms — (1) Ethanamine, 2-[4-(2-chloro-1,2-diphenylethenyl) phenoxy]-*N,N*-diethyl-, 2-hydroxy-1,2,3-propanetricarboxylate (1:1); (2) 2-[*p*-(2-chloro-1,2-diphenylvinyl)phenoxy]triethylamine citrate (1:1); CAS-50-41-9; CAS-911-45-5(clomiphene).

Uses — Clomiphene is a nonsteroidal compound with estrogenic and antiestrogenic properties. It has been used to induce ovulation or increase fertility in anovulatory or oligoovulatory women with adequate endogenous estrogens. Patients who have been hypoestrogenic for long periods may require pretreatment with estrogen to provide for ovum implantation. Estrogen therapy should be discontinued prior to the initiation of clomiphene therapy.

Administration and dosage — Usual oral adult dose: 50 mg daily for 5 days beginning on the 5th day of the menstrual cycle if bleeding occurs or at any time in the patient who had no recent uterine bleeding. If ovulation occurs without conception, this cycle is repeated until conception, or for three or four cycles. If ovulation does not occur, the dose is increased to 100 mg daily for 5 days, and repeated if ovulation without conception occurs. Some patients require up to 250 mg daily to induce ovulation.

Dosage forms and strengths usually available — Tablets: 50 mg.

Proprietaries — Clomid (Merrell-National Labs).

TAMOXIFEN CITRATE

Tamoxifen citrate is a white crystalline powder; mp 140 to 142°C; $C_{26}H_{29}NO \cdot C_6H_8O_7$; mol wt 563.65. The free base, tamoxifen, is a white crystalline solid; mp 96 to 98°C (petroleum ether); $C_{26}H_{29}O$; mol wt 371.53. Elucidation of structure and separation of isomers were reported in 1966 by Bedford and Richardson,[119] and in British patent 1,064,629. The bioactivity[98] and pharmacology[104,105,120] of the isomers have also been reported.

Uses — Tamoxifen citrate is a nonsteroidal, antiestrogenic agent which competes for cytosolic estrogen binding sites in target tissues such as breast tissue. It is used in the treatment of advanced breast cancer in postmenopausal women.

Chemical names and synonyms — (1) Ethanamine, 2-[4-(1,2-diphenyl-1-butenyl)-phenoxy]-*N,N*-dimethyl-, (Z), 2-hydroxy-1,2,3-propanetricarboxylate (1:1); (2) (Z)-2-[*p*-(1,2-diphenyl-1-butenyl)phenoxy]-*N,N*-dimethylethylamine citrate (1:1); CAS-54965-24-1; CAS-10540-29-1 (tamoxifen).

Administration and dosage — Advanced breast carcinoma in postmenopausal women, usual oral adult dose: 10 to 20 mg, the equivalent of tamoxifen twice daily (once in the morning and evening); stimulation of ovulation, usual oral adult dose: 5 to 40 mg, the equivalent of tamoxifen, twice daily for 4 days.

A response to cancer chemotherapy usually occurs within 4 to 10 weeks of therapy, but can take much longer in patients with bone metastases. Estrogen antagonism may persist for several weeks following a single dose.

Dosage forms and strengths usually available — 10 mg (the equivalent of tamoxifen).

Proprietaries — Nolvadex (Stuart).

ANTIOVULATORY AGENTS

Introduction

Improvements in nutrition and the rapid advances in the medical sciences during the past fifty years have extended life expectancy and contributed significantly to the current explosion in world population growth. The earth's capacity to support the population with food and essential materials is not unlimited. Accordingly, certain parts of the world are severely overpopulated at the present time. Thus, fertility and population control is essential to the future development of mankind. For these reasons, the development of antiovulatory agents has been the object of a considerable amount of research and pharmaceutical development.

In the late 1950s Rock, Pincus, Garcia, and associates[121,122] examined the antiovulatory activity of orally active progestational agents. It was later found that norethynodrel, the original progestational preparation used in these studies, was contaminated with estrogenic activity. The orally active estrogen contaminant, mestranol, serendipitously enhanced the antiovulatory effectiveness of the preparation and eventually led to the general use of the combination estrogen-protestin oral contraceptive. The combination contraceptive agent was found to be approximately 100% effective if taken properly. This agent contains both an orally active estrogen and orally active progestin which is taken daily from day 5 to day 25 of the menstrual cycle (day 1 is the first day of menses). To simplify administration, some preparations are taken on a monthly basis to provide 3 weeks of continuous medication and 1 week off per month, while other preparations are taken continuously on a calendar basis and contain 21 active pills and 7 blank pills.

Later, a modification of the steroidal contraceptive was developed. The new preparation was termed a sequential oral contraceptive since an estrogen alone was used for the first 14 to 16 days of the menstrual cycle and a combination of estrogen and progestin employed for the last 5 to 6 days. The sequential agent was developed to more closely duplicate the normal menstrual cycle. However, this preparation is less effective than the combination antiovulatory agents and has been reported to cause a higher incidence of endometrial cancer. Therefore, the use of the sequential agents has been discontinued in the U.S.

Mechanism of Action

Several of the chemical contraceptive agents which are on the market today do not act primarily as an antiovulatory agents. For example the "minipill" (continuous low-dose progestin) and the postcoital contraceptive (highdose estrogen) agents cause an alteration of the uterine endometrium and/or cervical mucous secretions and thereby prevent union of the sperm and ovum and subsequent implantation of the fertilized ovum. However, the combination oral contraceptives, which are the most widely used contraceptives, act as antiovulatory agents.

The combination contraceptive contains both an orally active estrogen and an orally active progestin which is taken from day 5 to 25 of the menstrual cycle (the first day of menses is day 1). The estrogen-progestin combination produces several contraceptive actions; however, its primary mechanism of action is the inhibition of gonadotropin (LH and FSH) secretion from the anterior pituitary. The estrogen inhibits the secretion of follicle stimulating hormone (FSH) which causes the growth and maturation of ovarian follicles. The progestin administered early in the cycle inhibits the mid-cycle surge of leutenizing hormone (LH) secretion which is thought to induce ovulation. In addition, the progestin will produce a viscous cervical secretion which will inhibit sperm migration and conception if ovulation does occur. Further, the estrogen and progestin-induced alterations in uterine endometrium would make implantation of a fertilized ovum very unlikely.

Pharmacokinetics

The synthetic estrogens (e.g., ethinyl estradiol and mestranol) and progestins (e.g., norethindrone and norethynodrel) which are commonly used in oral contraceptive agents are readily absorbed through the gastrointestinal tract. Further, they are less labile to metabolic inactivation by the liver. Following the oral administration of 50 µg of mestranol or ethinyl estradiol maximal blood levels in the range of 2 to 4 pg/mℓ have been reported to occur within 1 to 4 hr.[123-125] Mestranol is known to be biologically inactive; however, it is rapidly demethylated in the liver to its active metabolite ethinyl estradiol.[125,126]

An oral dose of 1 mg of norethindrone produced maximal plasma levels of 10 to 12 ng/mℓ within 102 hr.[127] The halflife of this drug in human subjects is in the range of 3 to 5 hr.[128] The halflife of norethindrone metabolites is in the range of 60 to 70 hr.[129] The major metabolites of norethindrone are glucuronide and sulfate conjugates which are excreted primarily in the urine.[130] It has been shown that norethynodrel and other structurally related progestins are biologically inactive and require prior metabolic conversion to norethindrone.[127]

Uses

In addition to their use as contraceptive agents in both parous and nulliparous women, the contraceptives, a combination of estrogen and progestin, are also sometimes utilized for the supplemental effect of the estrogen and progestin ingredients specifically.

Precautions

See estrogens for DES precautions. See estrogens and progestins precaution sections. Contraceptive use by nursing mothers is not recommended due to the potential for adverse effects in the nursing infant. Use of contraceptives has been shown to be associated with an increased risk of liver tumors. Risk of gall bladder disease is twofold in contraceptive users. Disturbances in normal tryptophan metabolism may result in a pyridoxine deficiency due to contraceptive therapy. Megaloblastic anemia has also been reported.

Cigarette smoking during contraceptive therapy increases the risk of serious cardiovascular disease, increasing with age and with heavier smoking. These effects are more marked in women over 35 years of age.

Use of contraceptives has been reported to increase the risk of both venous and arterial thromboembolism, thrombotic and hemorrhagic stroke, myocardial infarction, hepatic tumors, gall bladder disease, hypertension, visual disorders, and fetal abnormalities.

Prediabetic and diabetic patients should be observed carefully during contraceptive therapy due to a reported decrease in glucose tolerance, and an increase in trigylcerides and total phospholipids.

Oral contraceptives interfere with lactation, resulting in a decrease in both quality and quantity of breast milk. Small quantities of the contraceptives are also found in breast milk although the effects on the breast-fed child have not yet been determined. It is recommended that contraceptive use be deferred until the infant is weaned.

The onset of climacteric may be masked due to treatment with contraceptives.

Contraindications

Contraceptives should not be used during preganncy or suspected pregnancy, due to reported congenital malformations or in persons who have had a previous ectopic pregnancy. The presence or history of pelvic inflammatory disease, venereal disease, including gonorrhea, syphilis, or chlamydial infections of the genital tract are also points for contraindications. Contraceptives are contraindicated in the case of previous pelvic surgery, postpartum endometritis, or infected abortion. Abnormalities of the uterus resulting in distortion of the uterine cavity or suspected uterine or cervical malignancy are reasons not to use contraceptive therapy. See also the Estrogens and Progestins sections for contraindications.

Toxicity

Contraceptives are suspected of resulting in pyridoxine (vitamin B_6), folic acid, and cyanocobalamin (vitamin B_{12}) deficiencies.

Many side effects are related to the dominance of either the estrogen or progestin in the preparation. The adverse side effects tend to vary both in incidence and severity depending on the preparation. Side effects of combination contraceptives are due to the effects of the estrogens. See Estrogens and Progestins Toxicity sections for specific side effects. Changing types and ratios of preparations of estrogens and progestins often lessen or totally eliminate the side effects.

Impairment of fertility has been reported in women discontinuing oral contraceptive therapy which appears to be independent of the use of the preparations. This impairment diminishes with time, although there is still appreciable difference in the results in nulliparous women when tested up to 30 months following discontinuation of contraceptive therapy. In parous women however, the difference is not apparent 30 months after cessation of therapy.

No serious ill effects in young children have been reported as a result of acute overdosage of oral contraceptives. Following overdosage, nausea may occur in both males and females, and withdrawal bleeding may occur in females.

Physical-Chemical and Other Data (Combined Estrogens and Progestins)

See specific progestins and estrogens for physical-chemical and other data.

Preparations

- Ethynodiol diacetate and ethinyl estradiol tablets
- Ethynodiol diacetate and mestranol tablets
- Norethindrone and ethinyl estradiol tablets
- Norethindrone and mestranol tablets
- Norethindrone acetate and ethinyl estradiol tablets
- Norethynodrel and mestranol tablets
- Norgestrel and ethinyl estradiol tablets
- "Minipills"
- Postcoital contraceptives

Refer to the introductory section on antiovulatory agents. The uses of each component in the combined preparations listed below can be found in earlier sections, i.e., see the section on progestins and estrogens.

The progestin-estrogen preparations are used for either 20 or 21 days out of the normal 28-day cycle. Day 1 of the cycle is the first day of the menstrual flow. Some tablets are packaged in compaks (e.g., memorette, dialpak) to be taken serially by number for 28 days, and supply the user with 7 or 8 placebo or iron tablets for continuous daily dosage, so she will not have to count the days between cycles. Usually these tablets are of a different color.

ETHYNODIOL DIACETATE AND ETHINYL ESTRADIOL TABLETS

Administration and dosage — Usual oral adult dose: 21-day cycle, one tablet daily for 21 days beginning on day 5 of the menstrual cycle, or on the 8th day after taking the last tablet in the previous cycle; 28-day cycle, one tablet for 28 days beginning on the 5 day of the menstrual cycle, or on the day after taking the last tablet in the previous cycle.

Dosage forms and strengths usually available — 1 mg of ethynodiol diacetate and 50 µg of ethinyl estradiol.

Proprietaries — Demulen and Demulen-28 (Searle)

ETHYNODIOL DIACETATE AND MESTRANOL TABLETS

Administration and dosage — Usual oral adult dose: 20-day cycle, one tablet daily for

20 days beginning on day 5 of the menstrual cycle or on the 8th day after taking the last tablet of the previous cycle; for 21-day cycle and 28-day cycle: see the above dosing for ethynodiol diacetate and ethinyl estradiol.

Dosage forms and strengths usually available — Tablets: available as 20-, 21-, and 28-day cycles; 1 mg of ethynodiol diacetate and 100 μg of mestranol.

Proprietaries — Ovulen, Ovulen-21, and Ovulen-28 (Searle).

NORETHINDRONE AND ETHINYL ESTRADIOL TABLETS

Administration and dosage — Usual oral adult dose: 21- and 28-day cycles; see the above dosing for ethynodiol diacetate and ethinyl estradiol.

Dosage forms and strengths usually available — Tablets: several strengths, 400 μg norethindrone per 35 μg ethinyl estradiol; 500 μg/35 μg; 1 mg/35 μg and 1 mg/50 μg.

Proprietaries — Ovcon-50 and Ovcon-35 (Mead Johnson); Brevicon-21-Day and Brevicon-28-Day (Syntex); Modicon and Modicon 28 (Ortho); Ortho-Novum 1/35 21 and Ortho Novum 1/35 28 (Ortho); Norinyl 1 + 35 21-day and Norinyl 1 + 35 28-day (Syntex).

NORETHINDRONE AND MESTRANOL TABLETS

Administration and dosage — Usual oral adult dose: 20-, 21-, and 28-day cycles; see the above section on ethynodiol diacetate and mestranol tablets.

Dosage forms and strengths usually available — Tablets: several strengths: 1 mg norethindrone per 50 μg mestranol; 1 mg/80 μg; 2 mg/100 μg.

Proprietaries — Norinyl 2 mg (Syntex); Ortho-Novum 2 mg 21-Day (Ortho); Norinyl 1 + 50 21-day and Norinyl 1 + 50 28-day (Syntex); Norinyl 1 + 80 21-day and Norinyl 1 + 80 28-day (Syntex); Ortho-Novum 1/50 + 21-day and Ortho-Novum 1/50 + 28-day (Ortho); Ortho-Novum 1/80 21-day and Ortho-Novum 1/80 28-day (Ortho).

NORETHINDRONE ACETATE AND ETHINYL ESTRADIOL TABLETS

Administration and dosage — Usual oral adult dose: 21- and 28-day cycles; see the section on ethynodiol diacetate and ethinyl estradiol tablets.

Dosage forms and strengths usually available — Tablets: 1 mg norethindrone acetate/20 μg ethinyl estradiol; 1 mg/50 μg; 1.5 mg/30 μg; 2.5 mg/50 μg.

Proprietaries — Loestrin Fe 1.5/30, Loestrin 21 1.5/30 (Parke-Davis); Loestrin Fe 1/20, Loestrin 21 1/20 (Parke-Davis); Norlestrin 21 1/50, Norlestrin 28 1/50, Norlestrin-Fe 1/50, Norlestrin 21 2.5/50, Norlestrin-Fe 2.5/50 (Parke-Davis).

NORETHYNODREL AND MESTRANOL TABLETS

Administration and dosage — Usual oral adult dose: 21- and 28-day cycles see the above section on ethynodiol diacetate and ethinyl estradiol tablets.

Dosage forms and strengths usually available — Tablets: 2.5 mg norethynodrel and 100 μg of mestranol; 5 mg/75 μg.

Proprietaries — Enovid-E and Enovid-E 21 (Searle); Enovid 5 mg (Searle).

NORGESTREL AND ETHINYL ESTRADIOL TABLETS

Administration and dosage — Usual oral adult dose: 21- and 28-day cycles. See the above section on ethynodiol diacetate and ethinyl estradiol tablets.

Dosage forms and strengths usually available — 300 μg of norgestrel/30 μg of ethinyl estradiol; 500 μg/50 μg.

Proprietaries — Lo/Ovral and Lo/Ovral-28 (Wyeth); Ovral and Ovral-28 (Wyeth).

MINIPILL

The "Minipills" containing 0.35 mg of norethindrone, Micronor (Ortho) and Nor-Q-D (Syntex), or 0.075 mg of norgestrel, Ovrette, (Wyeth) are taken continuously on a daily basis. Pregnancy is possible during their administration, since they are less effective. If one or more pills have been missed and the patients have amenorrhea for more than 45 days, they should be examined for pregnancy.

TESTING METHODS

Receptor Binding Assay

The receptor binding activity of the test compounds is determined by use of the basic methodology developed by Korenman[131] and Layne.[132] An estrogen receptor fraction is obtained from the uteri of immature rats 21 days old. The uteri are homogenized (using a Polytron homogenizer) in 3 volumes of 0.01 M Tris HCl buffer pH 7.4 containing 0.001 M EDTA and 0.25 M sucrose, and 0.5 mM dithiothreitol. The homogenate is then centrifuged at 5000 × g for 15 min to bring down the particulate matter and cell debris; the supernatant is then centrifuged at 100,000 × g for 90 min. The supernatant of the second centrifugation containing the estrogen receptors is used immediately for assay preparation. Assay reaction mixtures are composed of the following:

1.   2000 to 5000 CPM tritiated 17β-estradiol (specific activity 100 mCi/mM).
2.   Sufficient uterine receptor cytosol (high speed supernatant) to produce 50 to 60% binding of the tritiated estradiol.
3.   Aliquot of standard (10^{-6} to 10^{-9} M 17β-estradiol) or unknown (10^{-3} to 10^{-6} M).
4.   Volume is increased to 0.5 mℓ with the Tris buffer (described above) in the presence and absence of excess DES to determine binding specificity.

The reaction mixtures are incubated for 4 hr at room temperature. Separation of receptor, bound and free fractions is accomplished by the addition of 0.5 mℓ of an ice cold activated charcoal suspension (0.25% Norit A and 0.025% dextran in 0.01 M Tris-HCl, pH 7.4). The incubation tubes are shaken at 4°C for 30 min and centrifuged at 500 × g for 10 min at 4°C. The supernatant containing the receptor bound estradiol is counted by liquid scintillation spectrometry. Sample quenching is determined by use of the counter external standard and counting times automatically adjusted to obtain a counting error of less than 1%. A curve for the standard and unknown is plotted as percent of the initial bound ³H-estradiol vs. the concentration of standard or unknown added.

The relative estrogen receptor binding activity of each test compound is calculated as follows:

Concentration of compound which displaced 50% ³H-estradiol ÷
Concentration of estradiol which displaced 50% ³H-estradiol × 100

The relative binding activity of each test compound is expressed as percent estradiol activity.

Estrogenic Assay

The relative estrogenic activity of test compounds can be determined using the uterotropic assay of Dorfman.[133] Immature female Sprague-Dawley rats 21 days old weighing 40 to 50 g are used in the assay system. The animals are randomly distributed into dosage groups which contain six rats per groups. Each assay contains one control group, three standard estradiol dosage groups (0.05, 0.10, and 0.20 μg) and three dosage groups for each compound to be tested (e.g., 5, 10, and 20 μg). Individual dosage groups are maintained in separate stainless steel hanging wire cages with food and water available *ad libitum*.

The assay standard, estradiol-17β and test compounds are prepared in sesame oil. The compounds are administered subcutaneously in a volume of 0.1 mℓ or an equal volume of diluent in the control group, daily on three consecutive days. On the 4th day the animals are sacrificed by cervical dislocation and the uteri dissected through a midline incision. The uteri are drained, blotted, and weighed to the nearest 0.1 mg. The animal body weight at the time of sacrifice is determined to the nearest 0.1 g. The uterotropic response of each group is reported as total uterine weight or uterine weight in mg per body weight in grams.

Antiestrogenic Assay

The anitestrogenic assay involves a slight modification of the estrogenic assay.[134] In this assay system groups of immature (21 days old) rats (6 rats per groups) are injected with both a standard dose of estradiol (0.2 μg) and a dose of test compound. The control groups receive the standard dose of estradiol alone or diluent. Three dosage levels of the compounds are tested in each antiestrogenic assay. The animals are injected daily for three consecutive days and the uterotropic response determined as described above. The antiestrogenic activity will be described as the dose of test compound required to produce a 50% reduction in uterotropic response to the standard dose of estradiol.

Uterine Histological Examination

Histological tissue sections of uteri from control rats or rats treated with the test compounds and estradiol are fixed in 10% formaldehyde, embedded in paraffin, sectioned on a microtome, and stained with hematoxylin-eosin. Slides are examined with a compound light microscope and various measurements of uterine horn cross sections are made microscopically. Measurements, to be made on each cross section at several levels along the uterine horn include: (1) total uterine horn diameter or thickness, at two different points, (2) endometrial thickness at two different points as measured from endometrial-myometrial border to maximum invagination of the endometrium into the lumen of the uterine horn. Photomicrographs of uterine horn cross section and epithelial linings are taken with a camera attached to a compound light microscope.[91]

Antifertility Assay

Adult (8-week-old) Swiss-Webster mice are used in the antifertility assay, which is a modification of the method of Wani et al.[135] The female mice are randomized into dosage groups containing eight mice per group. The test compounds are dissolved in sesame oil and administered by s.c. injection in a total volume of 0.1 mℓ. The control group receives an equal volume of sesame oil.

The female mice are dosed daily for 23 consecutive days. Males of known fertility are caged with the females (one male per four females) from treatment days 8 to 20. During this period, the females are checked for vaginal plugs; body weights are recorded weekly. The females are sacrificed on day 27, and the uterine horns are examined for the number of fetuses and any gross malformation. In addition, the fetal weights are recorded.

Antineoplastic Assay

In this study, 50-day-old female Sprague-Dawley rats receive a single oral dose of 10 mg of 7,12-dimethyl benz(*a*)anthracene dissolved in 1 mℓ of corn oil via a stomach tube. The animals are examined and palpated for tumors at weekly intervals until tumors are detected.

Animals that displayed tumors of 1 to 3 cm in their largest diameter are included. The rats are distributed into experimental groups on the basis of the total tumor volume and number so that each group contains approximately the same mean tumor volume and mean number at the beginning of treatment. Rats in an ovariectomized group have both ovaries removed 1 day prior to treatment.

The test compounds are dissolved in an appropriate solvent at a concentration of 1.2 mg/ mℓ. The treatment group receives 0.6 mg (0.5 mℓ s.c.) three times per week, and the control group receives an equal volume of the solvent. Tumor size is determined twice weekly in all groups using a vernier caliper to measure the major and minor diameters of each tumor. Tumor volume is calculated based on an ellipsoid tumor shape (V $= 4/3\pi r_1^2\, r_2$, where r_1 is the minor tumor radius).[110]

REFERENCES

1. **Knauer, E.,** Die ovarien-transplantation, *Arch. Gynaekol.,* 60, 322, 1900.
2. **Doisy, E. A., Veler, C. D., and Tayer, S. A.,** Folliculin from the urine of pregnant women, *Am. J. Physiol.,* 90, 329, 1929.
3. **Doisy, E. A., Veler, C. D., and Thayer, S. A.,** The preparation of the crystalline ovarian hormone from the urine of pregnant women, *J. Biol. Chem.,* 86, 499, 1930.
4. **White, A., Handler, P., Smith, E. L., Hill, R. L., and Lehman, I. R.,** *Principles of Biochemistry,* 6th ed., McGraw-Hill, New York, 1978, chap. 44.
5. **Murad, F. and Haynes, R. C.,** Estrogens and progestins, in *The Pharmacological Basis of Therapeutics,* 6th ed., Gilman, A. G., Goodman, L. S., and Gilman, A., Eds., MacMillan, 1980, chap. 61.
6. **Dao, T. L.,** Metabolism of estrogens in breast cancer, *Biochim. Biophys. Acta,* 560, 397, 1979.
7. **Paulsen, C. A.,** *Estrogen Assays in Clinical Medicine: Basis and Methodology,* University of Washington Press, Seattle, 1965, 162.
8. **Meldrum, D. R., Davidson, B. J., Tataryn, I. V., and Judd, H. L.,** Changes in circulating steroids with aging in postmenopausal women, *Obstet. Gynecol.,* 57, 624, 1981.
9. **Landau, R. L.,** Endocrine management of malignancies of the prostate, breast, endometrium, kidney, and ovary, in *Endocrinology,* Vol. 3, DeGroot, L. J., et al., Eds., Grune & Stratton, New York, 1979, 2111.
10. **Ziel, H. K. and Finkle, W. D.,** Increased risk of endometrial carcinoma among users of conjugated estrogens, *N. Engl. J. Med.,* 293, 1167, 1975.
11. **Smith, D. C., Prentice, R., Thompson, D. J., and Herrmann, W. L.,** Association of exogenous estrogen and endometrial carcinoma, *N. Engl. J. Med.,* 293, 1164, 1975.
12. **Thomas, D. B.,** Role of exogenous female hormones in altering the risk of benign and malignant neoplasms in humans, *Cancer Res.,* 38, 3991, 1978.
13. **Gasbert, S. B.,** Hormonal dependence of endometrial cancer, *Obstet. Gynecol.,* 30, 287, 1967.
14. **Anon.,** Estrogens and endometrial cancer *F.D.A. Drug Bull.,* 6, 18, 1976.
15. **Herbst, A. L., Ulfelder, H., and Poskanzer, D. C.,** Adenocarcinoma of the vagina: association of maternal stilbestrol therapy with tumor appearance in young women, *N. Engl. J. Med.,* 284, 878, 1971.
16. **Herbst, A. L., Scully, R. E., and Robboy, S. J.,** Prenatal diethylstilbestrol exposure and human genital tract abnormalities, *Natl. Cancer Inst. Monogr.,* 51, 25, 1979.
17. **Shapiro, S. and Slone, D.,** The effects of exogenous female hormones of the fetus, *Epidemiol. Rev.,* 1, 110, 1979.
18. **Bern, H. A., Jones, L. A., Mills, K. T., Kohrman, A., and Mori, T.,** Use of the neonatal mouse in studying longterm effects of early exposure to hormones and other agents, *J. Toxicol. Environ. Health Suppl.,* 1, 103, 1976.
19. **Crane, M. G., Harris, J. J., and Winsor, W.,** Hypertension, oral contraceptive agents and conjugated estrogens, *Ann. Intern. Med.,* 74, 13, 1971.
20. **Lauritzen, C.,** Neue Ergebuisse auf dem Geibiet der Hormonalen Kontrazeptiva, *Med. Welt.,* 26, 486, 1975.
21. **Neugebauer, H.,** Gesamtoestrogene und das Wachstum Junger Madchen, *Padietr. Padol.,* 9, 40, 1974.
22. **Crawford, J. D.,** Excessively tall stature in adolescent girls, in *Current Pediatric Therapy,* Vol. 5, Gellis, S. S. and Kagan, B. M., Eds., W. B. Saunders, Philadelphia, 1971, 311.

23. **Sartwell, P. E., Masi, A. T., and Arthes, F. G.,** Thromboembolism and oral contraceptives: an epidemiological case-control study, *Am. J. Epidemiol.,* 90, 365, 1969.

24. **Baran, J. S.,** A synthesis of 11B-hydroxyestrone and related 16-and 17-hydroxyestratrienes, *J. Med. Chem.,* 10, 1188, 1967.

25. **Schueler, F. W.,** Sex hormonal action and chemical constitution, *Science,* 103, 221, 1946.

26. **Grundy, J.,** Artificial estrogens, *Chem. Rev.,* 57, 305, 1957.

27. **Zielen, F. J. and Bergink, E. W.,** Structure-activity relationships of steroid estrogens, in *Cytotoxic Estrogens in Hormone Receptor Tumors,* Raus, J., Martens, H., and Leclercq, G., Eds., Academic Press, New York, 1980, 39.

28. **Fanchenko, N. D., Sturchak, S. V., Schchedrina, R. N., Pivnitsky, K. K., Novikov, E. A., and Ishkov, V. L.,** The specificity of the human uterine receptor, *Acta Endocrinol.,* 90, 167, 1979.

29. **Dodds, E. C., Goldberg, L., Lawson, W., and Robinson, R.,** Oestrogenic activity of alkylated stilboestrols, *Nature (London),* 142, 34, 1938.

30. **Keasling, H. H. and Schueler, F. W.,** The relationship between estrogenic action and chemical constitution in a group of azomethine derivatives, *J. Am. Pharm. Assoc.,* 39, 87, 1950.

31. **Fullerton, D. S.,** Steroid and therapeutically related compounds, in *Textbook of Organic Medicinal & Pharmaceutical Chemistry,* 7th ed., Wilson, C. O., Gisvold, O., and Doerge, R. F., Eds., J. B. Lippincott, Philadelphia, 1977, chap. 20.

32. **Solmssen, U. V.,** Synthetic estrogens and the relation between their structure and their activity, *Chem. Rev.,* 37, 481, 1945.

33. **Blanchard, E. W., Stuart, A. H., and Tallman, R. C.,** Studies on a new series of synthetic estrogenic substances, *Endocrinology,* 32, 307, 1943.

34. **Baker, B. R.,** Some analogs of hexestrol, *J. Am. Chem. Soc.,* 65, 1572, 1943.

35. **Rubin, M. and Wishinsky, H.,** Functional variants of diethylstilbestrol, *J. Am. Chem. Soc.,* 66, 1948, 1944.

36. **Katzenellenbogen, J. A., Heiman, D. F., Carlson, K. E., Payne, D., and Lloyd, J. E.,** Optimization of the binding selectivity of estrogens, in *Cytotoxic Estrogens in Hormone Receptive Tumors,* Raus, J., Martens, H., and Leclercq, G., Eds., Academic Press, New York, 1980, 3.

37. **MacCorquodale, D. W., Thayer, S. A., and Doisy, E. A.,** The isolation of the principal estrogenic substance of liquor folliculi, *J. Biol. Chem.,* 115, 435, 1936.

38. **Butenandt, A. and Goergens, C.,** Uber and B-oestradiol, *Z. Physiol. Chem.,* 248, 129, 1937.

39. **Inhoffen, H. H. and Zuhlsdorff, G.,** Ubergang von Sterinen in Aromatische Verbindungen, VI. Mitteil'. (Die darstellung des Follikelhormons oestradiol aus cholesterin), Bergakademie, 74, 1911, 1941.

40. **Butenandt, A.,** Uber "Progynon," ein Crystallisiertes, Weibliches Sexual-Hormon, *Naturwissenschaften,* 17, 879, 1929.

41. **Anner, von G. and Miescher, K.,** Die Synthese de Naturlichen oestrons. Total Synthesen in der Oestronreihe III, *Helv. Chim. Acta,* 31, 2173, 1948.

42. **Sih, J. C., Lee, S. S., Tsone, Y. Y., Wang, K. C., and Chang, F. N.,** An efficient synthesis of estrone and 19-norsteroids from cholesterol, *J. Am. Chem. Soc.,* 87, 2765, 1965.

43. **Johnson, W. S., David, I. A., Dehm, H. C., Highet, R. J., Warnhoff, E. W., Wood, W. D., and Jones, E. T.,** Configuration of the estrones. Total synthesis of the remaining stereoisomers, *J. Am. Chem. Soc.,* 80, 661, 1958.

44. **Fieser, L. F. and Fieser, M.,** Synthesis of estrone, in *Steroids,* Rheinhold, New York, 1959, 495.

45. **Windholz, T. B. and Windholz, M.,** Progress in the synthesis of 19-norsteroids, *Angew. Chem. Int. Ed. Engl.,* 3, 353, 1964.

46. **Taub, D.,** Naturally occurring aromatic steroids, in *Total Synthesis of Natural Products,* Vol. 2, ApSimon, J., Ed., John Wiley & Sons, New York, 1973, 670.

47. **Inhoffen, H. H., Logemann, W., Hohlweg, W., and Serini, A.,** Utersuchungen in der Sexualhormon-Reihe, *Bergakademia,* 71, 1024, 1938.

48. **Stuart, A. H., Shukis, A. J., Tallman, R. C., McCann, C., and Trenes, G. R.,** Synthetic estrogenic compounds. III. Trialkyl derivatives of 1,3-di-(p-hydroxyphenyl) propane. Benzestrol, *J. Am. Chem. Soc.,* 68, 729, 1946.

49. **Derkosch, J., Friederich, G.,** Zur frage der cis-trans-isomerie des Diathylstilbostrols und Ahnlicher Verbendungen, *Monatsh.,* 84, 1146, 1953.

50. **Kharasch, M. S. and Kleiman, M.,** Synthesis of polyenes. III. A new synthesis of diethylstilbestrol, *J. Am. Chem. Soc.,* 65, 11, 1943.

51. **Grundy, J.,** Artificial estrogens, *Chem. Rev.,* 57, 281, 1957.

52. **Dodds, E. C., Goldberg, L., Lawson, W., and Robinson, R.,** Synthetic oestrogenic compounds related to stilbene and diphenylethane. I, *Proc. R. Soc. London Ser. B.,* 127, 140, 1939.

53. **Hobday, G. J. and Short, W. F.,** Dienoestrol, *J. Chem. Soc.,* 609, 1943.

54. **Koch, H. P.,** Configuration of synthetic oestrogens, *Nature (London),* 161, 309, 1948.

55. **Lane, J. F. and Spialter, L.,** Studies of the pinacol rearrangement. III. The determination of products resulting from the dehydration of 3,4-bis (p-acetoxyphenyl)-3,4-hexanediol, *J. Am. Chem. Soc.,* 73, 4408, 1951.

56. **Colton, F. B., Nysted, L. N., Riegel, B., and Raymond, A. L.,** 17-alkyl-19-nortestosterones, *J. Am. Chem. Soc.,* 79, 1123, 1957.

57. **Ercoli, A. and Gardi, R.,** Cyclopentyl ethers of oestrogenic steroids, *Chem. Ind. (London),* 1037, 1961.

58. **Chan, L. and O'Malley, B. W.,** Mechanism of action of sex steroid hormones, *N. Engl. J. Med.,* 294, 1322, 1976.

59. **Fotherby, K. and James, F.,** Metabolism of synthetic steroids, *Adv. Steroid Biochem. Pharmacol.,* 3, 67, 1972.

60. **Colton, F. B.,** U.S. Patents 2,691,028 (1954) and 2,725,389 (1955).

61. **Djerassi, C., Miramontes, L., Rosenkrantz, G., and Sondheimer, F.,** Steroids. LIV. Synthesis of 19-nor-17α-ethynyltestosterone and 19-nor-17α-methyltestosterone, *J. Am. Chem. Soc.,* 76, 4092, 1954.

62. **Salhanick, H. A., Holmstrom, E. G., and Zarrow, M. X.,** Biological activity of 17α-hydroxyprogesterone in the mouse, rabbit and human being, *J. Clin. Endocrinol. Metabl.,* 17, 667, 1957.

63. **Davis, M. E. and Wied, G. L.,** 17-Alpha-hydroxyprogesterone-caproate: a new substance with prolonged progestational activity. A comparison with chemically pure progesterone, *J. Clin. Endocrinol. Metab.,* 15, 923, 1955.

64. **Siegel, I.,** Conception control by long-acting progestogens: preliminary report, *Obstet. Gynecol.,* 21, 666, 1963.

65. **Westerhof, P. and Reerink, E. H.,** Investigations on sterols. XV. The synthesis and properties of 9β, 10α-protesterone and 6-dehydro-9β, 10α-progesterone, *Rec. Trav. Chim.,* 79, 771, 1960.

66. **Rappoldt, M. P. and Westerhof, P.,** Investigations on sterols. XIX. 6-dehydro-9β, 10α-progesterone from pregnenolones, *Rec. Trav. Chim.,* 80, 43, 1961.

67. **Klimstra, P. D. and Colton, F. B.,** The synthesis of 3β-hydroxyestra-4-en-17-one and 3β-hydroxyandrost-4-en-17-one, *Steroids,* 10, 411, 1967.

68. **Elton, R. L., Nutting, E. F., and Saunders, F. J.,** Effects or reduction of the 3-ketone of 17α-ethynyl-19-nortestosterone on its endocrine properties, *Acta Endocrinol.,* 41, 381, 1962.

69. **Elton, R. L., Klimstra, P. D., and Colton, F. B.,** Induction of deciduoma in rabbits without uterine trauma by treatment with ethynodiol diacetate: a synthetic progestogen, *Proc. Soc. Exp. Biol. Med.,* 121, 1194, 1966.

70. **Babcock, J. C., Gutsell, F. S., Herr, M. E., Hogg, J. A., Stucki, J. C., Barres, L. E., and Dulin, W. E.,** 6α-Methyl-17α-hydroxyprogesterone 17-acylates; a new class of potent progestins, *J. Am. Chem. Soc.,* 80, 2904, 1958.

71. **Ringold, H. J., Ruelas, J. P., Batres, E., and Djerassi, C.,** Steroids. CXVIII. 6-Methyl derivatives of 17α-hydroxyprogesterone and of Reichstein's substance "S", *J. Am. Chem. Soc.,* 81, 3712, 1959.

72. **Liisberg, S., Godtfredsen, O., and Vangedal, S.,** Reaction of polyhalomethanes with enolethers of Δ⁴-3-ketosteroids (a new pathway to 6α-methyl-steroids), *Tetrahedron,* 9, 149, 1960.

73. **Smith, H., Hughes, G. A., Douglas, G. H., Hartley, D., McLoughlin, B. J., Siddell, J. B., Wendt, G. R., Buzby, Jr., G. C., Heobsh, D. R., Ledig, K. W., McMenamin, J. R,, Pattison, T. W., Suida, J., Tokolici, J., Edgren, R. A., Jausen, A. B. A., Godsby, B., Watson, D. H. R., and Phillips, P. C.,** Totally synthetic (±)-13-alkyl-3-hydroxy and methoxy-gona-1,3,5(10)-trien-17-ones and related compounds, *Experientia,* 19, 394, 1963.

74. **Smith, H., Hughes, G. A., Douglas, G. H., Wendt, G. R., Buzby, G. C., Edgren, R. A., Fisher, J., Foell, T., Gadsby, B., Hartley, D., Herbst, D., Jansen, A. B. A., Ledig, J. K., McLoughlin, B. J., McMenamin, J., Pattison, T. W., Phillips, P. C., Rees, R., Siddal, J., Sueda, J., Smith, L. L., Takolics, J., and Watson, D. H. P.,** Totally synthetic steroid hormones. II. 13β-alkylgona-1,3,5(10)-trienes, 13β-alkylgon-4-en-3-ones, and related compounds, *J. Chem. Soc.,* 4472, 1964.

75. **Butenandt, A. and Westphal, U.,** Zur Isolierung und Charakterisierung des Corpus-Luteum-Hormons, *Bergakademie,* 67, 1440, 1934.

76. **Wintersteiner, O. and Allen, W. M.,** Crystalline progestin, *J. Biol. Chem.,* 107, 321, 1934.

77. **Butenandt, A., Westphal, U., and Cobler, H.,** Uber einen abbau des Stigmasterins zu Corpus-Luteum-Wichsamen Stoffen; ein beitrag zur Konstitution des Corpus-Theeum-Hormons, *Bergakademie,* 67, 1611, 1934.

78. **Johnson, W. S., Gravestock, M. B., and McCarry, B. E.,** Acetylenic bond participation in biogenetic-like olefinic cyclization. II. Synthesis of dl-progesterone, *J. Am. Chem. Soc.,* 93, 4332, 1971.

79. **Strain, W. H.,** The steroids, in *Gilman's Organic Chemistry,* Vol. 2, 2nd ed., John Wiley & Sons, New York, 1943, 1487.

80. **Chang, C. C. and Kincl, F.A.,** Sustained release of hormonal preparations. III. Biological effectiveness of 6-methyl-17α-acetoxy-pregna-4,6-diene-3,20-dione, *Steroids,* 12, 689, 1968.

81. **Cooper, J. M. and Kellie, A. E.,** The metabolism of megestrol acetate (17α-acetoxy-6-methylpregna-4,6-diene-3,20-dione) in women, *Steroids,* 11, 133, 1968.

82. **Segal, S. J. and Thompson, C. R.,** Inhibition of estradiol-induced pituitary hypertrophy in rats, *Proc. Soc. Exp. Biol. Med.,* 91, 623, 1956.

83. **Korenman, S. G.,** Relation between oestrogen inhibiting activity and binding to cytosol of rabbit and human uterus, *Endocrinology,* 87, 1119, 1970.

84. **Skidmore, J. R., Walpole, A. L., and Woodburn, J.,** Effect of some triphenylethylenes on oestradiol binding *in vitro* to macromolecules from uterus and anterior pituitary, *J. Endocrinol.,* 52, 289, 1972.

85. **Jordan, V. C., Dix, C. J., Naylor, K. E., Prestwich, G., and Rowsby, L.,** Nonsteroidal antiestrogens: their biological effects and potential mechanisms of action, *J. Toxicol. Environ. Health,* 4, 363, 1978.

86. **Jordan, V. C., Collins, M. M., Rowsby, L., and Prestwich, G.,** A monohydroxylated metabolilte of tamoxifen with potent antioestrogenic activity, *J. Endocrinol.,* 75, 305, 1977.

87. **Clark, J. H., Peck, E. J., Hardin, J. W., and Eriksson, H.,** The biology and pharmacology of estrogen receptor binding: relationship to uterine growth, in *Receptors and Hormone Action,* Vol. 2, O'Malley, B. W. and Birnbaumer, L., Eds., Academic Press, New York, 1978, chap. 1.

88. **Clark, J. H., Peck, E. J., and Anderson, J. N.,** Oestrogen receptor antioestrogen complex-atypical binding by uterine nuclei and effects on uterine growth, *Steroids,* 22, 707, 1973.

89. **Capony, F. and Rochefort, H.,** *In vitro* effect of anti-oestrogens on localization and replenishment of oestrogen receptors, *Mol. Cell Endocrinol.,* 3, 233, 1975.

90. **Boccardo, F., Bruzzi, P., Rubagotti, A., Nicolo, G., and Rosso, R.,** Estrogen-like action of tamoxifen on vaginal epithelium in breast cancer patients, *Oncology,* 38, 281, 1981.

91. **Pento, J. T., Magarian, R. A., Wright, R. J., King, M. M., and Benjamin, E. J.,** Nonsteroidal estrogens and antiestrogens: biological activity of a series of analogs of stilbene and stilbenediol, *J. Pharm. Sci.,* 70, 399, 1981.

92. **Black, L. J. and Goode, R. L.,** Uterine bioassay of tamoxifen, trioxifene and a new estrogen antagonist (LY 117018) in rats and mice, *Life Sci.,* 26, 1453, 1980.

93. **Pento, J. T., Magarian, R. A., and King, M. M.,** A comparison of the efficacy for antitumor activity of the nonsteroidal antiestrogens analog II and tamoxifen in DMBA-induced rat mammary tumors, *Cancer Lett.,* 15, 261, 1982.

94. **Borgna, J. L. and Rochefort, H.,** Hydroxylated metabolites of tamoxifen are formed *in vivo* and bound to estrogen receptors in target tissues, *J. Biol. Chem.,* 256, 859, 1981.

95. **Palopoli, F. P., Feil, V. J., Allen, R. E., Holtkamp, D. E., and Richardons, A.,** Substituted aminoalkoxy-triaryl haloethylenes, *J. Med. Chem.,* 10, 84, 1967.

96. **Harger, M. T. K. and Walpole, A. L.,** Contrasting endocrine activities of cis and trans isomers in a series of substituted triphenylethylenes, *Nature (London),* 212, 87, 1966.

97. **Holtkamp, D. E., Greslin, J. G., Root, C. A., and Lerner, L. J.,** Gonadotrophin and anti-fertility effects of chloramiphene, *Proc. Soc. Exp. Biol. Med.,* 105, 197, 1960.

98. **Van Maanen, E. F., Greslin, J. G., Holtkamp, D. E., and King, W. M.,** Endocrine and other biological effects of chloramiphene, *Fed. Proc. Fed. Am. Soc. Exp. Biol.,* 20, 419, 1961.

99. **Greenblat, R. B., Barfield, W. E., Jungck, E. C., and Ray, A. W.,** Induction of ovulation with MRL 41, *JAMA,* 178, 101, 1961.

100. **Duncan, G. W., Lyster, S. C., Clark, J. J., and Lednicer, D.,** Antifertility activity of two diphenyl-dihydronaphthalene derivatives, *Proc. Soc. Exp. Biol. Med.,* 112, 439, 1963.

101. **Lednicer, D., Lystel, S. C., and Duncan, G. W.,** Mammalian anti-fertility agents. IV. Basic 3,4-dihydrophthalenes and 1,2,3,4,-tetrahydrol-1-naphthols, *J. Med. Chem.,* 10, 78, 1967.

102. **Callantine, M. R., Humphrey, R. R., Lee, S. L., Windsor, B. L., Schattin, N. H., and O'Brien, O. P.,** Action of an oestrogen antagonist on reproductive mechanism in the rat, *Endocrinology,* 79, 153, 1966.

103. **Dipietro, S. L., Sanders, F. J., and Goss, D. A.,** Effect of cis and trans isomers of clomiphene citrate on uterine hexokinase activity, *Endocrinology,* 84, 1404, 1969.

104. **Harper M. J. K. and Walpole, A. L.,** A new derivative of triphenylethylene: effect on implantation and of action in rats, *J. Reprod. Fertil.,* 13, 101, 1967.

105. **Harper, M, J. K. and Walpole, A. L.,** Mode of action of ICI 46,474 in preventing implantation in rats, *J. Endocrinol.,* 37, 83, 1967.

106. **Jordan, V. C.,** Antitumor activity of the Anti-oestrogen ICI 46,474 (tamoxifen) in dimethylbenzanthracene (DMBA) induced rat mammary carcinoma model, *J. Steroid Biochem.,* 5, 354, 1974.

107. **Jordan, V. C.,** Effect of tamoxifen (ICI 46,474) on inhibition and growth of DMBA-induced rat mammary carcinoma, *Eur. J. Cancer,* 12, 419, 1976.

108. **Terenius, L.,** Anti-oestrogens and breast cancer, *Eur. J. Cancer,* 7, 57, 1971.

109. **Schultz, K. D., Haselmayer, B., and Holzel, F.,** The influence of clomid and its isomers on dimethyl-benzanthracene-induced rat mammary tumours, in *Basic Action of Sex Steroids on Target Organs,* Hubinont, P. O., Ed., Phiebig, White Plains, N.Y., 1971, 274.

110. **DeSombre, E. R. and Arbogast, L. Y.,** Effect of anti-oestrogen CI 628 on the growth of rat mammary tumors, *Cancer Res.,* 34, 1971, 1974.

111. **Nicholson, R. I. and Golder, M. P.,** Effect of synthetic anti-oestrogen on the growth and biochemistry of rat mammary tumours, *Eur. J. Cancer,* 2, 571, 1975.

112. **Heuson, J. C., Coune, A., and Stoquet, M.,** Clinical trial of nafoxidine, an oestrogen antagonist in advanced breast cancer, *Eur. J. Cancer,* 8, 387, 1972.

113. **Herbst, A. L., Griffiths, C. T., and Kistner, R. W.,** Clomiphene citrate (NSC-35770) in disseminated mammary carcinoma, *Cancer Chemother. Rep.,* 43, 39, 1964.

114. **Cole, M. P., Jones, C. T. A., and Todd, I. D. H.,** A new anti-oestrogenic agent in late breast cancer, *Br. J. Cancer,* 25, 270, 1971.

115. **Ward, H. W. C.,** Anti-oestrogen therapy for breast cancer: a trial of tamoxifen at two dose levels, *Br. Med. J.,* 1, 13, 1973.

116. **Lednicer, D., Lystel, S. C., and Duncan, G. W.,** Mammalian anti-fertility agents. IV. Basic 3,4-dihydronaphthalene and 1,2,3,4-tetrahydrol-1-naphthols, *J. Med. Chem.,* 10, 78, 1967.

117. **Abbott, A. C., Clark, E. R., and Jordan, V. C.,** Inhibition of oestradiol binding to oestrogen receptor proteins by a methyl substituted analogue of tamoxifen, *J. Endocrinol.,* 69, 445, 1976.

118. **Ernst, S., Hite, G., Cantrell, J. S. and Richardson, Jr., A.,** Stereochemistry of geometric isomers of clomiphene: a correction of the literature and a reexamination of structure-activity relationships, *J. Pharm. Sci.,* 65, 148, 1976.

119. **Bedford, G. R. and Richardson, D. N.,** Preparation and identification of cis and trans isomers of a substituted triarylethylene, *Nature (London),* 212, 733, 1966.

120. **Terenius, L.,** Two modes of interaction between oestrogen and anti-estrogen, *Acta Endocrinol. (Copenhagen),* 64, 47, 1970.

121. **Rock, J., Garcia, C. M., and Pincus, G.,** Synthetic progestins in the normal human menstrual cycle, *Rec. Progr. Hormone Res.,* 13, 323, 1957.

122. **Pincus, G.,** *The Control of Fertility,* Academic Press, New York, 1965, 217.

123. **Goldzieher, J. W., Dozier, T. S., and de la Pena, A.,** Plasma levels and pharmacokinetics of ethynyl estrogens in various populations. I. Ethynyl estradiol, *Contraception,* 21, 1, 1980.

124. **Goldzieher, J. W., Dozier, T. S., and de la Pena, A.,** Plasma levels and pharmacokinetics of ethynyl estrogens in various populations. II. Mestranol, *Contraception,* 21, 17, 1980.

125. **Siekmann, L., Siekmann, A., and Brewer, H.,** Measurement by isotope dilution mass spectrometry of 17α-ethynyloestradiol-17β and norethisterone in serum of women taking oral contraceptives, *Biomed. Mass Spectrom.,* 7, 511, 1980.

126. **Kappus, H., Bolt, H. M., and Remmer, H.,** Affinity of ethynylestradiol and mestranol for the uterine estrogen receptor and for the microsomal mixed function oxidase of the liver, *J. Steroid. Biochem.,* 4, 121, 1973.

127. **Forchielli, E.,** Metabolism of norethindrone in the human, in *Norethindrone: The First Three Decades,* Pramik. M. J., Ed., Syntex Laboratories, Palo Alto, 1978, chap. 4.

128. **Warren, R. T. and Fotherhy, K.,** Radioimmunoassay of synthetic progestogens, norethisterone and norgestrel, *J. Endocrinol.,* 62, 605, 1974.

129. **Mahesh, V. B., Mills, T. M., Lin, T. J., Ellegood, J. D., and Braselton, W. E.,** Metabolism, metabolic clearance rate, blood metabolites and blood half-life of norethindrone and mestranol, in *Pharmacology of Steroid Contracepline Drugs,* Garatlini, B., Ed., Raven Press, New York, 1977.

130. **Gerhards, E., Hecher, W., Hitze, H., Nieweboer, B., and Bellman, O.,** The metabolism of norethindrone and norgestrel in man (alkyl-substituted steroid VIII), *Acta Endocrinol.,* 68, 219, 1971.

131. **Korenman, S. G.,** Radio-ligand binding assay of specific estrogens using a soluble uterine macromolecule, *J. Clin. Endocrinol. Metab.,* 28, 127, 1968.

132. **Layne, E.,** Spectrophotometric and turbidimetric methods for measuring proteins, *Meth. Enzymol.,* 3, 447, 1957.

133. **Emmens, C. W, II,** Steroid hormones and related substances. Estrogens, in *Methods in Hormone Research,* Vol. 2A, Dorfman, R. I., Ed., Academic Press, New York, 1969, 69.

134. **Dorfman, R. I., Kimel, F. A., and Ringold, H. J.,** Anti-estrogen assay of natural steroids administered by subcutaneous injection, *Endocrinology,* 68, 17, 1961.

135. **Wani, M. C., Rector, D. H., Christensen, H. D., Kimel, G. L., and Cook, C. D.,** Flavinoids. VIII. Synthesis and antifertility and estrogen receptor binding activities on coumarins and delta 3-isoflavenes, *J. Med. Chem.,* 18, 982, 1975.

THYROID AND ANTITHYROID DRUGS

D. Ellis, J. C. Emmett, P. D. Leeson, and A. H. Underwood

INTRODUCTION

The thyroid was first recognized as an endocrine organ towards the end of the 19th century when it was shown that the symptoms of surgical thyroidectomy and the naturally occurring disease, myxoedema, were not only very similar but could also be alleviated by treatment with extracts of the gland. Shortly afterwards it was established that thyroidal extracts enhanced nitrogen excretion and basal metabolic rate, actions which provided assay procedures to facilitate the chemical characterization of the active principle.[1] Baumann[2] (1896) was the first to recognize that the thyroid contained iodine and he obtained from thyroidal extracts a product, iodothyronin. This contained up to 10% of iodine, and mimicked the activity of whole thyroid. Later Kendall[3] isolated a fraction containing 65% of iodine which he called thyroxin and suggested it had the structure 4,5,6-trihydro-4,5,6-triiodo-2-oxy-β-indole propionic acid. Subsequently Harington[1] showed that this was incorrect and that the true structure of thyroxine was 3,5,3′,5′-tetraiodo-L-thyronine (T_4, Figure 1). Although it could mimic the effects of thyroidal extract the glandular content of thyroxine was recognized to be insufficient to account for all of its activity. Harington himself thought that this was because thyroxine was merely part of a larger, more active molecule, possibly a peptide, but Gross and Pitt-Rivers were to show much later that the thyroid, in fact, contained another more potent thyromimetic 3,5,3′-triiodo-L-thyronine (T_3, Figure 1).[4] It is now recognized that the effects of the thyroid are mediated by both of these hormones.

Recent work has concentrated on the synthesis of the hormones within the gland and the mechanism by which they exert their characteristic physiological effects. The most generally accepted theory rests on two key observations: that thyroid hormones, after a latent period, promote an increase in protein synthesis preceded by an increase in RNA synthesis;[5] and that the nuclei of cells sensitive to thyroid hormones contain a chromatin-bound protein which binds thyromimetics with affinities proportional to their thyromimetic potencies.[6] It is thought that the occupation of these receptor proteins by thyromimetics promotes the synthesis of new species of mRNA which in turn code for a new population of proteins within the cell. It is the appearance of these new proteins which causes the characteristic physiological effects of thyroid hormones.

Despite the recent advances in understanding the mechanism of action of thyroid hormones no truly novel drugs have emerged for the treatment of diseases of the thyroid since the introduction of the thionamide drugs some 30 years ago. Recent work has shown that these drugs act by a variety of mechanisms including their inhibition of thyroid-autoantibody production in Graves' disease. Other drugs such as β-blockers and deiodinase inhibitors are now also being used to reduce the peripheral effects of thyroid hormones in the absence of competive receptor antagonists and we have referred to these studies in this review.

FORMATION, DISTRIBUTION, AND METABOLISM OF THYROID HORMONES

The thyroid in humans is a highly vascular organ with two lobes which are found on either side of the trachea. The functional units responsible for the manufacture of thyroid hormones are the follicles or acini which are spherical structures consisting of a central lumen surrounded by an epithelium of follicular cells. The apical surface of these cells is covered with microvilli which project into the lumen; the opposite, basal surface is separated

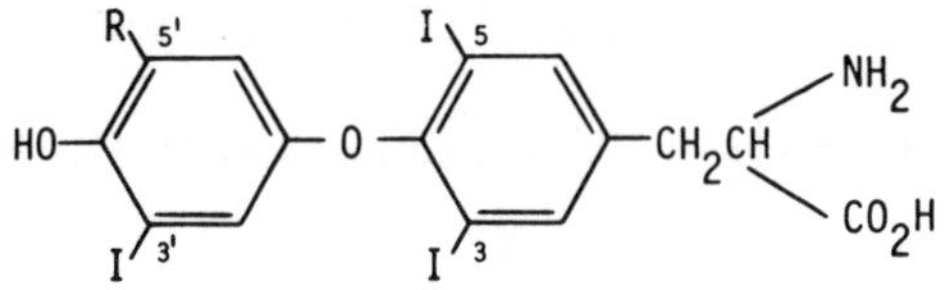

FIGURE 1.   Structures of thyroxine, 3,3′,5,5′-tetraio-
dothyronine (T_4, R = I) and 3,3′5-triiodothyronine (T_3,
R = H).

from the interfollicular space by a basement membrane. In addition to these acini the thyroid contains parafollicular cells whose function is to synthesize and secrete thyrocalcitonin.[7]

Biosynthesis of Thyroid Hormones

Thyroid hormones are synthesized via a glycoprotein precursor molecule, thyroglobulin. This is manufactured within the follicular cells, prior to iodination and coupling of some of the tyrosyl residues to give an iodinated thyroglobulin containing both T_4 and T_3 as constituent, amino-acyl residues. The thyroglobulin is then stored within the lumen of the acini. Release of thyroid hormones from this stored colloid is achieved by proteolytic degradation to its constituent amino acids within the follicular cells.

From the above brief outline it is obvious that thyroglobulin plays a central role in the function of the thyroid; and in fact accounts for 75% of the protein content of the normal gland.[8] Thyroglobulin is a large glycoprotein with a mol wt of 660,000[8] containing at least four peptide chains.[9] Under denaturing conditions the molecule can be dissociated into two subunits (mol wt 330,000).[10] About 10% of the mass of thyroglobulin is carbohydrate.[11] There are about 250 mol of half cystine per mole of thyroglobulin; about 200 of these exist in the form of disulfide bonds in the native protein.[9] The tyrosine content at 3% (140 residues per mole of protein) is not especially high.[8] The degree of iodination of thyroglobulin is variable, depending on such factors as the activity of the gland and the iodine content of the diet, but under normal conditions 10 to 25 tyrosine residues per molecule are iodinated.[12]

The metabolism of the thyroid gland is most conveniently discussed in terms of the synthesis of noniodinated thyroglobulin, the metabolism of iodine, the coupling of iodotyrosyl residues, and the proteolysis of thyroglobulin.

Synthesis of Noniodinated Thyroglobulin

An mRNA species, which codes for a protein with an approximate mol wt of 300,000, has been isolated from bovine thyroid. This protein is chemically and immunologically related to thyroglobulin and probably corresponds to the half thyroglobulin formed by mild denaturing conditions.[13] The implication of these observations is that thyroglobulin is a dimer of the primary transcription product.

After synthesis, the nascent thyroglobulin molecule is transferred to the cisternae of the endoplasmic reticulum and then to the Golgi apparatus where it is sequestered in exocytotic vesicles and finally expelled into the follicular lumen.[14] Glycosylation is also thought to occur during this series of events.[8]

Thyroidal Iodide Metabolism

The thyroid has a remarkable capacity to accumulate iodide from plasma by active transport. In rats in which organification of iodide has been blocked with propylthiouracil (PTU) the ratio of thyroidal to serum iodide is about 100. However, the great majority of the free iodide within the gland is derived from deiodination of iodotyrosine and iodothyronine molecules released by proteolysis of thyroglobulin. This "second pool" of iodide is kinetically, and perhaps functionally, distinct from that of the plasma.[15]

The transport of iodide into the thyroid is blocked by a number of inorganic ions such as perchlorate or thiocyanate. This property is the basis of their use in the treatment of hyperthyroidism (see below).[16]

Iodination and Coupling

The iodination of thyroglobulin, at the apical border of the lumen, is catalyzed by a specific thyroid peroxidase, which requires hydrogen peroxide as a cosubstrate. The enzyme is synthesized with thyroglobulin in the follicular cell and transported to the lumen in the same exocytotic vesicles.[17] Iodination does not take place randomly: the reactivity of each tyrosyl residue (presumably determined by its microenvironment within the protein molecule) is such that iodination occurs in a rigid sequential order.[18]

The formation of iodothyronines occurs when an iodophenol moiety is transferred from one iodotyrosine to another leaving behind a dehydroalanine residue.[19] This coupling is also catalyzed by thyroid peroxidase in the presence of hydrogen peroxide, although a different enzyme-H_2O_2 species, from that catalyzing iodination, is involved.[20]

The proportion of the various iodotyrosines and iodothyronines depends upon the iodine content of the thyroglobulin: the higher this is, the greater is the proportion of 3,5-diiodo-L-tyrosine (DIT) and T_4 relative to 3-iodo-L-tyrosine (MIT) and T_3. Even when the total iodine content is 70 mol/mol thyroglobulin, the T_4 content does not exceed 3 mol/mol thyroglobulin.[21] This apparent inefficiency emphasizes the importance of thyroglobulin as a store of iodine, as well as a precursor of T_4.

Release of Thyroid Hormones

Thyroglobulin is taken up into the follicular cells by endocytosis. These endocytotic vacuoles then fuse with lysosomes which contain the enzymes necessary for proteolytic degradation. This latter process is thought to be preceded by the reduction of some of the many intramolecular disulfide bridges of thyroglobulin. Hydrolysis to the component amino acids is then accomplished by a protease with an acidic pH optimum.[22]

The iodotyrosines released are completely and rapidly deiodinated by a specific enzyme: the iodide so released forms the so-called "second pool" and is reutilized. The iodothyronines are also deiodinated to a lesser extent by a second enzyme which is more active towards T_4 than T_3. A consequence of this is that the ratio of T_3:T_4 secreted by the gland is higher than would be expected from the composition of thyroglobulin.[23] In addition to T_4 and T_3 some immunologically reactive thyroglobulin is released from the normal, human gland. Its function, if any, is unknown.[24]

Control of Thyroid Function

The thyroid is stimulated to release T_4 and T_3 by the pituitary hormone, thyrotropin (thyroid-stimulating hormone — TSH). The secretion of TSH is, in turn, inhibited by thyroid hormones. These two elements constitute a negative feedback system which maintains a constant circulating level of thyroid hormones. Various other factors are able to modify this basic mechanism including the autonomic nervous system and biogenic amines from thyroidal mast cells.[25]

The principal controlling agent, however, is TSH, which rapidly (within minutes) stimulates the secretion of T_4 and T_3 by increasing colloid resorption and hydrolysis. TSH is thought to exert these effects on the thyroid by binding to a specific receptor on the plasma membrane. Activation of this receptor causes an increase in calcium uptake and adenylate cyclase activity. The consequent increase in intracellular cAMP promotes the phosphorylation of key enzymes or proteins resulting in stimulation of thyroidal function in a manner which is as yet obscure.[26]

TSH secretion is modified by two hypothalamic hormones; somatostatin, which is inhibitory, and thyrotropin releasing hormone (TRH), which rapidly stimulates secretion, and subsequently synthesis, of TSH by a cAMP-dependent mechanism.[27] TRH appears to maintain a tonic stimulation of the pituitary thyrotrophs. This can be modified by various factors, such as the ambient temperature and by circulating thyroid hormone levels.[27] The principal factors controlling TSH levels are the concentrations of thyroid hormones in plasma. Thyroid hormones administered acutely or chronically diminish plasma TSH levels. Long term treatment leads to total depletion of pituitary TSH presumably due to a reduction in TSH mRNA. The mechanism of the acute reduction of plasma TSH by thyroid hormones is not yet fully understood although it may be a result of an inhibition of the stimulation of TSH release by TRH. This effect apparently involves protein synthesis since it is blocked by inhibitors of protein and polynucleotide synthesis.[28]

Transport and Peripheral Distribution of Thyroid Hormones

In normal euthyroid, human blood the total concentration of T_4 is 50 to 100 times greater than that of T_3. The vast majority of both hormones is reversibly bound to plasma proteins: only 0.03% of T_4 and 0.3% of T_3 exist in the free (unbound) state. In human blood three proteins are responsible for thyroid binding; thyroxine-binding globulin (TBG), thyroxine-binding prealbumin (TBPA), and serum albumin (SA). All three proteins bind both T_3 and T_4 but the affinity for T_3 is 10 to 100 times less than for T_4. The affinity of TBG for T_4 and T_3 is greater than that of TBPA which in turn has a higher affinity than albumin. The concentrations of these proteins, however, are in the reverse order to their affinities. As a consequence, in normal human plasma, about half of the T_3 and about 67% of the T_4 are bound to TBG and 1% of T_3 and 20% of T_4 are bound to TBPA. The majority of the remaining hormones is bound to albumin.[29] This pattern of plasma binding proteins does not occur in all species. The rat for instance has a low level of TBG and TBPA is the principal carrier of thyroxine.[30]

The properties of this complex system are such that an increase in total T_4 causes a proportionately greater increase in free T_4, while free T_3 is directly related to total T_3. Free T_4 is not affected by variations in total T_3 but free T_3 is a nonlinear function of total T_4. It is clear, however, that in all species the plasma thyroid hormone binding proteins act not as a buffer for the free hormones but as a reservoir. The rate of dissociation from the binding proteins is so rapid that it does not constitute a rate-limiting step in the pharmacokinetics of thyroid hormones.[29]

Despite the fact that only a minute fraction of the hormones is free it is clear that this is the physiologically significant portion. Thyroid status is related to the free level of these hormones and not the total level. It is the unbound fraction which is transported into the cells, where its action is manifested.[29] Experiments in rats have shown that some organs (e.g., liver and kidney) have a higher concentration of thyroid hormones than does the plasma.[31,32] It has also been shown, in rats at least, that the ratio of T_3 to T_4 in various organs is much greater than that in the plasma.[31]

A number of factors can alter the concentration of thyroid hormones in the blood, not by modifying their synthesis or metabolism, but by altering the degree of plasma binding. Some agents, such as salicylate, can compete with thyroid hormones for the relevant binding site on the binding protein.[33] In other cases the absolute level of a binding protein can be changed. For instance estradiol is known to increase the level of TBG.[34] In these various cases thyroid status is not altered, presumably because the free level of the hormone remains constant.

Metabolism and Excretion of Thyroid Hormones

The principal route of metabolism in both rat and humans, accounting for 70 to 90% of T_4, is by deiodination from either the tyrosyl or phenolic ring, to give, in the first instance, 3,3′,5′-L-thyronine (reverse T_3-rT_3) or T_3, respectively. It has been estimated that 38% of

T_4 is converted to T_3 and that this represents about 90% of the total amount of T_3 formed. Almost all circulating rT_3 also arises from T_4. T_3 and rT_3 may be further deiodinated, first to the various, isomeric diiodothyronines (T_2), then to monoiodothyronines (T_1), and finally to thyronine itself. The halflife of rT_3 is less than that of T_3 which in turn is shorter than that for T_4. This accounts partly for the differences in plasma concentrations of these iodothyronines. The circulating levels of T_2 and T_1 are very low because they are very rapidly metabolized.[35]

The number of different rat tissue enzymes capable of deiodinating iodothyronines is currently uncertain. Two types of deiodinase activities which remove phenolic ring iodine atoms (5'-deiodinases) have been defined operationally and there is some evidence to suggest that an inner ring deiodinase enzyme can exist independently of 5'-deiodinating activity in some tissues but possibly not in the liver.[36a,b]

Type I 5'-deiodinase (5'-DI), characterized mainly from rat liver and kidney, prefers rT_3 to T_4 as substrate, requires a sulfhydryl containing cofactor (e.g., glutathione, mercaptoethanol, or dithiothreitol), and is inhibited noncompetitively by PTU. 5'-DI exhibits ping-pong type reaction kinetics, consistent with the requirement for the two substrates, iodothyronine and thiol cofactor, and suggesting that at least two forms of the enzyme are likely to be in equilibrium. It has been proposed that in the first stage, the enzyme interacts with T_4 (or rT_3) leading to T_3 (or $3,3'$-T_2) production and an enzyme sulfenyl-iodide (E-SI) intermediate. In the second stage, the E-SI complex would be reduced by the thiol cofactor to regenerate the enzyme (E-SH) and iodide, or react with PTU to produce an inactive (dead-end) complex.[37b,c] The participation of an enzyme SH group is supported by the observation that pretreatment with thiol reagents such as N-ethylmaleimide and iodoacetate results in irreversible loss of catalytic activity,[37a,d] and T_4 and rT_3 protect against inhibition by iodoacetate.[37d]

Type II 5'-deiodinase (5'-DII) also requires a thiol cofactor, is PTU insensitive, accepts rT_3 and T_4 as equally good substrates, has apparent K_m's and K_i's for rT_3 and T_4 in the 0.5 to 5 nm range (considerably lower than those in type I reactions), and exhibits sequential type reaction kinetics.[36b,38a-e] A mechanism has not been clearly proposed, but the kinetic pattern suggests that both the iodothyronine and the thiol combine with the enzyme before reaction takes place.[38e] To date, type II 5'-deiodinating activity has been identified only in rat brain, pituitary, and brown adipose tissue. These organs also have some type I activity, which is mainly found in liver and kidney.[36b]

The plasma concentrations of T_3 and rT_3 are affected by physiological status. Thus, in starvation and systemic illness the level of T_3 diminishes and that of rT_3 increases, while T_4 is unaltered. This situation occurs mainly because 5'-deiodination is diminished with a consequent reduction in T_3 generation and rT_3 degradation.[36a]

Since T_3 is more active as a thyromimetic than T_4, while rT_3 has essentially no activity, the concentration of T_4 to T_3 represents a metabolic activation, and the production of rT_3, an inactivating step. Teleologically it makes sense for an animal with a restricted food intake, or indeed a sick human, to diminish metabolism by diverting some T_4 to the inactive rT_3, rather than to T_3. Interestingly, the circulating level of TSH is not altered by starvation suggesting that plasma T_3 is not as important in the feedback control of thyroid function as is T_4.[28] This is because the local generation of T_3 from T_4 within the pituitary is more important in controlling TSH secretion than is circulating T_3, which is principally derived from the liver and kidney.[29,36a] Furthermore, the reduction in 5'-deiodination in the liver caused by starvation does not alter pituitary 5'-deiodination perhaps because different enzymes are involved.

In addition to deiodination, the various iodothyronines undergo a number of other metabolic transformations. Both glucuronide and sulfate conjugation of the phenolic hydroxyl occur. The liver is the principal site of glucuronidation and the great majority of the glucuronides is excreted via the bile, although some appear in the urine. Sulfo-conjugates are produced mainly by the kidney and are eliminated in both bile and urine. The alanine side chain is also subject to degradation. Deamination leads to pyruvic, lactic, and acetic acid derivatives and it is also possible that a small amount of decarboxylation to thyronamine derivatives take place. The quantitative importance of these reactions is not known.[29]

THE EFFECTS AND MECHANISM OF ACTION OF THYROID HORMONES

Although the thyroid is not essential for life, its hormones profoundly affect the physiology and biochemistry of most of the organs of the body. In the adult mammal the principal effect of thyroid hormones is to enhance metabolism. This is normally measured as an increase in whole body oxygen consumption (the thermogenic effect) but the metabolism of most substrates (e.g., carbohydrate and lipid) is also modified. Accompanying this effect on metabolism are other alterations in the physiology of the animal, notably in its cardiovascular system. In the fetal or immature mammal these hormones also stimulate growth and differentiation. The induction of metamorphosis in amphibians may represent a special aspect of the latter effect.

One of the most singular aspects of thyroid hormones is the relatively slow onset, and prolonged duration, of their effects. Thus, an increase in total body oxygen consumption did not occur for at least 12 hr after the injection of a low dose of T_3 into thyroidectomized rats. A maximum effect was not seen until 3 or 4 days after treatment and some elevation of oxygen consumption was still detectable 1 week after a single injection of T_3.[39] Most other physiological effects of thyroid hormones show a similar "latent period" and prolonged duration.

The challenge has been to devise a unifying hypothesis to explain the numerous effects of thyroid hormones on metabolism, physiology, and growth, and also the unique time-course of these responses. Tata et al.,[39] in a key paper, proposed that the hormones' central action is to modify protein metabolism. Clearly, growth and differentiation must involve protein synthesis. However, it was also hypothesized that the effects on the metabolism and physiology of mature animals are not direct, but are a consequence of the ability of these hormones to modify the concentration of key proteins and rate-limiting enzymes. It is envisaged that the latent period, at least in part, is due to the time necessary to initiate a change in the protein synthetic machinery of the cell, and for this to manifest itself as changes in protein concentration. In support of this hypothesis Tata et al.[39] showed that the time-course of changes in the rate of protein synthesis in the liver, caused by T_3, paralleled changes in the oxygen consumption of the whole rat. Furthermore, inhibitors of protein synthesis were shown to prevent the increase in whole body oxygen consumption caused by thyroid hormones.[40]

It is now generally accepted that effects on protein synthesis play a central role in the action of thyroid hormones. More recently, interest has centered on the way in which thyroid hormones control protein synthesis (mechanism of action), and the elucidation of the enzymic changes underlying the various physiological actions of thyroid hormones, particularly the thermogenic and cardiovascular effects. Some selected effects are discussed in more detail below, but others, such as those on calcium, phosphorous, nitrogen, fat, and carbohydrate metabolism, are fully described in recent review articles.[41-45]

Mechanism of Action

The long latent period, before thyroid hormone effects become manifest has meant that, with the exception of cell culture techniques (see below), it has not proved possible to demonstrate hormonal effects (e.g., on oxygen uptake or heart rate) in vitro. For this reason any proposed mechanism of action must rely upon indirect evidence. Nevertheless, some effects of thyroid hormones in vitro have been observed and attempts to relate these to their physiological actions (especially the thermogenic effect) have been made. For instance the observation that T_4 can uncouple isolated mitochondria led to the hypothesis that the increase in whole body oxygen consumption could also be due to an uncoupling action. This view is no longer regarded as tenable since (1) the uncoupling occurs almost instantaneously whereas the in vivo thermogenic effects occurs after a latent period, (2) the concentrations of hormone needed to uncouple are far greater than required to increase oxgyen consumption, (3) the structure-activity relationships for the two effects are dissimilar, and (4) isolated mitochondria from rat liver, which showed a thermogenic response after treatment with low doses of T_3, were as tightly coupled as those from untreated animals.

RNA Metabolism

The recognition that thyroid hormones modify protein synthesis directed attention to their effects on RNA metabolism. Obviously, an increase in protein synthesis could be due to a stimulation of either transcription or translation. In fact, Tata and Widnell[5] showed that the effects of T_3 on protein synthesis in the liver were preceded by an increase in RNA synthesis, and the activity of the enzymes catalyzing this synthesis (RNA polymerases).

In addition to thyroid hormone induction of these generalized increases in RNA synthesis, and higher levels of RNA in euthyroid than in hypothyroid rats, stimulation of the synthesis of mRNA for specific products has also been seen. Thyroid hormones, together with androgens and glucocorticoids, induce, and estrogens suppress,[46] α_{2u}-globulin mRNA production. Growth hormone, and growth hormone mRNA production, are stimulated by thyroid hormones in a thyroid hormone sensitive, pituitary, tumor cell line (GH_1).[47] Again T_3 acts synergistically with glucocorticoids which can also increase growth hormone mRNA by themselves. It is interesting that the response of T_3 is specific and there is no general increase in mRNA in this system, neither does T_3 elevate other mRNA species which are increased by glucocorticoids.[47]

These effects on RNA metabolism occur at doses (or concentrations, where cell culture has been used) of hormone similar to those which elicit changes in metabolism or physiology. This, and the time-course of the response, make it likely that changes in RNA metabolism are an obligatory step in the action of thyroid hormones, although no investigations of the relationship between structure and activity have been carried out. This conclusion is supported by the fact that actinomycin D, which inhibits transcription, also inhibits the thermogenic effects of thyroid hormones.[40]

2. Nuclear Receptors

The alteration, by thyroid hormones, of the amount of mRNA coding for specific proteins strongly suggested that the hormone receptor is located in the cell nucleus, and, in 1972,[48] a site capable of binding T_3 with high affinity was identified in nuclei isolated from rats previously given an i.v. injection containing radiolabeled T_3. Later, specific binding of T_3 analogs was demonstrated in vitro by incubation of radiolabeled T_3 with isolated nuclei, or the proteins extracted from them.[49] Nuclear membranes and cytoplasmic proteins are not needed to effect binding. A considerable body of evidence suggests that this binding site satisfies most of the criteria required of the thyroid hormone receptor.

The sites have limited capacity, and an affinity, such that, at physiological levels of hormone, they will be partially occupied (40 to 50%)[50] and therefore able to respond to any fluctuation of hormone levels with a change in their degree of saturation. Nuclear binding sites have been found in all responsive tissues so far examined but few are present in the insensitive spleen and testis.[50] The brain, which is usually considered metabolically unresponsive to thyroid hormones but affected during development, has an intermediate level of specific thyroid hormone binding sites.[50] Similar sites have been found in other species, including man,[51] where thyroid hormones are active, but not in *Drosophila,* which is not affected by thyroid hormones. In man, reduced nuclear thyroid hormone binding has been reported in cases of familial resistance to thyroid hormones.[52,53] When account is taken of some metabolic and pharmacokinetic factors (see below) there is a good correlation between biological activity and affinity for the binding site of full agonist analogs of T_3 and T_4.[6]

The relationship between receptor occupation and response has also been studied. In cultured GH_1 cells the response to thyroid hormones (a stimulation of the rate of growth hormone synthesis) is proportional to receptor occupancy.[54] This is consistent with an obligatory role for this binding site in the action of thyroid hormones. It is relatively simple, in such in vitro experiments, to maintain a constant degree of receptor occupancy, and to measure rates of protein synthesis. In vivo such experiments are complicated by metabolism of the hormone with a consequent continuous variation in receptor occupancy. Nevertheless, the relationship between protein synthesis (hepatic GPDH induction) and receptor occupancy in the rat, has been examined by one group[55] and a nonlinear relationship found, suggesting that postreceptor amplification of the signal had occurred. However, the use of other, lower estimates of initial occupancy in euthyroid rat liver (16 vs. 50%)[56] and allowance for possible induction of new binding sites,[57,58] could invalidate this conclusion.

Maximal occupation of the nuclear binding site occurs about 1 hr after parenteral administration of hormone. This is much earlier than any other relevant biochemical or physiological responses and is, therefore, consistent with its role as a receptor. The ability of the nuclear site to satisfy the most stringent test of a receptor, that is to initiate the response in vitro, cannot be checked until more is known of early events in thyroid hormone action.

The Nature and Location of the Nuclear Binding Site

The protein responsible for the binding of T_3 by nuclei can be extracted by 0.4 *M* KCl and is an acidic nonhistone protein.[59] Some purification of the site has been achieved using molecular sieve columns or, more recently, by affinity chromatography. The binding protein is asymmetric and the inhibition of T_3 binding by *p*-chloromercuribenzoate and iodoacetamide suggest that cysteine or lysine residues may be important components of the site.

Equilibration of ^{125}I-T_3 or ^{125}I-T_3-receptor complexes with nuclei or chromatin has shown that all of the binding sites are located on chromatin. Preferential binding to DNA, rather than RNA, has been shown, and there is some evidence that the protein is bound to segments of DNA which are undergoing active transcription. Recent evidence (reviewed by Samuels et al.)[60] suggests that the T_3-binding protein is attached to the internucleosomal ''linker'' DNA, possibly in association with another unspecified protein. Some preference for transcriptionally active chromatin is also likely.

Numbers and Classes of Binding Site

Estimates of rat liver binding site numbers vary up to 10,000 per cell. Binding site capacity was reported to be unaffected by thyroid status[61] with no evidence of autoregulation. However, these experiments failed to take into account occupancy by endogenous hormone and recently an increased receptor number was measured after thyroid hormone treatment of rats.[57,58] In starvation,[62] and various disease states, a direct relationship between receptor number and circulating T_3 levels is also seen.

Studies with GH_1 cells[63] in culture have shown that the receptors are continually synthesized and degraded with a halflife of about 5 hr, implying that receptors do not remain fixed to any specific regions of the chromatin. Occupation of the receptor by T_3 diminishes the rate of synthesis and enhances the rate of degradation of receptor, resulting in a diminution of their concentration within the cell.

Identical capacities for T_3 and T_4, and quantitative structure-activity/affinity relationship (QSAR) studies (see below), indicated that both natural hormones are bound by the same protein. However, heating nuclear extracts, or reducing their pH, dramatically reduced the binding of T_3 but had no effect on their affinity for T_4.[64] Furthermore, the loss of affinity for T_3, caused by partial purification of the receptor, could be restored by histones. These observations led to the hypothesis that the receptor consisted of a "core" subunit which bound T_4 more avidly than T_3 and that the affinity of T_3 but not T_4 could be increased by the association of the core receptor with histones to give a "holoreceptor".[65] More recently, these authors have abandoned this hypothesis as they have shown that heating of nuclear extracts inactivated a protein binding both T_4 and T_3 but generated or exposed another low affinity binding site which bound only T_4.[66] It is still thought, however, that histones play an important role in protecting and stabilizing the nuclear receptor.

A number of reports of a specific rT_3 binding site have appeared.[67] However, very recently, it has been suggested that these observations are an artefact due to the presence, in isolated nuclei, of a deiodinase.[68]

The Steroid Hormone Analogy

The discovery of thyroid hormone nuclear binding sites and known effects of thyroid hormones on protein synthesis prompted the proposal that thyroid and steroid hormones act by similar receptor mechanisms. However, nuclear T_3 binding occurs in vitro in the absence of cytoplasm.[69] Thus, in contrast to the action of steroid hormones, cytoplasmic binding proteins do not carry thyroid hormones into the nucleus so forming part of the receptor. Such cytoplasmic, thyroid hormone binding proteins will influence receptor function by controlling the intracellular, free, hormone concentration.

Alternative Receptors

The binding of thyroid hormones by a specific nuclear protein is firmly established as an obligatory step in their action. This does not, however, exclude the possibility that other receptors and mechanisms are operative, and alternatives have been proposed.

Because of the effect of thyroid hormones on oxygen uptake, the mitochondrion has often been regarded as a likely site for a receptor. Uncoupling is no longer regarded as a feasible mechanism of action of thyroid hormones but alternative effects are of possible significance. For instance very rapid effects on ATP formation have been found both in vivo[70] and in vitro,[71] using physiological doses (concentrations) of T_3. Mitochondrial protein synthesis is also stimulated shortly (3 hr) after T_3 administration in vivo.[72] Furthermore, the mitochondrial protein profile is specifically dependent upon thyroid status.

Sterling[73] has identified a high affinity, low capacity thyroid hormone binding site on the inner aspect of the mitochondrial membrane, which is also the site of oxidative phosphorylation. Tissue distribution, occupancy, and structure-activity correlations which support the hypothesis that this is a functional receptor have been reviewed recently.[45] Other authors have also reported evidence in favor of this binding site,[74] but some have been unable to confirm its existence.[75] The reported affinity of the mitochondrial T_3-binding site, in vitro, is significantly higher than that of the nuclear binding site, suggesting that it could be almost fully occupied by euthyroid, thyroid hormone levels. While direct effects on mitochondrial function could have a permissive role in the thermogenic and other actions of thyroid hormones it is difficult to see how an enhanced ability to generate ATP could cause the principal effects of these hormones.

Specific binding of T_3 and T_4 by isolated plasma membranes has been found.[76,77] Thyroid hormones have also been shown to enhance amino acid and deoxyglucose accumulation by isolated cells.[78,79] While these effects occur at physiological hormone concentrations the limited structure-activity work shows a lack of correspondence with the thermogenic effects of hormone analogs. These effects have not yet been demonstrated to occur in vivo, and their significance in the overall economy of the cell is obscure.

It has also been pointed out[80] that T_3 and T_4, as amino acids, could conceivably be incorporated into proteins or, as tyrosine analogs, could give rise to catecholamine analogs with biological activity. This hypothesis has yet to be proven.

Selected Effects of Thyroid Hormones

For a more detailed discussion of the alleged actions of thyroid hormones the reader is referred to a number of excellent reviews.[41-45] Some of the more important aspects are outlined below.

Energy Metabolism

The stimulation of whole body oxygen consumption has been recognized as a primary thyroid hormone action in man since 1895.[81] Oxygen consumption is reduced by thyroidectomy and restored by thyroid hormones in the intact rat or in tissue slices from treated rats.[82]

Under normal circumstances the rate of oxygen consumption by the cell is controlled by the rate of conversion of ADP to ATP. This, in turn, depends on the rate of production of ADP from ATP by the various energy requiring reactions of the cell. It is, therefore, reasonable to suppose that thyroid hormones increase oxygen consumption by stimulating the generation of ADP. Viewed in this light the increased capacity to generate ATP, found in mitochondria from thyroid hormone-treated animals, is part of a pleiotypic response designed to support increased energy utilization. The identity of the energy utilizing reaction is not known. Ismail-Beigi and Edelman[83] have suggested that the principal effect of thyroid hormones is to increase the amount of energy expended in translocating ions across the cell membrane. Other authors, however, have found that only a minor proportion of the cell's oxygen requirement is needed for ion translocation.[84,85] Moreover, since most of the effects of the hormone are energy utilizing, the overall increase in oxygen consumption may simply reflect the sum of many processes rather than one single effect.

The Cardiovascular System

Thyroid hormone effects on the heart (reviewed by Smallridge)[86] may be both direct and indirect. The increase in metabolic rate caused by thyroid hormones generates a demand for more oxygen and this is met in the whole organism by increasing cardiac output via effects on both heart rate and contractility.[87-89] While this effect could be achieved by the normal reflex neural mechanisms it has been shown that thyroid hormones, administered in vivo, can also increase intrinsic rate and contractility of hearts subsequently isolated and perfused.[90] This suggests a direct action of the hormones in the heart. In the rat this change in contractility is related to the proportions of two cardiac myosin isozymes with different ATPase activities.[91] Although this has not been demonstrated in some other species it could be a direct effect of thyroid hormones in selectively affecting protein synthesis. The increased heart size in hyperthyroidism could be caused by direct stimulation of protein synthesis or be a response to the prolonged increase in workload of the heart in satisfying the tissue demand for oxygen.

Brain

Thyroid hormones affect both the development of the immature brain and the function of the adult brain. The developmental effects of thyroid hormones in the human brain have been known since the association between fetal hypothyroidism and cretinism was first recognized. In the rat, postnatal brain development can be considered equivalent to late fetal brain development in the human[92] and has been used as a model to study the effects of thyroid hormone on brain differentiation. There is a 10-day period when thyroid hormones are essential for the development of adaptive responses[93] and learning ability. Later, thyroidectomy or substitution therapy has little effect, whereas normal development of these responses can be achieved by earlier thyroid hormone substitution in hypothyroid rats. Fetal hypothyroidism is accompanied by a reduced brain weight and cell size but not cell numbers.[94] Protein synthesis and the protein: DNA ratio are reduced. There is reduced growth of perikarya and axons, myelination is delayed, and total brain cholesterol, sulfatides, phospholipids, lipoproteins, gangliosides, and cerebrosides are lower in hypothyroid rats. Eayrs[95] has suggested that retarded development results from the reduction in axio-dendritic connections.

Cholesterol Metabolism

In man, hypothyroidism is associated with elevated serum levels of cholesterol and its low density lipoprotein (LDL) carrier, whereas the reverse situation is seen in the hyperthyroid state. Evidence from studies in the rat suggests that thyroid hormones stimulate both cholesterol synthesis and degradation. Synthesis is enhanced in vivo by increasing the activity of liver β-hydroxy-β-methylglutaryl-CoA reductase,[96] though high concentrations of T_3 and T_4 may inhibit the activity of this enzyme in vitro.[97] In hyperthyroidism breakdown of cholesterol by the liver, and excretion of metabolites as bile salts overrides the increased synthesis due to thyroid hormones. The lower serum LDL levels of hyperthyroidism result from a higher fractional clearance rate as seen in the intact rat.[98] T_3 has also been shown to increase the degradation of LDL by cultured human skin fibroblasts.[99] Both the effect of cholesterol metabolism and LDL clearance could be mediated by increased acid cholesterol ester hydrolase found in rat liver and adipocytes of T_3-treated thyroidectomized rats.[100]

The Endocrine and Nervous System

Thyroid hormones can interact with the endocrine system by modifying secretion, metabolism, or action of the various agents involved.

The similarity between the actions of catecholamines and thyroid hormones[101] led to the suggestion that the latter might potentiate the effects of the former, and this theory has been substantiated by the observation that the number of β-receptors in various systems[102,103] is dependent upon thyroid status. Some authors have also observed potentiation of the effect of catecholamines, but others have not.

Thyroid hormones and growth hormone act synergistically in the control of body size. Thyroid hormones can also stimulate the secretion of growth hormone by the rat pituitary leading to an increase in the circulating levels of this hormone.[104] By contrast, thyroid hormones stimulate both the synthesis and degradation of cortisol but without modifying circulating hormone levels.[105]

PROCEDURES FOR ASSAYING THE BIOLOGICAL ACTIVITY OF THYROID HORMONE ANALOGS

Any one of the multitudinous effects of thyroid hormones could, theoretically, be used as an endpoint in a bioassay. A number of these assays, such as the elevation of metabolic rate, goiter prevention, depression of thyroidal ^{131}I uptake by the thyroid gland, and the induction of tadpole metamorphosis have been widely used for many years in relating the variation in net response of a particular parameter to analog structure.[106] However, the latent period before action is observed, and the long duration of the experiments preclude the use of these assays in the characterization of the receptor mediated primary effects of thyroid hormones and their analogs.

The initial direct responses to thyroid hormones appear to be the variation in rates of synthesis of specific proteins, including a number of enzymes, although other direct effects on mitochondria and membranes cannot be excluded. Since a cascade of actions may follow this and be further complicated by interactions with other hormones, direct effects cannot be identified with certainty in the whole animal. Isolated organ preparations could be used to overcome the problems of hormonal interaction but unfortunately responsive organs, such as the heart, cannot be maintained in a viable state for a sufficient time (up to 48 hr) to demonstrate effects. Tissue culture of isolated thymocytes,[79] fetal chick heart cells,[78] and pituitary tumor cell lines[47,54] has allowed the demonstration of thyroid hormone effects on amino acid uptake, deoxyglucose uptake, and growth hormone secretion respectively in the absence of other hormones. Although the membrane transport effects may be direct thyroid hormone actions, they have not been demonstrated in vivo and the structure-activity relationships of these and whole body responses are dissimilar. They are therefore of doubtful use as general models of thyroid hormone actions. The measurement of growth hormone synthesis in pituitary tumor cells is a potentially useful assay, but the pituitary trophic hormone secreting cells are highly specialized and may not respond in a manner representative of other sensitive tissues. For this reason suppression of TSH secretion in the intact animal also may be less valuable than other assays.

More recently the induction of specific enzymes, has been used to assay hormone activity in vivo. Mitochondrial *sn* glycerol-1-phosphate-cytochrome c oxido-reductase (GPDH) is particularly useful in this respect, since it is induced specifically by thyromimetics in a dose-related manner in responsive tissues.[107] Unlike other bioassay procedures the changes in GPDH activity can be very large — the maximum hepatic activity after T_3 treatment being about 15 times greater than that in thyrodectomized rats. As with other assays the response is delayed with no measurable effects before 12 hr. Despite having numerous advantages this assay has been underused in structure activity studies and most reported studies have used the goiter prevention assay or elevation of metabolic rate.

Attempts to define the mechanism of thyroid hormone action before measurable biological response have met with some success. Of particular interest in the context of potential bioassays are the findings of the induction of specific mRNAs for growth hormone[47] in growth hormone secreting pituitary tumor cell lines and $\alpha2_\mu$ globulin mRNA[46] by liver cells. This type of response could well provide an extremely useful assay for direct effects of thyroid hormones in vitro.

The search for highly active novel agonists or antagonists is likely to involve the design of compounds with high receptor affinity. Consequently, the direct measurement of this property will greatly assist the medicinal chemist in correlating molecular properties and structure with receptor affinity. The discovery of a specific nuclear protein,[48] which is responsible for initiating some, if not all, thyroid hormone effects has provided the basis for measuring the relative receptor affinities of thyroid hormone analogs either in vivo[48,50] or in vitro.[49] In in vitro assays intact isolated cell nuclei, or salt extracted nuclear proteins, are incubated with ^{125}I-T_3 together with buffer, or various concentrations of nonradioactive T_3 or analog and the amount of ^{125}I-T_3 specifically bound to the T_3 receptor is determined. The concentrations of competing ligand which displace 50% of the specifically bound ^{125}I-T_3 are inversely related to their affinities for the T_3 receptor, which are usually expressed as a percentage of that of T_3. In the in vivo binding assay the rat is injected with ^{125}I-T_3 and competing ligand before the nuclei are isolated and their ^{125}I content determined. This is corrected for the DNA content of the extract and then related to the ^{125}I-T_3 content of the plasma before relative affinity is calculated as it was in vitro.

In vitro nuclear binding affinities of analog can be used to identify the structural features necessary for receptor recognition. In vivo nuclear binding affinities, however, are influenced not only by receptor binding, but also by pharamcokinetic and metabolic effects which control the concentration of hormone or analog available for receptor binding. Comparison of in vitro with in vivo affinities can permit the extent of these pharmacokinetic and metabolic phenomena to be evaluated. Use of the in vivo binding assay is especially important in accounting for those analogs where in vivo activity does not correlate with in vitro affinity. Most reported structure-activity work has utilized the correlation of the affinity of analogs for the liver binding site with activity in the goiter prevention assay. Since enzyme induction can be measured in the organ used to supply nuclei we believe that it would be more appropriate in future studies to relate affinity to activity in the same organ.

STRUCTURE-ACTIVITY AND STRUCTURE-AFFINITY RELATIONSHIPS WITH THYROID HORMONE ANALOGS

Introduction and Conformational Aspects

The physical properties of the naturally occurring thyroid hormones have been reviewed.[108] T_3 and T_4 (Figure 1) are high melting, sparingly soluble (2.5 to $5 \times 10^{-5} M$ for T_4 at pH 7.4, 38°C) compounds. Ionization of the carboxyl and amino groups, would, by analogy with other aromatic amino acids, be expected to be virtually complete at physiological pH. The acidic pK_as of the phenolic 4' hydroxyls of T_3 (pK_a 8.45) and T_4 (pK_a 6.73) mean that at physiological pH the hormones exist to the extent of 8.2 and 82.4% respectively, as 4'-phenolate anions. The alanine side chain exists as a single optically active L enantiomer, which has the S configuration. Crystallographic and spectral properties of the hormones and their analogs are presented where relevant in the following discussions on conformational aspects and structure activity/affinity relationships.

Since Harington and Barger's characterization and synthesis[109] of thyroxine (Figure 1) over half a century ago, several hundred thyroid hormone analogs have been prepared.[110-112] The biological activities determined for these analogs come from several types of assays performed in different laboratories. The most consistent sets of biological data, which have been used by Jorgensen in comprehensive discussions[112,113] of structure-activity relationships, are those derived from the in vivo rat antigoiter assay and the in vitro rat liver nuclear binding assay. In considering structure-activity/affinity studies, it is apparent that substituent variation, especially at the 3'- and 5'-positions, and to a certain extent with 3,5-positions (i.e., replacement of iodine atoms in Figure 1), is insufficient to allow the separation of such fundamental substituent properties as lipophilicity and size. The colinearity of 3,5,3',5'-substituent properties is especially serious when attempts are made to construct quantitative structure-activity/affinity relationships (QSARs). As a result, even the most extensive of QSARs in this field[114] actually gives rise to some ambiguous conclusions. An additional shortcoming of this work is that the correlation between receptor affinity and biological activity relies on measurements in different organs(i.e., rat liver nuclear binding vs. rat antigoiter activity). In our work, we have derived in vitro affinities and in vivo thyromimetic activities from the same organ, rat liver, and some of our data are included in this review.

It is not the aim of this review to give a comprehensive account of thyroid hormone structure-activity relationships. Rather, we intend to provide a critical summary of the principal findings, pointing out possible shortcomings where necessary. To aid this task, we have included biological data on some new compounds, in particular several belonging to the 3'-substituted 3,5-diiodothyronine series, in an attempt to re-evaluate the effects on receptor affinity and in vivo activity of 3'-substituent size, lipophilicity, and interactive effects with the 4'-hydroxyl.

Detailed conformational properties of thyroid hormones have been discussed previously by Cody[115,116] and Jorgensen.[112,113] In the following sections of this review we will refer to those pertinent aspects which relate to specific substituent effects.

The importance of diphenylether conformation in determining the correct spatial disposition of the substituents in T_3 and its analogs has been stressed.[112] The original working model (Figure 2), proposed by Zenker and Jorgensen,[117] in which the 3,5-iodines maintain

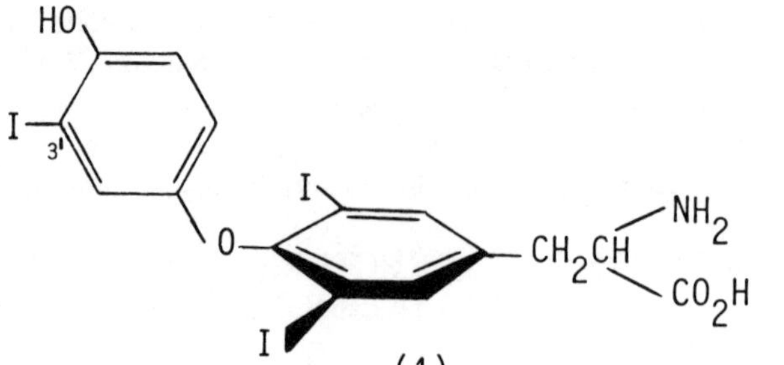

FIGURE 2. Structures of 3,3′,5-triiodothyronine (T_3), showing the orthogonal arrangement of the aromatic rings with the 3′-iodine atom positioned distally (1) and proximally (2).

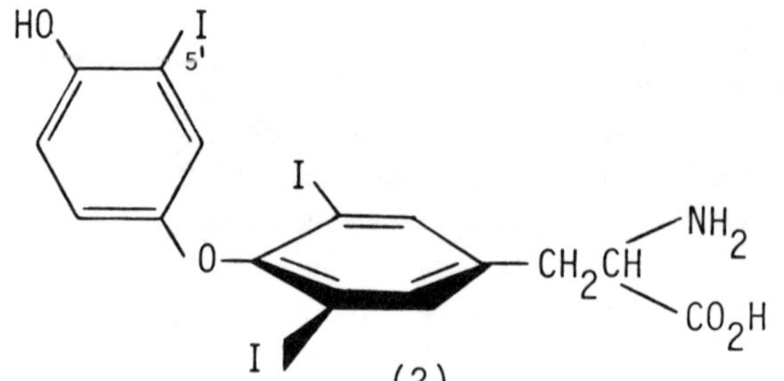

a preferred orthogonal conformation of the two rings and the 3′-substituent is positioned distally relative to the 3,5-diiodophenyl ring in the active conformation, has stood the test of time. Evidence for the orthogonal arrangement, coupled with a significant barrier to rotation, has been derived subsequently from a wealth of X-ray data,[115,116] NMR studies in solution,[118] and theoretical calculations.[119] These studies show that a barrier to rotation of 8 to 9 kcal/mol exists in 3,5-diiododiphenylethers and that the distal and proximal forms of T_3 are expected to have similar energy.

The favored receptor recognition of a distally positioned over a proximally positioned 3′-substituent is shown by a comparison of the 3,5-diiodo-2′,3′- and 5′-dimethyl-DL-thyronines[6] (Figure 3) in which the energetically favored distal positioning of a 2′-methyl group ensures the predominance of a single conformation. The former has activity at least an order of magnitude greater than the latter in the antigoiter test, the induction of liver GPDH, and the in vitro nuclear binding site assay.

The binding of thyroid hormones to transport proteins plays a crucial part in the expression of overall activity in vivo.[112] Recently, the determination[120] of the three-dimensional structure of TBPA has stimulated the study of analog-binding using computer generated models.[121] The role of TBPA in providing a model for the nuclear receptor binding site is discussed in this review.

The Phenol-Bearing Ring

The 4′-Substituent

Significant thyromimetic activity is only seen in analogs where the phenolic hydroxyl is located at the 4′-position and 2′- and 3′-isomers are inactive.[122] Removal of the 4′-hydroxyl gives 4′-unsubstituted analogs with much reduced receptor affinity in vitro (Table 1, 9 to 14) but with substantial in vivo activity. Metabolic activation has been suggested[112] to explain this difference since 4′-hydroxylation is known to occur with certain 4′-unsubstituted com-

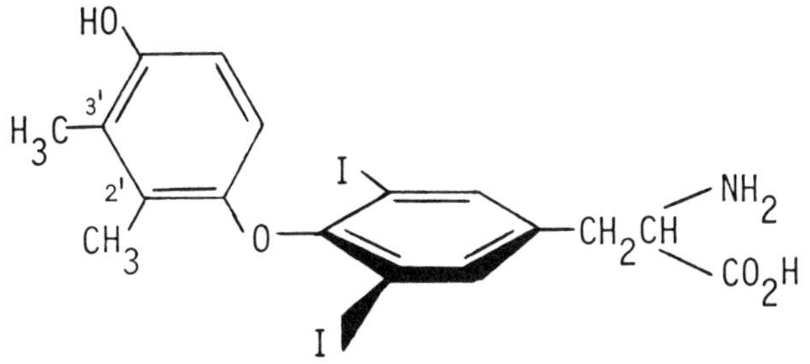

FIGURE 3. Structures of the conformationally fixed analog, 2',3'-dimethyl-3,5-diiodothyronine ([1], 3'-methyl group distally fixed) and 2',5'-dimethyl-3,5-diiodothyronine ([2], 5'-methyl group proximally fixed).

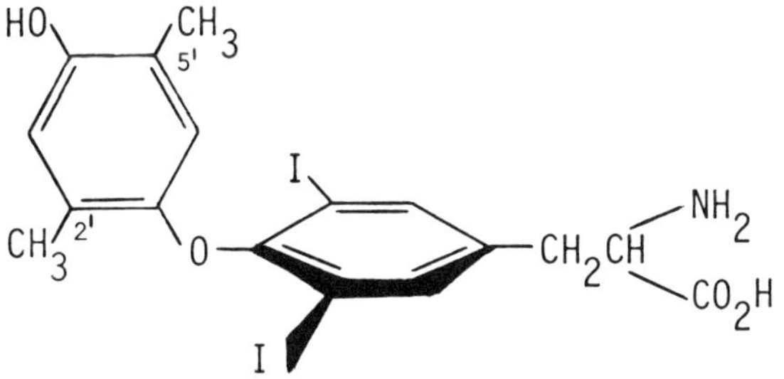

pounds.[123] 4'-Methyl ethers of active thyromimetics (Table 1, 15 to 17) also have weak in vitro affinities, but are active in vivo. This activity could also arise as a result of metabolic activation via cleavage of the ether function in in vivo binding. Analogs with 4'-groups which block metabolic hydroxylation, e.g., 4'-methyl and 4'-chloro are inactive in vivo[112] and possess very weak in vitro affinities.

Replacement of the 4'-hydroxyl group by 4'-amino[124] retains some activity, especially when a 3'-iodo substituent is present (Table 1, compare 1 to 4). The general observation that the contribution of a particular 3'-substituent to both receptor affinity and activity is dependent upon the nature of the 4'-substituent is clearly illustrated from a comparison of the effects of 3'-ethyl and 3'-iodo in thyronines and their 4'-amino analogs. Thus, with a 4'-hydroxyl substituent present 3'-ethyl and 3'-iodine substituents are almost equivalent (compare 7 and 8) whereas in the aniline derivatives the 3'-iodo analog (Figure 4) shows a much greater affinity than the 3'-ethyl analog. This difference could be due to different interactions of the 3'-iodine and 3'-ethyl groups with the adjacent 4'-amino group.

If it is assumed that the 4'-hydroxyl and 4'-amino groups utilize a similar mode of receptor binding, then the model proposed by Andrea et al.[119] for receptor binding of thyronines serves as a basis for a comparison of anilines and phenols. In this model the 4'-hydroxyl group acts as a hydrogen bond donor to an acceptor group (A) on the receptor positioned *trans* to the 3'-substituent (i.e., [1] in Figure 4). The aniline 4 could interact similarly via an intramolecularly hydrogen bonded species ([2] in Figure 4). Receptor affinity would then be dependent on the strength of the NH–A hydrogen bond and this would, in turn, depend on 4'-amino acidity and the Ar-NH-A torsion angle in 4. In contrast, the amino group in 3 is likely to suffer repulsion from the 3'-ethyl substituent rather than hydrogen bonded attraction and this could lead to an increase in the Ar-NH-A torsion angle. In addition, the

Table 1
4'-SUBSTITUTED ANALOGS

No.[a]	R_4'	R_3'	Activity in vivo		Nuclear binding in vitro	
			Antigoiter[d]	GPDH[e]	Intact[f]	Solubilized[g]
1	NH_2	H	<0.04	LM[i]	0.002	0.01
2[c]	NH_2	Cl		LM[i]	0.1	
3[c]	NH_2	Et		LM[i]	0.2	
4	NH_2	I	>0.3	9.9	12 (0.8[h])	
5	OH	H	0.8	1.1	0.08	0.1
6	OH	Cl	4.9	2.8	5.1	4.1
7	OH	Et	93.5	139	56	13
8	OH	I	100	100	100	100
9	H	F	1.4			0.01
10	H	Cl	7.8			0.1
11	H	Br	18			0.2
12[b]	H	I	>27	116	0.8	4.6
13[b]	H	CH_3	2.7		0.2[d]	0.2
14[b]	H	CF_3	14		0.2[d]	
15	OCH_3	I	11			1.3
16	OCH_3	iPr	19	111	1.8	6.8
17	OCH_3	tBu	2.4			0.3

[a]   All compounds are L-alanine derivatives unless otherwise indicated.
[b]   DL-.
[c]   SK & F (Smith, Kline & French Research LTD.), unpublished compounds.
[d]   References 111, 112, T_3 = 100.
[e]   SK & F, unpublished data; in this and in subsequent tables the activity of liver GPDH in thyroidectomized rats as measured 48 hr after a single injection of analog is given. Dose-response curves were fitted to a hyperbolic curve using a nonlinear curve fitting procedure, and ED_{50}s calculated. Figures given are relative to T_3 = 100; ED_{50} for T_3, 154 nmol/kg.
[f]   SK & F, unpublished data; intact rat liver nuclei, T_3 = 100.
[g]   Reference 134, solubilized rat liver nuclei, T_3 = 100.
[h]   Reference 113.
[i]   Low maximum response.

4'-amino group in 3 will be less acidic than the 4'-amino group in the 3'-iodo analog 4. These differences could, therefore, account for the different binding affinities and in vivo activities of 3 and 4.

The 3',5'-Substituents

Replacement of the 3'-iodo substituent in T_3 by other halogens and alkyls results in derivatives which retain varying degrees of in vivo agonist activity and in vitro receptor affinity (Table 2, 1 to 17). These analogs have provided much of the impetus for the recent derivation of quantitative structure-activity/affinity relationships[114] (QSARs) describing in

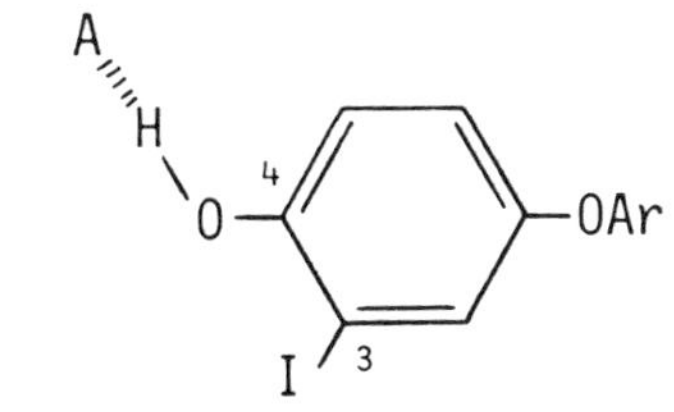

(1)

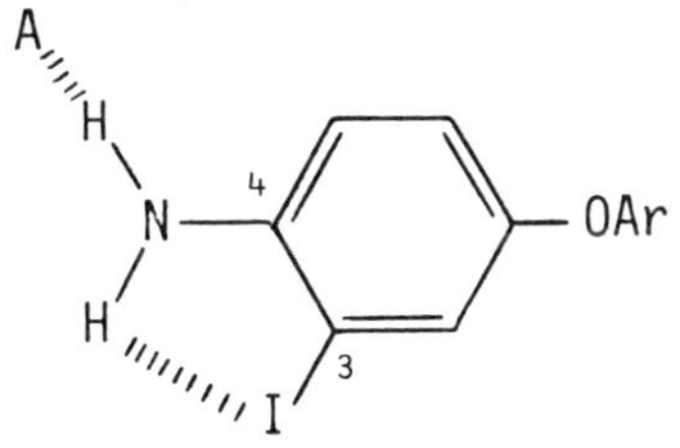

(2)

FIGURE 4. Proposed interactions of 3'-iodo-4'-hydroxyl (1) and 3'-iodo-4'-amino (2) analogs with a putative receptor electron donor, A.

vivo rat antigoiter activity and in vitro rat hepatic nuclear binding affinity. Earlier QSAR studies[125-130] have been discussed in detail by Jorgensen,[112] and will not be dealt with here.

In the most recent and extensive QSAR study by Jorgensen et al.,[114] indicator variables for 2'- and 4'-substitution and lipophilicity terms for the 3,5,5'-substituents were used to merge sets of compounds with the same variation in the 3'-substituent. Essentially identical QSAR equations resulted for the predictions of in vivo rat antigoiter activity, and in vitro affinity for intact, and solubilized, rat hepatic nuclei. The high correlation between in vivo activity and in vitro affinities provides good evidence for the nuclear receptor hypothesis of thyroid hormone action.

The QSAR studies by Jorgensen et al.[114] however, suffer from the shortcomings which are always inherent when attempts are made to construct QSARs from data sets in which substituent properties are covariables.[131] Thus, substituent lipophilicity, as measured by the Hansch π values,[132] and substituent bulk, estimated by molar refractivity (MR)[132] are colinear for the 3,5,3',5'-substituted analogs utilized in these studies. The method of estimating size used by Jorgensen et al. masks the high correlation between 3'-substituent size and lipophilicity, but the lack of the orthogonality for 3,5,5'-substituents was noted.

In the following discussion, we consider alternative QSAR equations describing relative in vitro affinities (SB, relative to $T_3 = 100$) of 3,5-diiodothyronines (Figure 5) for solubilized rat hepatic nuclear receptor. In Figure 5 $R_{3'}$ is H, Me, Et, Pr^n, Pr^i, Bu^t, Bu^s, F, Cl, Br, I, and NO$_2$; $R_{4'}$ is H, OH, and OCH$_3$; $R_{5'}$ is H, Me, Pr^i, Cl, Br. and I. With both $R_{3'}$ and $R_{5'}$ variation, two 3'-nitro derivatives are the only analogs which deviate from the size/lipophilicity colinearity, the correlation between π and MR for this group of 3'-substituents being 0.914.

In Equation 1, derived by Jorgensen et al.,[114] $\pi_{3'}$ and $\pi_{5'}$ are the Hansch lipophilicity constants 3' SIZE > I is an estimate of the distance

Table 2
3′-SUBSTITUTED 3,5-DIIODOTHYRONINES

No.[a]	R$_{3'}$	Activity in vivo		Nuclear binding in vitro		
		Antigoiter[d]	GPDH[e]	Intact[k]	Intact[f]	Predicted[l]
1	H	0.8	1.1	0.3	0.08	0.05
2	CH$_3$	14.5	7.5	13.5	0.6	1.6
3	Et	93.5	139	21	56	18
4	iPr	142	290	104	87	55
5	nPr	39.5	89		45	55
6	sBu	80				
7	tBu	22	26	38.5	25	63
8	iBu	7.7	F[m]	20	20.5	63
9[b]	cHex			1.4		
10[b]	Ph	3.5	6.6	2	7.3	9.5
11	CH$_2$Ph		2.1		10	5.2
12	OH	0.3	LM[i]		0.04	0.09
13	NO$_2$	0.2	0.3		0.13	—[n]
14	F	1.1	F[m]			
15	Cl	4.9	2.8	6.2	5.1	2.6
16	Br	24	20		13	11
17	I	100	100	100	100	38
18[c]	nBu		117		44	63
19[bc]	nPen		6.2		32	43
20[c]	nHex		5.0		60	24
21[c]	nHep		LM[i]		8.7	12.5
22[c]	CH$_2$cHex		LM[i]		36	15
23[c]	CH$_2$CH=CH$_2$		34		32	35
24[c]	(CH$_2$)$_2$Ph		LM[i]		1.8	2.7
25[c]	PhOH-p		LM[i]		0.8	3.0
26[c]	CH$_2$OCH$_3$		25		2.6	3.1
27[c]	CH$_2$OH		LM[i]		0.4	0.4
28[c]	CH$_2$CO$_2$H		LM[i]		0.03	0.01
29[c]	CH$_2$NH$_2$		0		0.01	0.03
30[j]	COCH$_3$		121		0.3	—[n]
31[c]	CO$_2$H		0		0.004	0.004
32[c]	(CH$_2$)$_4$OCH$_3$		0.8		8.6	3.4

[a] All compounds are L-alanine derivatives unless otherwise indicated.

[b] DL-.

[c] SK & F, unpublished compounds.

[d] References 112, 113, T$_3$ = 100.

[e] See Table 1.

[f] SK & F, unpublished data; intact rat liver nuclei, T$_3$ = 100.

[g] % Of maximum nuclear occupation achieved.

[h] % Of maximum response achieved.

[i] Low maximum response.

[j] Reference 135.

[k] Reference 114.

[l] From Equation 5.

[m] Full agonist.

[n] Not used in the derivation of Equation 5.

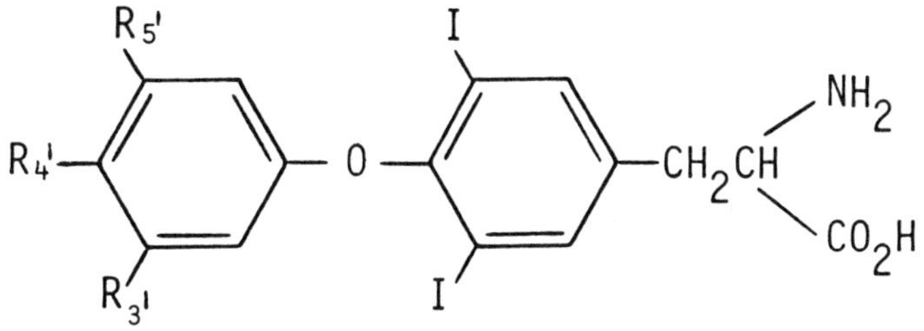

FIGURE 5. Structural variants ($R_{3'}$, $R_{4'}$, and $R_{5'}$) used by Jorgensen in a QSAR analysis of binding affinities to solubilized rat liver nuclei.

$$\log\ (SB) = -\ 0.222 + 1.55\pi_{3'} - 1.90\ 3'\ SIZE > I$$
$$-\ 0.780\pi_{5'} - 1.55I(4'\text{--}H)$$
$$-\ 1.32I(4'\text{--}OCH_3) + 0.958\sigma_{3'5'}$$
$$-\ 0.114\ INTERACT_{3'5'}$$

$$n = 31,\ r = 0.960,\ s = 0.364 \qquad (1)$$

each 3'-substituent extends out further than an iodo-substituent (3'-substituents smaller than iodine being assigned a value of zero); I(4'-H) and I(4'-OCH$_3$) are indicator variables for 4'-H and 4'-OCH$_3$ substitution respectively; $\sigma_{3'5'}$ is the sum of σ_p values for 3'- and 5'-substituents in analogs where a 4'-hydroxyl is present; INTERACT$_{3'5'}$ is an estimate[133] of the energy (in kcal/mol) required to orient the 4'-hydroxyl from a conformation *cis* to the 3'-substituent to a conformation *cis* to the 5'-substituent. In compounds with different 3'- and 5'-substituents, the larger substituent is assumed to reside in a distal 3'-position, on the basis of the conformational requirements for activity and affinity (see above). Equation 1 predicts that (a) increasing 3'-substituent lipophilicity will increase affinity until 3'-substituent "size" is equal to iodine; further increase in 3'-substituent "size" then reduces affinity, (b) 5'-substitution decreases affinity in proportion to 5'-substituent lipophilicity or bulk, (c) 4'-H and 4'-OCH$_3$ substitution cause considerable loss of affinity, suggesting an important role for the 4'-hydroxyl, and (d) 3'- and 5'-substituents which are electron withdrawing, and can orient the 4'-hydroxyl *cis* to the 5'-substituent, will increase affinity.

Prediction (d) rests upon the effectiveness of the $\sigma_{3'5'}$ and INTERACT$_{3'5'}$ terms in Equation 1; these terms make only a marginal contribution being statistically significant at p $\sim$ 0.05.[114] Inspection of the parameters used in Equation 1 reveals that a single analog, the 3'-NO$_2$-4'-OH derivative, has the largest $\sigma_{3'5'}$ and INTERACT$_{3'5'}$ terms and that this derivative *alone* makes $\sigma_{3'5'}$ and INTERACT$_{3'5'}$ statistically relevant in Equation 1. The use of the 3' SIZE $>$ I parameter masks the close correlation between π and size terms and allows affinities of analogs with 3'-substituents smaller than iodine to be accounted for by $\pi_{3'}$.

We have derived new QSAR equations in order to re-examine the value of $\pi_{3'}$, 3' SIZE $>$ I, $\sigma_{3'5'}$ and INTERACT$_{3'5'}$ in predicting affinities. We have utilized the most recent and extensive compilation by Jorgensen and Bolger[134] of reported affinities of 37 analogs (Figure 5) for the solubilized rat hepatic receptor, which include all of the compounds used in Equation 1, and six additional closely related congeners. Equation 2 uses the same parameters[114] as in Equation 1, and is very similar

$$\log (SB) = -0.437 + 180\pi_{3'} - 2.30\ 3'\ SIZE > I$$

$$- 0.712\pi_{5'} - 1.33I(4'-H)$$

$$- 1.10I(4'-OCH_3) + 0.898\sigma_{3'5'}$$

$$- 0.0793\ INTERACT_{3'5'}$$

$$n = 37,\ r = 0.954,\ s = 0.354 \tag{2}$$

to Equation 1, except that the $\sigma_{3'5'}$ and $INTERACT_{3'5'}$ terms are now *not* significant ($p > 0.05$). We have also shown that the terms $\pi_{3'}$, $3'\ SIZE > I$ and $\pi_{5'}$ in Equation 2 can be replaced by $MR_{3'}^I$ and $MR_{5'}$ to give Equation 3. $MR_{3'}^I$ is a steric difference term, being defined as the

$$\log (SB) = 1.88 - 1.67\ MR_{3'}^I - 0.709\ MR_{5'}$$

$$- 1.42I(4'-H) - 1.03I(4'-OCH_3)$$

$$+ 1.56\sigma_{3'5'} - 0.276\ INTERACT_{3'5'}$$

$$n = 37,\ r = 0.958,\ s = 0.332 \tag{3}$$

magnitude of the difference in molar refractivity[132] between each 3'-substituent and a 3'-iodo substituent. $MR_{5'}$ is the molar refractivity of the 5'-substituent. Equation 3 demonstrates that bulk parameters for 3'- and 5'-substituents can equally as well account for affinities as the lipophilicity parameters of Equations 1 and 2. In Equation 3, inclusion of the $\sigma_{3'5'}$ and $INTERACT_{3'5'}$ terms is statistically significant ($p < 0.01$), but, as in Equation 1, *only* because of the 3'-NO$_2$-4'-OH analog. Removal of this analog from the analysis gives Equation 4. Equation 4

$$\log (SB) = 1.96 - 1.80\ MR_{3'}^I - 0.576\ MR_{5'}$$

$$- 1.43I(4'-H) - 1.07I(4-OCH_3)$$

$$n = 36,\ r = 0.951,\ s = 0.349 \tag{4}$$

predicts affinities in terms of requirements for optimal 3'-substituent size, and minimal 5'-substituent size; the trend being the same for 4'-OH, -H, and -OCH$_3$ derivatives. Because of the ambiguous conclusions which result from Equations 1 to 4 *it is not possible from this data set to ascertain the lipophilic (or hydrophilic) nature of both 3'- and 5'-substituent binding sites.*

The 3'-NO$_2$-4'-OH derivative has weaker affinity than predicted by Equation 4. This could be due to (a) the strong intramolecular H-bond between the 4'-hydroxyl and 3'-nitro groups (Jorgensen et al.[114] used a calculated $INTERACT_{3'5'} = 8.29$ kcal/mol), (b) the hydrophilicity of the nitro group, or (c) the high acidity of the 4'-hydroxyl group ($pk_a = 6.85$),[135] leading to substantial ionization under the conditions of the assay. Clearly this analog is yielding important information about the interaction of 3'-substituents and the 4'-hydroxyl with the nuclear receptor. The best means of helping to establish which properties of the 3'-NO$_2$-4'-OH analog are influencing receptor affinity is to examine additional hydrophilic 3'-substituents with differing interactive effects with the 4'-hydroxyl.

We have synthesized and tested the additional 3′-substituted-3,5-diiodothyronines in Table 2 (i.e., compounds 18 to 32) specifically in order to examine the effects on in vitro affinity (and also in vivo activity) of 3′-substituent size, lipophilicity, and interactive effects with the 4′-hydroxyl. Our measurements of in vitro binding affinity to intact rat liver nuclei and in vivo thyromimetic GPDH activity of these new analogs, and of the known 3′-substituted-3,5-diiodothyronines, are given in Table 2. The in vitro affinities of the homologous alkyl series from ethyl (3) to n-hexyl (20) change little as the series is ascended. The next member, n-heptyl (21) has reduced affinity, but the cyclohexylmethyl derivative (22) maintains approximately the same affinity as the lower members of the series. Phenyl (10) and phenylalkyl (11, 24) substituents have weaker affinities than seen in the alkyl series. These data suggest that the 3′-substituent binding site must be capable of accepting substituents somewhat larger than an iodo-substituent.

The nuclear binding affinities observed with the compounds 25 to 32 indicate that the 3′-substituent binding site is probably lipophilic. The carboxylic acids 28 and 31, and the aminomethyl derivative 29 in particular have extremely weak affinities. These compounds will be almost completely ionized and hence highly hydrophilic, under the conditions (pH 7.8) of the in vitro nuclear binding assay. In addition, neutral hydrophilic 3′-substituents containing hydroxyl and methoxyl groups, i.e., 25, 26, 27, and 32, have markedly weaker receptor affinities than lipophilic 3′-substituents of the same size.

Using the in vitro affinity data in Table 2 (nuclear binding — NB) we have generated QSAR Equations 5 and 6. In these equations, $f_{3'}$ is the hydrophobic

$$\log NB = -1.49 + 0.568f_{3'} + 3.45MR_{3'} - 4.74\log (\alpha\, 0.10MR_{3'} + 1)$$

$$n = 27, r = 0.967, s = 0349, \alpha = 0.10$$

$$\text{optimal } MR_{3'} = 1.46 \tag{5}$$

$$\log NB = 1.07 + 0.535f_{3'} + 1.67\, MR_{3'} < I - 0.996\, MR_{3'} > I$$

$$n = 27, r = 0.964, s = 0.361$$

$$MR_{3'}\,(I) = 1.394 \tag{6}$$

fragmental constant for the 3′-substituent, calculated according to Rekker's[136,137] method. (For all practical QSAR purposes, $f_{3'}$ and $\pi_{3'}$ are colinear). $MR_{3'}$ is the molar refractivity[132] of the 3′-substituent, and $MR_{3'} < I$ and $MR_{3'} > I$ are the differences in $MR_{3'}$ between iodine and the smaller and larger 3′-substituents, respectively. Although $f_{3'}$ and $MR_{3'}$ are still somewhat colinear (r = 0.671), Equations 5 and 6 provide good support for a lipophilic 3′-substituent binding site. The $MR_{3'}$ terms in Equation 5 use the bilinear model[138] to describe an optimal 3′-substituent size requirement. The ascending and descending parts of the bilinear function have different slopes. The initial slope for the ascending curve is 3.45 and the descending curve has a slope of −1.29. This indicates that decreasing substituent size from the optimum causes a more rapid loss of affinity than increasing it over the optimum value. The calculated optimum $MR_{3'}$ from Equation 5 is 1.46, being very close to the value for an iodo substituent, (1.394). Using iodine as a size limiter gives Equation 6. The different coefficients in $MR_{3'} < I$ and $MR_{3'} > I$ in Equation 6 reflect the relative sensitivity to $MR_{3'}$ variations seen in Equation 5.

The 3′-nitro (13) and 3′-acetyl (30) compounds were not used in the derivation of Equations 5 and 6. These compounds possess strong intramolecular H-bonds between the 3′-substituent

Table 3
STRENGTH OF 4'-
HYDROXYL
INTERACTION WITH
SOLUBLE NUCLEAR
RECEPTOR IN 3'-
SUBSTITUTED 3,5-
DIIODOTHYRONINES

$R_{3'}$	$\Delta G(OH)$[a] Kcal/mol
H	−1.24
F	−1.56
Me	−1.60
Et	−2.03
Cl	−2.04
Br	−2.48
iPr	−2.54
I	−1.83, −3.60[b]
NO₂	−1.05
tBu	−1.95

[a]   Reference 134.
[b]   Reference 114.

and 4'-hydroxyl, of approximately 7 to 8 kcal/mol,[133] and their affinities are considerably overestimated by Equations 5 and 6. The other 3'-substituents in Table 2 would be expected to form intramolecular hydrogen bonds with the 4'-hydroxyl with energies of ∼3 to 4 kcal/mol (-CH₂OH, -CH₂OCH₃),[139] ∼2 kcal/mol (halogens, -OH, phenyl),[133] ∼ 0 kcal/mol (benzyl, allyl)[140] and ∼ −1 kcal/mol (alkyls)[133] based on published data for the parent phenols. These weaker interactions, when substituent lipophilicity and bulk are taken into consideration, do not affect affinity to any appreciable extent. These findings support the suggestion[119] that the 4'-hydroxyl interacts with the receptor via hydrogen bond donation. The strong intramolecular hydrogen bonds seen in 3'-acetyl and 3'-nitro analogs presumably inhibit interaction with the receptor and consequently these compounds have lower affinities than expected. It has been suggested from theoretical studies[119] that the 4'-hydroxyl is likely to be oriented *trans-* to the 3'-substituent, and in the plane of the aromatic ring, when interacting with the receptor. This model would account for the negative contribution to affinity of 5'-substitution[114] through steric inhibition of 4'-hydroxyl-receptor hydrogen bonding. This is supported by X-ray crystallographic findings with T_3 analogs[141] and model *ortho*-substituted phenols.[142] These studies show that the donor hydrogen is located *trans-* to the substituent of 2-substituted phenols and weaker hydrogen bonds occur in hindered 2,6-disubstituted phenols. There is, however, no direct experimental evidence to support any particular orientation of the *receptor bound* 4'-hydroxyl group.

The free energy contributions to binding affinity made by the 4'-hydroxyl, ($\Delta G(OH)$) can be determined from the difference in nuclear binding affinities between the 4'-deoxy analog and the corresponding 4'-hydroxyl compound.[114,134] These values of $\Delta G(OH)$ for ten 3'-substituents[134] have been calculated and are given in Table 3. In separate publications, Jorgensen and co-authors have correlated these $\Delta G(OH)$ values with 3'-substituent 4'-hydroxyl interactive and electronic effects,[114] 3'-substituent steric or lipophilic effects,[134] and a combination of steric, electronic, and interactive effects.[119] However, the different values quoted for $\Delta G(OH)$ for the 3'-iodo analog (T_3) (−3.60[114,119] and −1.83 kcal/mol[134]) add some confusion to the presented arguments.

From Table 3, it is apparent that −$\Delta G(OH)$ increases linearly with increasing 3'-substi-

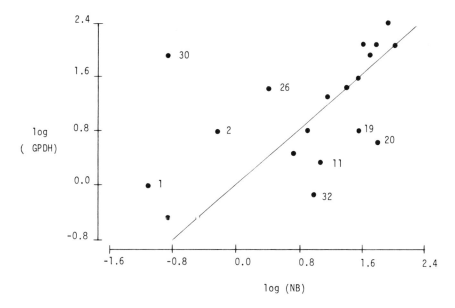

FIGURE 6. Correlation between rat liver thyromimetic potency in vivo (GPDH) and rat liver intact nuclear binding affinity in vitro (NB) for the fully active 3′-substituted-3,5-diiodothyronines in Table 2.

tuent size,[134] up to 3′-isopropyl, then decreases with the bulkier 3′-t-butyl and with 3′-nitro. A similar relationship is observed between 3′-substituent size and receptor affinities of the 3′-substituted thyronines used[134] to derive the ΔG(OH) values, and therefore ΔG(OH) and affinity are colinear. One explanation of these results is that the 4′-hydroxyl-receptor inter-action becomes more favorable as a result of subtle diphenyl ether conformational changes arising from increasingly beneficial 3′-substituent-receptor contacts. The weak ΔG(OH) for the 3′-nitro derivative is consistent with the presence of an intramolecular hydrogen bond in this compound and the 3′-t-butyl derivative could, additionally, sterically interfere with 4′-hydroxyl-receptor hydrogen bonding.

In vivo GPDH activities in the 3′-substituted series (Table 2) are best examined by first considering the correlation with affinity in vitro. The hydroxyl substituted compounds 12, 25, and 27 and the ionized (at physiological pH) compounds 28, 29, and 31 have the weakest in vitro affinities and are either inactive as agonists in vivo or are incapable of giving full agonist responses. Also, some compounds with high affinities in vitro, the 3′-n-heptyl (21) and 3′-cyclohexylmethyl (22) analogs, are not full agonists. The relationship between potency in vivo and affinity in vitro for the full agonists in Table 2 is given in Figure 6. Four compounds, 3′-H (1), 3′-CH$_3$ (2), 3′-CH$_2$OCH$_3$ (26), and especially 3′-COCH$_3$ (30), have higher potencies than affinities. Another four compounds, 3′-CH$_2$Ph (11), 3′-(CH$_2$)$_4$CH$_3$ (19), 3′-(CH$_2$)$_5$CH$_3$ (20), and 3′-(CH$_2$)$_4$OCH$_3$ (32) have higher affinities than potencies. Three of the compounds in Table 2 which show the greatest discrepancy between in vitro affinity and in vivo activity were selected for in vivo affinity measurements, and this study shows (Table 4) that in vivo activity correlates with in vivo affinity, supporting the nuclear receptor hypothesis[41] for thyroid hormone action. The discrepancies seen between in vitro affinity and in vivo activity could be due to the operation of pharmacokinetic effects, such as relative solubility, metabolic conversion, plasma protein binding,[112,113] transport to nuclear receptors,[143] or a combination of these. Figure 7 shows that these pharmacokinetic phenomena are apparently related to 3′-substituent bulk; as 3′-substituent MR increases, there is an increasing tendency for the ratio of in vivo potency to in vitro affinity to decrease. Excluding compound 30, an obvious outlier, Equation 7 is obtained, and analysis of 3′-alkyl and aryl compounds alone, gives Equation 8. Use of Equations

Table 4
COMPARISON OF AFFINITIES IN VITRO
AND IN VIVO WITH IN VIVO GPDH
ACTIVITIES

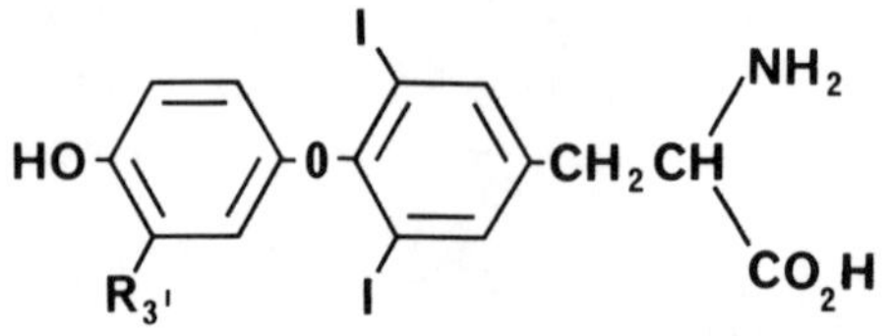

		Nuclear binding		
No.[a]	**$R_{3'}$**	**In vitro[d]**	**In vivo[e]**	**Activity in vivo GPDH[c]**
30[j]	$COCH_3$	0.3	47	121
20[b]	$(CH_2)_5CH_3$	60	>1[f]	5
21[b]	$(CH_2)_6CH_3$	8.7	(63)[g]	(38)[h]

[a] All compounds are L-alanine derivatives unless otherwise in-
    dicated; numbered as in Table 2.
[b] SK & F, unpublished compounds.
[c] See Table 1.
[d] SK & F, unpublished data; intact rat liver nuclei, $T_3 = 100$.
[e] Measured in rat liver after 1 hr in vivo; $T_3 = 100$, ED_{50} for
    T_3, 31 nmol/kg.
[f] Approximate figure.
[g] % Of maximum nuclear occupation achieved.
[h] % Of maximum response achieved.
[i] Low maximum response.
[j] Reference 135.

$$\log (GPDH) = 1.05 + 0.959 \log (NB) - 0.585 \, MR_{3'}$$

$$n = 18, r = 0.872, s = 0.447 \tag{7}$$

$$\log (GPDH) = 1.33 + 0.957 \log (NB) - 0.671 \, MR_{3'}$$

$$n = 12, r = 0.932, s = 0.313 \tag{8}$$

7 and 8 in conjunction with Equations 5 and 6 permits the prediction of in vitro affinities
and in vivo potencies of untested 3'-substituted analogs.

The Ether Link

The limited studies to date with analogs containing linking groups other than oxygen
between the aromatic rings have supported the notion that the ether link serves primarily to
maintain a specific orthogonal (skewed or twist-skewed) diphenyl ether conformation. Accordingly, sulfur (Table 5, 4 to 6) and methylene (3) analogs retain substantial in vitro
affinity and in vivo activity. Attempts[144] to prepare amino linked analogs were unsuccessful.
Removal of the linking atom with retention of the orthogonal arrangement, as in biphenyl
derivatives (2) leads to a complete loss of activity and a large reduction in affinity. This
underlines the necessity for the specific spatial positioning of the 4'-hydroxyl and 3'-iodo
groups relative to the remainder of the molecule since it is this aspect of structure which is
not retained in biphenyl compounds.

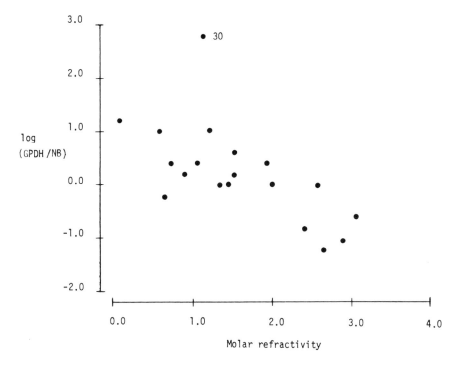

FIGURE 7. Correlation between the ratio rat liver potency in vivo to affinity in vitro (GPDH/NB) and molar refractivity of the 3′-substituent for the fully active 3′-substituted-3,5-diiodothyronines in Table 2.

Table 5
ETHER LINK ANALOGS

No.[a]	X	$R_{3'}$	Activity in vivo Antigoiter[d]	GPDH[e]	Nuclear binding in vitro[f]
1	0	I	100	100	100
2[b]	—	I	0	LM[g]	0.9
3[b]	CH_2	I	54	F[h]	183 (250[i])
4	S	I	14	4.5	185 (100[i])
5[c]	S	iPr		639	291
6[c]	S	H		0.2	7.4
7	0	H		1.1	0.08 (0.3[i])

[a] All compounds are L-alanine derivatives unless otherwise indicated.

[b] DL-.

[c] SK & F, unpublished compounds.

[d] References 112 and 113, $T_3 = 100$.

[e] See Table 1.

[f] SK & F, unpublished data; intact rat liver nuclei, $T_3 = 100$.

[g] Low maximum response.

[h] Full agonist.

[i] Reference 112.

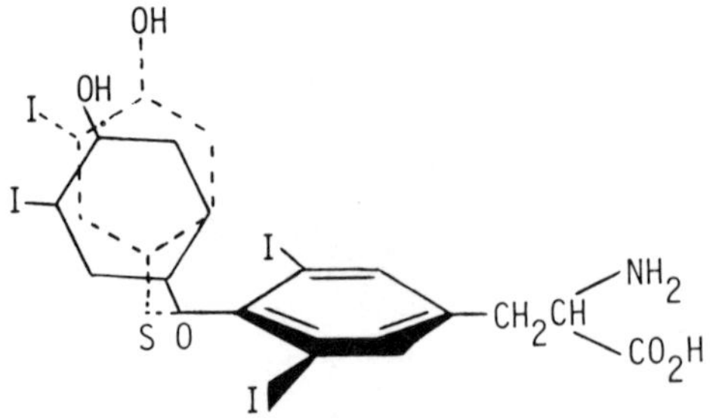

FIGURE 8. Superimposition of the phenolic rings of T_3 (solid lines) and the proposed structure for thio-T_3 (dotted lines), showing the relative positions of 3'-iodo and 4'-hydroxyl groups; both molecules are assumed to adopt the same skewed diphenyl ether conformation.

It has been suggested,[145] on the basis of a comparison of the crystal structures of triiodothyroacetic acid with 2,4-dinitrodiphenylsulfide, that diphenyl thioether substitution might cause displacements of the 3',4',5'-substituents relative to the same substituents in diphenyl ethers (Figure 8). These differences are a consequence of the lengthening of the bridge bonds (1.397 Å → 1.774 Å) with a concomitant decrease in bridge angle (120° → 104°) in going from ether to thioether. Use of molecular graphics showed that the sulfur analog of thyroxine would be expected to show similar large displacements compared with thyroxine. As a result, Cody[145] suggested that 2'-,3'-, and 4'-substituents in diphenylthioethers may be capable of interacting with the same parts of the receptor as 3',4'-, and 5'-substituents in diphenylethers with the implication that a 2',4'-diiodo-3'-hydroxy sulfur analog may bind. However, more structural information of sulfur bridged thyronines is necessary since this suggestion is based on the use of the geometry of 2,4-dinitrodiphenylsulfide, in which the nitro substituents are likely to cause a reduction in the nitrophenyl C-S bond length compared with other diarylsulfides.

In this context it is notable that we find a 100-fold difference in in vitro affinity between T_2 and thio-T_2 (Table 5, compare 6 and 7). The 2'- and 3'-hydrogens in thio-T_2 could be interacting more favorably with the receptor than in T_2 as a consequence of a change in the relative position of the phenolic ring in the receptor bound conformation. This large difference in affinity is not seen, however, with the 3'-iodo analogs (compare 1 and 4), and raises the possibility that thio-T_2 and thio-T_3 analogs bind to the receptor with different conformations of the diphenylthioether.

The in vivo potencies of thio-T_2 and thio-T_3 are considerably weaker than would be expected from in vitro binding affinities, in contrast to the 3'-isopropyl thio-T_2 (Table 5, 5). The reasons for these discrepancies are unclear.

The Alanine-Bearing Ring

The 3,5-Substituents

The 3,5-iodo substituents in the natural hormones play an important role in establishing the diphenyl ether conformation. Maintenance of the correct mutually perpendicular arrangement of the aromatic rings in thyroid hormone analogs is an essential requirement for in vivo activity and in vitro affinity.[112,113] Andrea et al.[119] have calculated the free energy required to "lock" the aromatic rings in the favored orthogonal conformation. In a series of 3,5-dialkyl and dihalo derivatives, this free energy requirement correlates with in vitro binding affinity to the solubilized rat liver nuclear receptor.

X-ray crystal structure analyses[146] have revealed that an analog with 3,5-groups as small as methyl can adopt the identical orthogonal diphenyl ether conformation as seen with 3,5-

Table 6
3,5-SUBSTITUTED ANALOGS

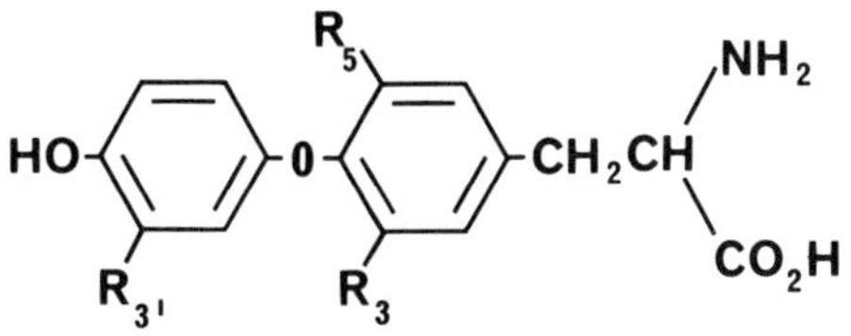

No.[a]	R_3	R_5	$R_{3'}$	Activity in vivo Antigoiter[d]	GPDH[e]	Nuclear binding in vitro[f]
1	I	I	I	100	100	100
2[b]	Br	Br	iPr	30		36[j]
3[b]	Cl	Cl	Cl	0.09		
4	CH_3	CH_3	iPr	3.6	16	0.4 (0.7[i])
5[b]	Et	Et	I			0.65[g]
6[b]	iPr	iPr	iPr		LM[h]	0.2
7[b]	sBu	sBu	I	0		
8[c]	CN	CN	iPr		LM[h]	0.04
9[b]	NH_2	NH_2	CH_3	0		
10	NO_2	NO_2	H	0		
11	SEt	SEt	iPr	0		
12	SPh	SPh	iPr	0		
13[b]	I	H	I	0.06	0	0.35 (0.75[g])
14[b]	I	CH_3	I	3.6		
15[b]	I	Br	I	41		
16	H	H	I	<0.006		0.0004[g]

[a]   All compounds are L-alanine derivatives unless otherwise indicated.

[b]   DL-.

[c]   SK & F, unpublished compounds.

[d]   References 112 and 113, $T_3 = 100$.

[e]   See Table 1.

[f]   SK & F, unpublished data; intact rat liver nuclei, $T_3 = 100$.

[g]   Reference 134, solubilized rat liver nuclei, $T_3 = 100$.

[h]   Low maximum response.

[i]   Reference 114.

[j]   Reference 112.

diiodo substitution. It might be expected therefore that 3,5-dialkyl substitution with other alkyl groups would also lead to retention of the correct conformation. Making the assumption that 3,5-dialkyl and 3,5-dihalogen analogs possess similar conformations, the higher affinities and activities seen with 3,5-halogens compared with 3,5-alkyls of approximately the same size and lipophilicity (e.g., Table 6, I vs. iPr, Br vs. Me or Et), imply that halogens exert an additional beneficial direct effect upon affinity. It has been suggested[134] that this could arise as a result of the greater polarizability of halogen atoms. Another possibility is an electronic effect arising from electron withdrawal from the aromatic ring. The weak in vitro affinity of the dicyano derivative (Table 6, 8) suggests that the 3,5-binding sites could be lipophilic, but it is not certain whether the 3,5-dicyano groups are bulky enough to constrain the diphenyl ether in the correct conformation.

If a single iodine atom is retained at the 3-position, activity increases as the 5-position is substituted with increasingly larger groups (Table 6, 1, 13, 14, 15). The high activity of the 3,5-dimethyl analog, DIMIT (4),[147] is apparently caused by in vivo pharmacokinetic effects, since this analog has weak in vitro affinity. Other 3,5-dialkyl, dicyano, diamino, dinitro, and dithioether analogs (Table 6, 6 to 12) are inactive in vivo.

Table 7
SIDE CHAIN ANALOGS

No.	R_1	$R_{3'}$	Activity in vivo Antigoiter[b]	GPDH[c]	Nuclear binding in vitro[d]
1	L-CH$_2$CH(NH$_2$)CO$_2$H	I	100	100	100
2	D-CH$_2$CH(NH$_2$)CO$_2$H	I	7.5	44	36 (63.8[e])
3	CO$_2$H	I	0.05		8.5[e]
4	CH$_2$CO$_2$H	iPr		58	154
5	CH$_2$CO$_2$H	I	6.5	F[f]	421 (282.5[e])
6	(CH$_2$)$_2$CO$_2$H	I	4.5	1.9	624 (234.5[e])
7[a]	(CH$_2$)$_2$CO$_2$H	iPr		2.4	402
8	(CH$_2$)$_3$CO$_2$H	I	1		14[e]
9	NH$_2$	I	0.2		
10	(CH$_2$)$_2$NH$_2$	I	2		
11[a]	(CH$_2$)$_2$NH$_2$	iPr		21	0.3
12[a]	L-CH$_2$CH(NHAc)CO$_2$H	iPr		234	0.5

[a]   SK & F, unpublished compounds.
[b]   References 112 and 113, T_3 = 100.
[c]   See Table 1.
[d]   SK & F, unpublished data; intact rat liver nuclei, T_3 = 100.
[e]   Reference 134, solubilized rat liver nuclei, T_3 = 100.
[f]   Full agonist.

The Alanine Side Chain

A large number of thyronine derivatives in which the L-alanine side chain has been modified have been reported.[110-113] For the purpose of this review only those compounds with a 3'-iodo or 3'-isopropyl substituent, i.e., close analogs of T_3 will be discussed. The L-alanine side chain is not essential for thyromimetic activity. The D-enantiomer (Table 7, 2) has slightly reduced GPDH activity and affinity, but markedly reduced antigoiter activity. The N-acetyl L-alanine derivative (Table 7, 12) which has a weak in vitro affinity, is also substantially active in vivo, presumably due to hydrolysis to the free L-alanine. Perhaps the most important observation with side-chain thyroid hormone analogs is the lack of an absolute requirement for the amino group. Thus, carboxylic acid derivatives (Table 7, 3 to 8) possess substantial in vitro affinities, suggesting that ion-pairing of the carboxylate anions with a positively charged receptor group may be involved. The requirement for location of the carboxylate within the side chain substituent appears to be quite flexible. Only with the lowest and highest members of the series (Table 7, 3 and 8) is weaker affinity in vitro observed. These observations could indicate that there is a degree of flexibility in the receptor structure, or that the receptor is large enough to allow the carboxylic side chains to adopt the best conformations to interact with a specifically located positive charge or hydrogen bonding group. Despite their high affinities in vitro, the carboxylic acid derivatives, notably 6, 7, and 8 (Table 7) have relatively weak activities in vivo compared with their receptor affinities in vitro. This is likely to be due to shorter halflives of these compounds in vivo compared with T_3, since Oppenheimer et al.[148] have observed a relatively rapid turnover for

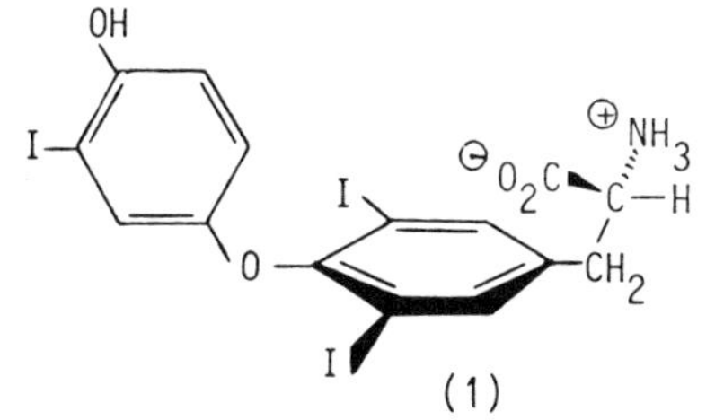

FIGURE 9. Structures of T$_3$, showing side chain *cis* (1) and *trans* (2) conformations.

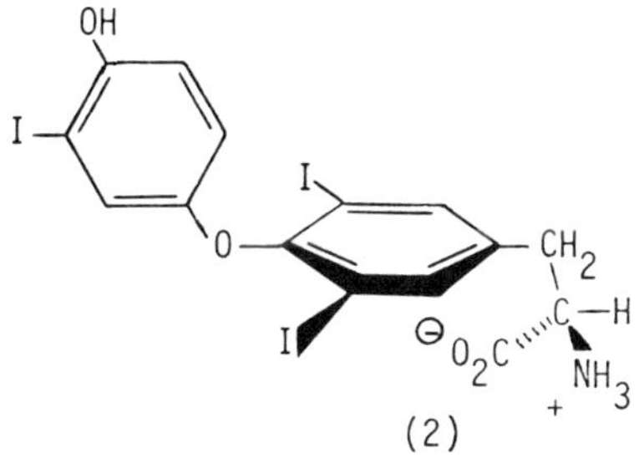

Triac (5) in vivo, and we have observed a halflife of 90 min for nuclear occupation of 7, compared with 11 hr for T$_3$.

The decarboxylated alanine derivatives (Table 7, 10 and 11) bind only weakly in vitro, yet are more active in vivo. This is reminiscent of several other analogs already mentioned, and could result from a higher effective nuclear concentration of active species as a result of pharmacokinetic effects. This is supported by the observation that 3'-isopropyl-3,5-diiodothyronamine (11) depresses in vivo T$_3$ binding to liver nuclear receptors effectively at 1 hr (EC$_{50}$ ~5% T$_3$).

The conformation of the L-alanine side-chain when receptor bound is unknown. Cody[115,116] has discussed the side-chain conformations seen in X-ray crystal structures of thyroid hormones and analogs. The CH$_2$-CH bond lies perpendicular to the aromatic ring, resulting in overall cisoid or transoid conformations (Figure 9). In addition, rotamers are observed where either H, CO$_2^-$, or NH$_3^+$ groups are fully extended with respect to the aromatic ring.

Binding to Plasma Proteins

General Aspects

An understanding of the structural requirements for binding to plasma proteins (TBG, TBPA, and SA) is essential in the consideration of the relationship between in vitro nuclear binding and in vivo activities.[112] Structure-affinity relationships with plasma proteins have been discussed at length by Jorgensen,[112,113] and can be compared with structure-affinity relationships with the nuclear receptor.[149,150] Relative affinities of some representative analogs for TBG, TBPA, SA, and nuclear receptor are given in Table 8. The principal trends can be summarized as follows.

1. 3',5'-Dihalosubstitution is the most important structural requirement for high affinity to all three plasma proteins; it is probable that this binding occurs via the 4'-phenolate anion.[149] Minor effects of bulk and lipophilicity of 3',5'-substituents are also seen. This contrasts with structure-affinity relationships to nuclear receptors, where bulk and lipophilic effects of 3',5'-substituents are dominant, and the unionized 4'-hydroxyl binds (see above).

Table 8
RELATIVE BINDING AFFINITIES OF THYROID
HORMONE ANALOGS TO TBG, TBPA, SA, AND
NUCLEAR RECEPTOR

Analog	TBG[a]	TBPA[b]	SA[a]	Nuclear receptor[c]
T_4	100	100	100	100
D-T_4	54	3.7	100	
T_3	9	9.2	4.9	694
D-T_3		0.25		436
3,3′,5′-T_3(rT_3)	38	33	3	1.3
3′-iPr-T_2	3.5	0.8		643
3′-iPr-3,5-Me_2-T_2	0.05			3.3
3′-I-3,5-Me_2-T_2		0.8		3.75
Tetrac[d]	1.7	676	20	
Triac[e]	0.3	20		1983
Thyroxamine[f]		0.4	6.4	<0.03

[a]   Reference 112.
[b]   Reference 149.
[c]   Reference 134, solubilized rat liver nuclei.
[d]   3,3′,5,5′-Tetraiodothyroacetic acid.
[e]   3,3′,5-Triiodothyroacetic acid.
[f]   Descarboxy-T_4.

2.   An intact diphenyl ether nucleus is important for binding to TBG, but some single
      ring *ortho*-diiodophenols have been shown to possess high affinities for TBPA[151] and
      SA.[152]
3.   Binding of L-alanine side chain analogs to TBG utilizes both ammonium and carbox-
      ylate ions, whereas both TBPA and nuclear receptor require the carboxylate ion only
      for high affinity.[149] Nuclear receptor and TBG[112] show slight preference and TBPA[149,153]
      shows greater preference for L-alanine groups, whereas SA[112] is not enantioselective.

Thyroxine Binding Prealbumin (TBPA) and the Nuclear Receptor

     Establishment of structure-affinity relationships with plasma proteins has received con-
siderable impetus recently from the determination of the X-ray crystal structure of TBPA.[120,154]
The structures of both TBPA and TBPA with T_4 bound, have been determined at 1.8 Å
resolution. This has permitted, for the first time, a detailed description of a protein-hormone
interaction.[121] TBPA is a tetramer, composed of identical subunits held together by hydrogen
bonding and hydrophobic interactions. A cylindrical channel, approximately 8 Å wide and
50 Å long, runs right through the center of the molecule, and two deep semi-cylindrical
grooves are seen on its outer surface. Because of the symmetry of the molecule, the central
channel gives rise to two identical hormone binding sites. The affinities of T_4 for these two
sites are 1×10^{-8} mol^{-1} and, when the first site is occupied, about 1×10^{-6} mol^{-1},[154]
suggesting negative cooperativity. The hormone binding site in TBPA has also been examined
in solution, by observation of ESR spectra of spin labeled nitroxide side chain T_4 analogs;[155]
this work suggested that the overall lengths of the binding channel of TBPA in solution and
in the crystal are similar, and slightly smaller than the hormone binding sites in TBG and
SA.

     The T_4 binding site in TBPA has been described in some detail (Figure 10).[121] T_4 binds
into the central channel with the 4′-hydroxyl near the center and the alanine side chain near
the opening. The 4′-hydroxyl or 4′-phenoxide ion is seemingly hydrogen bonded to a water
molecule, which in turn is hydrogen bonded to Ser and Thr hydroxyls, and the alanine side
chain ammonium and carboxylate groups are ion-paired with Lys and Glu residues. The

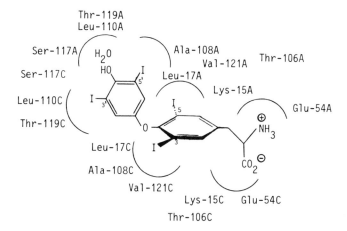

FIGURE 10. A schematic representation of the T_4 binding site in prealbumin, showing some of the amino acid residues which form the site.
Adapted from References 121 and 154.

3,5-iodines interact with identical essentially hydrophobic pockets, composed of the methyls
of Leu, Thr, Ala, and Val residues and possibly a Lys side chain and the hydroxyl of the
Thr residue. The 3′-iodine, *distal* to the inner ring, binds into a pocket with some hydrophilic
character, made up of amide backbone and hydroxyl groups, and the methyls of Ala and
Leu residues. The 5′-iodine, *proximal* to the inner ring, binds to a site not symmetrically
related to the 3′-binding site, consisting of a Lys carboxyl, and amide backbone group, and
the methyls of Ala and Leu residues. The 3,5,3′,5′-iodo binding sites for T_4 seem to be
tailored to make use of different physical properties of iodine, i.e., mainly lipophilic binding
at the 3,5-positions, and mainly polarizability/charge transfer binding at the 3′,5′-positions.
The greater contribution to binding of the 3′,5′-iodines relative to the 3,5-iodines[149] could
be a result of the effect of the 3′,5′-iodines on the acidity of the adjacent 4′-hydroxyl, (i.e.,
ionization) in addition to the more polarizable nature of the 3′,5′-binding sites relative to
the 3,5-binding sites.

Computer generated models of the T_4 binding site have been used to model the binding
of T_4 analogs.[121] A colored representation of the hydrophilic and hydrophobic surfaces of
the binding site permitted unfilled binding "pockets" to be visualized. The prediction was
made that 2′-substituted thyronines would interact profitably with an empty pocket in the
binding site near the 2′-position. The qualitative prediction of relative binding affinities
which resulted was conformed when the affinities of four previously untested 2′,3′-naphthyl
derivatives were measured. This study confirms the expectation that molecular modeling of
hormone-protein (or drug-receptor) interactions can provide a powerful means of designing
new, tightly bound analogs.

A QSAR study of analog-binding to prealbumin, using a distance geometry technique,
has been reported.[156] This method gave rise to a proposed binding site closely matching the
observed site seen in the crystal structure.

The surface grooves on TBPA have been shown to be structurally complementary to the
DNA double helix,[120,154] although experimentally DNA-TBPA binding has not been observed. It has been shown[157] that this putative DNA binding site of TBPA is probably not
electrostatically complementary to DNA. Since the nuclear receptor is known to bind DNA,
and have a similar mol wt (ca. 55,000) to TBPA, speculation has arisen that both proteins
could be derived from the same evolutionary precursor and may have much in common
structurally. Evidence supporting the structural similarity of nuclear receptor and TBPA,
based on analog binding affinities to a purified or "core" form of the receptor,[154] is no

longer valid, since this form of the receptor[65] (with a high affinity for T_4) is now known to be an artefact.[66]

The relationship between TBPA and nuclear receptor has been examined by comparisons of binding affinities, and structure-affinity relationships, with a variety of analogs.[112,149,150] These studies have revealed differences, which, in the light of the known structure of TBPA, have led some authors to suggest components of nuclear receptor structure. These studies are outlined below.

Outer Ring Substituents

Comparisons of the free energy contributions to binding affinities made by the 4'-hydroxyl in the presence of different 3'-substituents showed that the 4'-hydroxyl contributes about -2 kcal/mol to nuclear receptor binding (see Table 3), but negligibly to TBPA binding.[150] The small contribution of the 4'-hydroxyl to TBPA binding was considered unsurprising[150] since the hydrogen bonds between solvent water and the 4'-hydroxyl must be broken at the onset of binding, but then reformed between the 4'-hydroxyl and the crystallographically observed water molecule and Ser and Thr hydroxyls in the binding site. If the number of hydrogen bonds broken and reformed are identical, and entropy changes are negligible, then the net free energy change on 4'-hydroxyl binding should be close to zero. The higher contribution of the 4'-hydroxyl to nuclear receptor binding suggests that a different sort of interaction occurs. This could involve hydrogen bonding to nonhydroxylic moieties, e.g., carbonyl, amino, or carboxylate groups. This analysis[150] applies only to 3'-substituted 3,5-diiodothyronines, which might be expected to bind in the unionized form. 5'-Halo substitution in 3'-halo compounds leads to a decrease in nuclear receptor affinity, but to an increase in TBPA affinity.[149] The increase in TBPA affinity could be due to increased 4'-hydroxyl acidity, or 4'-hydroxyl ionization, or to a direct binding effect[121] of a 5'-halogen; testing of appropriate 4'-deshydroxyl-3'-5'-substituted compounds would help to differentiate between these possibilities. In nuclear receptor binding, an unionized 4'-hydroxyl is essential; the reduced affinity seen in 5'-substituted compounds is associated with steric interference of 5'-substituents with 4'-hydroxyl hydrogen bonding or directly with the receptor. The 3',5'-binding sites in TBPA have some hydrophilic character which could be responsible for the higher affinity of halogen atoms for these sites via polarization and charge transfer effects. With the nuclear receptor, the 3'-binding site in particular could be more lipophilic than in TBPA, the equal affinities of 3'-alkyl and halogen derivatives being explicable in terms of hydrophobic binding.

Inner Ring Substituents

With both nuclear receptor and TBPA,[149] replacement of the 3,5-iodines by alkyl groups of similar bulk leads to a loss in affinity. The effect is more pronounced with the nuclear receptor. This might mean that the nuclear receptor has somewhat more hydrophilic 3,5-iodine binding sites than in TBPA. This would support the proposal that 3,5-substituents contribute to nuclear receptor binding by polarization and/or charge transfer,[119,134] in addition to hydrophobic binding. However, the direct effects of 3,5-substitution in both TBPA and nuclear receptor are difficult to separate from the indirect effects on diphenyl ether conformational requirements.

Alanine Side Chain

TBPA and nuclear receptor are apparently similar in that carboxylate side chains have higher affinity and ammonium side chains have lower affinity, than the L-alanine side chain.[149] These results suggest that in TBPA the principal L-alanine side chain interaction is the carboxylate group ion-pairing with a Lys ammonium group at the mouth of the binding channel. Affinity labeling studies[158,159] have supported this concept. Both TBPA and nuclear receptor are enantioselective and bind L-alanine side chains better than D-alanine side chains;[149,153] the effect however is marginal with the nuclear receptor and is more pronounced with TBPA. The accommodation of side chain bulk has been examined by comparison of TBPA and nuclear receptor affinities for a series of N-acyl D- and L-T_3 and T_4 derivatives.[150] In the case of nuclear receptor, all N-acyl derivatives of D and L-T_3 showed no enantiose-lection, and 100 to 700-fold reductions in affinity. In contrast, binding to TBPA of N-acyl derivatives of D- and L-T_4 showed only 2 to 30-fold decreases in affinity, with some en-antioselection (2 to 4-fold) in favor of D-alanine derivatives being observed. These results suggested that TBPA is more tolerant than nuclear receptor to side chain bulk, and is also more discriminating with respect to location of charge. The higher affinity of TBPA for D-T_4 after acylation was explained[150] by loss of steric repulsion resulting from overall ligand-acceptor charge neutralization.

DISEASES OF THE THYROID

Various disease states are associated with the thyroid. Overproduction of thyroid hormones leads to hyperthyroidism, a syndrome of metabolic and pathological changes due to the action of elevated circulatory hormone levels on peripheral tissue. Hypothyroidism is usually caused by low circulating concentrations of thyroid hormones due to an underactive gland but can rarely be caused by end-organ resistance to the action of the hormones. The thyroid can also become enlarged to form a goiter. This may or may not be associated with a change in thyroid status.

Various laboratory tests are used to confirm diagnoses of thyroid diseases. Protein-bound iodine (PBI) is related to thyroid hormone concentration since normally at least 90% of the blood iodine is thyroxine.[29] It is however a nonspecific measure as iodine-containing drugs and other agents such as radioopaque contrast media can increase blood PBI. Some im-provement in specificity can be achieved by measuring the iodine content of acid butanol extracts of plasma (BEI). Total T_4 or T_3 can be measured by radioimmunoassay (RIA) or competitive protein binding. These measurements are not affected by other iodine-containing compounds of plasma but are altered by treatments which change the concentration of thyroid hormone binding proteins. Estimates of T_4 levels can be made using the T_3 resin uptake test, which measures the degree of saturation of plasma hormone binding sites. Again this test is subject to misinterpretation if TBG levels are abnormal. Free T_4 can now be measured by RIA.

TSH can also be measured by RIA either in the basal state or after stimulation with exogenous TRH. The function of the thyroid gland can be assessed from its capacity to accumulate and release radioactivity, after an oral dose of ^{131}I.

Hyperthyroidism

Hyperthyroidism[160] (or thyrotoxicosis) is a disease predominantly of women. The clinical signs are those which would be expected of hypermetabolism. Thus, the patients feels warm, heart rate is high, and cardiac output frequently elevated. If measured, basal metabolic rate (BMR) is greater than normal, whereas plasma cholesterol is likely to be lower than normal. Weight loss frequently occurs despite a good appetite.

A number of different diseases can cause the thyroid to be overactive. The principal cause, in the U.S. and U.K. is Graves' disease (toxic diffuse goiter). In addition to the normal symptoms of hyperthyroidism, Graves' disease is often accompanied by an extrathyroidal manifestation such as exopthalmos and pretibial myxoedema. Goiter is almost always present. Another important cause of hyperthyroidism is Plummer's disease (toxic nodular goiter). In this, the thyroid is irregularly enlarged due to the presence of nodules, which are actively secreting hormones. This accumulation is not inhibited by exogenous T_3 showing that the nodules function autonomously. Much more rarely hyperthyroidism is caused by tumors which secrete either thyroid hormone or thyroid stimulators such as TSH or human chorionic and molar thyrotrophin from the placenta.

In Graves' disease the overactivity of the thyroid is caused by abnormal IgG immunoglobulins, which bind to and activate the TSH receptor. The presence of these thyroid stimulating immunoglobulins, (TSI), in the plasma of patients, can be detected from their ability to prevent the binding of TSH to its receptor on human thyroidal plasma membranes. It can also be shown that the plasma of many patients with Graves' disease contains a component which will stimulate the mouse thyroid in vivo. This component is called the long acting thyroid stimulator (LATS) since its onset of action is slower than that of TSH but its duration is longer. In patients with detectable TSI but no LATS activity it is often possible to show that their serum will prevent LATS activity in the mouse: this is termed LATS-protector activity. These findings are interpreted as meaning that TSI are a family of immunoglobulins which are antibodies to the human TSH receptor but which, because of phylogenetic differences, may stimulate mouse thyroid TSH receptors, (i.e., have LATS activity) or inhibit their response to LATS.[161]

The sources of TSI are probably lymphocytes within the gland but why the TSH receptor should be, or become, antigenic is not known. Graves' disease is, therefore, a receptor-antibody disease like myasthenia gravis in which antibodies to the acetyl choline receptor are found.

Plasma T_4 and T_3 are usually elevated, but in rare instances an elevated T_3 level coupled with normal T_4 is found (T_3-thyrotoxicosis). Plasma TSH would be expected to be low but since many RIA methods for TSH are not sufficiently sensitive to detect levels much below normal this is sometimes difficult to prove. The response of plasma TSH to TRH stimulation is also suppressed. The presence of TSI, LATS, or LATS suppressor is also diagnostic of hyperthyroidism due to Graves' disease. Radioiodine uptake by the thyroid is elevated but is usually only used in the diagnosis of hyperfunctioning nodules or to locate ectopic or metastatic hyperfunctioning tissue.

Hypothyroidism

Hypothyroidism[162] is less common than thyrotoxicosis probably occurring in less than 0.5% of the population. The clinical features of the disease are those to be expected from a hypometabolic state. The patient is lethargic and susceptible to the cold; BMR and pulse rate are reduced, and plasma cholesterol is often elevated. In addition to these, a characteristic edema (myxoedema) is often seen due to the presence of unusual amounts of mucopolysaccharides in the skin.

Primary hypothyroidism is due to inability of the thyroid gland to produce thyroid hormones. This can be caused by a number of factors including Hashimoto's disease (see below), destructive therapy, such as radioiodine or surgery, or biosynthesis defects. These latter are discussed below in the section on goiter. Primary hypothyroidism is associated with a high circulating level of TSH.

In secondary hypothyroidism, the failure of thyroid is due to low circulating levels of TSH. This may be due to pituitary failure or in its turn, secondary to a reduced secretion of TRH by the hypothalamus. The TRH stimulation test distinguishes between these two causes.

Hypothyroidism *in utero* leads, if uncorrected at birth, to cretinism, a disease characterized by severe retardation, both physical and mental. Replacement therapy at birth can offset many of these disabilities.

Goiter

Simple goiter[163] is probably the most common disease of the thyroid, having been estimated as affecting some 200 million people throughout the world. Although it does occur sporadically, in certain parts of the world the incidence within a given population is very much higher than normal. It is then referred to as endemic goiter. Most frequently these areas provide a diet which is deficient in iodine, causing a hypothalamic-pituitary response resulting in intense thyrotropic stimulation. The consequent increase in activity of the iodide pump and size of the gland ensures that the iodide is sequestered from the blood in the most efficient manner possible. Other causes of simple goiter are dietary goitrogens and perhaps an excess of calcium in drinking water. Areas where endemic goiter occurs also suffer from a high incidence of cretinism. Simple goiters may or may not be associated with hypothyroidism.

Hashimoto's thyroiditis is an inflammation of the thyroid gland caused by circulating antibodies to either thyroglobulin or thyroidal microsomes. As with Graves' disease the reason for this antibody formation is unknown. In one series of patients suffering from this goiter 78% were euthyroid, 18% hypothyroid, and 4% hyperthyroid.[164] Other causes of goiter are infections and dyshormonogenesis due to congenital defects in the enzymatic machinery for synthesizing thyroid hormones. Again, there is no predictable effect of these diseases on thyroid status.

REPLACEMENT THERAPY AND THE USE OF THYROMIMETICS

The two major indications for the therapeutic use of thyroid hormones are hypothyroidism or myxedema and simple goiter and their use in these diseases represents true replacement therapy.[165] In addition, thyromimetics have been given to euthyroid individuals for a number of diverse conditions including obesity, hyperlipidemia, infertility, and psychiatric disorders. The majority view among clinicians at the present time is that nonthyroidal disorders should not be treated with thyroid hormones unless there is proved thyroid deficiency, largely because of the risk from adverse cardiac effects.[166,167]

Hypothyroidism and Simple Goiter[165,167-169]

Thyroid extract, as well as T_4 and T_3, are approved preparations. Variable potency of thyroid extract is a serious problem since the standard set by USP is based on total iodine content (0.17 to 0.23%) although RIA is used by some manufacturers to establish T_3 and T_4 content. In most clinical situations T_4 (levothyroxine sodium) is the preferred form of replacement and is dispensed in tablets containing 25 to 500 μg.[165] T_3 or liothyronine sodium may occasionally be preferred to T_4 when a quicker action is desired or in patients who are athyreotic, and in whom hormone therapy has been discontinued for a short while. T_4 is usually given as a single daily dose of 0.1 to 0.2 mg and T_3 is given in doses of 20 to 25 μg three times daily. The most important criteria for the final replacement dose are clinical, but T_4, T_3, and TSH levels should be assayed to ensure normality.[167]

Overtreatment with thyroid hormones causes features of hyperthyroidism and can produce cardiac complications such as angina or cardiac failure.[167,169]

Thyroid Hormone Therapy in Nonthyroid Disorders
Obesity

The recognition that weight loss occurs in hyperthyroidism, and hypothyroid patients lose weight when given thyroid hormones, led to the use of thyroid hormones for the treatment of obesity. Relatively little attention has been paid to the particular thyroid hormone analog given to obese patients. Recent evidence has suggested that T_4 conversion to T_3 is decreased in starvation with increased formation of T_3 and, therefore, whether T_3 or T_4 is given may significantly affect the amount of metabolically active hormone available in starved patients.[166]

Pharmacological doses of thyroid hormone undoubtedly result in increased weight loss and this is due to increased oxygen consumption and increased protein catabolism.[170] Doses of T_3 (100 μg/day) consistently increase metabolic rate of hospitalized obese patients, and the loss of nitrogen associated with lean body mass can be avoided if the dietary intake of protein is increased.[170] Unfortunately, weight loss may be readily and rapidly reversed after discharge from hospital unless diet is strictly controlled.[166] In addition to this difficulty in maintaining weight loss, there is a risk of cardiovascular complications and it is this side effect which has restricted the use of thyroid hormones for the treatment of obesity.

Hyperlipidemia

D-T_4 has been used as a lipid-lowering agent because its effects on serum lipids are claimed to be greater than its calorigenic effects.[166,168] It was envisaged that this selectivity would lead to a reduction in serum lipids such as cholesterol without adverse effects on the heart. Recent evidence indeed suggests that D-T_4 may increase both the conversion of cholesterol to bile acids and the uptake of low density lipoprotein (LDL) by cells.[171] However, when D-T_4 was used in the U.S. Coronary Drug Project it was necessary to terminate the study due to a high rate of cardiac deaths and nonfatal infarcts.[168] The possibility still exists, however, that this drug could be useful in patients free of coronary artery disease.

In the 1960s several groups attempted to design novel thyromimetics with an improved profile of activity as selective hypocholesterolemic agents. In particular, methyl ethers of 3,3',5-triiodo- and 3,5-diiodo-3'-isopropyl thyroacetic acids were shown to be much more active in lowering cholesterol than in increasing metabolic rate in rats.[172] However, no compounds emerged as useful therapeutic agents from these studies.

Psychiatric Disease[166]

The disturbed mental state associated with both hyper- and hypothyroidism has attracted investigators to the study of thyroid function in psychiatric patients. It has been observed that low doses of thyroid hormone potentiate the antidepressant effects of imipramine without incurring signs of hypermetabolism. Similar results were also obtained in patients who had previously been resistant to tricyclic antidepressants. These effects appear to be more marked in women than men. Thyroid hormones have been used occasionally to treat autistic and emotionally disturbed children but these reports are largely anecdotal.

Thyromimetic Therapy of the Fetus

Thyroid hormones do not pass through the placenta from maternal to fetal circulation. As a consequence the majority of intrauterine development takes place in the presence of very low concentrations of thyroid hormone until the final stages of pregnancy when the fetus starts to produce its own thyroid hormones. Among other actions these hormones stimulate the lung to produce phospholipids (surfactant) which allow it to function efficiently after birth. Failure of this maturation process leads to respiratory distress syndrome (RDS). Babies who are premature, or delivered of diabetic mothers, are particularly prone to RDS. Unlike the natural hormones, 3,5-dimethyl-3'-isopropyl-L-thyronine (L-DIMIT) has been shown to produce thyromimetic effects in the fetus when administered to the mother,[173] and it has been suggested that RDS could be prevented by prophylactic treatment of the mothers of babies at risk with DIMIT.[174] In support of this hypothesis it has been shown that treatment of diabetic, pregnant rabbits with DIMIT increased fetal lung surfactant synthesis, prolonged the survival time of prematurely delivered fetuses, and reduced fetal blood glucose and insulin levels.[175] This method of alleviating fetal hypothyroidism has not yet been used in humans.

In summary it may be said that (1) the majority of these nonthyroidal disorders, where thyroid hormone therapy has been tried, also tends to occur in the hypothyroid patient, (2) definitive results are lacking in the euthyroid patient, (3) the results of therapy are often difficult to determine, and (4) the risk of cardiac complications will necessarily limit the use of thyroid hormones.

TREATMENT OF HYPERTHYROIDISM

The therapeutic options available for the treatment of hyperthyroidism can be categorized as follows:[167,176]

1. Inhibition of thyroid hormone synthesis and/or secretion
2. Reduction of the mass of functioning thyroid tissue
3. Reduction of the peripheral effects of thyroid hormones

Attention has largely focused on method (1) in recent years and this involves the main approach of drug therapy. Method (3) is being considered more seriously as a practical proposition, especially with the increasing use of β-blockers.

Until recently, none of these options was thought to treat the underlying cause of thyroid hormone overproduction. However, it has become apparent since 1980 that, in addition to their inhibitory effect on thyroid hormone synthesis, the thionamide class of antithyroid drugs, typified by methimazole (MMI) and propylthiouracil (PTU), may have an immunomodulating effect in the control of autoimmune hyperthyroid states such as Graves' disease.[177] Consequently, renewed interest in these well-established drugs has been stimulated, with investigations emphasizing their possible effects on autoimmune mechanisms in general.[178]

Inhibition of Thyroid Hormone Synthesis and/or Secretion — Antithyroid Drugs

The term antithyroid should by definition refer to any agent which acts as an intrathyroidal inhibitor in blocking the synthesis and/or secretion of thyroid hormones. This broad definition is rarely adopted, however, since iodide and other ionic inhibitors are generally considered as a separate class from the thionamides, and in clinical practice the antithyroid drugs usually refer mainly to the thionamide group of inhibitors and other goitrogens such as aniline and phenol derivatives.[165,167,176] Recent studies have shown that most intrathyroidal inhibitors cannot be classified in precise mechanistic terms since they often act by more than one mechanism. Therefore the term antithyroid drug will be used synonymously with intrathyroidal inhibitor in this review.

The Thionamides

Following the initial discovery of the goitrogenic effect of phenylthiourea in rats by Richter and Clisby[179] in 1942 a family of antithyroid drugs containing the common thionamide group (-NHCS-) emerged as the most widely used drugs in the treatment of hyperthyroidism. Despite the difficulties in assessing relative antithyroid activity in animals (see below) the most potent compounds generally possess a thiourea group (-NHCSNH-) and this is preferably part of a cyclic structure. The testing of a wide range of heterocyclic thiones led to the development of the four drugs: methyluracil (1a), propylthiouracil (1b), methimazole (2a), and carbimazole (2b) (Figure 11) as the main thionamides currently in use. Carbimazole is generally considered to act merely as a pro-drug for methimazole.[165,180]

Mechanism of Action
Inhibition of Thyroid Peroxidase

It is now recognized that the efficacy of the thionamide drugs in the treatment of hyperthyroidism depends on more than one mechanism of action.[165,177] There is wide agreement,

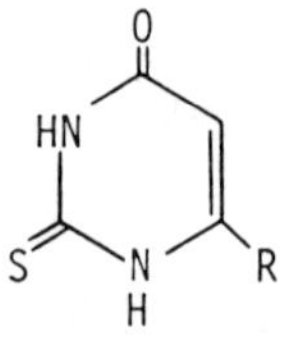

(1) 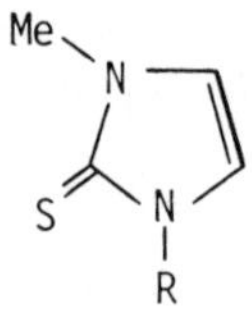   (2)

a, R = Me,   Methylthiouracil   a, R = H,   Methimazole
b, R = n-Pr, Propylthiouracil   b, R = CO$_2$Et, Carbimazole

FIGURE 11.   Structures of the thionamide drugs.

however, that a primary common action is inhibition of thyroid peroxidase, the enzyme involved in iodide oxidation, iodination of tyrosine, and the coupling of iodotyrosines to form iodothyronines.[181] Since Astwood[182] first suggested in 1949 that inhibition of thyroid peroxidase might account for their antithyroid action several of the thionamides have been shown to inhibit the oxidation of various substrates by several peroxidases, including those isolated from thyroid tissue.

The detailed mechanism of peroxidase inhibition by the thionamides remains to be elucidated. It is generally considered that inhibition is achieved by competition between the drug and tyrosine for a common intermediary complex formed between the enzyme and an oxidized form of iodide. This complex has been designated (E-I$^+$), (E-SI$^+$), or (E-I) but no direct evidence exists to support this.[179,182,183] Taurog[185] depicted the iodinating species as (E-I) and suggested that at low concentrations the drug is rapidly oxidized and no peroxidase inhibition is seen, but at higher drug/iodide ratios irreversible inactivation of thyroid peroxidase occurred by inhibiting the formation of the (E-I) complex. In order to explain the more recent finding that thionamides inactivate thyroid peroxidase in the absence of iodide but are themselves oxidized when iodide is present the scheme has been further refined (Figure 12). It is now suggested that the oxidized enzyme (E*) either oxidizes the drug and is itself inactivated or combines with iodide to form E-I* which oxidizes the drug via a sulfenyl iodide intermediate to a disulfide and regenerates active enzyme.[186] More concrete evidence to support this scheme is required, however.

Recent experiments by Ohtaki et al.[187] with purified hog thyroid peroxidase have provided spectroscopic evidence of an inactivated complex between the enzyme and MMI, which has been shown to inactivate various peroxidases at much lower concentrations than PTU.[185,186,188]

Studies in rats have established that PTU and MMI not only inhibit the oxidation of iodine and the resulting iodination of tyrosine but they also inhibit coupling of iodotyrosyl residues.[180] Before the significance of thyroid peroxidase was widely recognized it was shown that in intact rats T$_4$ formation in the thyroid is more sensitive than 3,5-diiodotyrosine formation to inhibition by PTU, suggesting a selective inhibitory effect of thionamides on coupling.[189] Engler et al. have confirmed this selectivity in an in vitro study of the effects of PTU and MMI on the iodination of thyroglobulin catalyzed by purified thyroid peroxidase.[190] Under certain incubation conditions a significant inhibitory effect on T$_4$ and T$_3$ formation without any decrease in diiodotyrosine formation was observed. It was suggested that this difference in sensitivity could be due to the sole involvement of the oxidized form of the enzyme (E*), the form inactivated by thionamide drugs (Figure 12). This would be consistent with the observation that iodine is not required in the coupling reaction and thyroid peroxidase is more sensitive to inhibition at low iodide concentrations.

Effects of Thionamides on Thyroid-Autoantibody Production

The observations that LATS levels are often reduced during long-term treatment with

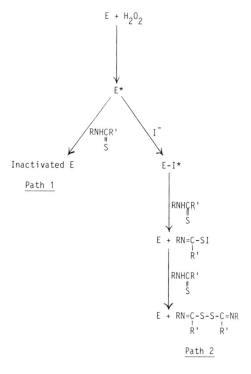

FIGURE 12. Irreversible inactivation (path 1) and reversible inhibition (path 2) of thyroid peroxidase.[186]

thionamides,[191] and lymphocytic infiltration of the thyroid is reduced in patients treated with carbimazole,[192] provided the first clues that these drugs may inhibit thyroid autoantibody production. Recently, in an elegant study, McGregor et al.[193] showed that in patients the serum concentrations of thyroid auto-antibodies, measured by a TSH radioreceptor assay, decreased during carbimazole treatment independently of changes in serum thyroid hormone concentrations.[193] In vitro studies of cultured lymphocytes have also shown that MMI (the active metabolite of carbimazole) inhibits auto-antibody synthesis.[178] Similar in vitro results were obtained with PTU. This immunosuppressive effect of thionamides seems to be specific to thyroid antibody production since gastric parietal cell antibody activity remained unchanged in patients who showed reductions in thyroid stimulating immunoglobulins.[194]

Peripheral Effects of the Thionamides

PTU, but not MMI, also inhibits the peripheral conversion of T_4 to T_3 by a deiodinase in both animal and man.[195] This action reduces the biological effectiveness of T_4 as measured by a decrease in metabolic rate or induction of oxidative enzymes, but not of T_3 — possibly because of compensatory increased fecal excretion. Thionamides which inhibit T_4 deiodination in vivo also inhibit microsomal deiodinase in vitro while MMI has no effect in either test. The practical significance of the inhibition of deiodinase activity by PTU is unclear since it has not been shown to ameliorate thyrotoxicosis more rapidly than MMI.[176,180]

As the enzyme requires a soluble cofactor, possibly glutathione, and thiouracils react with the enzyme and bind to microsomes only in the presence of iodothyronines, Visser et al.[196,197] suggested that thiouracils form a dead-end complex with an enzyme-sulphenyl iodide intermediate (E-SI) formed from reaction of enzyme (E-SH) with substrate. In the absence of thiouracil, E-SI is reduced by the thiol cofactor to regenerate enzyme.

Structure-Activity Relationships

The studies aimed at defining the structural features necessary for the antithyroid activity of thionamides were carried out largely prior to 1950 and the results have been reviewed.[198,199] The main test used involved measuring the effect of compounds in preventing thyroidal iodide uptake over a 10-day period. Subsequent studies showed a poor correlation between the rat assay and clinical efficacy, and therefore an assay measuring ^{131}I-labeled iodine incorporation as protein-bound iodine over a short period of time was devised.[200] The two assays gave widely differing estimates of relative activities (Table 9), underlining the inherent problems involved in structure-activity comparisons using in vivo data obtained from chronic administration, when metabolic and pharmacokinetic effects can play a major role in determining overall activity. In addition, it is evident from the forgoing discussion on mechanism of action that the antithyroid activity of these compounds is likely to be due to several discrete molecular events for which separate structure-activity studies are required.

Since most structure-activity studies have concentrated on cyclic derivatives related to PTU and MMI only broad general observations can be made in attempting to identify the essential chemical features required for activity in the thionamides. In the simple prototype, thiourea, addition of alkyl substituents has little effect on activity whereas the incorporation of additional polar groups leads to loss of activity. The most active compounds which have emerged are cyclic thioureas, PTU being the most active in the rat, and MMI the most active in man, when a different assay is used (Table 9).

There have been no systematic structure-activity studies of the inhibitory effects of thionamides on the thyroid peroxidases involved in iodination and coupling of tyrosine residues. The inactivation of peroxidase coupled with the oxidation of thionamides in the inhibitory process have complicated the analysis and difficulties in obtaining pure thyroid peroxidase appear to have caused a dearth of studies with this enzyme. Generally, however, MMI has proved to be more potent than PTU as an inactivator of thyroid peroxidase.[185]

A limited series of compounds have been studied as potential inhibitors of iodothyronine deiodinase using rT_3 as the substrate (Table 9).[197] This shows that in thiouracils (1) a thione group is essential, (2) removal or replacement of the 4-hydroxyl group abolishes activity, (3) alkyl groups at C_5 and C_6 increase activity, and (4) methylation at N^1 abolishes activity. A similar pattern is evident with the 5-membered rings, confirming the need for the -NHCSNH- system, with optimum activity associated with lipophilic substituents at positions remote from the thiourea system. The lack of in vitro activity of MMI is consistent with in vivo results and highlights the difference between thyroid peroxidase and iodothyronine deiodinase, implying a different mechanism of inhibition of the two enzymes, as suggested by Visser and Hennemann.[196]

With evidence emerging of several distinct molecular mechanisms associated with thionamide action it would be timely and appropriate to study the effect of drug structure on each of these mechanisms. Any attempt to predict overall activity in vivo should also consider metabolic factors, and in particular the oxidative effects of the target enzymes thyroid peroxidase and iodothyronine deiodinase.

Pharmacokinetics

A useful review of the clinical pharmacokinetics of thionamide drugs has appeared recently.[202]

MMI and PTU can be assayed accurately in serum using gas liquid chromatography (GLC), high performance liquid chromatography (HPLC), and radioimmunoassay (RIA). After extraction and derivatization to the S-methyl compound, MMI can be detected at a limit of 30 ng/mℓ in plasma by GLC alone,[203] and, in combination with mass spectrometry (S-benzyl derivative) this was improved to 2 ng/mℓ.[204] Plasma concentrations of carbimazole have not been detected due to rapid and complete conversion to methimazole.[205] HPLC is preferable to GLC for the assay of PTU, but the method of choice is a recently developed RIA with a detection limit of 2.5 ng/mℓ.[206]

Table 9

**RELATIVE ANTITHYROID ACTIVITIES (MAN AND RAT) AND
DEIODINASE INHIBITORY ACTIVITIES (RAT LIVER) OF
SELECTED THIONAMIDES**

Compound	Structure	Antithyroid action[a] (% thiouracil)		Deiodinase action[c] (% thiouracil) Rat liver
		Man	Rat	
Thiourea	NH_2CSNH_2	100	10	—
1-Isopropylthiourea	$NH_2CSNHPr$	100	40	—
Pyrimidine-2-thione		—	—	<0.1

4-Amino-	$4-NH_2$	<0.2	—	0.1
2-Thiouracil		100	100	100

5-Carboxy-	$5-CO_2H$	—	10	35
5-Propyl-	5-Pr	—	200	200
6-Hydroxy-	6-OH	—	<10	8
6-Methyl-	6-Me	200	100	71
6-n-Propyl- (PTU)	6-Pr	80	1100	125
6-n-Hexyl-	$6-n-C_6H_{13}$	50	20	—
6-Benzyl	$6-CH_2Ph$	80	1000	—
1-Methyl-6-propyl	1-Me-6-Pr	—	—	<0.1
6-Amino-	$6-NH_2$	<10	<0.1	—
Imidazole-2-thione		1000	200	18

1-Methyl- (MMI)	1-Me	10000	166[b]	<0.1
Thiohydantoin		250	40	3.5

Table 9 (continued)
RELATIVE ANTITHYROID ACTIVITIES (MAN AND RAT) AND
DEIODINASE INHIBITORY ACTIVITIES (RAT LIVER) OF
SELECTED THIONAMIDES

| Compound | Structure | Antithyroid action[a] (% thiouracil) | | Deiodinase action[c] (% thiouracil) |
		Man	Rat	Rat liver
Triazole-2-thione	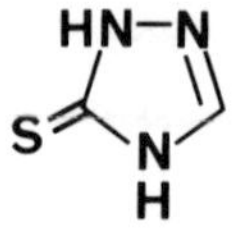	200	30	35
Benzimidazole-2-thione	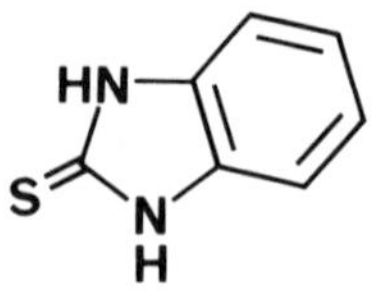	250	50	316
Benzthiazole-2-thione	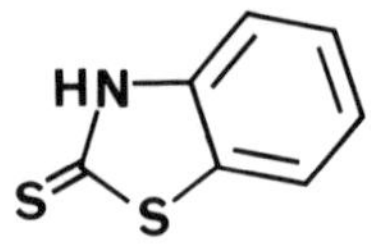	10	0.5	3.2
Benzoxazole-2-thione	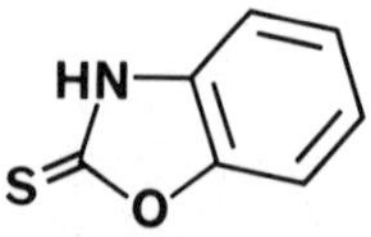	—	—	0.35

[a]   Data from Anderson[198] unless otherwise noted.
[b]   From Iiono.[201]
[c]   From Visser et al.[197]

Bioavailability of MMI and PTU varies from 80 to 95%, with PTU 80% protein-bound and MMI nonprotein-bound. These drugs are rapidly absorbed, particularly carbimazole due possibly to its greater lipophilicity. MMI and PTU are concentrated in the thyroid gland and less than 10% of each is excreted unchanged in urine. MMI has a half-life of 3 to 5 hr and PTU 1 to 2 hr. Little is known about the metabolic fate of these drugs; the glucuronide is the major metabolite of PTU in urine but the major metabolite of MMI is unknown. Except for the formation of sulfate, the oxidation products of both PTU and MMI have not been determined, despite their relevance to the mechanism of drug inactivation by thyroid peroxidase.[180,202]

Uses and Doses

There have been several recent reviews on the clinical use of thionamides and other

Table 10
CHEMICAL PROPERTIES OF THIONAMIDE DRUGS

	Propylthiouracil (PTU)	Methimazole (MMI)	Carbimazole
Structure			

	Propylthiouracil (PTU)	Methimazole (MMI)	Carbimazole
Chemical name	6-n-propyl-2-thiouracil	1-methyl-1,3-dihydro-2H-imidazole-2-thione	1-carbethoxy-3-methyl-1,3-dihydro-2H-imidazole-2 thione
Chemical formula	$C_7H_{10}N_2OS$	$C_4H_6N_2S$	$C_7H_{10}N_2O_2S$
Mol Wt	170.2	114.2	186.2
Melting point (°C)	218—219[207]	146—148[208]	122—123[209,210]
pK$_a$ (°C)	7.76 (25)[211]	11.64 (25)[212]	
	7.48 (35)[211]		
	8.25 (21)[213]	11.22 (25)[214]	
Solubility in water	7.1×10^{-3} M/ℓ[211]		
	(0.1 M HClO$_4$)		
	1 Part in 700[215]	1 Part in 5[215]	1 Part in 500[215]

antithyroid agents.[165,167,176] The thionamides are used in the treatment of hyperthyroidism in three ways:

1. Primary treatment of hyperthyroidism
2. In conjunction with radioiodine
3. To control the disorder in preparation for surgery

A proportion of patients with Graves' disease (30 to 50%) will have a lasting remission when thionamides are discontinued whereas spontaneous remissions are infrequently seen in toxic nodular goiter. Consequently, in the latter disease thionamides are best used for preparation of patients for surgical or radioiodine therapy.

PTU is available in 50-mg tablets, methimazole and carbimazole in 5- and 10-mg tablets. The standard dose of methimazole or carbimazole is 30 mg daily and PTU 300 mg daily. It is usually recommended that the drugs be given in three equal doses because of their rapid metabolism, but some clinicians have found that a single daily dose is just as effective.[176]

Side Effects

PTU is used widely in the U.S. where carbimazole is difficult to obtain; carbimazole is the drug of choice in the U.K. These differences have been fostered, in part by the belief that one or other of the drugs is less toxic. In comparably effective doses, there is little or no difference in side effects. The most common reaction, occurring in 3 to 5% of patients, is a mild papular rash, which may subside spontaneously. The most serious, although rare, side effect is agranulocytosis, which may develop within a few hours, but leukocyte production spontaneously recovers within 1 to 2 weeks after stopping the drug. This particular side effect is a common property of nearly all thioureas.[165,167,176]

Chemical Properties of Propylthiouracil, Methimazole, and Carbimazole

The important properties of the three main thionamide drugs are given in Table 10. PTU is considerably more acidic than MMI and will be significantly ionized at physiological pH (7.4) and temperature (35°C). In addition, PTU is much less soluble than MMI and, although carbimazole is also only sparingly soluble in water, it is well absorbed orally as a result of its greater lipophilicity. There appear to be no published partition coefficients on any of these drugs.

Inorganic Anions
Iodide
The effect of large doses of iodide to decrease thyroid secretion and vascularity has been employed since its introduction for the preoperative management of hyperthyroid patients. Except in this latter situation when propranolol may be used as an alternative treatment, iodide should not be used alone in thyrotoxicosis since it can result in increased synthesis of thyroid hormones. Stable iodide following adequate antithyroid or radioiodine therapy may improve symptoms of hyperthyroidism more rapidly.[176]

Other Monovalent Anions
A number of anions act as competitive inhibitors of iodide transport in the thyroid. The most effective are pertechnetate (TcO_4^-), perchlorate (ClO_4^-), thiocyanate (SCN^-), and fluoroborate (BF_4^-) in that order. Thiocyanate differs from the other anions in not being concentrated by thyroid tissue, in being metabolized by the thyroid gland, and as an inhibitor of organic iodinations. None of these drugs is used widely due to serious toxic effects.[181]

Lithium
The antithyroid effect of lithium became apparent when goiter and/or hypothyroidism developed in about 4% of patients treated with lithium carbonate for affective disorders. Although there has been debate about how it acts, the weight of evidence indicates that it prevents the release of formed hormones. Side effects such as visual disturbances, nausea, vomiting, and tremor severely limit the use of lithium salts, but, in patients for whom rapid improvement of hyperthyroidism is necessary, a combination of lithium and thionamides may be useful.[167,176]

Thyroid Ablation
Radioactive iodine provides a simple, effective, and relatively safe treatment for hyperthyroidism and remains the most successful treatment for Graves' disease. The thyroid cells do not differentiate between radioactive and natural iodine and therefore a source of radiation can be localized within the colloid of the gland leading to destruction of thyroid tissue, without affecting other local organs. ^{131}I is the only isotope of iodine currently in wide use, and patients are usually limited to those over the age of 40 in the U.K. and over 30 in the U.S. The main disadvantage is the increasing incidence of hypothyroidism in the years following therapy.[167]

Surgical treatment of hyperthyroidism has become progressively less popular. However, thyroidectomy is still an effective and safe approach which provides lasting alleviation in most patients, especially if propranolol is used as a preoperative drug.

Reduction of the Peripheral Effects of Thyroid Hormones
Antithyroid drugs and radioiodine require several weeks to return hyperthyroid patients to a euthyroid state and drugs which inhibit thyroid hormone secretion (e.g., iodide and lithium) require days to produce an effect because of the long half-life of T_4. Consequently, any method which results in a decrease in the binding of thyroid hormones to intracellular receptor sites or which reduces the physiological response induced by thyroid hormones should provide a more rapid clinical improvement. Currently, no thyroid hormone receptor antagonists are available, but the peripheral effects of thyroid hormones can be inhibited by the inhibition of T_4 to T_3 conversion. In addition to the thionamides, other effective inhibitors

of peripheral deiodinase enzymes, such as the radiocontrast agent, sodium ipodate are being investigated clinically for the treatment of Graves' disease.[216]

Since many of the cardiovascular, metabolic, and neuromuscular features of hyperthyroidism resemble those of catecholamine excess, propranolol has also become an important adjunct in the treatment of thyrotoxicosis.[176]

ACKNOWLEDGMENTS

We thank our colleagues Mr. R. Novelli, Mr. H. D. Prain, Mr. V. P. Shah, and Mr. G. A. Showell in Medicinal Chemistry and Mr. G. M. Benson, Ms. E. Brush, and Mr. N. J. Pearce in Pharmacological Biochemistry for permission to disclose new compounds and unpublished results. In addition, we thank Drs. C. R. Ganellin and S. B. Flynn for helpful discussions and Mrs. C. A. Hallgren for invaluable secretarial assistance.

ADDENDUM

Since this review was written an important report concerning the mechanisms controlling cellular and intracellular thyroid hormone distribution has been published (Oppenheimer, J. H. and Schwartz, H. L., *J. Clin. Invest.*, 75, 147, 1985). This paper suggests that there is a stereospecific transport mechanism which causes selective accumulation of the L- isomer of T_3 from cytoplasm to nucleus in liver, kidney, heart, and brain. Previously it was believed that entry of thyroid hormones to the nucleus was by passive diffusion. The importance of this new component to our overall understanding of the mechanism of action of thyroid hormones remains to be determined.

REFERENCES

1. **Harington, C. R.**, *The Thyroid Gland*, Oxford University Press, London, 1933.
2. **Baumann, E.**, Uber das normale Vorkommen von Jod im Thierkorper, *Z. Physiol. Chem.*, 21, 319, 1896.
3. **Kendall, E. C.**, The thyroid hormone, *Collect. Pap. Mayo. Clin. Mayo. Found.*, 9, 309, 1917.
4. **Pitt-Rivers, R.**, The thyroid hormones: historical aspects, in *Hormonal Proteins and Peptides*, Vol. 6, Li, C. H., Ed., Academic Press, New York, 1978, chap. 7.
5. **Tata, J. R. and Widnell, C. C.**, Ribonucleic acid synthesis during the early action of thyroid hormones, *Biochem. J.*, 98, 604, 1966.
6. **Koerner, D., Schwartz, H. L., Surks, M. I., Oppenheimer, J. H., and Jorgensen, E. C.**, Binding of selected iodothyronine analogues to receptor sites of isolated rat hepatic nuclei, *J. Biol. Chem.*, 250, 6417, 1975.
7. **Nadler, N. J.**, Anatomy and histochemistry of the thyroid: comparative anatomy, in *The Thyroid*, 3rd ed., Werner, S. C. and Ingbar, S. H., Eds., Haper and Row, New York, 1971, chap. 2.
8. **Van Herle, A. J., Vassart, G., and Dumont, J. E.**, Control of thyroglobulin synthesis and secretion, *N. Engl. J. Med.*, 301, 239, 1979.
9. **Spiro, M. J.**, Studies on the protein portion of thyroglobulin, *J. Biol. Chem.*, 245, 5820, 1970.
10. **Edelhoch, H.**, The properties of thyroglobulin, *J. Biol. Chem.*, 235, 1326, 1960.
11. **Arima, T., Spiro, M. J. I., and Spiro, R. G.**, Studies on the carbohydrate units of thyroglobulin, *J. Biol. Chem.*, 247, 1825, 1972.
12. **Dunn, J. T.**, The amino acid neighbors of thyroxine in thyroglobulin, *J. Biol. Chem.*, 245, 5954, 1970.
13. **Vassart, G., Refetoff, S., Brocas, H., Dinsart, C., and Dumont, J. E.**, Translation of thyroglobulin 33S messenger RNA as a means of determining thyroglobulin quaternary structure, *Proc. Natl. Acad. Sci. U.S.A.*, 72, 3839, 1975.
14. **Bjorkman, V., Ekholm, R., Elmqvist, L.-G., Ericson, L. E., Melander, A., and Smeds, S.**, Induced unidirectional transport of protein into the thyroid follicular lumen, *Endocrinology*, 95, 1506, 1974.
15. **Halmi, N. S. and Pitt-Rivers, R.**, The iodide pools of the rat thyroid, *Endocrinology*, 70, 660, 1962.

16. **De Groot, L. J.,** Current views on formation of thyroid hormones, *N. Engl. J. Med.,* 272, 243, 1965.

17. **De Groot, L. J. and Niepomniszcze, H.,** Biosynthesis of thyroid hormone: basic and clinical aspects, *Metabolism,* 26, 665, 1977.

18. **Gavaret, J. M., Deme, D., and Nunez, J.,** Sequential reactivity of tyrosyl residues of thyroglobulin upon iodination catalysed by thyroid peroxidase, *J. Biol. Chem.,* 252, 3281, 1977.

19. **Gavaret, J. M., Cahnmann, H. J., and Nunez, J.,** Thyroid hormone synthesis in thyroglobulin: the mechanism of the coupling reaction, *J. Biol. Chem.,* 256, 9167, 1981.

20. **Virion, A., Pommier, J., Deme, D., and Nunez, J.,** Kinetics of thyroglobulin iodination and thyroid hormone synthesis catalyzed by peroxidases: the role of H_2O_2, *Eur. J. Biochem.,* 117, 103, 1981.

21. **Deme, D., Gavaret, J. M., Pommier, J., and Nunez, J.,** Maximal number of hormonogenic iodotyrosine residues in thyroglobulin iodinated by thyroid peroxidase, *Eur. J. Biochem.,* 70, 7, 1976.

22. **Deiss, W. P., Jr. and Peake, R. L.,** The mechanism of thyroid hormone secretion, *Ann. Int. Med.,* 69, 881, 1968.

23. **Laurberg, P.,** Iodothyronine release from the perfused canine thyroid, *Acta Endocrinol.,* Suppl. 26, 1, 1980.

24. **Van Herle, A. J., Vassart, G., and Dumont, J. E.,** Control of thyroglobulin synthesis and secretion, *N. Engl. J. Med.,* 301, 307, 1979.

25. **Yamada, T.,** Control of thyroid secretion, in *International Encyclopedia of Pharmacology and Therapeutics,* Section 101, Hershman, J. M. and Bray, G. A., Eds., Peragamon Press, Oxford, 1979, chap. 3.

26. **Smith, B. R. and Hall, R.,** Pituitary thyroid-stimulating hormone and thyroid-stimulating immunoglobulins, in *Peptide Hormones,* Parsons, J. A., Ed., MacMillan, New York, 1976, chap. 12.

27. **Demeestre-Mirkine, N. and Dumont, J. E.,** The hypothalamo-pituitary thyroid axis, in *The Thyroid Gland,* De Visscher, M., Ed., Raven Press, New York, 1980, chap. 7.

28. **Larsen, P. R.,** Thyroid-pituitary interaction, *N. Engl. J. Med.,* 306, 23, 1982.

29. **DiStefano, J. J. and Fischer, D. A.,** Peripheral distribution and metabolism of the thyroid hormones: a primarily quantitative assessment, in *International Encyclopedia of Pharmacology and Therapeutics,* Section 101, Hershman, J. M. and Bray, G. A., Eds., Pergamon Press, Oxford, 1979, chap. 2.

30. **Davis, P. J., Spaulding, S. W., and Gregerman, R. I.,** The three thyroxine-binding proteins in rat serum: binding capacities and effects of binding inhibitors, *Endocrinology,* 87, 978, 1970.

31. **Heninger, R. W., Larson, F. C., and Albright, E. C.,** Iodine-containing compounds of extrathyroidal tissue, *J. Clin. Invest.,* 42, 1761, 1963.

32. **Obregon, M. J., Morreale del Escobar, G., and Escobar del Rey, F.,** Concentrations of triiodo-L-thyronine in the plasma and tissue of normal rats, as determined by radioimmunoassay: comparison with results obtained by an isotopic equilibrium technique, *Endocrinology,* 103, 2145, 1978.

33. **Larson, P. R.,** Salicylate-induced increases in free triiodothyronine in human serum: evidence of inhibition of triiodothyronine binding to thyroxine-binding globulin and thyroxine-binding prealbumin, *J. Clin. Invest.,* 51, 1125, 1972.

34. **Robbins, J., Cheng, S.-Y., Gershengorn, M. C., Glioner, D., Cahnmann, H. J., and Edelhoch, H.,** Thyroxine transport proteins of plasma. Molecular properties and biosynthesis, *Rec. Progr. Horm. Res.,* 34, 477, 1978.

35. **Burger, A. G.,** Qualitative and quantitative aspects of thyroxine metabolism, in *Proc. VI Int. Congr. Endocrinol.,* Cumming, I. A., Funder, J. W., and Mendelsohn, F. A. O., Eds., Australian Academy of Science, Canberra, 1980, 223.

36. **Visser, T. J.,** A tentative review of recent in vitro observations of the enzymatic deiodinations of iodothyronines and its possible physiological implications, *Mol. Cell. Endocrinol.,* 10, 241, 1978.

36a. **De Groot, L. J., Larsen, P. R., Refetoff, S., and Stanbury, J. B., Eds.,** *The Thyroid and its Diseases,* 5th ed., Robert. E. Krieger, Melbourne, Fla., 1984, 75.

36b. **McCann U. D., Shaw, E. A., and Kaplan, M. M.,** Iodothyronine deiodination reaction types in several rat tissues: effects of age, thyroid status and glucocorticoid treatment, *Endocrinology,* 114, 1513, 1984.

37a. **Leonard, J. L. and Rosenberg, I. N.,** Thyroxine 5'-deiodinase from rat kidney. Iodothyronine substrate specificity and the 5'-deiodination of reverse triiodothyronine, *Endocrinology,* 107, 1376, 1980.

37b. **Visser, T. J.,** Mechanism of action of iodothyronine 5'-deiodinase, *Biochim. Biophys. Acta,* 569, 302, 1979.

37c. **Visser, T. J. and Van Overmeeren, E.,** Substrate requirement for inactivation of iodothyronine 5'-deiodinase activity by thiouracil, *Biochim. Biophys. Acta,* 658, 202, 1981.

37d. **Leonard, J. L. and Visser, T. J.,** Selective modification of the active center of renal iodothyronine 5'-deiodinase by iodoacetate, *Biochim. Biophys. Acta,* 787, 122, 1984.

38. **Chopra, I. J., Solomon, D. H., Chopra, U., Wu, S.-Y., Fisher, D. A., and Nakamura, Y.,** Pathways of metabolism of thyroid hormones, *Rec. Progr. Horm. Res.,* 34, 521, 1978.

38a. **Visser, T. J., Leonard, J. L., Kaplan, M. M., and Larsen, P. R.,** Different pathways of iodothyronine 5'-deiodination in rat cerebral cortex, *Biochem. Biophys. Res. Commun.,* 101, 1297, 1981.

38b. **Visser, T. J., Leonard, J. L., Kaplan, M. M., and Larsen, P. R.,** Kinetic evidence suggesting two mechanisms for iodothyronine 5'-deiodination in rat cerebral cortex, *Proc. Natl. Acad. Sci. U.S.A.,* 79, 5080, 1982.

38c. **Kaplan, M. M.,** Thyroxine 5'-deiodination in rat anterior pituitary homogenate, *Endocrinology,* 106, 567, 1980.

38d. **Leonard, J. L., Mellen, S. A., and Larsen, P. R.,** Thyroxine 5'-deiodinase activity in brown adipose tissue, *Endocrinology,* 112, 1153, 1982.

38e. **Visser, T. J., Kaplan, M. M., Leonard, J. L., and Larson, P. R.,** Evidence for two pathways of iodothyronine 5'-deiodination in rat pituitary that differs in kinetics, propylthiouracil sensitivity and response to hypothyroidism, *J. Clin. Invest.,* 71, 992, 1983.

39. **Tata, J. R., Ernster, L., Lindberg, O., Arrhenius, E., Pederson, S., and Hedman, R.,** The action of thyroid hormones at the cell level, *Biochem. J.,* 86, 408, 1963.

40. **Tata, J. R.,** Inhibition of the biological action of thyroid hormones by actinomycin D and puromycin, *Nature (London),* 197, 1167, 1963.

41. **Eberhardt, N. L., Apriletti, J. W., and Baxter, J. D.,** The molecular biology of thyroid hormone action, in *Biochemical Actions of Hormones,* Vol. 7, Litwack, G., Ed., Academic Press, New York, 1980, 311.

42. **Schwartz, H. L. and Oppenheimer, J. H.,** Physiologic and biochemical actions of thyroid hormone, *Pharmacol. Ther. B.,* 3, 349, 1978.

43. **Oppenheimer, J. H.,** Thyroid hormone action at the cellular level, *Science,* 203, 971, 1979.

44. **Sterling, K.,** Thyroid hormone action at the cell level, *N. Engl. J. Med.,* 300, 117, 1979.

45. **Sterling, K.,** Thyroid hormone action at the cell level, *N. Engl. J. Med.,* 300, 173, 1979.

46. **Kurtz, D. T., Sippel, A. E., Ansah-Yiadom, R., and Feigelson, P.,** Effects of sex hormones on the level of the messenger RNA for the rat hepatic protein, $\alpha_2\mu$ globulin, *J. Biol. Chem.,* 251, 3594, 1976.

47. **Samuels, H. H., Klein, D., Stanley, F., and Casanova, J.,** Evidence for thyroid hormone-dependent and independent glucocorticoid actions in cultured cells, *J. Biol. Chem.,* 253, 5895, 1978.

48. **Oppenheimer, J. H., Koerner, D., Schwartz, H. L., and Surks, M. I.,** Specific nuclear triiodothyronine binding sites in rat liver and kidney, *J. Clin. Endocrinol. Metab.,* 35, 330, 1972.

49. **Samuels, H. H., Tsai, J. S., Casanova, J., and Stanley, F.,** *In vitro* characterisation of solubilised nuclear receptors from rat liver and cultured GH₁ cells, *J. Clin. Invest.,* 54, 853, 1974.

50. **Oppenheimer, J. H., Schwartz, H. L., and Surks, M. I.,** Tissue differences in the concentration of triiodothyronine nuclear binding sites in the rat: liver, kidney, pituitary, heart, brain, spleen and testis, *Endocrinology,* 96, 897, 1974.

51. **Schuster, L. D., Schwartz, H. L., and Oppenheimer, J. H.,** Nuclear receptors for 3,5,3'-triiodothyronine in human liver and kidney: characterization, quantitation and similarities to rat receptor, *J. Clin. Endocrinol. Metab.,* 48, 627, 1979.

52. **Liewendahl, K., Rosengard, S., and Lamberg, B. A.,** Nuclear binding of triodothyronine and thyroxine in lymphocytes from subjects with hyperthyroidism, hypothyroidism and resistance to thyroid hormones, *Clin. Chim. Acta,* 83, 41, 1978.

53. **Bernal, J., Refetoff, S., and DeGroot, L. J.,** Abnormalities of triiodothyronine binding to lymphocyte and fibroblast nuclei from a patient with peripheral tissue resistance to thyroid hormone action, *J. Clin. Endocrinol. Metab.,* 47, 1266, 1978.

54. **Samuels, H. H., Stanley, F., and Shapiro, L. E.,** Dose-dependent depletion of nuclear receptors by L-triiodothyronine: evidence for a role in induction of growth hormone synthesis in cultured GH₁ cells, *Proc. Natl. Acad. Sci. U.S.A.,* 73, 3877, 1976.

55. **Oppenheimer, J. H., Coulombe, P., Schwartz, H. L., and Gulfield, N. W.,** Nonlinear (amplified) relationship between nuclear occupancy by triiodothyronine and the appearance rate of hepatic α-glycerophosphate dehydrogenase and malic enzyme in the rat, *J. Clin. Invest.,* 61, 987, 1978.

56. **DeGroot, L. J., Robertson, M., and Rue, P. A.,** Triiodothyronine receptors during maturation, *Endocinology,* 100, 1511, 1977.

57. **Hamada, S., Nakamura, H., Nanuo, M., and Imura, H.,** Triiodothyronine-induced increase in rat liver nuclear thyroid hormone receptors associated with increased mitochondrial α-glycerophosphate dehydrogenase activity, *Biochem. J.,* 182, 371, 1979.

58. **Nakamura, H., Hamada, S., and Imura, H.,** Sequential changes in rat liver nuclear triiodothyronine receptors and mitochondrial α-glycerophosphate dehydrogenase activity after administration of triiodothyronine, *Biochem. J.,* 182, 377, 1979.

59. **Latham, K. R., Ring, J. C., and Baxter, J. D.,** Solubilized nuclear "receptors" for thyroid hormones, *J. Biol. Chem.,* 251, 7388, 1976.

60. **Samuels, H. H., Perlman, A. J., Raaka, B. M., and Stanley, F.,** Organization of the thyroid hormone receptor in chromatin, *Res. Progr. Horm. Res.,* 38, 557, 1982.

61. **DeGroot, L. J., Torresani, J., Carrayon, P., and Tirard, A.,** Factors influencing triiodothyronine binding properties of liver nuclear receptors, *Acta Endocrinol.,* 83, 293, 1976.

62. **Burman, K. D., Lukes, Y., Wright, F. D., and Wartofsky, L.,** Reduction in hepatic triiodothyronine binding capacity induced by fasting, *Endocrinology,* 101, 1331, 1977.

63. **Raaka, B. M. and Samuels, H. H.,** Regulation of thyroid hormone nuclear receptor levels in GH₁ cells by 3,5,3'-triiodo-L-thyronine, *J. Biol. Chem.,* 256, 6883, 1981.

64. **Eberhardt, N. L., Ring, J. C., Latham, K. R., and Baxter, J. D.,** Thyroid hormones receptors, *J. Biol. Chem.,* 254, 8534, 1979.

65. **Eberhardt, N. L., Ring, J. C., Johnson, L. K., Latham, K. R., Apriletti, J. W., Kitsis, R. N., and Baxter, J. D.,** Regulation of activity of chromatin receptors for thyroid hormone: possible involvement of histone-like proteins, *Proc. Natl. Acad. Sci. U.S.A.,* 76, 5005, 1979.

66. **Apriletti, J. W., David-Inouye, Y., Eberhardt, N. L., and Baxter, J. D.,** Interactions of the nuclear thyroid hormone receptor with core histone proteins, *Abstracts of the 58th Meeting of the American Thyroid Association,* T-24, 1982.

67. **Smith, H. C. and Eastman, C. J.,** Sulfhydryl groups regulate thyroid hormone binding at nuclear receptor sites: further evidence for a separate binding site for reverse T_3, *Biochem. Biophys. Res. Commun.,* 96, 1178, 1980.

68. **Cutten, A. E., Smith, H. C., Rashford, V. E., Waite, K. V., and Eastman, C. J.,** Does the cell nucleus contain iodothyronine deiodinases?, *Abstracts of the 12th Int. Congr. of Biochemistry,* 281, 1982.

69. **Surks, M. I., Koerner, D. H., and Oppenheimer, J. H.,** Kinetics of binding, extraction properties, and lack of requirement for cytosol proteins, *J. Clin. Invest.,* 55, 50, 1975.

70. **Bronk, J. R.,** Thyroid hormone: effects on electron transport, *Science,* 153, 638, 1966.

71. **Bronk, J. R.,** Some actions of thyroxine on oxidative phosphorylation, *Biochim. Biophys. Acta,* 37, 327, 1960.

72. **Herd, P., Kaplay, S. S., and Sanadi, D. R.,** On the origin and mechanism of action of a thyroxine-responsive protein, *Endocrinology,* 94, 464, 1974.

73. **Sterling, K.,** The mitochondrial route of thyroid hormone action, *Bull. N.Y. Acad. Med.,* 53, 260, 1977.

74. **Goglia, F., Torresani, J., Bugli, P., Barletta, A., and Liverini, G.,** *In vitro* binding of triiodothyronine to rat liver mitochondria, *Pflugers Arch.,* 390, 120, 1981.

75. **Greif, R. L. and Sloane, D.,** Mitochondrial binding sites for triiodothyronine, *Endocrinology,* 103, 1899, 1978.

76. **Pliam, N. B. and Goldfine, I. D.,** High affinity thyroid hormone binding sites on purified rat liver plasma membranes, *Biochem. Biophys. Res. Commun.,* 79, 166, 1977.

77. **Gharbi, J. and Torresani, J.,** High affinity thyroxine binding to purified rat liver plasma membranes, *Biochem. Biophys. Res. Commun.,* 88, 170, 1979.

78. **Segal, J. and Gordon, A.,** The effects of actinomycin D, puromycin, cycloheximide and hydroxyurea on 3',5,3-triiodo-L-thyronine stimulated 2-deoxy-D-glucose uptake in chick embryo heart cells *in vitro, Endocrinology,* 101, 150, 1977.

79. **Segal, J. and Ingbar, S. H.,** Effects of triiodothyronine on calcium metabolism in rat thymocytes and their relation to triodothyronine-stimulated uptake of 2-deoxy-glucose, *Clin. Res.,* 26, 312, 1978.

80. **Dratman, M. B.,** On the mechanism of action of thyroxine, an amino acid analogue of tyrosine, *J. Theor. Biol.,* 46, 255, 1974.

81. **Magnus-Levy, A.,** Ueber den respiratorischen Gaswechsel unter dem Einfluss der Thyreoidea sowie unter verschiedenen pathologische Zustanden, *Berl. Klin. Woch.,* 32, 650, 1895.

82. **Nielson, R. R., Loizzi, R. F., and Klitgaard, H. M.,** Metabolic changes in the intact rat and excised tissues after thyroidectomy, *Am. J. Physiol.,* 200, 55, 1961.

83. **Ismail-Beigi, F. and Edelman, I. S.,** Mechanism of thyroid calorigenesis: role of active sodium transport, *Proc. Natl. Acad. Sci. U.S.A.,* 67, 1071, 1970.

84. **Folke, M. and Sestoft, L.,** Thyroid calorigenesis in isolated, perfused rat liver: minor role of active sodium-potassium transport, *J. Physiol. (London),* 269, 407, 1977.

85. **Chinet, A., Clausen, T., and Giradier, L.,** Microcalorimetric determination of energy expenditure due to active sodium-potassium transport in the soleus muscle and brown adipose tissue of the rat, *J. Physiol. (London),* 265, 43, 1977.

86. **Smallridge, R. C.,** Thyroid hormone effects on the heart, in *Hearts and Heart-Like Organs,* Vol. 2, Academic Press, New York, 1980, 93.

87. **Funatsu, T.,** Hemodynamics of hyperthyroidism: the effects of autonomic nervous blocking and anti-thyroid drug treatment, *Jpn. Heart. J.,* 17, 12, 1976.

88. **Marillon, J. P., Passa, Ph., Chastre, J., Wolf, A., and Gowgon, R.,** Left ventricular function and hyperthyroidism, *Br. Heart J.,* 46, 137, 1981.

89. **Rutherford, J. D., Vatner, S. F., and Braunwald, E.,** Adrenergic control of myocardial contractility in conscious hyperthyroid dogs, *Am. J. Physiol.,* 237, 590, 1979.

90. **Brooks, I., Flynn, S. B., and Underwood, A. H.,** Effects of L-T_3 on rat cardiac function, *Br. J. Pharmacol.,* 73, 198P, 1981.

91. **Ebrecht, G., Rupp, H., and Jacob, R.,** Alterations of mechanical parameters in chemically skinned preparations of rat myocardium as a function of isozyme pattern of myosin, *Basic Res. Cardiol.,* 77, 220, 1982.

92. **Balazs, R.,** Effects of hormones and nutrition on brain development, *Adv. Exp. Med. Biol.,* 30, 385, 1972.

93. **Eayrs, J. T.,** Effect of neonatal hyperthyroidism on maturation and learning in the rat, *Anim. Behav.,* 12, 195, 1964.

94. **Hamburgh, M.,** An analysis of the action of the thyroid hormone on development based on *in vivo* and *in vitro* studies, *Gen. Comp. Endocrinol.,* 10, 198, 1968.

95. **Eayrs, J. T.,** Thyroid and developing brain: anatomical and behavioural effects, *Hor. Dev.,* 345, 355, 1971.

96. **Guder, W., Nolte, I., and Wieland, O.,** The influence of thyroid hormones on β-hydroxy-β-methylglutaryl-coenzyme A reductase of rat liver, *Eur. J. Biochem.,* 4, 273, 1968.

97. **Eskelson, C. D., Cazee, C. R., Anthony, W., Towne, J. C., and Walske, B. R.,** *In vitro* inhibition of cholesterolgenesis by various thyroid hormone analogues, *J. Med. Chem.,* 13, 215, 1970.

98. **Walton, K. W., Scott, P. J., Dykes, P. W., and Davies, J. S.,** The significance of alterations in serum lipids in thyroid dysfunction. II. Alterations of the metabolism and turnover of ^{131}I low-density lipoproteins in hypothyroidism and thyrotoxicosis, *Clin. Sci.,* 29, 217, 1965.

99. **Chait, A., Bierman, E. L., and Albers, J. J.,** Regulatory role of triiodothyronine in the degradation of low density lipotrotein by cultured human skin fibroblasts, *J. Clin. Endocrinol. Metab.,* 48, 887, 1979.

100. **Severson, D. L. and Fletcher, T.,** Effect of thyroid hormones on acid cholesterol ester hydrolase activity in rat liver, heart and epididymal fat pads, *Biochim. Biophys. Acta,* 675, 256, 1981.

101. **Fregby, M. J., Nelson, E. L., Jr., Resch, G. E., Field, F. P., and Lutherer, L. O.,** Reduced β-adrenergic responsiveness in hypothyroid rats, *Am. J. Physiol.,* 229, 916, 1975.

102. **Banerjee, S. P. and Kung, L. S.,** β-Adrenergic receptors in rat heart: effects of thyroidectomy, *Eur. J. Pharmacol.,* 43, 207, 1977.

103. **Stiles, G. L. and Lefkowitz, R. J.,** Thyroid hormone modulation of agonist-beta-adrenergic receptor interactions in the rat heart, *Life Sci.,* 28, 2529, 1981.

104. **Hervas, F., Morreale de Escobar, G., and Escobar del Ray, F.,** Rapid effects of single small doses of L-thyroxine and triiodo-L-thyronine on growth hormone as studied in the rat by radioimmunoassay, *Endocrinology,* 97, 91, 1975.

105. **Gordon, G. G. and Southern, A. L.,** Thyroid-hormone effects on steroid-hormone metabolism, *Bull. N.Y. Acad. Med.,* 53, 241, 1977.

106. **Money, W. L.,** Biological activity of iodo compounds, in *Endocrinologia Experimentalis: Estimation of Iodo Compounds in Biological Material,* Stoec, V., Ed., Publishing House of the Slovac Academy of Sciences, Bratislava, 1966, 265.

107. **Lee, Y-P., Takemori, A. E., and Lardy, H.,** Enhanced oxidation of α-glycerophosphate by mitochondria of thyroid-fed rats, *J. Biol. Chem.,* 234, 3051, 1959.

108. **Jorgensen, E. C.,** Thyroid hormones and analogues. I. Synthesis, physical properties and theoretical calculations, in *Hormonal Peptides and Proteins,* Vol. 6, Li, C. H., Ed., Academic Press, New York, 1978, Chap 2.

109. **Harington, C. R. and Barger, G.,** Chemistry of thyroxine. III. Constitution and synthesis of thyroxine, *Biochem. J.,* 21, 169, 1927.

110. **Selenkow, H. A. and Asper, S. P.,** Biological activity of compounds structurally related to thyroxine, *Physiol. Rev.,* 35, 426, 1955.

111. **Money, W. L., Kumaoka, S., Rawson, R. W., and Kroc, R. L.,** Comparative effects of thyroxine analogues in experimental animals, *Ann. N.Y. Acad. Sci.,* 86, 512, 1960.

112. **Jorgensen, E. C.,** Thyroid hormones and analogues. II. Structure-activity relationships, in *Hormonal Proteins and Peptides,* Vol. 6, Li, C. H., Ed., Academic Press, New York, 1978, chap. 3.

113. **Jorgensen, E. C.,** Thyromimetic and antithyroid drugs, in *Burger's Medicinal Chemistry,* 4th ed., Part 3, Wolff, M. E., Ed., John Wiley & Sons, New York, 1981, 103.

114. **Dietrich, S. W., Bolger, M. B., Kollman, P. A., and Jorgensen, E. C.,** Thyroxine analogues. XXIII. Quantitative structure-activity correlation studies of *in vivo* and *in vitro* thyromimetic activities, *J. Med. Chem.,* 20, 863, 1977.

115. **Cody, V.,** Thyroid hormones-receptor interactions: binding models from molecular conformation and binding affinity data, in *Computer Assisted Drug Design,* Am. Chem. Soc. Symp. Ser. 112, Olson, E. C. and Christoferson, C., Eds., American Chemical Society, Washington, D.C., 1979, 281.

116. **Cody, V.,** Thyroid Hormones: crystal structure, molecular conformation, binding and structure-function relationships, *Rec. Progr. Horm. Res.,* 34, 437, 1978.

117. **Zenker, N. and Jorgensen, E. C.,** Thyroxine analogues. I. Synthesis of 3,5-diiodo-4-(2' alkylphenoxy)-DL-phenylalanines, *J. Am. Chem. Soc.,* 81, 4643, 1959.

118. **Emmett, J. C. and Pepper, E. S.,** Conformation of thyroid hormone analogues, *Nature (London),* 257, 334, 1975.

119. **Andrea, T. A., Dietrich, S. W., Murray, W. J., Kollman, P. A., Jorgensen, E. C., and Rothenberg, S.**, A model for thyroid hormone-receptor interactions, *J. Med. Chem.*, 22, 221, 1979.

120. **Blake, C. C. F. and Oatley, S. J.**, Protein DNA and protein-hormone interactions in prealbumin: a model of the thyroid hormone nuclear receptor?, *Nature (London)*, 268, 115, 1977.

121. **Blaney, J. M., Jorgensen, E. C., Connolly, M. L., Ferrin, T. E., Langridge, R., Oatley, S. J., Burridge, J. M., and Blake, C. C. F.**, Computer graphics in drug design: molecular modelling of thyroid hormone-prealbumin interactions, *J. Med. Chem.*, 25, 785, 1982.

122. **Jorgensen, E. C. and Berteau, P. E.**, Thyroxine analogs. XXI. o- and m-L-thyroxine and related compounds, *J. Med. Chem.*, 14, 1199, 1971.

123. **Barker, S. B. and Shimada, M.**, Some aspects of metabolism of thyroxine and of analogues devoid of the phenolic group, *Proc. Mayo Clin.*, 39, 609, 1964.

124. **Jorgensen, E. C. and Slade, P.**, Thyroxine analogues. VI. Synthesis and antigoitrogenic activity of 3,5-diiodo-4-(4'-aminophenoxyl)-L-phenyl-alanines, including the 4'-amino analogues of 3,5,3'-triiodo-L-thyronine, *J. Med. Chem.*, 5, 729, 1962.

125. **Bruice, T. C., Kharasch, N., and Winzler, R. J.**, A correlation of thyroxine-like activity and chemical structure, *Arch. Biochem. Biophys.*, 62, 305, 1956.

126. **Hansch, C. and Fujita, T.**, -σ-π Analysis. A method for the correlation of biological activity and chemical structure, *J. Am. Chem. Soc.*, 86, 1616, 1964.

127. **Jorgensen, E. C., Dietrich, S. W., Koerner, D., Surks, M. I., and Oppenheimer, J. H.**, Thyroid hormones: comparative structural requirements for activity *in vivo* and for binding to rat liver nuclei, *Proc. West. Pharmacol. Soc.*, 18, 389, 1975.

128. **Ahmad, P. A., Fyfe, L. A., and Mellors, A.**, Parachors in drug design, *Biochem. Pharmacol.*, 24, 1103, 1975.

129. **Kubinyi, H. and Kehrhahn, O-H.**, Quantitative structure-activity relationships. I. The modified Free-Wilson approach, *J. Med. Chem.*, 19, 578, 1976.

130. **Kubinyi, H.**, Quantitative structure-activity relationships. II. A mixed approach, based on Hansch and Free-Wilson analysis, *J. Med. Chem.*, 19, 587, 1976.

131. **Martin, Y. C.**, *Quantitative Drug Design*, Marcel Dekker, New York, 1978.

132. **Hansch, C. and Leo, A. J.**, *Substituent Constants for Correlation Analysis in Chemistry and Biology*, John Wiley & Sons, New York, 1979.

133. **Dietrich, S. W., Jorgensen, E. C., Kollman, P. A., and Rothenberg, S. W.**, A theoretical study of intramolecular hydrogen bonding in ortho-substituted phenols and thiophenols, *J. Am. Chem. Soc.*, 98, 8310, 1976.

134. **Bolger, M. B. and Jorgensen, E. C.**, Molecular interactions between thyroid hormone analogs and the rat liver nuclear receptor, *J. Biol. Chem.*, 255, 10271, 1980.

135. **Ellis, D., Emmett, J. C., Pearce, N. J., Shah, V. P., and Underwood, A. H.**, 3'-Acetyl-3,5-diiodo-L-thyronine: a novel highly active thyromimetic with lower receptor affinity, *Abstracts of the 58th Meeting of the American Thyroid Association*, 1982.

136. **Rekker, R. F.**, *The Hydrophobic Fragmental Constant*, Elsevier, Amsterdam, 1977.

137. **Rekker, R. F. and de Kort, H. M.**, The hydrophobic fragmental constant, an extension to a 1000 data point set, *Eur. J. Med. Chem. Chim. Ther.*, 14, 479, 1979.

138. **Kubinyi, H.**, Quantitative structure-activity relationships. VII. The bilinear model, a new model for nonlinear dependence of biological activity on hydrophobic character, *J. Med. Chem.*, 20, 625, 1977.

139. **Takesuka, M. and Matsui, Y.**, Experimental observations and CNDO/2 calculations for hydroxy stretching frequency shifts, intensities, and hydrogen bond energies of intramolecular hydrogen bonds in *ortho*-substituted phenols, *J. Chem. Soc. Perkin Trans:2*, 1743, 1979.

140. **Schaefer, T., Sebastian, R., and Wildman, T. A.**, The allyl and benzyl groups as hydrogen bond acceptors in derivatives of 2-allylphenol and 2-benzylphenyl, *Can. J. Chem.*, 57, 3005, 1979.

141. **Cody, V.**, Structure of thyroxine: role of thyroxine hydroxyl in protein binding, *Acta Cryst.*, B37, 1685, 1981.

142. **Fail, J., Prout, C. K., and Emmett, J. C.**, Structural properties of thyroid hormones and related derivatives, Abstracts of the British Crystallographic Association Meeting, Durham, April 1982.

143. **Rao, G. S.**, Mode of entry of steroid and thyroid hormones into cells, *Mol. Cell. Endrocrinol.*, 21, 97, 1981.

144. **Mukherjee, R. and Block, P., Jr.**, Thyroxine analogues: synthesis and nuclear magnetic resonance spectral studies of diphenylamines, *J. Chem. Soc. C*, 1596, 1971.

145. **Cody, V.**, Conformational effects of ether bridge substitution in thyroid hormone analogs, *Endocrinol. Res. Commun.*, 9, 55, 1982.

146. **Cody, V.**, Role of iodine in thyroid hormones; molecular conformation of a halogen-free hormone analogue, *J. Med. Chem.*, 23, 584, 1980.

147. **Jorgensen, E. C., Murray, W. J., and Block, P., Jr.**, Thyroxine analogues. XXII. Thyromimetic activity of halogen-free derivatives of 3,5-dimethyl-L-thyronine, *J. Med. Chem.*, 17, 434, 1974.

148. **Oppenheimer, J. H., Schwartz, H. L., Dillman, W., and Surks, M. I.,** Effect of thyroid hormone analogues on the displacement of ^{125}I-L-triiodothyronine from hepatic and heart nuclei *in vivo:* possible relationship to hormonal activity, *Biochem. Biophys. Res. Commun.,* 55, 544, 1973.

149. **Andrea, T. A., Cavieri, R. R., Goldfine, I. D., and Jorgensen, E. C.,** Binding of thyroid hormone analogues to the human plasma protein prealbumin, *Biochemistry,* 19, 55, 1980.

150. **Somack, R., Andrea, T. A., and Jorgensen, E. C.,** Thyroid hormone binding to human serum prealbumin and rat liver nuclear receptor: kinetics, contribution of the hormone phenolic hydroxyl group, and accommodation of hormone side-chain bulk, *Biochemistry,* 21, 163, 1982.

151. **Cheng, S-Y., Pages, R. A., Saroff, H. A., Edelhoch, H., and Robbins, J.,** Analysis of thyroid hormone binding to human serum prealbumin by 8-anilinonaphthalene-1-sulphonate fluorescence, *Biochemistry,* 16, 3707, 1977.

152. **Tabachnik, M., Downs, F. J., and Giogio, N. A., Jr.,** Thyroxine-protein interactions. VI. Structural requirements for binding of benzene derivatives to thyroxine-binding sites on human serum albumin, *Arch. Biochem. Biophys.,* 136, 467, 1970.

153. **Andrea, T. A., Jorgensen, E. C., and Kollman, P. A.,** Differentiation of D- and L-thyroxine by the plasma protein prealbumin, *Int. J. Quant. Chem. Quant. Biol. Symp.,* 5, 191, 1978.

154. **Blake, C. C. F.,** Prealbumin and the thyroid hormone nuclear receptor, *Proc. R. Soc. London,* B2H, 413, 1981.

155. **Cheng, S-Y., Rakhit, G., Erard, F., Robbins, J., and Chignell, C. F.,** A spin label study of thyroid hormone-binding sites in human plasma thyroxine transport proteins, *J. Biol. Chem.,* 256, 831, 1981.

156. **Crippen, G. M.,** Quantitative structure-activity relationships by distance geometry: thyroxine binding site, *J. Med. Chem.,* 24, 198, 1981.

157. **Weiner, P. K., Langridge, R., Blaney, J. M., Schaefer, R., and Kollman, P. A.,** Electrostatic potential molecular surfaces, *Proc. Natl. Acad. Sci. U.S.A.,* 79, 3754, 1982.

158. **Cheng, S-Y., Cahnmann, H. J., Wilchek, M., and Ferguson, R. N.,** Affinity labeling of the thyroxine binding domain of human serum prealbumin with dansyl chloride, *Biochemistry,* 14, 4132, 1975.

159. **Cheng, S-Y., Wilchek, M., Cahnmann, H. J., and Robbins, J.,** Affinity labeling of human serum prealbumin with N-bromoacetyl-L-thyroxine, *J. Biol. Chem.,* 252, 6076, 1977.

160. **Geffner, D. L. and Hershman, J. M.,** Hyperthyroidism causes, etiology of Graves' disease, clinical features, general aspects of treatment, in *International Encyclopedia of Pharmacology and Therapeutics,* Section 101, Hershman, J. M. and Bray, G. A., Eds., Pergamon Press, Oxford, 1979, chap. 6.

161. **Hall, R.,** Thyroid stimulators, in *Proc. VI Int. Congress Endocrinol.,* Cummings, I. A., Funder, J. W., and Mendelsohn, F. A. O., Eds., Australian Academy of Science, Canberra, 1980, 9.

162. **Ibbertson, H. K.,** Hypothyroidism, in *International Encyclopedia of Pharmacology and Therapeutics,* Section 101, Hershman, J. M. and Bray, G. A., Eds., Pergamon Press, Oxford, 1979, chap. 14.

163. **Delange, F. M. and Ermans, A. M.,** Endemic goiter and cretinism. Naturally occurring goitrogens, in *International Encyclopedia of Pharmacology and Therapeutics,* Section 101, Hershman, J. M. and Bray, G. A., Eds., Pergamon Press, Oxford, 1979, chap. 20.

164. **Fisher, D. A. and Beall, G. N.,** Hashimoto's thyroiditis, in *International Encyclopedia of Pharmacology and Therapeutics,* Section 101, Hershaman, J. M. and Bray, G. A., Eds., Pergamon Press, Oxford, 1979, chap. 24.

165. **Haynes, R. C. and Murad, F.,** Thyroid and antithyroid drugs, in *The Pharmacological Basics of Therapeutics,* Goodman, L. S. and Gilman, A., Eds., 6th ed., 1980, 1397.

166. **Burrow, G. N.,** Thyroid hormone therapy in nonthyroid disorders, in *The Thyroid,* Werner, S. C. and Ingbar, S. H., Eds., 4th ed., Harper and Row, New York, 1978, 974.

167. **McDougall, I. R.,** Treatment of hyper- and hypothyroidism, *J. Clin. Pharmacol.,* 21, 365, 1981.

168. **Von Eickstedt, K. W.,** *Meyler's Side Effects of Drugs,* Dutes, M. N. G., Ed., 9th ed., 1980, 695.

169. **Werner, S. C.,** Treatment of hypothyroidism, in *The Thyroid,* Werner, S. C. and Ingbar, S. H., Eds., 4th ed., Harper and Row, New York, 1978, 965.

170. **Bray, G. A.,** Obesity and thyroid hormone, in *International Encyclopedia of Pharmacology and Therapeutics,* Section 101, Hershman, J. M. and Bray, S. A., Eds., Pergamon Press, Oxford, 1979, chap. 28.

171. **Havel, R. J. and Kane, J. P.,** Therapy of hyperlipidemic states, *Ann. Rev. Med.,* 33, 417, 1982.

172. **Blank, B., Greenburg, C. M., and Kerwin, J. F.,** Thyromimetics. III. The synthesis and relative thyromimetic activities of some 4'-ethers of iodinated thyronines and thyroalkanoic acids, *J. Med. Chem.,* 7, 53, 1964.

173. **Comite, F., Burrow, G. N., and Jorgensen, E. C.,** Thyroid hormone analogues and fetal goiter, *Endocrinology,* 102, 1670, 1978.

174. **Ballard, P. L., Benson, B. J., Brehier, A., Carter, J. P., Kriz, B. M., and Jorgensen, E. C.,** Transplacental stimulation of lung development in the fetal rabbit by 3,5-dimethyl-3'-isopropyl-L-thyronine, *J. Clin. Invest.,* 65, 1407, 1980.

175. **Melmed, S. and Neufeld, N.,** personal communication.

176. **McClung, M. R. and Greer, M. A.,** Treatment of hyperthyroidism, *Ann. Rev. Med.,* 31, 385, 1980.

177. **Bouillon, R.,** Thyroid and antithyroid drugs, in *Side Effects Drugs Annu.,* 6, 363, 1982.
178. **Hallengren, B., Forsgren, A., and Melander, A.,** Effects of antithyroid drugs on lymphocyte function *in vitro, J. Clin. Endocrinol. Metab.,* 51, 298, 1980.
179. **Richter, C. P. and Clisby, K. H.,** Toxic effects of bitter-tasting phenylthiocarbamide, *Arch. Pathol.,* 33, 46, 1942.
180. **Marchant, B., Lees, J. F. H., and Alexander, W. D.,** Antithyroid drugs, *Pharmacol. Ther. B.,* 3, 305, 1978.
181. **Green, W. L.,** Mechanisms of action of antithyroid compounds, in *The Thyroid,* Werner, S. C. and Ingbar, S. H., Eds., 4th ed., Harper and Row, New York, 1978, 77.
182. **Astwood, E. B.,** Mechanisms of action of various antithyroid compounds, *Ann. N.Y. Acad. Sci.,* 50, 419, 1949.
183. **Morris, D. R. and Hager, L. P.,** Mechanism of the inhibition of enzymatic halogenation by antithyroid agents, *J. Biol. Chem.,* 241, 3582, 1966.
184. **Maloof, F., Smith, S., and Soodak, M.,** The mechanism of action of the thiocarbamide-type antithyroid drugs in inhibiting iodination in thyroid tissue, *Mech. React. Sulfur Comp.,* 4, 61, 1969.
185. **Taurog, A.,** The mechanism of action of thioureylene antithyroid drugs, *Endocrinology,* 98, 1031, 1976.
186. **Davidson, B., Soodak, M., Neary, J. T., Strout, H. V., Kieffer, J. D., Mover, H., and Maloof, F.,** The irreversible inactivation of thyroid peroxidase by methylmercaptoimidazole, thiouracil and propyl-thiouracil *in vitro* and its relationship to *in vivo* findings, *Endocrinology,* 103, 871, 1978.
187. **Ohtaki, S., Nakagawa, H., Nakamura, M., and Yamazaki, I.,** Reactions of purified hog thyroid peroxidase with H_2O_2, tyrosine, and methylmercaptoimidazole in comparison with bovine lactoperoxidase, *J. Biol. Chem.,* 257, 761, 1982.
188. **Edelhoch, H., Irace, G., Johnson, M. L., Michot, J. L., and Nunez, J.,** The effects of thiourylene compounds lactoperoxidase activity, *J. Biol. Chem.,* 11822, 254, 1979.
189. **Richards, J. B. and Ingbar, S. H.,** The effects of propylthiouracil and perchlorate on the biogenesis of thyroid hormone, *Endocrinology,* 65, 198, 1959.
190. **Engler, H., Taurog, A., and Dorris, M. L.,** Preferential inhibition of thyroxine and 3,5,3'-triiodothyronine formation by propylthiouracil and methylmercaptoimidazole in thyroid-peroxidase catalysed iodination of thyroglobulin, *Endocrinology,* 110, 190, 1982.
191. **Pinchera, A., Liberti, P., Martino, E., Fenzi, G. F., Grasso, L., Rovis, L., Baschieri, L., and Doria, G.,** Effects of antithyroid therapy on the long-acting thyroid stimulator and the antithyroglobulin antibodies, *J. Clin. Endocrinol. Metab.,* 29, 231, 1969.
192. **Beck, J. S., Young, R. J., Simpson, J. G., Gray, E. S., Nicol, A. G., Pegg, C. A. S., and Michie, W.,** Lymphoid tissue in the thyroid gland and thymus of patients with primary thyrotoxicosis, *Br. J. Surg.,* 60, 769, 1973.
193. **McGregor, A. M., Peterson, M. M., McLachlan, S. M., Rooke, P., Smith, B. R., and Hall, R.,** Carbimazole and the autoimmune response in Graves' disease, *N. Engl. J. Med.,* 303, 302, 1980.
194. **McGregor, A. M., Smith, B. R., Hall, R., Collins, P. N., Bottazzo, G. F., and Petersen, M. M.,** Specificity of the immunosuppressive action of carbimazole in Graves' disease, *Br. Med. J.,* 284, 1750, 1982.
195. **Oppenheimer, J. H., Schwartz, H. L., and Surks, M. I.,** Propylthiouracil inhibits the conversion of L-thyroxine to L-triiodothyronine, *J. Clin. Invest.,* 51, 2493, 1972.
196. **Visser, T. J. and Hennemann, G.,** Mechanism of thyroid hormone deiodination, *Proceedings of the VI International Congress of Endocrinology,* 227, 1980.
197. **Visser, T. J., Van Overmeeren, E., Fekhes, D., Docter, R., and Hennemann, G.,** Inhibition of iodothyronine 5'-deiodinase by thiourylenes; structure-activity relationships, *FEBS Lett.,* 103, 314, 1979.
198. **Anderson, G. W.,** *Medicinal Chemistry,* Vol. 1, Suter, C. M., Ed., John Wiley & Sons, 1951, 1.
199. **Greer, M. A., Kendall, J. W., and Smith, M.,** Antithyroid compounds, in *The Thyroid Gland,* Vol. 1, Pitt-Rivers, R. and Trotter, W. R., Eds., Butterworths, London, 1964, chap. 14.
200. **Stanley, M. M. and Astwood, E. B.,** Determination of the relative activity of antithyroid compounds in man using radioactive iodine, *Endocrinology,* 41, 66, 1947.
201. **Iiono, S.,** Comparison of the effects of various goitrogens on the biosynthesis of thyroid hormones *in vitro, Acta Endocrinol.,* 36, 312, 1965.
202. **Kampmann, J. P. and Hansen, J. M.,** Clinical pharmacokinetics of antithyroid drugs, *Clin. Pharmacokinet.,* 6, 401, 1981.
203. **Bending, M. R. and Stevenson, D.,** Measurement of methimazole in human plasma using gas-liquid chromatography, *J. Chromatogr.,* 154, 267, 1978.
204. **Floberg, S., Lanbeck, K., and Lindstrom, B.,** Determination of methimazole in plasma using gas chromatography-mass spectrometry after extractive alkylation, *J. Chromatogr.,* 182, 63, 1980.
205. **Melander, A., Hallengren, B., Rosendal-Helgesen, S., Sjoberg, A. K., and Wahlin-Boll, E.,** Comparative *in vitro* effects and *in vivo* kinetics of antithyroid drugs, *Eur. J. Clin. Pharmacol.,* 17, 295, 1980.

206. **Cooper, D. S., Saxe, V. C., Maloof, F., and Ridgway, E. C.,** Studies of propylthiouracil using a newly developed radioimmunoassay, *J. Clin. Endocrinol. Metab.,* 52, 204, 1981.
207. **Anderson, G. W., Halverstadt, L. F., Miller, W. H., and Roblin, O. R.,** Studies in chemotherapy. X. Antithyroid compounds. Synthesis of 5- and 6-substituted 2-thiouracils from β-oxoesters and thiourea, *J. Am. Chem. Soc.,* 67, 2197, 1945.
208. **Jones, R. G., Kornfield, E. C., McLaughlin, K. C., and Anderson, R. C.,** Studies on imidazoles. IV. The synthesis and antithyroid activity of some 1-substituted-2-mercaptoimidazoles, *J. Am. Chem. Soc.,* 71, 4000, 1949.
209. **Lawson, A. and Morley, H. V.,** 2-Mercaptoglyoscalises. X. The acylation of 2-Mercaptoglyoscalises, *J. Chem. Soc.,* 1103, 1956.
210. **Baker, J. A.,** The mechanism of N-acylation of 2-mercaptoglyoxalines, *J. Chem. Soc.,* 2387, 1958.
211. **Garrett, E. R. and Weber, D. J.,** Metal complexes of thiouracils. I. Stability constants by potentiometric titration studies and structures of complexes, *J. Pharm. Sci.,* 59, 1383, 1970.
212. **Sakurai, H. and Takeshima, S.,** Acid dissociation of 2-mercaptohistamine and its related compounds, *Talanta,* 24, 531, 1977.
213. **Stanovnik, B. and Tisler, M.,** Contribution to the structure of heterocyclic compounds with thioamide groups, *Arzneim Forsch,* 14, 1004, 1964.
214. **Foye, W. O. and Lo, J. R.,** Metal-binding abilities of antibacterial heterocyclic thioureas, *J. Pharm. Sci.,* 61, 1209, 1972.
215. **Martindale,** *The Extra Pharmacopoeia,* 27th ed., Wade, A., Ed., Pharmaceutical Press, Philadelphia, 1977.
216. **Wu, S., Shyh, T., Chopra, I. J., Soloman, D. H., Huang, H., and Chu, P.,** Comparison of sodium ipodate and propylthiouracil in early treatment of hyperthyroidism, *J. Clin. Endocrinol. Metab.,* 54, 630, 1982.

INSULIN AND ORAL HYPOGLYCEMIC AGENTS*

Edmund J. Hengesh

INTRODUCTION

Insulin and the oral hypoglycemic agents are used almost exclusively to treat patients suffering from various types of diabetes mellitus. Diabetes mellitus, or more commonly diabetes, is a major disease estimated by the National Institutes of Health (NIH) to afflict some 10.2 million Americans. It is believed to be increasing at the rate of 5 to 6% per year. In only 5.2 million of the 10.2 million cases has the disease actually been diagnosed. Of these diagnosed cases only 5 to 10% have been found to be completely dependent upon insulin for control of their disease. Of the remaining 90 to 95%, while some may use insulin, they do not demonstrate the same dependency on insulin to alleviate symptoms. Control in these noninsulin-dependent diabetic patients is often achieved through diet or a combination of diet and an oral hypoglycemic agent. In addition, virtually all of the undiagnosed cases, due to the mild nature of their symptoms, fall into the noninsulin-dependent category and are potential candidates for oral hypoglycemic therapy. An extensive five-volume handbook series on diabetes and its treatment has recently been published.[1]

DIABETES MELLITUS

Diabetes mellitus is a disease of long-standing having been described in the Ebers Papyrus around 1500 B.C. The name derives from the Greek words meaning ''to pass through'' and ''honey-sweet'' referring to the observations that sugar seemed to pass through the body unaltered and gave the urine a sweet taste. The all-important connection between the appearance of sugar in the urine of the diabetic and the presence of excess sugar in the blood was established by Mathew Dobson in the 17th century. Identification of the sugar as glucose occurred in 1815. Minkowski and von Mering implicated the pancreas as the site of the disorder in 1889 with attention turning to the islets of Langerhans in 1901. While scientists believed that the islets secreted a substance and proposed that this substance was lacking in the diabetic, its identity remained a mystery until the momentous discovery of insulin in 1921 by Banting and Best. It then became obvious that it was the lack of insulin that interfered with the normal metabolic disposition of glucose and resulted in the hyperglycemia and the glucosuria characteristic of the diabetic state.

Symptoms

The symptoms of diabetes are well-recognized. The osmotic effects of abnormally high quantities of glucose result in polyuria and polydipsia. Due to the loss of a major energy source to the insulin-dependent tissues, compensatory metabolic adjustments occur, and the body becomes more dependent on lipids and proteins to meet the demands. Polyphagia occurs and muscular weakness and weight loss ensue. Ultimately ketoacidosis and/or diabetic coma result in death. The mortality rate associated with an episode of ketoacidosis ranges from 1 to 19% with a worldwide average since 1950 of 10%. Ketoacidosis accounts for 14% of all hospital admissions for diabetes and is the most common cause for diabetic patients less than 20 years of age.[2]

Complications

Prior to the advent of insulin therapy, diabetic patients were placed on what amounted to

* Submitted for publication July 23rd, 1982.

Table 1
LONG-TERM COMPLICATIONS OF DIABETES

Kidney damage
Destruction of the retina
Cataracts
Premature atherosclerosis
Predisposition to gangrene
Neurological dysfunction

a starvation diet attempting to balance dietary caloric intake with energy usage. Consequently, diabetic patients had a shortened lifespan and generally did not live long enough to develop the chronic complications associated with diabetes of long duration. For example, for the period from 1914 to 1922 only 24.6% of diabetics died of cardiovascular and renal disease, whereas in the 2-year span from 1966 to 1968, 74.2% of diabetics died of these disorders.[3] The complications usually involve the noninsulin-dependent tissues, and, besides the cardiovascular and renal systems, affect the neural and visual systems. It is generally believed, although unproven, that these tissues are susceptible to the ravages of diabetes because of the wide fluctuations of blood glucose to which they are exposed. This overexposure to glucose is true even in patients taking daily injections of insulin.

Specific long-term complications are listed in Table 1. It has been estimated that approximately 50% of diabetics would show a pathological kidney lesion of some sort with microscopy. The first clinical evidence of nephropathy[4] is proteinuria which, however, is seldom recorded in young patients within the first 10 years. Edema appears when the protein loss approaches 5 g/day. Diabetic retinopathy[5] is the leading cause of new blindness among adults aged 20 to 65 years. It rarely occurs within the first few years, but by 10 years, 50% of patients exhibit some degree of retinopathy. After 20 to 25 years the problem is present in about 90% of patients although less than 5% actually become completely blind. Atherosclerosis, as with normal individuals, is a major cause of death in diabetic patients.[6] They, however, have about twice the incidence of cardiovascular episodes as compared to nondiabetics and suffer 2 to 3 times higher mortality. Peripheral vascular disease is found in 8% of patients at time of diagnosis,[7] it predisposes the diabetic to foot complications. This increased susceptibility to injury enhances the chances of infection and all too often results in gangrene. Gangrene is 40 to 50 times more common in the diabetic and often leads to amputation. Neuropathy[8] is probably the most common of the complications and is the source of severe discomfort for many patients. Sensations include numbness, coldness, tingling, and pain. Neurological dysfunction can result in abnormalities involving virtually every organ system. All factors totaled, the average diabetic has a life expectancy about one third less than the general population. The biochemistry of the complications of diabetes has been reviewed by Brownlee and Cerami.[9]

Diagnosis and Classification

Diabetes in the overt cases can be detected by measuring urinary glucose and ketone bodies using any of the readily available, selfadministered tests. In the less well-developed cases, urinary tests may be negative so other parameters are sought. A diagnosis of diabetes is consistent with any one of the following criteria:[10] (1) classic symptoms along with unequivocal hyperglycemia (>200 mg/dℓ), (2) a fasting venous plasma glucose $\geqslant140$ mg/dℓ on more than one occasion, and (3) fasting plasma glucose less than 140 mg/dℓ but a sustained venous plasma glucose $\geqslant200$ mg/dℓ during a 75-g oral glucose tolerance test (OGTT) demonstrated both at 2 hr after glucose injection and also at some other time between glucose ingestion and 2 hr. The OGTT is not needed when plasma glucose is >140 mg/dℓ as virtually all patients will exhibit responses that meet or exceed the established reference points.

Table 2
CLASSIFICATION OF DIABETES MELLITUS

Type	Acceptable terminology	Former terminology	Clinical features
Insulin-dependent	IDDM, type I	Juvenile diabetes, juvenile-onset diabetes, juvenile-onset-type diabetes, JOD, ketosis-prone diabetes, brittle diabetes	Abrupt onset of symptoms most often in juveniles, insulinopenia with dependence upon injected insulin to sustain life, proneness to ketosis, islet cell antibodies often present at diagnosis
Noninsulin dependent	NIDDM, type II	Adult-onset diabetes, maturity-onset diabetes, maturity-onset-type-diabetes, MOD, ketosis-resistant diabetes, stable diabetes	Onset may occur at any age but commonly after age 40, 60—90% of subjects are obese, insulin levels may be normal, increased, or decreased, not dependent upon injected insulin, not prone to ketosis

Other types associated with certain conditions and syndromes
  Pancreatic disease
  Hormonal
  Drug or chemical induced
  Insulin receptor abnormalities
  Certain genetic syndromes
  Other types
		Secondary diabetes	Diabetes Mellitus in addition to the presence of the specific condition or syndrome

The adequacy of diabetic therapy can be monitored by measuring the plasma concentration of glycosylated hemoglobin. Glucose can react nonenzymatically with the N-terminal amino group of the β-chain of hemoglobin as well as that of other proteins. The Schiff base initially formed can undergo an Amadori rearrangement to form a more stable ketoamine linkage. Hemoglobin modified in this manner can be detected by a microcolumn procedure and has been designated as being hemoglobin A_{1c} (Hb A_{1c}). Normal subjects have Hb A_{1c} levels of approximately 5% whereas uncontrolled and poorly controlled diabetics have levels 2 to 3 times normal. Since erythrocytes have lifespans of only 90 to 120 days, turnover is rapid and the Hb A_{1c} level reflects the extent of glycemia over the previous 4 to 6 weeks. See Bunn for a review of Hb A_{1c}.[11]

A systemic evaluation and revision of the nomenclature and classification of diabetes was sponsored by the National Diabetes Data Group of the NIH in 1978. Findings of this group as they relate to diabetes mellitus are presented in Table 2. For a more extensive discussion, as well as coverage of the other classes of glucose in tolerance, the reader is referred to the original reference.[10] It should be emphasized that a major thrust of the report is a streamlining of the nomenclature of diabetes by eliminating names based upon age or symptoms. Classification into type I or type II diabetes is based exclusively upon whether or not the patient is dependent upon injected insulin to sustain life. The recommended nomenclature will be used throughout the report.

Etiology

As addressed in the revised classification scheme, diabetes can occur in many different ways. However, despite an enormous amount of effort, the questions "Why does a person become diabetic?'' and ''How does a person become a diabetic?'' have remained largely unanswered. Currently, diabetes is considered to be an extremely heterogenous group of diseases, resulting from various combinations of genetic, environmental, and immunologic factors, that seemingly have only one thing in common — an inability to metabolize glucose properly.

Diabetes has a genetic connection that has been known for years.[12] There are at least 40 distinct genetic syndromes known to be associated with varying degrees of glucose intolerance, but they are rare and do not include type I and type II diabetes. The monozygotic twin studies of Pike and co-workers have helped to clarify the genetics of these disorders. Twin pairs (185) have been investigated for concordance (both becoming diabetic if one was diabetic) in regard to both types of diabetes. Concordance among type II twins approached 100% whereas concordance with type I diabetic twins was only about 50%. These results are interpreted as suggesting that the genetic linkage is stronger with type II diabetes and as implying that, although there is a genetic predisposition to type I diabetes, other factors are also of major importance. They also strongly support the separation of diabetes into at least two distinct entities.

Further genetic support for the separation comes from studies involving histocompatibility antigens (HLA). The HLA system represents a series of gene products from chromosome 6 that must be compatible for successful organ transplants and skin grafts. Certain of these antigens (B-8 and B-15) have a strong association with type I diabetes but not type II diabetes. These alleles are believed to serve as markers for closely linked ''diabetogenic'' genes that are responsible for susceptibility to insulin-dependent diabetes. Whatever the gene product, it is not insulin, as the insulin gene has recently been found to reside on the short arm of chromosome 11.[13]

Of the possible environmental factors that could cause diabetes, viruses have received the most attention. Support for this hypothesis comes from retrospective epidemiological studies done relating the onset of diabetes to the time of the year and to its temporal association with childhood viral infections such as mumps and rubella. While these lines of evidence are largely circumstantial, when combined with observations in animal model systems of viral β-cell cytotoxicity, they do become rather compelling.[14] In fact Nerup and collaborators have proposed that HLA genes may predispose individuals to diabetes by increasing their susceptibility to viruses that destroy β-cells, either directly or through the triggering of an autoimmune response.[15]

The concept of an autoimmune component in the pathogenesis of diabetes derives from the observation that different endocrinologic disorders of autoimmune character are four to five times more prevalent in type I diabetics than in the general population.[16] This is consistent with the finding that 60 to 70% of patients with insulin-dependent diabetes have islet cell cytoplasmic antibody at time of diagnosis or a few weeks thereafter. Disregarding the duration of the disease, 20 to 40% of patients demonstrate islet cell antibody with those who have the HLA-B-8 allele being preferentially affected. Noninsulin-dependent diabetics have a prevalence of islet cell antibody close to that of the control population.

Hormonal Interrelationships

Classically, diabetes mellitus has been considered to be a ''unihormonal'' disease with all of the metabolic defects thought to be primarily or secondarily due to a deficiency of effective insulin. More recently the concept of a ''bihormonal'' disease has been proposed[17,18] with the insulin deficiency occurring in the presence of an excess of glucagon. Such a relationship would not be expected because glucagon is normally present in the bloodstream during hypoglycemia and diabetes is characterized by hyperglycemia. However, in every form of spontaneous or experimentally induced diabetes examined to date, hyperglucagonemia has been found to coexist with the hyperglycemia.

Figure 1

Amino Acid Sequences of Pancreatic Hormones

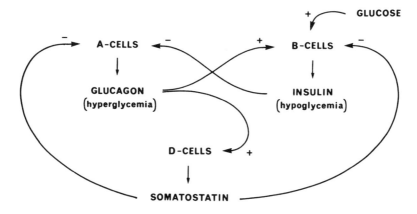

Ala-Gly-Cys-Lys-Asn-Phe-Phe
            | \
            S   Trp
            | |
            S   Lys
            | /
      Cys-Ser-Thr-Phe-Thr

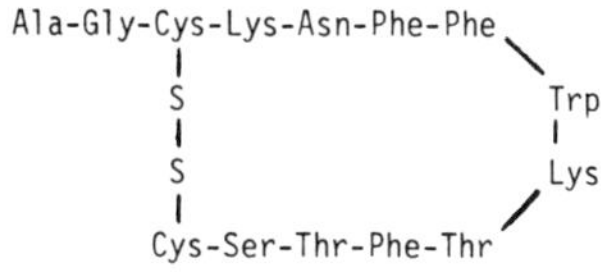

Somatostatin

His-Ser-Gln-Gly-Thr-Phe-Thr-Ser-Asn-Tyr-Ser-Lys-Tyr-Leu-Asn-Ser-Arg Ala Gln Asn Phe Val-Gln-Trp-Leu-Met-Asn-Thr

Glucagon

FIGURE 1. Amino acid sequences of pancreatic hormones.

DOUBLE TROUBLE HYPOTHESIS

FIGURE 2. Double trouble hypothesis.

Both glucagon and insulin originate from the islets of Langerhans in the pancreas; glucagon is a product of the α-cells and insulin is produced by the β-cells. In addition, the islets contain a third cell type, the δ-cells, which secrete somatostatin (see Figure 1 for the amino acid sequence of glucagon and somatostatin and Figure 3 for that of insulin). The islet cell distribution is 32% α, 57% β, and 11% δ. The hormones produced by these cells can alter the secretions of the others as summarized in Figure 2. Proponents of the "bihormonal" hypothesis argue that the primary defect of diabetes may be a loss of glucose-sensing ability by the β-cells. Since insulin normally suppresses the release of glucagon, a defect in insulin release would allow glucagon secretion to continue more or less unchecked. As it relates to diabetes, the hyposecretion of insulin would account for the under-utilization of insulin while the hypersecretion of glucagon would promote glucose production that would aggravate the existing hyperglycemia.

Support for this so-called "double trouble" hypothesis comes from studies done utilizing somatostatin, the δ-cell hormone that suppresses the release of both glucagon and insulin as well as others (see Figure 2). When somatostatin is administered to type I diabetics not receiving insulin, the hyperglycemia in both the fasting and postprandial states is attenuated. In addition, if a diabetic formerly receiving insulin is taken off insulin but infused with somatostatin, the onset of hyperglycemia is more gradual and the degree of hyperglycemia not nearly so extreme. Furthermore, the use of somatostatin in combination with insulin allows the dose of insulin to be decreased while maintaining the same level of glycemic control.

While there is controversy about the relative importance of the double trouble hypothesis in the development of diabetes, it is generally agreed that controlling glucagon levels could be beneficial. Consequently, a search for somatostatin-like compounds with selected biologic activity and a reasonable serum halflife is underway (see section on hypoglycemic agents, "Other Drugs — Past, Present, and Future").

DRUG MONOGRAPHS

INSULIN

Mechanism of Action

Although our knowledge of the molecular basis of insulin action is incomplete, significant insight was gained with the isolation and characterization of cell surface insulin receptors.[19] Binding of insulin to these receptors (1) is specific and has great affinity, (2) is rapid and reversible, (3) can be saturated, and (4) can be related to insulin activity.

The structure of the receptor for insulin appears to be highly conserved among vertebrates.[20] Czech has reviewed the available data and has proposed a minimal structure of approximately 300,000 molecular weight (mol wt).[21] Each of these structures is composed of four subunits of two different types designated α and β. The α-subunits are of mol wt 125,000 and the β-subunits are of mol wt 90,000. β-Subunits are extremely sensitive to proteolytic cleavage into approximately equal parts. The four subunits are linked together by disulfide bonds to give a symmetrical complex having the configuration (α-s-s-β)-s-s-(α-s-s-β). The similarity between this structure and that of the immunoglobin antibodies suggests the possibility of binding up to two insulin molecules.

Internalization of the insulin signal upon its initial binding occurs by means that are largely speculative at the current time.[22] Originally it was thought that insulin did not enter the cell itself,[23] but more recent evidence confirms that at least a portion of the bound insulin does enter the cell and in fact may associate with intracellular receptors.[24,25] In addition, Larner et al. have demonstrated the release by insulin of a chemical mediator that controls phosphorylation and dephosphorylation.[26] This is of significance because many of the enzyme systems regulated by insulin (glycogen synthetase, pyruvate dehydrogenase, pyruvate kinase, and acetyl CoA carboxylase) are controlled by phosphorylation-dephosphorylation reactions. Seals and Czech[27] have provided evidence that the mediator generated in response to insulin receptor interaction is a peptide or peptide-like substance. Czech postulates that the interaction of insulin with the receptor activates a plasma membrane protease and that this protease releases a low molecular weight peptide secondary messenger from a membrane protein precursor.[21] It is not known whether this precursor is part of the insulin-receptor complex, but the knowledge that the β-subunit is sensitive to proteolytic cleavage makes such a proposal attractive. It is further hypothesized that the peptide mediator modulates phosphorylation-dephosphorylation reactions by activating phosphatase activity.

All receptors studied so far have about the same affinity for a specific type of insulin, but the affinity does change with changes in insulin structure. Receptors prefer chicken insulin > pork = beef = human > fish > guinea pig > insulin-like growth factors.[28]

Table 3
METABOLIC EFFECTS
OF INSULIN

Metabolic Function	Effect
Glucose transport	↑
Amino acid transport	↑
Potassium transport	↑
Glucose oxidation	↑
Glucogenesis	↓
Glycogen formation	↑
Glycogen mobilization	↓
Fatty acid synthesis	↑
Lipid formation	↑
Lipolysis	↓
Ketogenesis	↓
Protein synthesis	↑
Proteolysis	↓

Note: ↑ Means the metabolic function is stimulated, ↓ means the metabolic function is antagonized.

The effects of insulin on carbohydrate, lipid, protein, and nucleic acid metabolism depend upon the tissue involved and its metabolic state. The main tissues affected by insulin are liver, adipose tissue, and skeletal muscles. Adipose tissue and skeletal muscles are dependent upon insulin for glucose uptake,[29,30] whereas the liver is penetrable by glucose but requires insulin for its metabolism. While the effect of insulin upon glucose transport is familiar to all, many other actions are ascribed to its use. It is difficult to determine which actions are primary and which are secondary, but in general, insulin favors anabolism and the formation of energy reserves. The major metabolic effects of insulin have been reviewed[31] and are summarized in Table 3.

Structure-Activity Relationships

In 1889 von Mering and Minkowski demonstrated that pancreatectomized dogs developed diabetes-like symptoms. To explain this phenomenon, investigators proposed that the pancreas must secrete a substance that was antidiabetic in nature. This then hypothetical substance was named "insuline" by de Meyer in 1909. Banting and Best eventually reversed the work of von Mering and Minkowski by demonstrating that a pancreatic extract could lower blood glucose levels in diabetic dogs. Less than one year later in Toronto in 1922, a pancreatic extract of insulin was administered to the first human patient — Leonard Thompson. It is interesting to note that Leonard Thompson was maintained with insulin therapy for approximately 13 years and died at age 27 of bronchopneumonia.[32]

Insulin was crystallized by Abel in 1926[33] and had its chemical structure (Figure 3) elucidated by Sanger and co-workers in the early 1950s.[34] Insulin is composed of two polypeptide chains designated as A and B. The A chain has 21 amino acid residues and the B chain has 30. The A chain has an intrachain disulfide bond spanning residues 6 and 11, and there are two interchain disulfide bonds located between residues A-7 and B-7 as well as between residues A-20 and B-19. A chain and B chain amino acid differences from a number of species are summarized in Table 4. When compared with human insulin, beef insulin differs at residues A-8, A-10, and B-30; pig insulin is more similar differing only at residue B-30. Due to the increased number of amino acid differences, beef insulin is more antigenic than pig insulin although their biologic activities are the same.

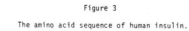

Figure 3

The amino acid sequence of human insulin.

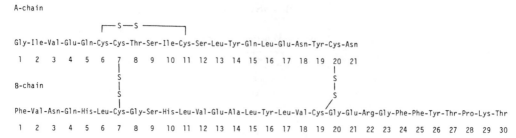

FIGURE 3.   The amino acid sequence of human insulin.

Table 4
AMINO ACID DIFFERENCES AMONG
VARIOUS SPECIES

	A chain			B chain
Source	**8**	**9**	**10**	**30**
Human	Threonine	Serine	Isoleucine	Threonine
Pig	Threonine	Serine	Isoleucine	Alanine
Beef	Alanine	Serine	Valine	Alanine
Horse	Threonine	Glycine	Isoleucine	Alanine
Sheep	Alanine	Glycine	Valine	Alanine

The chemical synthesis of insulin was achieved independently by three groups during the 1960s. All three groups separately synthesized the individual chains and then allowed for random disulfide bond formation. Yields of biologically active product were poor due to the large number of ways in which the disulfide bonds could spontaneously form. More recently, yields have been improved by treating the sulfhydryl form of one chain with the S-sulfonated form of the other. The formation of the correct disulfide bonds has been further enhanced through conformational-directed disulfide bond formation. This process involves crosslinking of amino acids known to be in juxtaposition in the three-dimensional structure, allowing the disulfide bond to form, and then reversing the amino acid linkage.[35] Kamber et al.[36] have found a way to avoid erroneous disulfide bond formation altogether. The correct disulfide bond is first formed between fragments of the A and B chains, then the fragments containing the proper disulfide bonds are condensed in an orderly fashion so as to form the final product. Human insulin synthesized in this manner has been shown to be biologically equivalent to the natural hormone.[37] Human insulin has also been synthesized using a semisynthetic method. Inouye et al.[38] coupled desoctapeptide insulin (insulin lacking the eight C-terminal amino acids of the B chain) with an octapeptide corresponding to positions B-23 to B-30 of human insulin using trypsin as the catalyst. Using a refinement of the same procedure, Morihara et al.[39] added a threonine to the C-terminal end of desalanine B-30 insulin. To obtain the desalanine B-30 insulin, porcine insulin was treated with carboxy-peptidase A. Consequently, porcine insulin was converted to human insulin in good yield (41%). The state of the art for the synthesis of human insulin utilizes cloned genes that are propagated in bacteria. So far, the genes are cloned separately, producing either A or B chains[40] that are purified and then combined by standard chemical methods[41] to yield a purified product.

The problems encountered in the chemical synthesis of insulin are overcome in vivo through the formation of a precursor protein known as proinsulin. Proinsulin, initially sequenced by Chance et al.[42] contains the A chain of insulin at its C-terminal end and the B chain of insulin at its N-terminal end. Between these two peptides is the connecting or C-peptide that has a pair of basic amino acids at each end. Human C-peptide within proinsulin allows the molecule to assume a conformational state that favors the formation of the correct disulfide bonds. Steiner and Clark[43] have reduced these disulfide bonds once formed and noted that their correct reformation in yields greater than 70%. The transformation of proinsulin into insulin occurs during the maturation of the storate granules. It requires protease activity similar to that of trypsin and carboxypeptidase B acting at the cleavage sites identified by the basic amino acids. The products of the conversion include one molecule of insulin, four basic amino acids, and one C-peptide from each proinsulin molecule processed. The halftime for conversion is about 1 hr. Gilbert and co-workers[44] are investigating the proinsulin approach to the production of cloned insulin. Reviews of the biosynthesis of insulin are available.[45-47]

The biological potency of all insulins and insulin analogs studied so far is proportional to their receptor binding affinity, which, however, can vary over a 1000-fold range. Porcine, bovine, and human insulins are considered to be equally potent; neither the A chain nor the B chain is active in the fully reduced form. There is no apparent loss of activity in the insulin molecule when the C-terminal alanine is removed from the B chain of porcine or bovine insulin, but the biologic activity is diminished appreciably when both the C-terminal alanine and the C-terminal asparagine are removed.[48] The removal of the second and third amino acids from the C-terminus of the B chain decreases the potency slightly, and desoctapeptide insulin (insulin minus eight amino acids from the C-terminal end of the B chain) has almost no activity and retains little ability to dimerize. Removing or chemically modifying the N-terminal glycine of the A chain substantially decreases biologic activity, but activity is retained if the B chain N-terminal phenylalanine is deleted. Chemical modification of the side chain carboxyl groups or the tyrosine residues also leads to inactivity.[49]

The receptor binding region of insulin has been deduced from these and other studies and is thought to involve invariant amino acids located in both the A and B chains.[50] Specific A chain residues include A-1 gly, A-5 gln, A-19 tyr, and A-21 asn; the adjacent B chain residues are B-24 phe, B-25 phe, B-26 tyr, B-12 val, and B-16 tyr. Located within this receptor binding region is an area believed to be responsible for negative cooperativity.[51] Negative cooperativity is the term applied to the loss of receptor affinity for insulin induced by the binding of insulin to other receptors. The observed effect is actually the result of an accelerated dissociation rate of the insulin-receptor complex. The area comprises some of the eight C-terminal residues of the B chain and the A-21 asparagine.

The three-dimensional structure of insulin has been determined by Hodgkin and co-workers,[35,52,53] and Blundell and Wood.[54] It presents as a remarkably complex small globular protein. Physiologically, insulin exists in the monomeric form but, when crystallized with zinc, insulin forms globular zine-stabilized hexamers. The hexamers consist of three identical, slightly asymmetric dimers arranged around a threefold axis. The dimers are held together by hydrophobic interactions and hydrogen bonds between the conserved regions of the B chains of each opposing monomer.[55] Presumably, insulin is stored in the granules of the β-cell as the hexamer.

Pharmacokinetics

The premise of insulin therapy is either the replacement of the insulin that is lacking or the supplementation of that which is inadequate in eliciting the biologic actions of insulin in the diabetic. To provide flexibility in meeting the demands of the patient, a large number of insulin preparations are available that differ in onset, peak, and duration of action. The pharmacology of these agents is summarized in Table 5. It is recognized that wide variations

Table 5
PHARMACOLOGY OF VARIOUS INSULIN PREPARATIONS[56]

Preparation	Onset (hr)	Peak (hr)	Duration (hr)
Rapid-acting			
Insulin injection (regular crystalline)	0.5—1	2—3	5—7
Prompt insulin zinc suspension (Semilente® insulin)	0.5—1	4—7	12—16
Intermediate-acting			
Insulin zinc suspension (Lente® insulin)	1—4	8—12	18—24
Isophane insulin suspension (NPH insulin)	1—2	8—12	18—24
Long-acting			
Protamine zinc insulin suspension (PZI)	4—8	14—20	36
Extended insulin zinc suspension (Ultralente® insulin)	4—8	16—18	36

in activity from a single preparation are possible; therefore all values should serve only as guidelines. An example of such a disparity has recently been reported by Roy et al.[57] In a study of the time action characteristics of regular and NPH insulin in diabetics treated with insulin for 13 years, they found the peak (5.7 ± 3 hr) and duration (16.2 ± 1.1 hr) of regular insulin were much longer than generally reported. They did, however, find that their results with NPH insulin confirmed the literature values.

The pharmacokinetics of exogenous insulin are generally those of endogenous insulin. In the normal individual[58,59] the insulin content of the pancreas is about 10 mg. Under fasting conditions approximately 20 μg of insulin per hour is released into the portal vein resulting in portal insulin concentrations ranging from 2 to 4 ng/mℓ. During the first pass through the liver 40 to 60% of the insulin is destroyed (model systems assume 47%). Consequently, the concentration of insulin in the systemic circulation is lower than that of the portal circulation ranging around 0.5 ng/mℓ (10 to 20 μU/mℓ). Insulin is small enough to be filtered at the glomeruli, but it is reabsorbed in the proximal convoluted tubules which also degrade approximately 60%.[60] Less than 2% of the daily insulin production is excreted unchanged in the urine. After a high carbohydrate meal plasma insulin levels rapidly increase to 100 to 140 μU/mℓ and then decrease as the blood glucose level falls. Normally only 1 to 2 mg of insulin are secreted on a daily basis. In the absence of insulin antibodies, insulin in the blood is unbound.

At the liver and kidney, the degradation of insulin can occur by either of two processes. Glutathione-insulin transhydrogenase (GIT) can reduce the disulfide bonds releasing the A and B chains.[61] These biologically inactive peptides then are broken down into amino acids by proteases. The other insulin-degrading mechanism involves its direct proteolytic cleavage by the enzyme insulin protease (insulinase). The initial cleavage occurs between residues 16 and 17 in the B chain resulting in a molecule consisting of three peptide chains held together by disulfide bonds.[62] Nonspecific proteases complete the destruction probably assisted by GIT.

Various models have been proposed to describe the kinetics of insulin disappearance in man. Bressler and Galloway[56] fit the data to a two-compartment open-ended model with a rapid halflife of 6.4 min and a slow halflife of 211 min. Three compartment models have been proposed by Silvers et al.[63] and Sherwin et al.[64] In addition to the plasma space (compartment 1, 4.5% body weight), there are fast equilibrating (compartment 2, 1.7% body weight) and slow equilibrating (compartment 3, 9.5% body weight) compartments. The combined insulin mass of the three compartments (expressed as plasma equivalent volume) is equal to the inulin space (15.7%). The distribution space of inulin is 157 mℓ/ kg and corresponds to the extracellular water compartment. The metabolic clearance rate (MCR) determined by Sherwin et al.[64] was 780 mℓ/min/1.73 m^2 and compares favorably with the MCR determined by Genuth[65] (861 mℓ/min) and Navalesi et al.,[66] 727 mℓ/min. The composite MCR also agrees with the sum (720 mℓ/min) of the clearance rates of various tissues. Hepatic clearance has been computed to be 400 mℓ/min, renal plasma clearance is estimated to be 190 mℓ/min, and peripheral tissue clearance is approximated to be 130 mℓ/ min.[64] The MCR of insulin has been found to be similar in both diabetic patients and normal subjects although the latter-onset patients had slightly lower MCR than the earlier-onset diabetics.[66]

Newer, more complex models incorporating high and low affinity receptor populations, partial insulin degradation, and delayed insulin degradation probably associated with internalization are available.[67,68]

Generally, exogenous insulin is administered subcutaneously in doses adequate to bring the blood glucose concentration into acceptable limits. To achieve this goal of near-normal glycemia, plasma insulin levels are practically always elevated above normal. However, since the exogenously administered insulin enters the systemic circulation rather than the portal circulation, the livers of insulin-dependent diabetics rarely experience normal insulin concentrations.

Numerous studies (see Galloway et al. for list[69]) have been done investigating the absorption of insulin from the injection site. A comparison of the data is difficult in that almost one half the studies no effort was made to establish the comparability of the biologic handling of the labeled hormone to the unlabeled, and, in the studies done with insulin-dependent diabetics, no effort was made to determine how the presence of insulin antibodies may have altered the disposition of the insulin. Nevertheless, by dividing the area under the serum insulin curve after the injection by the area under the serum insulin curve after an intravenous dose, the bioavailability index can be computed.[70] Bioavailability indexes correspond to the fraction absorbed and range around 50% for 10-hr studies done using neutral regular insulin.[69] Bioavailability indexes for the modified insulins are more difficult to determine due to their slower absorption rates. In a study of NPH insulin, 40% of the injected dose remained at the injection site 10 hr postinjection with 10% still remaining after 24 hr.[71] In addition, evidence suggests that at least some NPH insulin is absorbed unchanged and would not be detected by routine assays.[72] Both of these factors would tend to falsely decrease the observed bioavailability index. Similarly, the absorption of Lente® insulin is slow with 70% of the dose located at the injection site after 10 hr and 25% still remaining after 36 hr.[71] The disappearance of NPH followed first order kinetics while that of Lente® insulin is biphasic probably representing the crystalline mixture. Kølendorf and Bojsen[73] have correlated the disappearance of NPH insulin administered subcutaneously to its appearance in the plasma. A disappearance halflife of 6.6 hr was determined.

That there is a loss of insulin at the injection site is supported by a number of lines of evidence. Cases are known in which insulin-dependent diabetics, unsatisfactorily controlled with large doses of insulin given subcutaneously or intramuscularly, are adequately controlled with conventional doses administered intravenously.[74] Likewise, Stevensen et al.[75] have demonstrated in rats that the blood glucose response of 0.4 U/kg of insulin administered subcutaneously could be duplicated by an intravenous dose only half as large. Berger et al.[76] have presented data that 15 to 25% of administered semisynthetic insulin was degraded at the site with a disappearance halflife of 59 min. More recently they have reported that the insulin can be partially protected at the injection site by Trasylol, a pancreatic protease inhibitor.[77] It is speculated that the protease inhibitor blocks the action of insulin-degrading enzymes known to be present in adipose tissue.

Aside from the formulation of the insulin preparation and its degradation at the site, there are a number of other factors that influence its absorption. (1) *Site of injection:* Koivisto and Felig[78] have determined that the disappearance of insulin from injection sites in the abdominal wall is 86% greater than from the leg and 30% greater than from the arm. Absorption from the arm is 40% greater than from the leg. Abdominal absorption blunts the postprandial rise in blood glucose by 30 to 50 mg/dℓ as compared to leg. Peak serum insulin concentrations are reached most rapidly with abdominal injection and slowest with injection into the anterior thigh. Peak height is greatest with deltoid injection and lowest with injection into the buttock.[69] Absorption of insulin from the extremities is enhanced by exercise. (2) *Depth of injection:* the deeper insulin is injected, the quicker is its onset and the higher is its peak.[69] (3) *Concentration of insulin:* insulin disappearance from the injection site slows down as the concentration of insulin is increased.[79] However, insulin concentrations in the range of 40 to 100 U/mℓ do not significantly alter the bioavailability. (4) *Presence of antibodies:* insulin antibodies delay the onset and duration of injected insulin.[80]

Due to these factors and various other reasons, intrasubject and intersubject variations in insulin response are significant. Galloway et al.[69] report that the intrasubject coefficients of variation for peak response and time of peak for regular insulin were actually greater than those intersubject (63.6 vs. 50.4 for peak, 107.2 vs. 101.5 for time of peak). Results with NPH insulin were similar but less dramatic. Lauritzen et al.[81] in studies using NPH and Lente® insulins have reported an individual daily range of absorption of injected insulin label to be 19 to 104%. The magnitude of the coefficients of variation calls attention to the shortcomings of conventional insulin therapy.

Uses and Dosage

Insulin therapy is required by all patients in which the metabolic derangements associated with its lack cannot be controlled by agents that stimulate the secretion of endogenous insulin (e.g., sulfonylureas) or by procedures that balance the effectiveness of residual insulin with the demand (e.g., weight reduction and dietary control). Into this category fall all type I diabetics, some type II diabetics, and all diabetics who are ketosis-prone with or without the stress due to trauma, surgery, or infection. Some 5 to 10% of the 5.2 million diagnosed American diabetics are insulin-dependent. The insulin preparations available in the U.S. are summarized in Table 6.[82]

Various avenues to administer insulin have been investigated. Although the oral route would be the most desirable since it would introduce insulin into the portal circulation wherein it is normally secreted, it is not feasible. Insulin is a proteinaceous hormone and is subject to the action of the digestive enzymes. Studies, however, have demonstrated that insulin can be absorbed from the duodenum, but doses 20 times higher than those effective subcutaneously are required. Efforts have been made to enhance absorption through chemical means. Galloway and Root[83] have demonstrated that the plasma insulin concentration can be raised by administering 8 to 10 U insulin per kg body weight orally along with a surface-active substance such as polyoxethylene oleyl ether. The intrajejunal administration of water-in-oil-in-water insulin emulsions has also been tested in alloxan-diabetic rats.[84] Yet another potential route is by inhalation. Clinical evidence has indicated that insulin is absorbed through the respiratory mucosa.[85] In response to this observation, an aerosol dosage form containing insulin has been developed and subjected to physiochemical evaluation.[86] Perhaps a more normal approach has been the administration of insulin by rectal suppository. Yamasaki et al.[87] have found that diabetic subjects given a 100-U suppository 15 min after meals three times daily showed a significant improvement in postprandial hyperglycemia accompanied by a restoration of the normal circadian immunoreactive insulin profile and a

Table 6
INSULIN PREPARATIONS AVAILABLE IN THE U.S.[a]

Product (manufacturer)	Species source	Purity (ppm) proinsulin	Strength
Rapid-Acting			
Regular Iletin® I (Lilly)	Beef & pork	<50	U-40, U-100
Regular Iletin® II (Lilly)	Pork	<10	U-100, U-500
Regular Iletin® II (Lilly)	Beef	<10	U-100
Semilente® Iletin® I (Lilly)	Beef & pork	<50	U-40, U-100
Velosulin® Regular Insulin (Nordisk)	Pork	<10	U-100
Actrapid® Regular Insulin (Novo)	Pork	<10	U-100
Semitard® Insulin Zinc Susp. (Novo)	Pork	<10	U-100
Regular Insulin (Squibb)	Pork	<25	U-40, U-100
Regular Insulin Purified (Squibb)	Pork	<10	U-100
Semilente® Insulin (Squibb)	Beef	<25	U-100
Intermediate-Acting			
Lente® Iletin® I (Lilly)	Beef & pork	<50	U-40, U-100
Lente® Iletin® II (Lilly)	Beef or pork	<10	U-100
NPH Iletin® I (Lilly)	Beef & pork	<50	U-40, U-100
NPH Iletin® II (Lilly)	Beef or pork	<10	U-100
Insulatard® NPH (Nordisk)	Pork	<10	U-100
Mixtard®, NPH + regular insulin (Nordisk)	Pork	<10	U-100
Lentard® insulin zinc susp. (Novo)	Beef & pork	<10	U-100
Monotard® insulin zinc susp. (Novo)	Pork	<10	U-100
Protophane® NPH (Novo)	Pork	<10	U-100
Isophane NPH insulin (Squibb)	Beef	<25	U-40, U-100
Isophane NPH insulin purified (Squibb)	Beef	<10	U-100
Lente® insulin (Squibb)	Beef	<25	U-40, U-100
Lente® insulin purified (Squibb)	Beef	<10	U-100
Long-Acting			
Protamine zinc iletin I (Lilly)	Beef & pork	<50	U-40, U-100
Protamine zinc iletin II (Lilly)	Beef or pork	<10	U-100
Ultralente® iletin I (Lilly)	Beef & pork	<50	U-40, U-100
Ultratard® insulin zinc susp. (Novo)	Beef	<10	U-100
Protamine zinc insulin (Squibb)	Beef	<25	U-100
Ultralente® insulin (Squibb)	Beef	<25	U-100

[a] E. R. Squibb & Sons, and Novo Industries A/S have formed Squibb/Novo which market insulins produced by Novo and are sold in the U.S. by Squibb Operations since May 1, 1982.

reduction of urinary glucose from 26 ± 5.9 to 2.0 ± 1.0 g/day. It was estimated that about 30% of the insulin absorbed by the rectum was assigned directly to the portal vein. Questions over the long term safety of this method limit its clinical consideration. Currently, when one considers the size of the insulin dose needed in each of the above routes of administration and calculates the cost to the patient in dollars and cents, one must conclude that as yet they are not practical. This leaves the parenteral administration of insulin as the only reasonable option. Rapid-acting insulins may be administered intravenously, intramuscularly, or subcutaneously regardless of the pH of the solvent. Long- or intermediate-acting insulins, whether or not they are dissolved or suspended in the vial, should not be administered intravenously because of a risk of emboli. Even then to ensure accurate delivery, bottles containing NPH and Lente® insulins should be inverted several times before drawing the preparation into the syringe. The palatability of the parenteral route is improving with the development of automated insulin delivery systems of both open and closed loop design.[88,89]

In tailoring a course of insulin therapy to a patient, many factors must be considered. These include age, residual insulin secretion, diet, duration of diabetes, antibodies, physical activity, degree of obesity, intercurrent disease (particularly those affecting the metabolism and elimination of insulin, e.g., cirrhosis and uremia), degree of metabolic decompensation, and the presence of drugs and/or hormones that may affect insulin sensitivity.[90] In the uncomplicated, nonketotic diabetic an initial dose of 10 to 20 U of an intermediate acting insulin is recommended. This should be followed by weekly determinations of the extent of hyperglycemia with fractional urine tests 4 to 5 times daily. If all values obtained with the copper-reduction methods are in a 3 to 4+ range, the patient is instructed to increase the following day's dose of insulin by 4 U. If all values are in the range 0 to 2+, but all are not zero, then the insulin dose is left unchanged. On the other hand, if all values are 0 to 1+, the patient is instructed to reduce the next day's dose by 4 U. When the dose of insulin reaches 50 to 60 U daily, consideration is given to splitting the dose with two thirds given in the morning and the remaining one third before supper.[91] Of course, many other alternatives are possible to further refine the glycemic profile (see Galloway et al.[69] for a discussion of the bioavailability of combinations of regular and intermediate-acting preparations). For a more detailed discussion of insulin therapy as well as therapy of the more complicated cases, including diabetic ketoacidosis and insulin resistance, the reader is referred to therapeutic textbooks[92,93] (see also the following section on toxicity). One other point worth mentioning is that when converting patients to one of the more highly purified insulin preparations, a slight downward adjustment of dosage may be required.[94,95]

Toxicities

The major problem is hypoglycemia. Hypoglycemia induced by insulin can result from failure to agitate the vial subsequent to use, improper measurement of insulin, reduction of insulin requirement as a result of a spontaneous change in the course of the disease, and the chronic use of excess dosage. The majority of the signs and symptoms of hypoglycemia are the result of functional abnormalities of the CNS. They range from sweating, weakness, and tachycardia through headache, blurred vision, and mental confusion to coma, convulsions, and death. The symptoms reverse almost immediately with intravenous glucose unless brain deprivation of glucose was too prolonged. A particularly bothersome phenomenon associated with hypoglycemia is known as the Somoygi effect.[96] It usually occurs in poorly controlled patients and involves a counter-regulatory hormone-mediated increase in blood glucose. Although the response is caused by hypoglycemia, it often is misinterpreted as a sign of insulin deficiency thereby resulting in an increase in the insulin dose. Thus, a vicious cycle is established. Medication with beta blocking agents may eliminate or reduce the hypoglycemic warnings. Alcohol intake, in addition to masking the warnings, may promote hypoglycemia by reducing glucogenesis by the liver.

Other adverse reactions include local and systemic allergies.[97] The allergies are correlated with the formation of antibodies. It is not known how the insulin molecule is recognized by the immune system, but the formation of antibodies to insulin preparations is believed to be related to a number of factors: (1) the genetic composition of the individual; (2) the pattern of exposure-systemic allergies often associated with interrupted therapy; (3) the species source of the insulin — beef is more antigenic than pork; (4) the purity of the insulin preparation — the higher the proinsulin content, the greater the antigenicity; and (5) the formulation of the preparation — Lente® insulin is more immunogenic than regular insulin.[98]

Local allergic reactions occur most frequently in patients receiving insulin for the first time; the incidence has been estimated to be in the range of 20 to 50% of patients.[91] They appear as hard, indurated areas within a few minutes to several hours after an injection. About 80% of patients with persistent local allergy to mixed beef-pork insulin will improve if treated with monospecies pork insulin.[91] Approximately 15% of the remaining patients are less reactive to beef insulin than pork. A small percentage of patients require "single component" insulin.

In a study of patients with systemic allergies, a history of intermittent therapy was found in 60% of cases.[99] Systemic allergies are characterized by symptoms ranging from generalized hives to hypotension and death. Treatment of systemic allergies and a few local allergies refractory to other methods of treatment involves desensitization.[56] Desensitization to porcine insulin is more common since 80% of patients will tolerate pork insulin better than beef insulin. If desensitization cannot be achieved, steroid therapy has proved to be effective.[56]

Coexisting with local allergy in about 15% of cases is lipodystrophy; lipodystrophy may take the form of atrophy or hypertrophy.[56] Occasionally, both types are observed in the same patient. Lipoatrophy occurs at the site of the injections, most commonly in children and adolescent girls. It is considered a benign condition of unknown cause. Lipohypertrophy is most commonly found in the anterior or lateral thigh with an incidence slightly higher in males than females. Treatment involves rotating the site of injection and/or conversion to a more purified form of insulin. Virtually all patients with lipoatrophy improve when treated with purified pork insulin. In fact, lipodystrophy and allergy have not been reported in patients who have received only purified pork insulin.[98]

A rare complication of insulin therapy is insulin resistance defined as "hyporesponsiveness or a tolerance for at least 200 U of insulin daily over a period of time in the absence of injection and coma".[100] Obesity is perhaps the most common cause although a number of unrelated diseases — hyperthyroidism, acromegaly, Cushing's syndrome, chronic lymphocytic leukemia, and liver disease have also been implicated. Insulin resistance due to the formation of excess antibodies is of particular concern. Normally the serum of diabetic subjects will bind less than 10 U of insulin per liter, but serum from patients with immune insulin resistance may bind from 6 to 1000 times the normal amount.[91] Regular insulin preparations containing 500 U/mℓ are often required to treat insulin resistance with marked reductions in doses occurring in some instances with the purified forms. Large doses of corticosteroids may also be beneficial.[56]

Physical-Chemical and Other Data

Due to the diversity of the group of patients subject to insulin therapy, no single preparation is adequate. Consequently, many different preparations, classified according to their duration of action, have been developed (see Uses and Dosage section). The physical-chemical properties of these preparations are summarized in Table 7. All consist primarily of insulin and have the biologic effects of insulin.

The source for most insulin has been — and remains — the pancreata of animals, most commonly those of beef cattle and pigs. Current extraction and crystallization procedures are essentially modifications of the original methods used 60 years ago. In brief, pancreata are minced and extracted with acid ethanol at pH 1 to 3. The acid inhibits the proteolytic enzymes, and the insulin is freely soluble in the aqueous ethanol. The extract is filtered, neutralized, and then centrifuged to remove debris. The supernatant is slightly acidified and defatted by slowly evaporating the alcohol under vacuum. After filtration the raw insulin is salted out at weakly acidic pH. The crude insulin after isolation is redissolved in dilute acid and precipitated isoelectrically at pH 5.3 to 5.4 as required for purification. Crystallization is effected by precipitating the insulin as a zinc compound from an aqueous insulin solution at a pH slightly above the isoelectric point. The result is known as conventional or USP

Table 7

PHYSICAL-CHEMICAL PROPERTIES OF INSULIN PREPARATIONS[104,105]

Type	Description	Zinc content (mg/100 units)	pH	Buffer	Preservative (w/v)	Modifying protein	
						Type	Amount
Insulin injection (regular crystalline)	A sterile, acidified or neutral solution of insulin; when contained in each mℓ not more than 100 USP units, it is a colorless or almost colorless liquid; that containing 500 units may be strawcolored; substantially free from turbidity and from insoluble matter	0.01—0.04	2.5—3.5 for acidified 7.0—7.8 for neutral	—	Contains 0.1— 0.25% of either phenol or cresol and 1.4—1.8% of glycerin	None	None
Isophane insulin suspension (NPH insulin)	A sterile, white suspension of rod-shaped crystals approximately 30 μm in length and free from large aggregates of crystals following moderate agitation	0.01—0.04	7.1—7.4	Phosphate	Contains either 1.4—1.8% glycerin, 0.15—0.17% of metacresol, and 0.06—0.07% of phenol, or 1.4— 1.8% of glycerin and 0.20—0.25% of phenol	Protamine	0.3—0.6
Protamine zinc insulin suspension	A sterile, white, or almost white suspension free from large particles following moderate agitation	0.15—0.25	7.1—7.4	Phosphate	Contains 1.4— 1.8% of glycerin, and either 0.18— 0.22% of cresol or 0.22—0.28% of phenol	Protamine	1.0—1.5 mg

Globin zinc insulin injection	A sterile almost colorless liquid, substantially free from turbidity and insoluble material	0.25—0.35	3.4—3.8	—	Contains 1.3—1.7% of glycerin and either 0.15—0.20% of cresol or 0.20—0.26% of phenol	Globin	3.6—4.0 mg
Prompt insulin zinc suspension (SemiLente® insulin)	A sterile, almost colorless suspension of particles that have no uniform shape and the maximum dimension of which does not exceed 2 μm	0.2—0.5	7.2—7.5	Acetate	0.09—0.11% methylparaben	None	None
Insulin zinc suspension (Lente® insulin)	A sterile, almost colorless suspension of a mixture of crystals predominantly 10—40 μm in maximum diameter and many particles which have no uniform shape and do not exceed 2 μm in maximum dimension	0.12—0.25	7.2—7.5	Acetate	Contains 0.09—0.11% methylparaben	None	None
Extended insulin zinc suspension (Ultralente® insulin)	A sterile, almost colorless suspension of a mixture of characteristic crystals the maximum dimension of which is predominantly 10—40 μm	0.12—0.25	7.2—7.5	Acetate	0.09—0.11% methylparaben	None	None

insulin. Over the years, the yield of insulin has improved to approximately 150 mg/kg pork pancreas, 100 mg/kg beef pancreas, and about 50 mg/kg human pancreas.[90]

Interest in the further purification of insulin was aroused in 1968 by the finding[101] and identification[42] of proinsulin in commercial insulin preparations. Proinsulin elutes near insulin in the chromatographic procedures and has become recognized as an index of the purity of the insulin preparation. Conventional insulin contains between 10,000 and 40,000 parts per million (ppm) proinsulin. By subjecting conventional insulin to gel filtration and ion exchange chromatographic procedures, single peak, "improved" single peak, and purified (single component) insulin preparations are obtained. They contain 300 to 3000 ppm, <50 ppm, and <10 ppm proinsulin, respectively.[98] Immunoassays for glucagon, pancreatic polypeptide, vasoactive intestinal peptide, and somatostatin can also be used to assess the degree of purity.

The potency of all insulin preparations is determined by comparison to an absolute weight of insulin prepared from a recrystallized composite sample. The current standard contains 24 U/mg.[102] For years insulin was marketed in two different strengths; one contained 40 U of insulin per milliliter (U-40), and the other contained 80 U/mℓ (U-80). Then, in 1973 a U-100 product was placed on the market with the intent to gradually replace the others. The impetus for this change was concern expressed by the American Diabetes Association and the FDA over possibilities that diabetic patients may erroneously use the wrong strength or misinterpret the double scale on the barrel of the syringe. Consequently, decertification of U-80 insulin was completed on March 24, 1980.[103] However, U-40 insulin continues to be produced in response to demands for a less concentrated form of insulin. In addition, a U-500 preparation of regular insulin is available for the treatment of insulin resistance.

Until 1973, regular insulin was produced at a pH of 2.8 to 3.5 to prevent particles from forming in the vial. As insulin purification methods improved, it was found that the pH could be neutralized with sodium hydroxide with no effect upon the solution.[102] NRI is more stable than acid regular and will maintain nearly full potency when stored up to 18 months at 5 and 25°C. After 12 months of storage at 37°C, NRI still maintains 95% of its potency. Therefore, it is acceptable to store opened vials of insulin at room temperature.[102]

A desire to spare diabetic patients the anguish of having to inject four doses of regular insulin each day led to the development of the intermediate and long-acting insulin preparations. Protamine zinc insulin (PZI) was developed by Hagedorn and co-workers[106] in the laboratories of Nordisk in Copenhagen in 1936. In this preparation insulin is mixed with zinc and protamine, a basic protein, to yield a complex that has an isoelectric point (7.4) close to physiologic pH. Due to the decreased solubility, insulin release into the extracellular fluids is prolonged accounting for its increased duration of action. The protamine used is prepared from the sperm or from the testes of certain fish and is considered to be devoid of immunogenic properties. Globin, another basic protein, was found to combine with insulin in a similar manner with almost identical results. However, globin zinc insulin has never gained popularity in the U.S. Neutral protamine Hagedorn (NPH) insulin was derived from PZI in 1946[107] when it was discovered that, if the protamine and zinc were brought together in near stoichiometric proportions, a crystalline entity was obtained that had biologic properties similar to a 2:1 mixture of regular insulin and PZI. NPH insulin is also called isophane based upon the Greek *iso* and *phane* meaning "equal" and "appearance".

In 1951, Hallas-Møller et al.[108] working at Novo in Denmark observed that the solubility of insulin at neutral pH in acetate buffer is reduced by a surplus of zinc in the absence of a modifying protein.[108] By carefully adjusting the pH, two physical forms of the zinc insulin complex can be produced. One is crystalline (Ultralente®) and the other is microcrystalline or amorphous (Semilente®). Due to the greater amount of surface exposed to the extracellular fluids, the amorphous preparation is much more rapidly absorbed. A mixture of 70% Ultralente® and 30% Semilente®, known as Lente® insulin, is also available. It has action characteristics similar to those of NPH insulin.

Caution should be exercised when combining various insulin preparations. Since PZI has an excess of protamine, NRI must be added in a ratio greater than 1:1 otherwise the action characteristics remain essentially those of PZI. Phosphate buffers alter the solubility characteristics of Lente® crystals. Therefore NPH and PZI should not be mixed with the Lente® preparations. However, the Lente® insulin can be mixed with each other in any ratio desired. In addition, NRI can be added to either Lente® or NPH insulin with no adverse effects. Studies in rabbits disclose that the mixtures are stable for up to 3 months if they are kept refrigerated.[56]

SULFONYLUREAS

Mechanism of Action

The sulfonylureas reduce blood glucose levels in both normal[109] and type II diabetic man as well as in animals. They have been shown to be ineffective in reducing blood glucose levels in pancreatectomized[110] and alloxan diabetic animals,[111] and in type I diabetic man. Therefore, it is concluded that these compounds require functional pancreatic tissue in order to produce their hypoglycemic effect.

Several different mechanisms involving the pancreas have been proposed to account for the ability of these agents to lower blood glucose levels (see reviews).[112-116] A decrease in pancreatic glucagon secretion would be consistent with the antidiabetic effect of the sulfonylureas, but the results have been contradictory and appear to be dependent upon the concentration of the drug.[114] Currently, sulfonylurea-induced alterations in glucagon secretion are not considered to be significantly involved in the induction of hypoglycemia. At least part of the antidiabetic action of sulfonylureas can be attributed to their ability to stimulate the acute phase of insulin release from the pancreatic β-cells.[117] Just recently it was hypothesized that this insulinotropic action resulted from changes in the flow of ions through the cell membranes.[118] Hypoglycemic sulfonamides were found to promote calcium translocation whereas hyperglycemic sulfonamides were found to antagonize calcium flow. Such membrane effects are consistent with the observation that the sulfonylureas do not penetrate the β-cells.[119] However, while increasing the circulating levels of insulin would definitely be consistent with the hypoglycemic action of sulfonylureas, the mechanism is apparently more complex. The hyperinsulinemia has been shown to be temporary. Therapy with these agents for 6 months or more usually results in a return of insulin to levels equal to or less than those originally present in the untreated state even though the improvement in blood glucose control continues.[120] Glipizide may be an exception to this generalized observation as increased insulin secretory responses of 100 to 1500% have been maintained in some cases for longer than 2 years.[113,121] To explain the continuing control of sulfonylureas over blood glucose in the face of diminishing insulin levels, attention has turned towards unmasking extrapancreatic effects.

A variety of extrapancreatic actions of sulfonylureas have been identified over the years (see table in Lebowitz and Feinglos[112]). Perhaps of primary importance is the observation that chronic sulfonylurea therapy increases insulin sensitivity in insulin-independent patients. While the specifics as to how sulfonylureas promote this increased sensitivity remain speculative, attention has focused upon insulin receptors. Olefsky and Reaven[122] have demonstrated that chronic chlorpropamide therapy in type II diabetic patients restores the deficient number of insulin receptors on circulating monocytes towards normal.[122] Glipizide also has been shown to increase the number of plasma membrane insulin receptors in normal mice.[123] These observations and others[124,125] have resulted in the hypothesis that at least some of the antidiabetic effects of sulfonylureas are achieved through altering the membrane responsiveness of insulin-sensitive tissues by increasing the number of insulin receptors.[113]

In summary, although the mechanistic details remain to be elucidated, the net effect of the sulfonylureas on blood glucose levels appears to be the result of a combination of factors and depends upon the time course of therapy. Early in the course of treatment, insulin secretion is stimulated resulting in an increase in circulating insulin levels which promote a move towards hypoglycemia. Later on in the course of therapy, the hypoglycemic effect is maintained in the face of declining insulin levels by an increase in insulin effectiveness mediated through an enhancement of the membrane effects of the insulin.

Structure-Activity Relationships

The history of the sulfonylurea antidiabetic agents began in the Montpellier district of France during the German occupation in 1942.[126] Due to the conditions of war, food was scarce and infectious disease, particularly typhoid fever, was epidemic. An experimental sulfonamide drug, sulfathiadiazole, had been synthesized in 1941 by Von Kennel and Kimmig and had been shown to have an in vitro inhibitory effect on the multiplication of the typhoid bacillus. First attempts by Janbon to treat typhoid fever with sulfathiadiazole involved 30 patients and resulted in the deaths of 3 of them by "obscure causes" while other patients experienced convulsions and coma. In others, a lowering of blood sugars was casually noted. It was later elucidated by Loubatieres[126] that the deaths, convulsions, and comas could be attributed to hypoglycemia precipitated by the combination of sulfonamide and inadequate food intake. Loubatieres went on to systematically correlate the chemical structure of various sulfonamide derivatives with the intensity of their hypoglycemic action and to suggest that the hypoglycemic sulfonamides might be useful in the diagnosis and treatment of diabetes. In 1955 the first clinical findings on the hypoglycemic effect of sulfonamides were published.

Meanwhile in Germany, a group of researchers were reporting their results concerning the hypoglycemic effects of another sulfonamide, carbutamide, which was being used to treat respiratory infections. Carbutamide was found to have a more pronounced effect upon lowering blood sugar levels than sulfathiadiazole. Consequently, it was tested clinically in diabetes by C. F. Boehringer and Sons in Germany and by Eli Lilly in the U.S. but was found to have major toxic effects. However, in 1956, results of the replacement of the *p*-amino group of carbutamide with a methyl group were made public. The new drug (tolbutamide) lacked the antibacterial effects of sulfonamides, retained the antidiabetic effects, and was devoid of most of the adverse problems. Upjohn, under license from Hoechst, subjected tolbutamide to clinical testing in the U.S. and brought it to market in mid-1957. Since then, more than 12,000 sulfonylureas have been synthesized and tested, but, at present, only tolbutamide, chlorpropamide, acetohexamide, and tolazamide are commercially available in the U.S. It is anticipated that some of the more powerful "second generation" agents, for example, glyburide, glipizide, and glibornuride will be marketed at some later date.

The structure-activity relationships of these sulfonylureas are summarized in Tables 8 and 9. In general, for a compound to have hypoglycemic activity, the benzene ring should contain one substituent, preferably in the *para* position as represented by R_1 in the structural formula. Obvious choices are methyl, chloro, acetyl, and certain ρ-(β-arylcarboxyamidoethyl) groups. Other possibilities include bromo, iodo, methylthio, and trifluoromethyl groups.[128] Compounds containing the ρ-(β-arylcarboxyamidoethyl) substituents are newer and are orders of magnitude more powerful than the original or first generation compounds.[129] Hence, they are classified along with agents such as glibornuride as second generation agents. It is believed that the high activity of these derivatives is a function of the specific distance between the nitrogen atom of the substituent and the sulfonamide nitrogen atom.[130] These compounds have accordingly been termed "N-d-N" hypoglycemic sulfonylureas.[131]

It is worthy of note that the acyl-amino-alcyl benzoic acid moiety of glyburide has hypoglycemic activity of its own. The compound, HB699, has about one third of the activity of an equal amount of tolbutamide, with the hypoglycemic effect being more transitory. Like tolbutamide, HB699 stimulates the release of insulin.[132]

Table 8
FIRST GENERATION COMPOUNDS

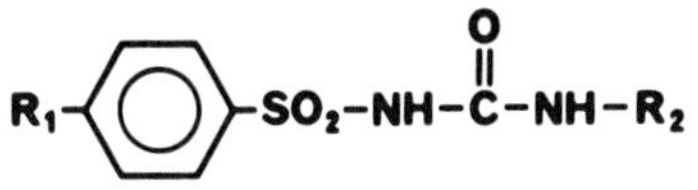

$$R_1 - \langle \bigcirc \rangle - SO_2 - NH - \overset{\overset{\textstyle O}{\|}}{C} - NH - R_2$$

Name	R_1	R_2	Equivalent therapeutic dose (mg)	Usual adult dose (mg)	Tablet size (mg)
Tolbutamide	CH_3-	$-CH_2-CH_2-CH_2-CH_3$	1000	500—3000	250,500
Chlorpropamide	$Cl-$	$-CH_2-CH_2-CH_3$	250	100—750	100,250
Tolazamide	CH_3-	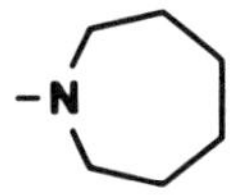 $-N\langle \text{(7-membered ring)} \rangle$	250	100—1000	100,250,500
Acetohexamide	$CH_3-\overset{\overset{\textstyle O}{\|}}{C}-$	(cyclohexyl ring)	500	250—1500	250,500

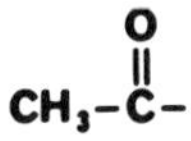

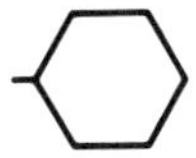

The groups attached to the terminal urea nitrogen, R_2 on the structural formula, should be a certain size and should impart lipophilic properties to the molecule. Consequently, optimal activity is usually found in compounds containing three to six carbons in an aliphatic side chain or five, six, or seven carbons in an alicyclic ring. Various heterocyclic ring systems, both unsubstituted and substituted, are also active.

Pharmacokinetics

Generally, the sulfonylurea hypoglycemic agents are well absorbed from the upper gastrointestinal tract, are transported protein-bound in the blood, are metabolized in the liver, and are excreted in the urine. The pharmacokinetic parameters — volume of distribution, percent serum protein binding, time to achieve peak plasma concentration, percent dose at peak concentration, elimination halflife, and usual number of daily doses of some of the first and second generation agents are summarized in Table 10. In addition, the usual adult dose range is available from Tables 8 and 9. Although steady state values determined in diabetics would potentially be of more value, most data are derived from single dose experiments using normal patients. Due to the large interindividual variations and the absence of some of the basic information in some of the earlier studies, values should serve only as indications of what to expect. Several recent reviews on the pharmacology of the sulfonylureas are available.[133-139]

It has been reported that concurrent intake of food with tolbutamide and chlorpropamide does not affect their bioavailability, absorption, or elimination.[140] However, the absorption of tolbutamide as well as acetohexamide can be improved by increasing the hydrophilicity of the compound.[141] Although the influence of food on tolbutamide is minimal, a 30-min delay in the effect of tolbutamide on blood glucose and insulin levels in normal subjects suggests that the drug might best be taken prior to meals. A similar conclusion was reached with glipizide but for a different reason. Unlike tolbutamide and chlorpropamide, concurrent intake of food with glipizide does significantly delay its absorption. Administration of

Table 9
SECOND GENERATION COMPOUNDS

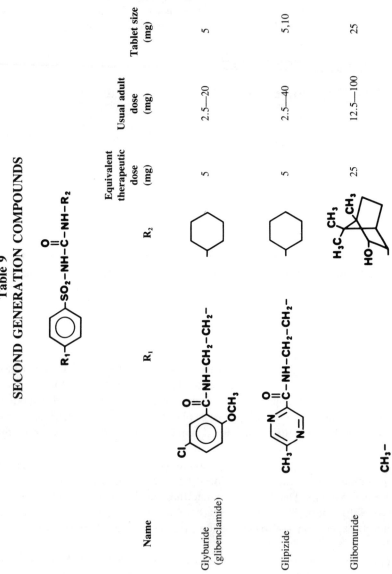

Name	R_1	R_2	Equivalent therapeutic dose (mg)	Usual adult dose (mg)	Tablet size (mg)
Glyburide (glibenclamide)			5	2.5—20	5
Glipizide			5	2.5—40	5,10
Glibornuride			25	12.5—100	25

Table 10
PHARMACOKINETIC PROPERTIES OF SULFONYLUREAS[133,135]

	Volume distribution (ℓ)	Serum protein binding (%)	Time to achieve peak plasma conc. (hr)	Dose at peak conc. (%)	Elimination halflife (hr)	Number of daily doses
Tolbutamide	10	95—97	2—4	9	7 (4—25)	2—3
Chlorpropamide	10	88—96	3—6	13	35 (25—60)	1
Tolazamide		94	4—8		7 (?)	1—2
Acetohexamide	15	65—88		5	6—8 (includes metabolites)	1—2
Glyburide	15	99	2—6	4.4—6.0	10 (6—12)	1—2
Glipizide	15	92—97	2	9—11	4 (3—7)	1—2
Glibornuride	18	95		5	8.2 (5.4—10.9)	1—2

glipizide 30 min before breakfast was found to maximize its metabolic impact.[142] Food did not affect either the rate or completeness of absorption of glyburide in nine healthy volunteers.[143]

Due to the fact that the sulfonylureas are weakly acidic (pK_a = 5.4), they bind moderately to strongly to plasma proteins; the most important protein in this regard is albumin although globulins may be involved to some extent. The binding sites of tolbutamide, chlorpropamide, and acetohexamide appear to differ from those of glipizide and glyburide.[144-146] In addition, glipizide and glyburide bind with greater affinity. It is not known whether the difference in binding between these two groups of agents is related to the vast difference in their potencies.

Efforts have been made to establish the plasma steady state concentrations of the sulfonylureas and to relate their plasma concentration to the dose response. Results are generally poor. Melander et al. found steady state tolbutamide concentrations to range from close to 0 to 370 μmol/ℓ (mean = 104 $\pm$ 15 μmol/ℓ) although the dosage variation was only sixfold. The fasting blood glucose concentrations in these patients varied from 4.8 to 15.5 mmol/ℓ (mean = 9.1 $\pm$ 0.04 mmol/ℓ). Steady state chlorpropamide concentration varied even more widely ranging from close to 0 to 882 μmol/ℓ (mean = 262 $\pm$ 24 μmol/ℓ) with only a fourfold variation in dosing. Fasting blood glucose levels varied from 3.3 to 17.1 mmol/ℓ although the mean did not differ significantly from that of the tolbutamide group.[147] Bergman et al. did find a significant dose vs. concentration relationship with chlorpropamide although there was a 30-fold interindividual variation in plasma clearance. A modest relationship between chlorpropamide serum concentration and extent of glycemic control was also noted.[148] Results of studies done utilizing second generation agents have also been nebulous. In one study involving 37 diabetics, no correlation could be found between serum glyburide levels and fasting blood glucose concentration.[143]

Most of the sulfonylureas undergo extensive metabolism by the liver, although metabolism is negligible during first-past. Specific biotransformations depend upon the chemical nature of the R groups and do differ from species to species. Referring to Figure 4, the compound can have R_1 oxidized or reduced at point A, can be hydrolyzed to a phenylsulfonylurea at point C, or could have R_2 hydroxylated at point D. Neither aromatic ring hydroxylation nor glucuronide or sulfate conjugation has been observed.

Tolbutamide is rapidly metabolized to p-hydroxytolbutamide (Figure 5) although there is a ninefold difference in the rate of transformation among individuals. There is evidence to suggest that the rate of oxidation of tolbutamide is under genetic control.[149] p-Hydroxytolbutamide has 35% of the hypoglycemic activity of the parent,[150] but it is further oxidized to p-carboxytolbutamide. Consequently, the blood concentration of p-carboxytolbutamide is

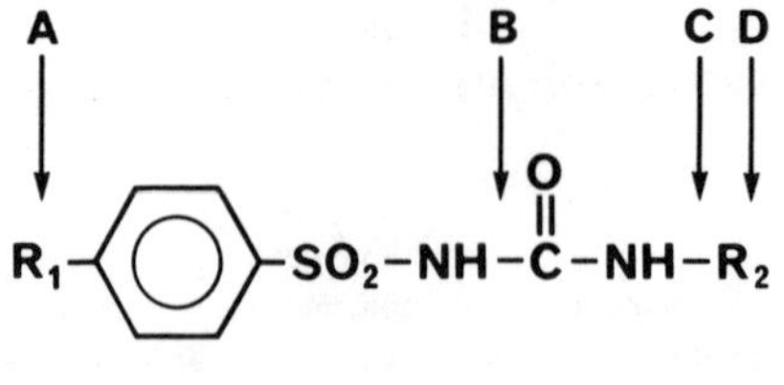

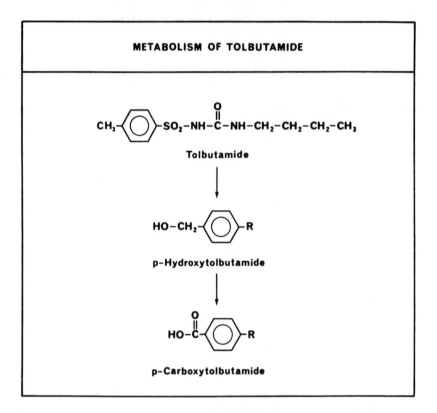

FIGURE 4. Transformations of sulfonylurea.

FIGURE 5. Metabolism of tolbutamide.

5%.[151] ρ-Carboxytolbutamide is the main excretory metabolite accounting for 60% of the administered dose in the 48-hr urine while ρ-hydroxytolbutamide accounts for only 30%.[152]

Chlorpropamide (CPA), despite continuing reports to the contrary, does undergo significant metabolism[153] (Figure 6). Eighty percent of the dose eventually is converted into three metabolites, 2-hydroxychlorpropamide (2-OH CPA), ρ-chlorobenzenesulfonylurea (CBSU), and 3-hydroxychlorpropamide (3-OH CPA).[154] The hypoglycemic activity of these compounds is uncharacterized. However, in the plasma 2 hr after dosing, chlorpropamide exists 95% unchanged, 3.5% in the form of CBSU, and 1.5% as the 2-hydroxy derivative.[155] This indicates that the metabolites are rapidly cleared by the kidney and that any inherent hypoglycemic activity would be of little consequence. Urinary analysis after prolonged collection of samples found 18% unchanged CPA, 21% CBSU, 55% 2-OH CPA, 2% ρ-chlorbenzenesulfonamide (CBSA), and 2% 3-OH CPA. The CBSA is believed to result from the nonbiological decomposition of CBSU in the urine. As a result of the long halflife of chlorpropamide, the drug will accumulate with continued dosing reaching a steady state in 7 to 10 days.

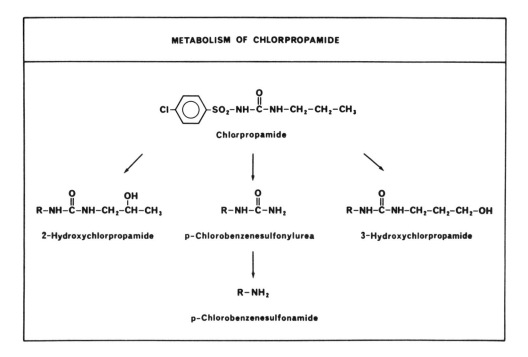

FIGURE 6.   Metabolism of chlorpropamide.

The metabolic fate of tolazamide is similar to that of tolbutamide but is more complex[156] (Figure 7). In addition to the two-stage oxidation, tolazamide can be hydroxylated and hydrolyzed as well as being converted into some unidentified metabolite. The 4-hydroxy and hydroxymethyl derivatives have less hypoglycemic activity than tolazamide but are more potent than tolbutamide. Carboxytolazamide is also active with about one third of the activity of tolbutamide. The peak hypoglycemic effect occurs about 1 hr after intravenous dosing and lasts about 10 hr.[157] Determination of the relative amounts of tolazamide and its metabolites in human urine during the 24-hr period immediately following dosing provides the following percentages: 7% tolazamide, 10% ρ-hydroxytolazamide, 17% carboxytolazamide, 25% 4-hydroxytolazamide, 26% ρ-toluenesulfonamide, and 15% uncharacterized metabolite.[158]

Acetohexamide differs in its metabolic conversion from the other sulfonylureas (Figure 8) in that one of its metabolites, L-hydroxyhexamide formed by the reduction of the ketone, has 2.5 times more hypoglycemic activity. The elimination halflife of acetohexamide is about 1.5 hr and that of L-hydroxyhexamide is about 5 hr.[159] Therefore, the hypoglycemic activity demonstrated in the blood represents the sum of the individual activities and yields a collective elimination halflife of 6 to 8 hr. Acetohexamide is also subject to parallel transformation to an hydroxylated form, 4-hydroxyacetohexamide, which lacks hypoglycemic activity. In turn, each of these monohydroxy forms can be converted to the dihydroxylated form. About 10% of acetohexamide is excreted unchanged in the urine while L-hydroxyacetohexamide accounts for 50% of the dose and 4-hydroxyacetohexamide accounts for another 15%.[160,161]

The second generation agent that has been studied the most is glyburide (glibenclamide). Glyburide is totally metabolized by the liver (Figure 9). The main metabolite in man is 4-transhydroxyglyburide although 3-*cis*-hydroxyglyburide is also formed. 4-Transhydroxyglyburide has approximately 15% of the hypoglycemic activity of glyburide.[162] While the elimination halflife of glyburide is reported to average 10 hr, Rupp et al.[163] found it took 5 days to recover 95% of a dose. In the urine he found 50% 4-transhydroxyglyburide, 8% 3-*cis*-hydroxyglyburide, and 6% unidentified metabolite.

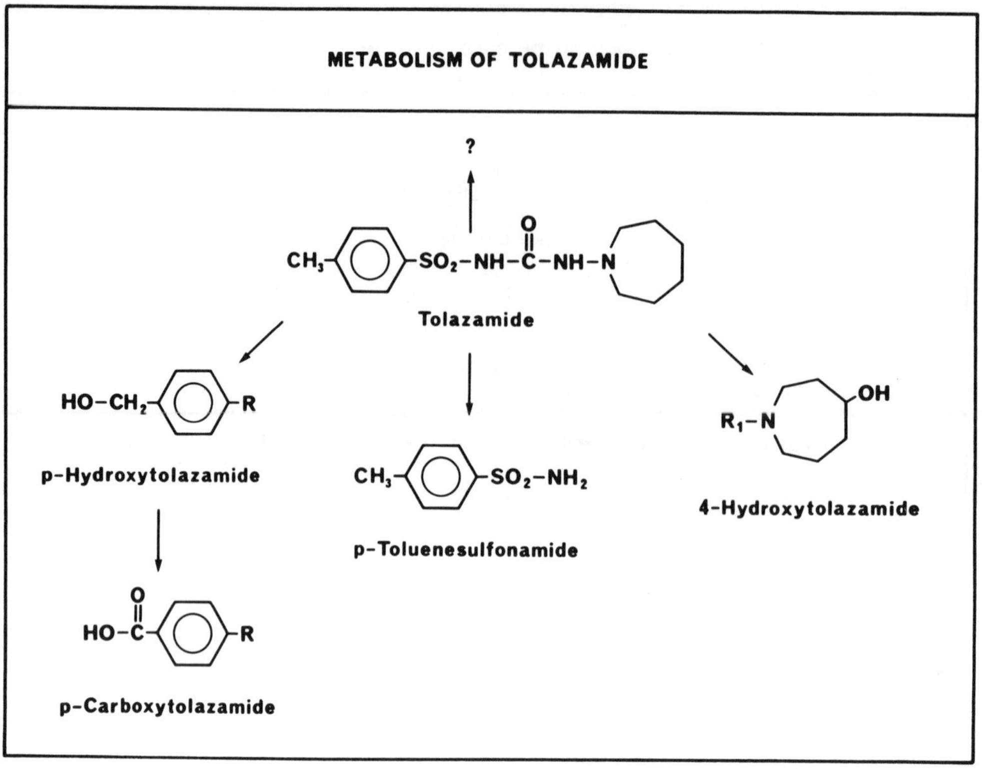

FIGURE 7.   Metabolism of tolazamide.

Glipizide is almost completely metabolized to a variety of metabolites that are essentially devoid of hypoglycemic activity[164] (Figure 10). In the first 24 hr, up to 65% of the dose administered is recovered in the urine as 4-transhydroxyglipizide while 3-*cis*-hydroxyglipizide appears to the extent of 14%. The N-acetyl derivative accounts for only 0.8 to 1.7% of the administered dose while 3 to 9% of glipizide is excreted unchanged.[165-167]

The second generation agent that is not of the n-d-n type is glibornuride. Glibornuride is totally metabolized by the liver into at least six different compounds one of which has not been characterized (Figure 11). Four of these metabolites have been synthesized and found to have from moderate to no hypoglycemic activity.[168] In plasma, the parent drug predominates to the extent of 85%. The major part of the metabolites (60 to 72%) are excreted in the urine with a minor portion (23 to 33%) excreted via the bile and feces.[169] While the urine was found to lack unchanged glibornuride, quantification of metabolite concentrations found 6% *p*-hydroxyglibornuride, 7% *p*-carboxyglibornuride, 37% hydroxyglibornuride, 24% exohydroxyglibornuride, and 7% endohydroxyglibornuride.

Uses and Dosage

Since the sulfonylureas rely on the presence of functional pancreatic tissue to achieve their hypoglycemic effect, only insulin-independent (type II) diabetics are candidates for their use. Even then, these agents are indicated only when diet alone fails to provide adequate control over blood glucose levels. It has been suggested that this qualification should limit their use to about one in ten diabetics if diet therapy were pursued intensively enough.[133] But be that as it may, the facts remain that nearly 2 million treatment years of oral hypoglycemic agents were prescribed in the U.S. in 1975[170] and that their clinical use continues to be widespread today.

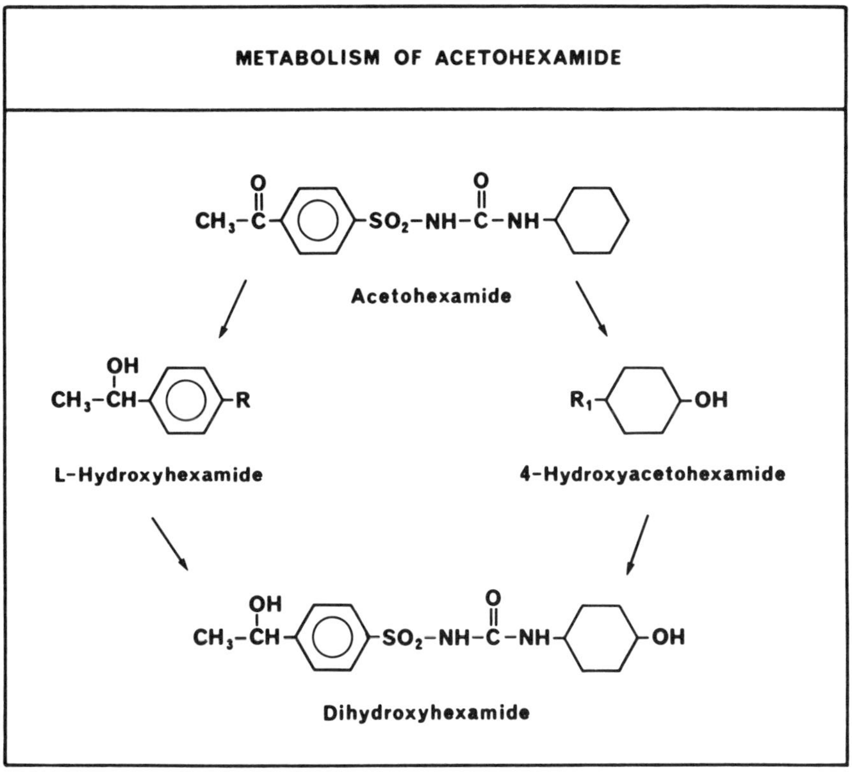

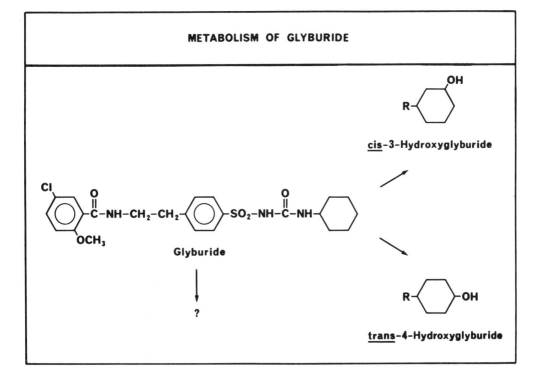

FIGURE 8.   Metabolism of acetohexamide.

FIGURE 9.   Metabolism of glyburide.

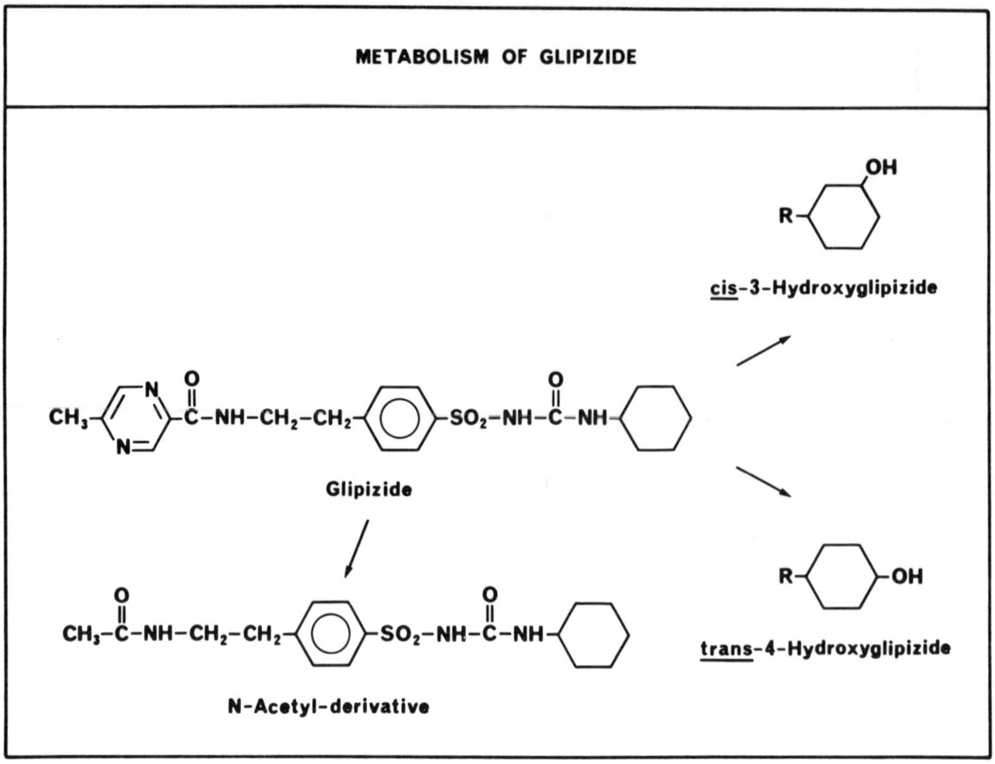

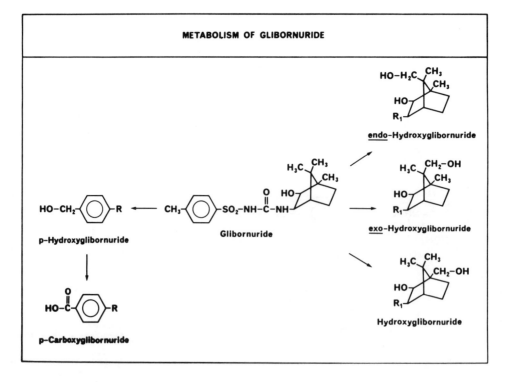

FIGURE 10. Metabolism of glipizide.

FIGURE 11. Metabolism of glibornuride.

To maximize the chances of obtaining beneficial responses with these agents, patients should be carefully selected and their blood glucose and urinary glucose levels constantly monitored. The treatment goal should be to achieve fasting and 2-hr postprandial blood glucose levels less than 130 mg/dℓ with no glucosuria.[112] Patients found to be particularly responsive to sulfonylureas tend to be age 40 or older, mildly to moderately obese, having had diabetes for less than 5 years, having never demonstrated ketosis, and having either no history of insulin therapy or a history with control being obtained with less than 20 insulin units per day. There is little indication for the simultaneous use of both insulin and a sulfonylurea. If these agents are administered to patients with either hepatic or renal disease, some caution should be exercised. Since most undergo conversion by the liver to metabolites which, depending upon the particular compound, may or may not have hypoglycemic activity and since most of these metabolites are excreted by the kidney, there is a good possibility that the pharmacological effects may be prolonged in the presence of disease.

A patient whose blood glucose level is never brought under satisfactory control with diet plus maximal sulfonylurea therapy is classified as a ''primary failure''. The reason for primary failure is largely unknown. Primary failure rates determined in earlier studies involving large numbers of patients treated with first generation agents were found to range from 5.3 to 36%.[171-174] Judicious application of the above patient selection criteria and better overall study design would be expected to result in primary failure rates of 5 to 15%.[133,175] This expectation receives some support from some of the newer studies done using second generation agents in which lower primary failure rates for glipizide[147] and glyburide[176] have been reported. Occasionally, a patient whose hyperglycemia cannot be controlled with one agent can be successfully treated with another agent.

Patients who become refractory to sulfonylurea therapy after being brought under good control are called ''secondary failures''. Secondary failure rates, like the primary failure rates determined in the earlier studies, are subject to the same criticisms and are reported to range from 15 to 25% (see references for primary failure rates). Perhaps a range of 15 to 20% would be more realistic if the appropriate safeguards were taken. Most secondary failures occur within 1 to 3 years of therapy. While the causes of these secondary failures remain largely unknown, inability of patients to adhere strictly to their diet may be a significant contributing factor. Occasionally, patients who suffer a secondary failure on one agent can be brought back under control by switching over to a more potent agent. Not long ago, secondary failures to sulfonylurea therapy often could be treated successfully by putting the sulfonylurea in combination with phenformin. However, with the removal of phenformin from the American market in 1977, such combination therapy is no longer a viable option.

Questions regarding the efficacy of the sulfonylureas surfaced in 1970 with the release of the observations of the University Groups Diabetes Project (UGDP)[177] (see Toxicity section for detailed discussion). One pertinent observation was that tolbutamide plus diet was no more effective than diet alone in prolonging life. More recently, Shen and Bressler[138] have observed that after one eliminates primary failures, secondary failures, and placebo successes from the patient population, continuous satisfactory control over the blood glucose level is achieved in only 20 to 30% of patients. They further conclude that much of this success is obtained with patients that could be equally well controlled with diet or placebo.[138] In this regard Hadden et al.[178] reported in 1975 that of a group of 57 patients only 6 remained candidates for oral hypoglycemic agents after 6 months of intensive dietary management. Boyden and Bressler[179] went on to conclude in 1979 that, since these agents have no predictable effect on serum lipids and do not decrease the frequency of diabetic complications, they are not suitable for the treatment of a chronic disease.[179] In contrast Seltzer[175] finds that the sulfonylureas are effective when correctly used in properly selected patients. He discounts the high secondary failure rates observed in most studies by questioning the lack of attention paid to patient weight gain. He further emphasizes the importance of dietary control and the use of the lowest effective dose of drug in achieving good long term success over the blood glucose concentration. To substantiate the effectiveness of sulfonylureas in treating type II diabetes, studies such as that of Tsalikian et al.[180] are often cited. When these investigators took a group of 19 patients off maintenance therapy they observed that, within a few weeks off therapy, 16 of the 19 became symptomatic with 3 becoming so severely hyperglycemic that they required hospitalization. Earlier, Tompkins and Bloom[181] in a similar experiment also found that, with the discontinuation of sulfonylurea therapy, 59% of patients relapsed into hyperglycemia. However, an interesting corollary to their study was the observation that 31% of the other patients remained in good control for at least 6 months. It has been postulated that these patients either were needlessly being treated as a diabetic or that some metabolic defect had been, at least temporarily, ameliorated.

Perhaps a reasonable compromise position on the effectiveness of sulfonylureas is that taken by Lebowitz and Feinglos.[112] They conclude that the sulfonylureas are effective in controlling hyperglycemia for at least several years in selected type II diabetic patients, but that the degree of effectiveness of chronic (greater than 5 years) sulfonylurea therapy in controlling hyperglycemia is unclear. Supportive of this position is that of Breidahl[182] who concludes that the sulfonylureas do appear to have a limited duration of the effective action which, from his experience, averages about $8^1/_2$ years with a range of 1 to 20 years. Perhaps in the future when the mechanisms of action of both the first and second generation agents are known at the molecular level, criteria for patient selection can be developed that will enhance the chances of successful therapy.

All sulfonylureas are available in tablet form with the size of the tablet related to the amount of drug necessary to obtain an equivalent therapeutic dose. Available tablet sizes (mg) and the usual adult dose range (mg) are summarized in Tables 8 and 9. Tolbutamide sodium is also available in a sterile solution for intravenous injection.

Toxicities

Hypoglycemia is probably the most frequent serious toxic effect of sulfonylureas occurring in about 1% of the patients who use the drugs. In a review of drug-induced hypoglycemia, Seltzer[183] reported 60% of cases (465) resulted from sulfonylurea use. Of these 465 cases, 10% died and another 3% suffered permanent neurological damage. Chlorpropamide, as a result of its long elimination halflife, was responsible for more than 50% of the hypoglycemic episodes and almost half of the deaths and other serious sequalae. The newer agent, glyburide, is becoming increasingly important as a causative agent being responsible for a jump from 7 cases of hypoglycemia to 78 cases in only 4 years. Patients especially prone to hypoglycemia tend to be over 60 years of age and living alone or poorly monitored in nursing homes. Other patients at risk are those who are malnourished or are suffering from hepatic or renal disease. Sulfonylurea-induced hypoglycemia is quite refractory to therapy persisting for several days. Patients undergoing treatment for hypoglycemia should be kept on continuous 10% glucose infusion for a period of time until the effects of the drug have worn off.

Another problem that has continued to cloud the issue of sulfonylurea use is its alleged cardiovascular toxicity. Although diabetics in general show an increased morbidity and mortality from all cardiovascular causes, findings of the University Groups Diabetes Project (UGDP) suggested the possibility that the sulfonylureas might aggravate underlying conditions thereby increasing the risk.[177] This long term study, begun in 1961 under the sponsorship of the NIH, had set among its objectives: (1) the evaluation of the efficacy of hypoglycemic treatments in the prevention of vascular complications and (2) the study of the natural history of vascular disease in insulin-independent diabetics.[184] Towards these goals eventually 1027 selected diabetic patients were assigned to one of five treatment schedules: (1) placebo, (2) tolbutamide, (3) insulin at a fixed dose, (4) insulin at a variable dose, and later (5) phenformin; all participants also were placed on a prescribed diet. Long term follow-up, in addition to posing questions concerning the efficacy of tolbutamide and the other courses of therapy, led to the conclusion that there was an excess cardiovascular mortality rate of nearly 1%/year in the tolbutamide group as compared to diet alone and diet plus insulin.[177] As a result, the tolbutamide group was discontinued in 1969 to be followed in 1971 by the discontinuation of the phenformin group for the same reason.[185] The response of the FDA was to propose a labeling change in the package insert to be included with all sulfonylurea agents that would warn of the potential cardiovascular toxicity and to recommend restricting their use to patients who require more than dietary control alone but in whom insulin was "impractical or unacceptable". The medical community has split pro and con on the UGDP cardiovascular issue, and the controversy continues yet today (see summary by Kolata).[186] Meanwhile the proposed labeling changes still have not been implemented by the FDA. However, while waiting for the resolution of the issue, it should be pointed out that another study has concluded cardiovascular toxicity at borderline statistical significance[187] and evidence has been presented that tolbutamide does have some direct effect upon the heart.[188-190] Such direct effects upon the heart may not be associated with glyburide. In fact, it has been demonstrated that glyburide reduces myocardial contractile force and arterial blood pressure.[191] Nevertheless, it seems rational to select patients for sulfonylurea therapy and to monitor their progress keeping in mind the potential for cardiovascular complications.

Potentially, toxic manifestations can occur from the effects of sulfonylureas on water metabolism.[192] Chlorpropamide produces an antidiuretic effect by stimulating the release of antidiuretic hormone ADH from the posterior pituitary and increasing the sensitivity of the renal tubules to the effects of the hormone. These effects are attributed to the chemical similarity between chlorpropamide and clofibrate — an effective antidiuretic.[193] On the other hand, acetohexamide, tolazamide, and glyburide tend to have a mild diuretic effect and are the agents of choice if water intoxication is a potential problem.

The incidence of reversible side effects resulting from sulfonylurea therapy is quite low. O'Donovan found a total incidence for tolbutamide of 3.2%.[194] Gastrointestinal side effects including anorexia, nausea, vomiting, diarrhea, and abdominal pain accounted for 1.4%. Skin reactions occurred in 1.1% of patients, and hematological reactions in 0.24%. Chlorpropamide has a slightly higher total incidence with 1.1% of patients experiencing essentially the same problems. While acetohexamide and tolazamide have not been studied as much as the other two more popular agents, it is generally conceded that the adverse effects expected with these agents are similar to those of tolbutamide and occur with approximately the same frequency. The incidence of side effects with second generation agents, glyburide specifically, exclusive of hypoglycemia, was found to be 3.9%.[178] Again, gastrointestinal disturbances predominated (2%) with dermatological reactions accounting for another 1.6%. In a study involving 1064 patients treated with glipizide, side effects occurred in 7.8% of patients.[195] Gastrointestinal complaints were found in 2.16% of patients with skin reactions occurring in 5 patients (0.47%). One other side effect worth noting is hyponatremia.[196] Hyponatremia was found to be associated with tolbutamide therapy but not with the frequency reported for chlorpropamide.

Another side effect found to occur in approximately one third of the patients on chlorpropamide therapy is called the antabuse syndrome.[197] The term refers to a facial flush that can develop when a patient receiving sulfonylureas drinks alcohol. Apparently, the reaction of acetaldehyde dehydrogenase is inhibited stalling the conversion of ethanol to acetic acid at the aldehyde stage. In fact, the increase in plasma acetaldehyde has been proposed to be an objective indicator of the chlorpropamide alcohol flush.[198] While chlorpropamide is most commonly the causative agent, glyburide has also been implicated. Leslie and Pyke[199] have suggested that the chlorpropamide alcohol flush may be a genetic marker for a subgroup of diabetics, but Kobberling et al.[200] have questioned this hypothesis with their observations that the facial flush occurred with almost equal frequency (16.9% in normals, 23.3% in insulin-dependent diabetics, 16.5% in noninsulin-dependent diabetics) regardless of the type of diabetes. The flush can be prevented by pretreatment with aspirin.[201]

Drug Interactions

The sulfonylurea drugs have been reported to interact with numerous drugs by a variety of different mechanisms. The subject has been recently reviewed by Hansen and Christensen[202] and Jackson and Bressler.[134] For a detailed discussion of mechanisms, clinical significance, and recommendations the reader is referred to publications such as Hansten's *Drug Interactions*[203] and the American Pharmaceutical Association's (APhA) *Evaluations of Drug Interactions.*[204]

In general, the mechanisms by which drugs alter the response to the sulfonylureas are divided into two classes; pharmacokinetic interactions and pharmacodynamic interactions. Each type can either increase or decrease the action of the sulfonylurea. Pharmacokinetic interactions include changes which affect the absorption, extent of protein binding, degree of hepatic metabolism, or the rate of elimination of the sulfonylurea. Pharmacodynamic interactions are more indirect in that they are the result of the interacting agent affecting glucose homostasis. Changes in insulin secretion and response fall into this category as do changes in glucogenesis, glycogen turnover, and peripheral glucose uptake.

Perhaps the most important interactions of the pharmacokinetic type are those affecting plasma protein binding. First generation agents such as tolbutamide and chlorpropamide are weakly acidic at physiological pH and are found bound to positive binding sites on serum albumin. In the presence of other anionic compounds such as aspirin, phenylbutazone, warfarin, or long-acting sulfa drugs, displacement of the sulfonylurea has been shown to occur.[205] Since it is the unbound fraction of drug that produces the pharmacological response, an increase in this fraction would be expected to increase the hypoglycemic effect. On the other hand, agents such as glyburide are less susceptible to displacement because they contain large hydrophobic groups. As a result of their molecular structure, the binding of glyburide and others to albumin is less dependent upon charge and more dependent upon nonpolar interactions that are not affected by charge. While the dose of chlorpropamide or tolbutamide may have to be decreased to compensate for the decrease in protein binding, such adjustments may not be as frequent with the use of second generation agents.

Pharmacodynamic interactions involving alterations in glycogen metabolism should be anticipated with agents that act at the β-receptor. Epinephrine, glucagon, isoproterenol, and other adrenergic agents mobilize liver glycogen stores and promote hyperglycemia whereas β-blockers, such as propanolol, potentiate hypoglycemia by preventing glycogenolysis. This interaction is of particular importance as β-blockers have been known to suppress the tachycardia of hypoglycemia. It is suggested that their concurrent use be avoided.[206]

Hormone therapy, including the use of oral contraceptives and glucocorticoids, is another source of pharmacodynamic interactions. Both categories of agents favor hyperglycemia and would antagonize the action of the sulfonylurea. An upward adjustment in the dose of sulfonylurea may be required to offset the additional glucose load.

Monoamine oxidase (MAO) inhibitors and thiazide diuretics are two other classes of drugs that directly affect insulin secretion. MAO inhibitors increase insulin secretion while the thiazides decrease insulin secretion if potassium depletion occurs. Prudent therapy will minimize the importance of these interactions.

The interaction of alcohol with sulfonylureas also deserves mention due to the social acceptability of drinking and the frequency of the diabetic encounter with liquor. Infrequent ingestion of alcohol potentiates hypoglycemia while chronic consumption prematurely ends the hypoglycemic response. The reason for such diverse effects is that chronic exposure to alcohol leads to induction of the enzymes responsible for metabolism of sulfonylureas. Consequently, their elimination halflives are significantly shortened.

Physical-Chemical and Other Data

The physical-chemical data of the sulfonylureas are summarized in Table 11. Tolbutamide is the reference compound, and it has a pK_a of 5.3. The Chemical Abstract Service (CAS) Registry Number for tolbutamide is 54-77-7, for chlorpropamide it is 94-20-2, for tolazamide it is 1156-19-0, and for acetohexamide it is 968-81-0.

The sulfonylureas are generally considered to be quite stable under normal conditions. However, under various experimental conditions, degradation can occur with hydrolysis serving as the major route.[210] Thermal dissociation in various solvents has also been reported.[211]

OTHER DRUGS — PAST, PRESENT, AND FUTURE BIGUANIDES — PHENFORMIN, METFORMIN, AND BUFORMIN

The biguanides (Figure 12) represent the outcome of an observation made in 1918 by Watanabe when he described the hypoglycemic action of guanidine (Figure 12).[212] Guanidine, *per se,* was too toxic for clinical use but led to the eventual marketing of two diguanides, Synthalin A and Synthalin B (Figure 12), in the 1920s. While these two agents were substantially less toxic than guanidine, they were capable of hepatic and renal toxicity with prolonged use. Due to their potential for toxicity and the introduction of insulin, they were withdrawn from use in the early 1930s. Interest in guanidine derivatives laid dormant until 1953 when it was renewed by the synthesis of a substituted biguanide (phenformin) that had hypoglycemic activity. Phenformin was first used to treat diabetes in 1956 and was approved for the American market in March of 1959. Due to the poor initial acceptance of phenformin as an outgrowth of the Synthalin experience, two other biguanides, metformin and buformin, never were accepted for marketing in the U.S. although all three compounds were put into common usage in other parts of the world.

Phenformin and the other biguanides are indicated for use in stable, insulin-dependent (type II) diabetic patients, particularly those tending towards the obese. They are also used in combination with sulfonylureas to stabilize blood glucose in patients who are secondary failures to sulfonylureas used alone. Improved control over insulin-dependent (type I) diabetics may occur if phenformin is used as an adjunct to insulin therapy.

In 1959 severe metabolic acidosis without ketosis was reported in diabetics being treated with biguanides.[213] It was soon discovered that the accumulation of lactic acid was the cause of the acidosis. Still, the clinical syndrome of lactic acidosis was considered to be a rare complication of phenformin therapy. However, an FDA review of the risks associated with the use of phenformin, concluded in 1976, found that lactic acidosis was much more prevalent than previously thought.[214] It was estimated that the incidence was between 0.25 and 4 cases per 1000 users per year with death occurring in approximately 50% of cases. Based upon the estimated number of American phenformin users at the time, perhaps 50 to 700 deaths per year were to be expected. As a result of these observations, phenformin use in the U.S. ended abruptly in 1977 when the Secretary of Health, Education, and Welfare (HEW) suspended the New Drug Application (NDA) and ordered an end to general marketing.[215] It was suggested that patients taking phenformin should be reevaluated and transferred over to insulin, sulfonylureas, or dietary control. Despite efforts by the Committee for Care of the Diabetic (CCD) and the various manufacturers to reverse the ruling, the decision was finalized on April 6, 1979. Although the American edict does not pertain to the use of phenformin in other countries, the impact has been worldwide. The relationship between biguanide use and lactic acidosis has been reviewed[216-218] and communications regarding the effect of the discontinuation of biguanide therapy are available.[219-221]

The appearance of lactate in the blood in unusually high concentrations in patients undergoing phenformin therapy appears to be correlated to the way in which the biguanides achieve their hypoglycemic effect. Although part of their hypoglycemic effect is postulated to result

Table 11

PHYSICAL-CHEMICAL DATA OF SULFONYLUREAS[207-209]

Generic name	Chemical name	Trade name	Chemical formula	Mol wt	Physical description	MP (C°)	Solubility data
Tolbutamide	Benzenesulfonamide, N-[(butylamino)carbonyl]-4-methyl-1-Butyl-3-(p-tolylsulfonyl)urea	Orinase (Upjohn), Diabetamid, Rastinon, Diabuton, Mobenol, Oterben, Toluina, Diaben, Diabesan, Ipoglicone, Orabet, Oralin, Artosin, Dolipol, Tolbet, Tarasina, Tolbusal, Pramidex, Tolbutone, Willbutamide	$C_{12}H_{18}N_2O_3S$	270.35	White to practically white, almost odorless, slightly bitter tasting, crystalline powder	128.5—129.5	Practically insoluble in water; soluble: 1 in 10 of alcohol, 1 in 3 acetone, chloroform, dilute solution alkali hydroxides
Chlorpropamide	Benzenesulfonamide, 4-chloro-N-[propylamino)carbonyl] 1-[(p-chlorophenyl)sulfonyl]-3-propylurea	Diabinese (Pfizer), Adiaben, Asucrol, Catanil, Chloronase, Diabechlor, Diabenal, Diabetoral, Melitase, Millinese, Oradian, Stabinol	$C_{10}H_{13}ClN_2O_3S$	276.74	White, odorless to almost odorless, almost tasteless, crystalline powder	126—130	Insoluble in water; soluble: 1 in 12 alcohol, 1 in 5 acetone, 1 in 9 chloroform, 1 in 200 ether, solutions of alkali hydroxides
Tolazamide	Benzenesulfonamide, N-[[(hexahydro-1H-azepin-1-yl)amino]carbonyl]-4-methyl 1-(Hexahydro-1H-azepin-1-yl)-3-(p-tolylsulfonyl)urea	Tolinase (Upjohn), Diabewas, Norglycin, Tolonase	$C_{14}H_{21}N_3O_3S$	311.40	White to almost white, odorless to almost odorless, crystalline powder	170—173	Very slightly soluble in water, slightly soluble in alcohol, soluble in acetone, freely soluble in chloroform

Name	Chemical name	Trade names / Manufacturer	Molecular formula	MW	Description	Melting point	Solubility
Acetohexamide	Benzenesulfonamide, 4-acetyl-N-[(cyclohexylamino)-carbonyl] 1-(p-Acetylphenyl)sulfonyl]-3-cyclohexylurea	Dymelor (Lilly), Dimelor, Dimelin, Ordimel	$C_{15}H_{20}N_2O_4S$	324.39	White, almost odorless, crystalline powder	188—190 (crystals from 90% aq. ethanol)	Practically insoluble in water and ether; soluble: 1 in 230 alcohol, 1 in 210 chloroform and pyridine
Glyburide	Benzamide, 5-chloro-N-[2-[4-[[[(cyclohexylamino) carbonyl]amino]sulfonyl]phenyl]-ethyl]-2-methoxy 1-[[p-[2-(5-Chloro-o-anisamido)-ethyl]phenyl]sulfonyl]-3-cyclohexylurea	Micronase (Upjohn), DiaBeta (Hoechst) Adiab, Daonil, Euglucon, Maninil, Lisaglucon, Glidiabet, Euclamin, Hemi-Daonil	$C_{23}H_{28}ClN_3O_5S$	494.00	White to almost white, odorless to almost odorless, tasteless crystalline powder	172—174 (crystals from methanol) 169—170 (crystals from alcohol-DMF)	Practically insoluble in water, alcohol, and chlorinated solvents, sparingly soluble in acetone
Glipizide	Pyrazinecarboxamide,N-[2-[4-[[[(cyclohexylamino) carbonyl]amino]sulfonyl]phenyl]ethyl]-5-methyl-1-Cyclohexyl-3-[[p-[2-(5-methylpyrazinecarboxamido)ethyl]phenyl]sulfonyl]urea	Glucotrol (Pfizer), Minidiab	$C_{21}H_{27}N_5O_4S$	445.54	White, odorless powder	208—209 (crystals from ethanol)	Insoluble in water and alcohols, soluble in 0,1N NaOH, freely soluble in dimethylformamide
Glibornuride	Benzenesulfonamide, N-[3-hydroxy-4,7,7-trimethylbicyclo[2.2.1]hept-2-yl]amino] carbonyl]-4-methyl-1S-(endo, endo)]-endo, endo-1-[(1R)-(2-hydroxy-3-bornyl)]-3-(p-tolylsulfonyl) urea	Glutril (Hoffman-LaRoche)	$C_{18}H_{26}N_2O_4S$	366.47	White crystalline powder	195	Insoluble in water at 20°C, soluble in alkali

GUANIDINE DERIVATIVES

$$NH$$
$$\|$$
$$H_2N-C-NH_2$$

Guanidine

$$NH \qquad\qquad NH$$
$$\| \qquad\qquad \|$$
$$H_2N-C-NH-(CH_2)_n-NH-C-NH_2$$

Synthalin A: n = 10
Synthalin B: n = 12

$$\begin{array}{c} H_3C \\ \\ H_3C \end{array} \!\!\! N-C-NH-C-NH_2$$

$$NH \quad NH$$
$$\| \quad \|$$

Metformin

$$NH \quad NH$$
$$\| \quad \|$$
$$\langle\bigcirc\rangle\!-CH_2-CH_2-NH-C-NH-C-NH_2$$

Phenformin

$$NH \quad NH$$
$$\| \quad \|$$
$$CH_3-CH_2-CH_2-CH_2-NH-C-NH-C-NH_2$$

Buformin

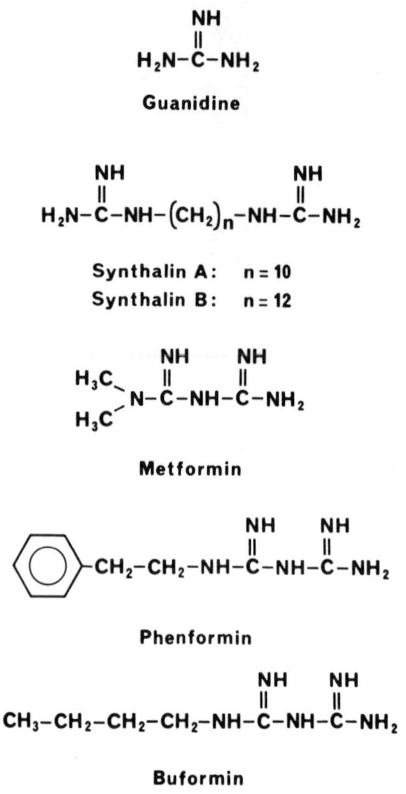

FIGURE 12.   Guanidine derivatives.

from the inhibition of glucose absorption from the intestinal lumen,[222] the majority of the hypoglycemic effects are generally thought to result from an increase in peripheral glucose uptake[223,224] and/or a decrease in hepatic glucose output.[225,226] Either impaired hepatic glucogenesis and/or increased peripheral glucose utilization could account for the elevations in lactate and the other glucogenic precursors, pyruvate and alanine, that are observed. In addition, the redox ratios of lactate/pyruvate and 3-hydroxybutyrate/acetoacetate are both increased[225,227] suggesting the presence of a more reduced energy state within tissues. For a long time it has been known that the biguanides do inhibit mitochondrial respiration, which is an action that would favor a more reduced state, but this effect is only observed with biguanide concentrations several orders of magnitude above those normally associated with therapeutic doses.[228] Nevertheless, the presence of such a reduced state in the tissues does promote glycolysis and would increase Cori cycle activity — the cycling of glucose-derived lactate produced in the periphery to the liver where it is converted back into glucose (see Cohen and Woods[217] for a discussion of the Cori cycle). Apparently Cori cycle activity is somewhat balanced in normal subjects receiving biguanides as there is little change in the net blood glucose concentration. However, in the diabetic, the compensatory increase in hepatic glucogenesis expected as a result of the increased lactate production seems not to occur.[226] This decrease in glucose production, combined with a potential impairment of glycogenolysis, restricts the supply of glucose from the liver to the circulation and may account for the observed hypoglycemic effect in the presence of elevated lactate levels. It is interesting to note that lactate levels in patients receiving sulfonylurea therapy in addition to a biguanide are no different from those receiving a biguanide alone.[229] If sulfonylureas had been found to suppress lactate production, combination therapy would have provided a method to circumvent this problem.

While most of the attention concerned with drug-induced lactic acidosis has been focused on phenformin, the other biguanides should not be ignored. This is particularly important since there is an increasing tendency in countries where biguanides are still used to substitute metformin for phenformin. However, while lactate elevations occur less frequently with the other agents, they do occur, and there are documented cases of both metformin and buformin inducing lactic acidosis.[227,229-232]

From an audit of 330 cases of lactic acidosis that met specific criteria, Luft et al.[233] have established guidelines to identify patients at risk for biguanide therapy. They suggest that biguanides should not be used (1) in patients over the age of 60, (2) in the presence of accompanying illnesses such as cardiovascular disease, renal disease, hepatic disease, or infectious processes, and (3) in pathological states that in themselves can result in an accumulation of lactate, for example, shock, ketoacidosis, pulmonary insufficiency, alcoholism, and weight reducing diets.

In patients undergoing phenformin therapy, attempts have been made to relate lactic acidosis to the serum level of phenformin and creatinine. However, no correlation was demonstrated nor was there any relationship between the severity of the lactic acidosis and the serum creatinine concentration.[234] Currently, it is extremely difficult to predict which diabetic patients will develop lactic acidosis when treated with phenformin.

Aside from the problem of lactic acidosis, the use of biguanides has also been questioned on the basis of potential cardiovascular toxicity. A little more than 1 year after withdrawing tolbutamide from the UGDP, phenformin use was discontinued and for the same reason — excessive cardiovascular toxicity.[185] The complete report filed in 1975 concluded that "the mortality from all causes and from cardiovascular causes for patients in the phenformin-treated group was higher than that observed in any of the other treatment groups".[235] Although this conclusion and the other observations of the UGDP continue to be disputed it seems safe to assume that the use of phenformin will never return to its pre-UGDP stature. It also seems apparent that the biguanides, particularly phenformin, should be reserved for use in only carefully selected patients.

Meanwhile, progress has been made in the elucidation of the molecular basis for the proposed mechanisms of action of the biguanides. Davidoff et al.[115,236] have found that phenformin enhances calcium ion uptake rates in liver mitochondria. Since one of the earliest measurable responses to glucagon stimulation of the perfused liver is a large outflow of calcium ions, it is thought that phenformin may block the full expression of the glucagon signal of the liver. Consequently, the glucagon-mediated stimulation of hepatic glucogenesis and glycogenolysis would be antagonized. Along the same line, phenformin has been shown to suppress plasma glucagon levels in insulin-requiring diabetics both alone and in combination with insulin.[237] The suppression of glucagon release as well as its expression would go far in explaining the net decrease in hepatic glucose output believed to result from biguanide therapy. To explain the peripheral actions of the biguanides, enhanced insulin effectiveness has been investigated. Biguanides have no direct stimulatory effect on the pancreas so there is no drug-induced increase in plasma insulin levels. In fact, there may actually be a reduction that is believed to be secondary to the decrease in the blood glucose concentration.[238] Therefore, any increase in glucose utilization by peripheral tissues cannot be explained on the basis of more insulin being present. However, Cohen et al.[239] have reported that phenformin increases insulin binding to human cultured breast cancer cells. The increase in binding is the result of an increase in the number of insulin receptors as insulin receptor affinity is not altered. While it is not known whether this observation can be extrapolated to the biguanide-treated human patient, it is interesting in light of the similar observations that have been made concerning the effects of sulfonylureas on insulin receptor populations.

The normal therapeutic dose of phenformin ranges from 25 to 150 mg/day with approximately 50% of the administered dose being absorbed from the gastrointestinal tract. Peak serum concentrations in the range of 102 to 240 ng/mℓ are reached within 2 to 4 hr after the last dose. Only about 20% or less of the phenformin in the plasma is protein bound. About one third of the drug reaching the circulation is converted to the parahydroxylated form by the liver. Both the metabolite and the unaltered drug are excreted by the kidney into the urine. The elimination halflife for phenformin is 3.7 hr while *p*-hydroxyphenformin has an elimination halflife of 3.8 hr.[240] The usual duration of action is 4 to 6 hr.

Metformin has about 1/20 of the potency of phenformin and is used in correspondingly larger doses. Gastrointestinal absorption is incomplete, plasma protein binding is negligible, and the drug is excreted unchanged in the urine. The elimination halflife is 1 to 2 hr.

SOMATOSTATIN ANALOGS

The observation that diabetics with rare exception have elevated plasma glucagon levels in combination with decreased or absent plasma insulin levels[241] has provided the impetus for the investigation of agents that can suppress glucagon release. While such agents most likely would not be used alone because the metabolic expression of insulin still would be deficient, they potentially would be beneficial when used as adjuncts with insulin due to their ability to mute the hyperglycemic contribution of glucagon.[242] Theoretically, this combination might allow the dose of insulin to be reduced. Since somatostatin was known to suppress glucagon release from the α-cells of the pancreatic islets, it represented a logical starting point for the development of this class of agents.

The shortcomings of somatostatin therapy are manifold. Aside from having a very short plasma halflife of 1.1 to 3 min and a metabolic clearance rate of 28.4 ± 4.2 mℓ/min kg body weight,[243] somatostatin suppresses the release of many other hormones besides glucagon. Unfortunately, one of these other hormones is insulin.[244] Obviously it would be undesirable to treat diabetic patients with an agent that would suppress whatever residual insulin-releasing ability that remained. Consequently, emphasis has been placed on the design of somatostatin analogs that retain the ability to suppress glucagon release but are devoid of suppressive effects on insulin release.

Towards this goal, the amino acid sequence of somatostatin (see Figure 1) is being systematically altered, and the selective effects against glucagon and insulin are being evaluated. D-cys^{14}-SS, D-trp^8-D-cys^{14}-SS, and ala^2-D-trp^8-D-cys^{14}-SS (the superscript refers to the amino acid position of somatostatin that has been altered or replaced) have all been shown to suppress arginine-induced glucagon release with a concomitant decrease in blood glucose. Insulin release was not affected.[245] When glucose was used to stimulate insulin release, the first two analogs had no effect while the third actually enhanced insulin release induced by the glucose. On the other hand, D-trp^8-SS has been shown to be 6 to 8 times more potent than somatostatin in suppressing both glucagon and insulin release,[246] and Des-Asn^5-SS (the asparagine residue in position 5 of somatostatin has been deleted) and D-ser^{13}-SS were both found to selectively reduce plasma insulin but not glucagon concentrations.[247] Des-asn^5-D-trp-^{8}-D-ser^{13}-SS has also been found to be more inhibitory towards β-cell function.[248] Another interesting finding is that some somatostatin analogs have a dramatic prolongation of effect. Des^{1,2,4,5,12,13} somatostatin has been shown to suppress glucagon release 65% for 3 hr resulting in a decrease in hyperglycemia. When the dose was increased from 2 to 5 or 10 mg, hormonal suppression was greater and was maintained for at least 12 hr.[249]

While the idea of somatostatin therapy in the treatment of diabetes is very futuristic at this point, the data taken together suggest that somatostatin binding sites on cells do differ and, potentially, are exploitable with analogs that have an acceptable duration of action.

ACKNOWLEDGMENTS

The author wishes to express his appreciation to the Upjohn Company for their financial assistance, to Dr. Marvin Pankaskie for drawing the figures, and to Ms. Linda Mondrella for the preparation of the manuscript.

ADDENDUM

Since the submission of this manuscript, many noteworthy changes and/or advancements have occurred pertaining to both the areas of insulin and the oral hypoglycemic agents. Human insulin products obtained from recombinant DNA technology using E. coli[250] and produced semisynthetically from porcine insulin[251] are now commercially available (see *Facts and Comparisons* for a current list of all insulin products[252]). The pharmacokinetics of insulin have been reviewed[253] and optimal insulin delivery systems have been investigated.[254] In addition, the long-awaited publication of the FDA sulfonylurea labelling requirements arising from the conclusions reached by the University Group Diabetes Program (UGDP) has occurred.[255] Consequently, glyburide,[256] and glipizide[257] have been approved for marketing in the U.S. Current research on the mechanism of action of the sulfonylureas has centered on their extrapancreatic effects,[258-260] and has resulted in the conjecture that sulfonylureas may facilitate the action of insulin when used concurrently.[261-262] Metformin, although still not available in America, has emerged as the biguanide of choice outside the U.S. Attention to its mechanism has focused upon its effect upon the binding of insulin to its receptor,[260] the structure of which has been updated.[260]

REFERENCES

1. **Brownlee, M., Ed.,** *Handbook of Diabetes Mellitus,* Vols. 1—5, Garland STPM Press, New York, 1980.
2. **Schade, D. S. and Eaton, R. P.,** Pathogenesis of diabetic ketoacidosis: a reappraisal, *Diabetes Care,* 2, 296, 1979.
3. **Marble, A.,** Late complications of diabetes. A continuing challenge, *Diabetologia,* 12, 193, 1976.
4. **Goetz, F. C. and Kjellstrand, C.-M.,** The treatment of diabetic kidney disease, *Diabetologia,* 17, 267, 1969.
5. **Palmberg, P. F.,** Diabetic retinopathy, *Diabetes,* 26, 703, 1977.
6. **Colwell, J. A., Lopes-Virella, M., and Halushka, P. V.,** Pathogenesis of atherosclerosis in diabetes mellitus, *Diabetes Care,* 4, 121, 1981.
7. **Melton III, L. J., Macken, K. M., Palumbo, P. J., and Elveback, L. R.,** Incidence and prevalence of clinical peripheral vascular disease in a population-based cohort of diabetic patients, *Diabetes Care,* 3, 650, 1980.
8. **Porte, D., Graf, R. J., Halter, J. B., Pfeifer, M. A., and Halar, E.,** Diabetic neuropathy and plasma glucose control, *Am. J. Med.,* 70, 195, 1981.
9. **Brownlee, M. and Cerami, A.,** The biochemistry of the complications of diabetes mellitus, in *Annu. Rev. Biochem.,* 50, 385, 1981.
10. National Diabetes Data Group, Classification and diagnosis of diabetes mellitus and other categories of glucose intolerance, *Diabetes,* 28, 1039, 1979.
11. **Bunn, H. F.,** Nonenzymatic glycosylation of protein: relevance to diabetes, *Am. J. Med.,* 70, 325, 1981.
12. **Rotter, J. I. and Rimoin, D. L.,** The genetics of the glucose intolerance disorders, *Am. J. Med.,* 70, 116, 1981.
13. **Owerbach, D., Bell, G. I., Rutter, W. J., Brown, J. A., and Shows, T. B.,** The insulin gene is located in the short arm of chromosome 11 in humans, *Diabetes,* 30, 267, 1981.
14. **Craighead, J. E.,** Viral diabetes mellitus in man and experimental animals, *Am. J. Med.,* 70, 127, 1981.
15. **Nerup, J., Ortven Anderson, O., Christy, M., Platz, P., Ryder, L., Thomsen, M., and Svejgaard, A.,** in *Immunological Aspects of Diabetes Mellitus,* Ortved Anderson, O., Deckert, T., and Nerup, J., Eds., A Lindgren and Söner, Mölndal, 1976, 167.

16. **Nerup, J. and Lernmark, A.,** Autoimmunity in insulin-dependent diabetes, *Am. J. Med.,* 70, 135, 1981.
17. **Unger, R. H. and Orci, L. O.,** The role of glucagon in the endogenous hyperglycemia of diabetes mellitus, in *Annu. Rev. Med.,* 28, 119, 1977.
18. **Unger, R. H., Dobbs, R. E., and Orci, L.,** Insulin, glucagon, and somatostatin secretion in the regulation of metabolism, in *Annu. Rev. Physiol.,* 40, 307, 1978.
19. **Cuatrecasas, P. and Hollenberg, M.,** Membrane receptors and hormone action, in *Advances in Protein Chemistry,* Anfinsen, C. B., Edsall, J. T., and Richards, F. M., Eds., Academic Press, New York, 1976, 251.
20. **Muggeo, M., Ginsberg, B. H., Roth, J., Kahn, C. R., DeMeyts, P., and Neville, D. M.,** The insulin receptor in vertebrates is functionally more conserved during evolution than insulin itself, *Endocrinology,* 104, 1393, 1979.
21. **Czech, M. P.,** Insulin action, *Am. J. Med.,* 70, 142, 1981.
22. **Czech, M. P.,** Molecular basis of insulin action, *Annu. Rev. Biochem.,* 46, 359, 1977.
23. **Pastan, I. H. and Willingham, M. C.,** The internalization of insulin and other hormones by fibroblastic cells, *Diabetes Care,* 4, 33, 1981.
24. **Bergeron, J. M., Posner, B. I., Josefsberg, Z., and Sikstrom, R.,** Intracellular polypeptide hormone receptors. The demonstration of specific binding sites for insulin and growth hormone in golgi fractions from the liver of female rats, *J. Biol. Chem.,* 253, 4058, 1978.
25. **Posner, B. I., Josefsberg, Z., and Bergeron, J. M.,** Intracellular polypeptide hormone receptors characterization of insulin binding sites in golgi fractions from the liver of female rats, *J. Biol. Chem.,* 253, 4067, 1978.
26. **Larner, J., Galasko, G., Cheng, K., De Paoli-Roach, A. A., Huang, L., Daggy, P., and Kellogg, J.,** Generation by insulin of a chemical mediator that controls protein phosphorylation and dephosporylation, *Science,* 206, 1408, 1979.
27. **Seals, J. R. and Czech, M. P.,** Evidence that insulin activates an intrinsic plasma membrane protease in generating a secondary chemical mediator, *J. Biol. Chem.,* 255, 6529, 1980.
28. **Roth, J.,** Insulin binding to the receptor: is the receptor more important than the hormone?, *Diabetes Care,* 4, 27, 1981.
29. **Morgan, H. E. and Whitfield, C. F.,** Regulation of sugar transport in eukaryotic cells, *Curr. Top. Membr. Transp.,* 4, 255, 1973.
30. **Czech, M. P.,** Insulin action and the regulation of hexose transport, *Diabetes,* 29, 399, 1980.
31. **Denton, R. M., Brownsey, R. W., and Belsham, G. J.,** A partial view of the mechanism of insulin action, *Diabetologia,* 21, 347, 1981.
32. **Burrow, G. N., Hazlett, B. E., and Phillips, M. J.,** A case of diabetes mellitus, *N. Engl. J. Med.,* 306, 340, 1982.
33. **Abel, J. J.,** Crystalline insulin, *Proc. Natl. Acad. Sci. U.S.A.,* 12, 132, 1926.
34. **Sanger, F.,** Chemistry of insulin, *Br. Med. Bull.,* 16, 183, 1960.
35. **Blundell, T. L., Dodson, G., Hodgkin, D., and Mercola, D.,** Insulin: the structure in the crystal and its reflection in chemistry and biology, in *Advances in Protein Chemistry,* 26th ed., Anfinsen, C. B., Ed., Academic Press, New York, 1972, 279.
36. **Kamber, B., Hartman, A., Jöhl, A., Märki, F., Riniker, B., Rittel, W., and Sieber, P.,** A new route towards the synthesis of human insulin, in *Peptides: Chemistry, Structure and Biology,* Walter, R. and Meienhofer, J., Eds., Ann Arbor Science, Ann Arbor, Mich., 1975, 477.
37. **Märki, F. and Albrecht, W.,** Biological activity of synthetic human insulin, *Diabetologia,* 13, 293, 1977.
38. **Inouye, K., Watanabe, K., Morihara, K., Tochino, Y., Kanaya, T., Emura, J., and Sakakibara, S.,** Enzyme-assisted semisynthesis of human insulin, *J. Am. Chem. Soc.,* 101, 751, 1979.
39. **Morihara, K., Oka, T., and Tsuzuki, H.,** Semi-synthesis of human insulin by trypsin-catalyzed replacement of ala-B30 by thr in porcine insulin, *Nature (London),* 280, 412, 1979.
40. **Goeddel, D. V., Kleid, D. G., Bolivar, F., Heyneker, H. L., Yansura, D. G., Crea, R., Hirose, T., Kraszewski, A., Itakura, K., and Riggs, A. D.,** Expression in *Escherichia coli* of chemically synthesized genes for human insulin, *Proc. Natl. Acad. Sci. U.S.A.,* 76, 106, 1979.
41. **Kaysoyannis, P. G. and Tometsko, A.,** Insulin synthesis by recombination of A and B chains: a highly efficient method, *Proc. Natl. Acad. Sci. U.S.A.,* 55, 1554, 1966.
42. **Chance, R. E., Ellis, R. M., and Broemer, W. W.,** Porcine proinsulin: characterization and amino acid sequence, *Science,* 161, 165, 1968.
43. **Steiner, D. F. and Clark, J. L.,** The spontaneous reoxidation of reduced beef and rat proinsulins, *Proc. Natl. Acad. Sci. U.S.A.,* 60, 622, 1968.
44. **Talmadge, K., Stahl, S., and Gilbert, W.,** Eukaryotic signal sequence transports an insulin antigen in *Escherichia coli, Proc. Natl. Acad. Sci. U.S.A.,* 77, 3369, 1980.
45. **Steiner, D. F.,** Insulin today, *Diabetes,* 26, 322, 1977.
46. **Track, N. S.,** Insulin biosynthesis, in *Insulin and Metabolism,* Bajaj, J. S., Ed., Elsevier/North Holland, Amsterdam, 1977, chap. 2.

47. **Chan, S. J., Kwok, S. C. M., and Steiner, D. F.,** The biosynthesis of insulin: some genetic and evolutionary aspects, *Diabetes Care,* 4, 4, 1981.

48. **Blundell, T. L., Cutfield, J. F., Cutfield, S. M., Dodson, E. J., Dodson, G. G., Hodgkin, D. C., and Mercola, D. A.,** Three-dimensional atomic structure of insulin and its relationship to activity, *Diabetes,* 21(Suppl. 2), 492, 1972.

49. **Zahn, H., Brandenburg, D., and Gattner, H. G.,** Molecular basis of insulin action: contributions of chemical modifications and synthetic approaches, *Diabetes,* 21(Suppl. 2), 468, 1972.

50. **Pullen, R. A., Lindsay, D. G., Wood, S. P., Tickle, I. J., Blundell, T. L., Wollmer, A., Krail, G., Brandenburg, D., Zahn, H., Gliemann, J., and Gammeltoft, S.,** Receptor-binding region of insulin, *Nature (London),* 259, 369, 1976.

51. **De Meyts, P., VanObberghen, E., Roth, J., Wollner, A., and Brandenburg, D.,** Mapping of the residues responsible for the negative cooperativity of the receptor-binding region of insulin, *Nature (London),* 273, 504, 1978.

52. **Hodgkin, D. C.,** The structure of insulin, *Diabetes,* 21, 1131, 1972.

53. **Blundell, T. L., Dodson, G. G., Dodson, E., Hodgkin, D. C., and Vijayans, M.,** X-ray analysis and the structure of insulin, in *Rec. Progr. Hormone Res.,* 27, 1, 1971.

54. **Blundell, T. L. and Wood, S. P.,** Is the evolution of insulin Darwinian or due to selectively neutral mutation?, *Nature (London),* 257, 197, 1975.

55. **Wood, S. P., Blundell, T. L., Wollmer, A., Lazarus, N. R., and Neville, R. W. J.,** The relation of conformation and association of insulin to receptor binding; x-ray and circular dichroism studies on bovine and hystricomorph insulins, *Eur. J. Biochem.,* 55, 531, 1975.

56. **Bressler, R. and Galloway, J. A.,** The insulins: pharmacology and uses, *Drug Therapy,* 8, 43, 1978.

57. **Roy, B., Chou, M. C. Y., and Field, J. B.,** Time-action characteristics of regular and NPH insulin in insulin-treated diabetics, *J. Clin. Endocrinol. Metab.,* 50, 475, 1980.

58. **Orten, J. M. and Neuhaus, O. W.,** *Human Biochemistry,* 10th ed., C. V. Mosby, St. Louis, Mo., 1982, 633.

59. **Lehninger, A. L.,** *Biochemistry,* 2nd ed., Worth Publ., New York, 1975, 817.

60. **Rubenstein, A. H. and Spitz, I.,** Role of the kidney in insulin metabolism and excretion, *Diabetes,* 17, 161, 1968.

61. **Varandani, P. T., Nafz, M. A., and Shroyer, L. A.,** Insulin degradation. VI. Feedback control by insulin of liver glutathione insulin transhydrogenase in rats, *Diabetes,* 23, 117, 1974.

62. **Duckworth, W. C., Stentz, F. B., Heinemann, M., and Kitabchi, A. E.,** Initial site of insulin cleavage by insulin protease, *Proc. Natl. Acad. Sci. U.S.A.,* 76, 635, 1979.

63. **Silvers, A., Sivenson, R. S., Farquhar, J. W., and Reaven, G. M.,** Derivation of a three compartment model describing disappearance of plasma insulin — [131]I in man, *J. Clin. Invest.,* 48, 1461, 1969.

64. **Sherwin, R. S., Kramer, K. J., Tobin, J. D., Insel, P. A., Liljenquist Berman, A., and Andres, R.,** A model of the kinetics of insulin in man, *J. Clin. Invest.,* 53, 1481, 1974.

65. **Genuth, S. M.,** Metabolic clearance of insulin in man, *Diabetes,* 21, 1003, 1972.

66. **Navalesi, R., Pilo, A., and Ferrannini, E.,** Kinetic analysis of plasma insulin disappearance in nonketotic diabetic patients and in normal subjects, *J. Clin. Invest.,* 61, 197, 1978.

67. **Berman, M.,** Insulin kinetics, models, and delivery schedules, *Diabetes Care,* 3, 266, 1980.

68. **Berman, M., McGuire, E. A., Roth, J., and Zeleznik, A. J.,** Kinetic modeling of insulin binding to receptors and degradation in vivo in the rabbit, *Diabetes,* 29, 50, 1980.

69. **Galloway, J. A., Spradlin, C. T., Nelson, R. L., Wentworth, S. M., Davidson, J. A., and Swarner, J. L.,** Factors influencing the absorption, serum insulin concentration, and blood glucose responses after injections of regular insulin and various insulin mixtures, *Diabetes Care,* 4, 366, 1981.

70. **Greenblatt, D. J. and Koch-Weser, J.,** Clinical pharmacokinetics. Part II, *N. Engl. J. Med.,* 293, 964, 1975.

71. **Deckert, T.,** Intermediate-acting insulin preparations: NPH and lente, *Diabetes Care,* 3, 623, 1980.

72. **Bauman, W. A. and Yalow, R. S.,** Differential diagnosis between endogenous and exogenous insulin-induced refractory hypoglycemia in a nondiabetic patient, *N. Engl. J. Med.,* 303, 198, 1980.

73. **Kølendorf, K. and Bojsen, J.,** Kinetics of subcutaneous NPH insulin in diabetics, *Clin. Pharmacol. Ther.,* 31, 494, 1982.

74. **Kitabchi, A. E., Stentz, F. B., Cole, C., and Duckworth, W. C.,** Accelerated insulin degradation: an alternate mechanism for insulin resistance, *Diabetes Care,* 2, 414, 1979.

75. **Stevenson, R. W., Tsakok, T. I., and Parsons, J. A.,** Matched glucose responses to insulin administered subcutaneously and intravenously, *Diabetologia,* 18, 423, 1980.

76. **Berger, M., Halben, P. A., Girardier, L., Seydoux, J., Offord, R. E., and Renold, A. E.,** Absorption kinetics of subcutaneously injected insulin. Evidence for degradation at the injection site, *Diabetologia,* 17, 97, 1979.

77. **Berger, M., Cuppers, H. J., Halban, P. A., and Offord, R. E.,** The effect of aprotinin on the absorption of subcutaneously injected regular insulin in normal subjects, *Diabetes,* 29, 81, 1980.

78. **Koivisto, V. A. and Felig, P.,** Alterations in insulin absorption and in blood glucose control associated with varying insulin injection sites in diabetic patients, *Ann. Intern. Med.,* 92, 59, 1980.

79. **Binder, C.,** Absorption of injected insulin, *Acta Pharmacol. Toxicol.,* 27(Suppl. 2), 1, 1969.

80. **Davidson, J. K. and DeBra, D. W.,** Immunologic insulin resistance, *Diabetes,* 27, 307, 1978.

81. **Lauritzen, T., Faber, O. K., and Binder, C.,** Variation in ^{125}I-insulin absorption and blood glucose concentration, *Diabetologia,* 17, 291, 1979.

82. **Anon.,** *Physicians' Desk Reference,* 36th ed., Medical Economics Co., Oradell, N.J., 1982.

83. **Galloway, J. A. and Root, M. A.,** New forms of insulin, *Diabetes,* 21(Suppl. 2), 637, 1972.

84. **Shichiri, M., Kawamori, R., Yoshida, M., Etani, N., Hoshi, M., Izumi, K., Shigeta, Y., and Abe, H.,** Short-term treatment of alloxan-diabetic rats with intrajejunal administration of water-in-oil-in-water insulin emulsions, *Diabetes,* 24, 971, 1975.

85. **Wigley, F. M., Londons, J. H., Wood, S. H., Shipp, J. C., and Waldman, R. H.,** Insulin across respiratory mucosae by aerosol delivery, *Diabetes,* 20, 552, 1971.

86. **Shin-Wei, L. and Sciarra, J. J.,** Development of an aerosol dosage form containing insulin, *J. Pharm. Sci.,* 65, 567, 1976.

87. **Yamasaki, Y., Shichiri, M., Kawamori, R., Kikuchi, M., Yagi, T., Arai, S., Tohdo, R., Hakui, N., Oji, N., and Abe, H.,** The effectiveness of rectal administration of insulin suppository on normal and diabetic subjects, *Diabetes Care,* 4, 454, 1981.

88. **Schade, D. S., Eaton, R. P., Carlson, G. A., Bair, R. E., Gaona, J. I., Love, J. T., Urenda, R. S., and Spencer, W. J.,** Future therapy of the insulin-dependent diabetic patient — the implantable insulin delivery system, *Diabetes Care,* 4, 319, 1981.

89. **Soeldner, J. S.,** Treatment of diabetes mellitus by devices, *Am. J. Med.,* 70, 183, 1981.

90. **Poulsen, J. E. and Deckert, T.,** Insulin preparations and the clinical use of insulin, *Acta Med. Scand.,* 601, 197, 1977.

91. **Anon.,** Clinical use of insulin, in *Diabetes Mellitus,* 8th ed., Waife, S. O., Ed., Lilly Research Laboratories, Indianapolis, Ind., 1979, chap. 7.

92. **Foster, D. W.,** Diabetes Mellitus, in *Harrison's Principles of Internal Medicine,* 9th ed., Isselbacher, K. J., Adams, R. D., Braunwald, E., Petersdorf, R. G., and Wilson, J. D., Eds., McGraw-Hill, New York, 1980, chap. 338.

93. **Marble, A., Selenkow, H. A., Rose, L. I., Dluhy, R. G., and Williams, G. H.,** Endocrine diseases, in *Drug Treatment,* 2nd ed., Avery, G. S., Ed., ADIS Press, New York, 1980, 498.

94. **Wright, A. D., Walsh, C. H., Fitzgerald, M. G., and Malins, J. M.,** Very pure porcine insulin in clinical practice, *Br. Med. J.,* 1, 25, 1979.

95. **Wentworth, S. M.,** Insulin dose change with increase purity, *Diabetes Care,* 4, 504, 1981.

96. **Somogyi, M.,** Exacerbation of diabetes by excess insulin action, *Am. J. Med.,* 26, 169, 1959.

97. **Kahn, C. R. and Rosenthal, A. S.,** Immunologic reactions to insulin: insulin allergy, insulin resistance, and the autoimmune insulin syndrome, *Diabetes Care,* 2, 283, 1979.

98. **Galloway, J. A.,** Insulin treatment for the early 80's: facts and questions about old and new insulins and their usage, *Diabetes Care,* 3, 615, 1980.

99. **Wentworth, S. M., Galloway, J. A., Davidson, J. A., Root, M. A., Chance, R. E., and Haunz, E. A.,** An update of the results of the use of "single peak" (SP) and "single component" (SC) insulin in patients with complications of insulin therapy, *Diabetes,* 25, 326, 1976.

100. **Smelo, L. S.,** Insulin resistance, *Proc. Am. Diabetes A,* 8, 75, 1948.

101. **Steiner, D. F. and Oyler, P. E.,** The biosynthesis of insulin and a probable precursor of insulin by a human islet cell adenoma, *Proc. Natl. Acad. Sci., U.S.A.,* 57, 473, 1967.

102. **Anon.,** Insulin, in *Diabetes Mellitus,* 8th ed., Waife, S. O., Ed., Lilly Research Laboratories, Indianapolis, Ind., 1979, chap. 4.

103. **Anon.,** Discontinuation of certification of all U-80 insulin products, *Fed. Reg.,* 44, 55169, 1979.

104. **Harvey, S. C.,** Hormones, in *Remington's Pharmaceutical Science,* 16th ed., Osol, A., Ed., Mack Publ., Easton, Pa., 1980, chap. 51.

105. **Anon.,** *U.S. Pharmacopeia National Formulary,* USPXX, NF XV, Mack Publ., Easton, Pa., 1979, 401.

106. **Hagedorn, H. C., Jensen, B. N., Krarup, N. B., and Wodstrup, I.,** Protamine insulinate, *JAMA,* 106, 177, 1936.

107. **Krayenbühl, C. and Rosenberg, T.,** Crystalline protamine insulin, *Rep. Steno Mem. Hosp. Nord. Insulinlab,* 1, 60, 1946.

108. **Hallas-Møller, K., Jersild, M., Petersen, K., and Schlichtkrull, J.,** Zinc insulin preparations for single daily injection, *JAMA,* 150, 1667, 1952.

109. **Haupt, V. C., Koberich, W., Cordes, U., Beyer, J., and Schoffling, K.,** Untersuchungen zu Dosis-Wirkungs-Relationen Werscheidener Sulfonylharnstoffderivate der alten und neuen Gencration, *Arzneim. Forsch.,* 22, 2203, 1972.

110. **Loubatieres, A.,** The hypoglycemic sulfonamides: history and development of the problem from 1942 to 1945, *Ann. N.Y. Acad. Sci.,* 71, 4, 1957.

111. **Mirsky, I. A., Perisutti, G., and Jinks, R.,** Ineffectiveness of sulfonylureas in alloxan diabetic rats, *Proc. Soc. Exp. Biol. Med.,* 91, 475, 1956.
112. **Lebowitz, H. E. and Feinglos, M. N.,** Sulfonylurea drugs: mechanism of antidiabetic action and therapeutic usefulness, *Diabetes Care,* 1, 189, 1978.
113. **Feinglos, M. N. and Lebovitz, H. E.,** Sulfonylurea treatment of insulin-independent diabetes mellitus, *Metabolism,* 29, 488, 1980.
114. **Grodsky, G. M., Epstein, G. H., Fanska, R., and Karam, J. H.,** Pancreatic action of the sulfonylureas, *Fed. Proc. Fed. Am. Soc. Exp. Biol.,* 36, 2714, 1977.
115. **Davidoff, F.,** Hepatic effects of oral hypoglycemic agents, *Fed. Proc. Fed. Am. Soc. Exp. Biol.,* 36, 2724, 1977.
116. **Levey, G. S.,** The effects of sulfonylureas on peripheral metabolic processes, *Fed. Proc. Fed. Am. Soc. Exp. Biol.,* 36, 2720, 1977.
117. **Henquin, J. C.,** Tolbutamide stimulation and inhibition of insulin release, *Diabetologia,* 18, 151, 1980.
118. **Couturier, E. and Malaisse, W. J.,** Insulinotropic effects of hypoglycaemic and hyperglycaemic sulfon-amides: the ionophoretic hypothesis, *Diabetologia,* 19, 335, 1980.
119. **Hellman, B., Sehlin, J., and Täljedal, I-B,** The pancreatic β-cell recognition of insulin secretagogues. II. Site of action of tolbutamide, *Biochem. Biophys. Res. Commun.,* 45, 1384, 1971.
120. **Duckworth, W. C., Solomon, S. S., and Kitabchi, A. E.,** Effect of chronic sulfonylurea therapy on plasma insulin and proinsulin levels, *J. Clin. Endocrinol.,* 35, 585, 1972.
121. **Fineberg, S. E. and Schneider, S. H.,** Glipizide versus tolbutamide, an open trial, *Diabetologia,* 18, 49, 1980.
122. **Olefsky, J. M. and Reaven, G. M.,** Effects of sulfonylurea therapy on insulin binding to mononuclear leukocytes of diabetic patients, *Am. J. Med.,* 60, 89, 1976.
123. **Feinglos, M. N. and Lebovitz, H. E.,** Sulfonylureas increase the number of insulin receptors, *Nature (London),* 276, 184, 1978.
124. **Prince, M. J. and Olefsky, J. M.,** Direct *in vitro* effect of a sulfonylurea to increase human fibroblast insulin receptors, *J. Clin. Invest.,* 66, 608, 1980.
125. **Beck-Nielsen, H., Pederson, O., and Lindskov, H. O.,** Increased insulin sensitivity and cellular insulin binding in obese diabetics following treatment with glibenclamide, *Acta Endocrinol.,* 90, 451, 1979.
126. **Loubatieres, A.,** History and development of the oral treatment of diabetes, in *Oral Hypoglycemic Agents,* Vol. 9, Campbell, G. D., Ed., Academic Press, New York, 1969, chap. 1.
127. **Anon.,** Glibornuride — another oral hypoglycemic agent, *Drug Ther. Bull.,* 14, 41, 1976.
128. **Bander, A.,** The relationship between chemical structure and hypoglycemic activity, in *Oral Hypoglycemic Agents,* Vol. 9, Campbell, G. D., Ed., Academic Press, New York, 1969, chap. 2.
129. **Biere, H., Rufer, C., Ahrens, H., Loge, O., and Schroder, E.,** Blood glucose lowering sulfonamides with asymmetric carbon atoms. II, *J. Med. Chem.,* 17, 716, 1974.
130. **Rufer, C., Biere, H., Ahrens, H., Loge, O., and Schroder, E.,** Blood glucose lowering sulfonamides with asymmetric carbon atoms. I, *J. Med. Chem.,* 17, 708, 1974.
131. **Balant, L.,** Les sulfonylurées hypoglycémiantes: un probléme de générations? Considérations pharmaco-cinétiques et pharmacodynamiques, *Diabete Metabol.,* 4, 135, 1978.
132. **Ribes, G., Trimble, E. R., Blayac, J. P., Wollheim, C. B., Puech, R., and Loubatieres-Mariani, M. M.,** Effect of a new hypoglycemic agent (HB699) on the in vivo secretion of pancreatic hormones in the dog, *Diabetologia,* 20, 501, 1981.
133. **Jackson, J. E. and Bressler, R.,** Clinical pharmacology of sulfonylurea hypoglycaemic agents. Part I, *Drugs,* 22, 211, 1981.
134. **Jackson, J. E. and Bressler, R.,** Clinical pharmacology of sulfonylurea hypoglycemic agents. Part 2, *Drugs,* 22, 295, 1981.
135. **Balant, L.,** Clinical pharmacokinetics of sulfonylurea hypoglycaemic drugs, *Clin. Pharmacokinet.,* 6, 215, 1981.
136. **Skillman, T. G. and Feldman, J. M.,** The pharmacology of sulfonylureas, *Am. J. Med.,* 70, 361, 1981.
137. **Shen, S. W. and Bressler, R.,** Clinical pharmacology of oral antidiabetic agents (first of two parts), *N. Engl. J. Med.,* 296, 493, 1977.
138. **Shen, S. W. and Bressler, R.,** Clinical pharmacology of oral antidiabetic agents (second of two parts), *N. Engl. J. Med.,* 296, 787, 1977.
139. **Stowers, J. M. and Borthwick, L. J.,** Oral hypoglycaemic drugs: clinical pharmacology and therapeutic use, *Drugs,* 14, 41, 1977.
140. **Sartor, G., Melander, A., Schersten, B., and Wahlin-Boll, E.,** Influence of food and age on the single-dose kinetics and effects of tolbutamide and chlorpropamide, *Eur. J. Clin. Pharmacol.,* 17, 285, 1980.
141. **Said, S. A. and Al-Shora, H. I.,** Hypoglycemic activity of oral hypoglycemics with increased hydro-philicity, *J. Pharm. Sci.,* 70, 67, 1981.
142. **Wahlin-Boll, E., Melander, A., Sartor, G., and Schersten, B.,** Influence of food intake on the absorption and effect of glipizide in diabetics and in healthy subjects, *Eur. J. Clin. Pharmacol.,* 18, 279, 1980.

143. **Sartor, G., Schersten, B., and Melander, A.,** Serum glibenclamide in diabetic patients, and influence of food on the kinetics of glibenclamide, *Diabetologia,* 18, 17, 1980.

144. **Hsu, P. L., Ma, J. K. H., and Luzzi, L. A.,** Interactions of sulfonylureas with plasma proteins, *J. Pharm. Sci.,* 63, 570, 1974.

145. **Crooks, M. J. and Brown, K. F.,** Interactions of glipizide with human serum albumin, *Biochem. Pharmacol.,* 24, 298, 1975.

146. **Brogden, R. N., Heel, R. C., Pakes, G. E., Speight, T. M., and Avery, G. S.,** Glipizide: a review of its pharmacological properties and therapeutic use, *Drugs,* 18, 329, 1979.

147. **Melander, A., Sartor, G., Wahlin, E., Schersten, B., and Bitzen, P-O.,** Serum tolbutamide and chlorpropamide concentrations in patients with diabetis mellitus, *Br. Med. J.,* 1, 142, 1978.

148. **Bergman, U., Christenson, I., Jansson, B., Wilholm, B.-E., and Ostman, J.,** Wide variations in serum chlorpropamide concentration in outpatients, *Eur. J. Clin. Pharmacol.,* 18, 165, 1980.

149. **Scott, J. and Poffenbarger, P. L.,** Pharmacogenetics of tolbutamide metabolism in humans, *Diabetes,* 28, 41, 1979.

150. **Feldman, J. M. and Lebovitz, H. E.,** Biological activities of tolbutamide and its metabolites, *Diabetes,* 18, 529, 1969.

151. **Braselton, W. E. and Huff, T. A.,** Measurement of antidiabetic sulfonylureas in serum by gas chromatography with electron capture, *Diabetes,* 26, 50, 1977.

152. **Thomas, R. C. and Ikeda, G. J.,** The metabolic fate of tolbutamide in man and in the rat, *J. Med. Chem.,* 9, 507, 1966.

153. **Campbell, R. K. and Hansten, P. D.,** Metabolism of chlorpropamide, *Diabetes Care,* 4, 332, 1981.

154. **Brotherton, P. M., Grieveson, P., and McMartin, C.,** A study of the metabolic fate of chlorpropamide in man, *Clin. Pharmacol. Ther.,* 10, 505, 1969.

155. **Taylor, J. A.,** Pharmacokinetics and biotransformation of chlorpropamide in man, *Clin. Pharmacol. Ther.,* 13, 710, 1972.

156. **Forist, A. A. and Judy, R. W.,** 1-(Hexahydroazepin-1-yl)-3-p-carboxyphenylsulfonylurea-a metabolite of tolazamide in man, *J. Pharm. Pharmacol.,* 26, 565, 1974.

157. **McMahon, F. G., Upjohn, H. L., Carpenter, O. S., Wright, J. B., Oster, H. L., and Dulin, W. E.,** The comparative pharmacology of a variety of hypoglycemic drugs, *Curr. Ther. Res.,* 4, 333, 1962.

158. **Thomas, R. C., Duchamp, D. J., Judy, R. W., and Ikeda, G. J.,** Metabolic fate of tolazamide in man and in the rat, *J. Med. Chem.,* 21, 725, 1978.

159. **Smith, D. L., Vecchio, T. J., and Forist, A. A.,** Biological half-lives of the p-acetylbenezenesulfonylureas U-18536 and acetohexamide and their metabolites, *Metabolism,* 14, 229, 1965.

160. **McMahon, R. E., Marshall, F. J., and Culp, H. W.,** The nature of the metabolites of acetohexamide in the rat and in the human, *J. Pharmacol. Exp. Ther.,* 149, 272, 1965.

161. **Galloway, J. A., McMahon, R. E., Culp, H. W., Marshall, F. J., and Young, E. C.,** Metabolism, blood levels and rate of excretion of acetohexamide in human subjects, *Diabetes,* 16, 118, 1967.

162. **Balant, L., Fabre, J., Loutan, L., and Samimi, H.,** Does 4-transhydroxy-glibenclamide show hypoglycemic activity?, *Arzneim. Forsch.,* 29, 162, 1979.

163. **Rupp, W., Christ, O., and Heptner, W.,** Resorption, Ausscheidung und metabolismus nach intravenoser and oraler gabe von HB 419-^{14}C an menschen, *Arzneim. Forsch.,* 19, 1428, 1969.

164. **Tamassia, V.,** Pharmacokinetics and bioavailability of glipizide, *Curr. Med. Res. Opinion,* 3 (Suppl. 1), 20, 1975.

165. **Fuccella, L. M., Tamassia, V., and Valzelli, G.,** Metabolism and kinetics of the hypoglycemic agent glipizide in man — comparison with glibenclamide, *J. Clin. Pharmacol.,* 13, 68, 1973.

166. **Balant, L., Zahnd, G., Gorgia, A., Schwarz, R., and Fabre, J.,** Pharmacokinetics of glipizide in man: influence of renal insufficiency, *Diabetologia,* 9(Suppl.), 331, 1973.

167. **Schmidt, H. A. E., Schoog, M., Schweer, K. H., and Winkler, E.,** Pharmacokinetics and pharmacodynamics as well as metabolism following orally and intravenously administered C14-glipizide, a new antidiabetic, *Diabetologia,* 9(Suppl.), 320, 1973.

168. **Bigler, F., Quitt, P., Vecchi, M., and Vetter, W.,** Metabolism of glibornuride, a new hypoglycemic sulfonylurea derivative in man, *Arzneim. Forsch.,* 22(12a), 2191, 1972.

169. **Rentsch, G., Schmidt, H. A. E., and Rieder, J.,** Pharmacokinetics of glibornuride, *Arzneim. Forsch.,* 22(12a), 2209, 1972.

170. **Crosby, D. L.,** Oral Hypoglycemics: A Drug Use Analysis Report, U.S. Food and Drug Administration, Washington, D.C., 1977.

171. **Balodimos, M. C., Camerini-Davalos, R. A., and Marble, A.,** Nine years experience with tolbutamide in the treatment of diabetes, *Metabolism,* 11, 957, 1966.

172. **Singer, D. L. and Hurwitz, D.,** Long-term experience with sulfonylureas and placebo, *N. Engl. J. Med.,* 227, 450, 1967.

173. **Bernhard, H.,** Long-term observations on oral hypoglycemic agents in diabetes. The effect of carbutamide and tolbutamide, *Diabetes,* 14, 59, 1965.

174. **De Lawter, D. E. and Moss, J. M.,** A five year study of tolbutamide in the treatment of diabetes mellitus, *JAMA,* 181, 156, 1962.
175. **Seltzer, H. S.,** Efficacy and safety of oral hypoglycemic agents, in *Annu. Rev. Med.,* 31, 261, 1980.
176. **Gundersen, K., Molony, B. A., Crim, J. A., Hearron, A. E., and Maile, J. P.,** in *Micronase (Glyburide) Pharmacological and Clinical Evaluation,* Rifkin, H., Ed., Excerpta Medica, Amsterdam, 1975, 254.
177. University Groups Diabetes Program, A study of the effects of hypoglycemic agents on vascular complications in patients with adult-onset diabetes, *Diabetes,* 19(Suppl. 2), 789, 1970.
178. **Hadden, D. R., Mongomery, D. A. D., Skelly, R. J., Trimble, E. R., Weaver, J. A., Wilson, E. A., and Buchanan, K. D.,** Maturity onset diabetes mellitus: response to intensive dietary management, *Br. Med. J.,* 3, 276, 1975.
179. **Boyden, T. and Bressler, R.,** Oral hypoglycemic agents, *Adv. Intern. Med.,* 24, 53, 1979.
180. **Tsalikian, E., Dunphy, T. W., Bohannon, N. V., Lorenzi, M., Gerich, J. E., Forsham, P. H., Kane, J. P., and Karem, J. H.,** The effect of chronic oral antidiabetic therapy on insulin and glucagon responses to a meal, *Diabetes,* 26, 314, 1977.
181. **Tomkins, G. M. and Bloom, A.,** Assessment of the need for continued oral therapy in diabetes, *Br. Med. J.,* 1, 649, 1972.
182. **Breidahl, H. D.,** Control of long term antidiabetic therapy, *Drugs,* 21, 292, 1981.
183. **Seltzer, H. S.,** Severe drug-induced hypoglycemia: a review, *Compr. Ther.,* 5, 21, 1979.
184. **Klimt, C. R., Knatterud, G. L., Meinert, C. L., and Prout, T. E.,** A study of the effects of hypoglycemic agents on vascular complications in patients with adult-onset diabetes. I. Design, methods and baseline results, *Diabetes,* 19(Suppl. 2), 747, 1970.
185. **Knatterud, G. L., Meinert, C. L., Klimt, C. R., Osborne, R. K., and Martin, D. B.,** Effects of hypoglycemic agents on vascular complications in patients with adult-onset diabetes. IV. A preliminary report on phenformin results, *JAMA,* 217, 777, 1971.
186. **Kolata, G. B.,** Controversy over study of diabetes drugs continues for nearly a decade, *Science,* 203, 986, 1979.
187. Coronary Drug Project Research Group, The prognostic importance of plasma glucose levels and of the use of oral hypoglycemic drugs after myocardial infarctions in men, *Diabetes,* 26, 453, 1977.
188. **Lasseter, K. C., Levey, G. S., Palmer, R. F., and McCarthy, J. S.,** The effect of sulfonylurea drugs on rabbit myocardial contractility, canine purkinje fiber automaticity, and adenylate cyclase activity from rabbit and human hearts, *J. Clin. Invest.,* 51, 2429, 1972.
189. **Hildner, F. J., Yeh, B. K., Javier, P. J., Fenster, A., and Samet, P.,** Inotropic action of tolbutamide on human myocardium, *Cathet. Cardiovasc. Diagn.,* 1, 47, 1975.
190. **Pogatsa, G. and Dubecz, E.,** The direct effect of hypoglycemic sulfonylureas on myocardial contractile force and arterial blood pressure, *Diabetologia,* 13, 515, 1977.
191. **Pogatsa, G. and Nemeth, M.,** Electrophysiologic effects of hypoglycemic sulfonylureas on rabbit heart, *Eur. J. Pharmacol.,* 67, 333, 1980.
192. **David, F. B. and Davis, P. J.,** Water metabolism in diabetes mellitus, *Am. J. Med.,* 70, 210, 1981.
193. **Moses, A. M.,** Effect of sulfonylurea drugs on water metabolism, in *Micronase (Glyburide) Pharmacological and Clinical Evaluation,* Rifkin, H., Ed., Excerpta Medica, Amsterdam, 1975, 105.
194. **O'Donovan, C. J.,** Analysis of long-term experience with tolbutamide (Orinase) in the management of diabetes, *Curr. Ther. Res.,* 1, 69, 1959.
195. **Emaneuli, A., Molari, E., Pirola, L. C., and Caputo, G.,** Glipizide, a new sulfonylurea in the treatment of diabetes mellitus, summary of clinical experience in 1064 patients, *Arzneim. Forsch.,* 22, 1881, 1972.
196. **Weissman, P. N., Shenkman, L., and Gregerman, R. I.,** Chloropropamide hyponatremia. Drug-induced inappropriate anti-diuretic hormone activity, *N. Engl. J. Med.,* 284, 65, 1971.
197. **Skillman, T. G. and Feldman, J. M.,** The pharmacology of sulfonylureas, *Am. J. Med.,* 70, 361, 1981.
198. **Jerntorp, P., Ohlin, H., Bergstrom, B., and Almer, L-O.,** Increase in plasma acetaldehyde: an objective indicator of the chlorpropamide alcohol flush, *Diabetes,* 30, 788, 1981.
199. **Leslie, R. D. G. and Pyke, D. A.,** Chlorpropamide-alcohol flushing: a dominantly inherited trait associated with diabetes, *Br. Med. J.,* 2, 1519, 1978.
200. **Kobberling, J., Bengsch, N., Bruggeboes, B., Schwarck, H., Tillil, H., and Weber, M.,** The chlorpropamide alcohol flush, *Diabetologia,* 19, 359, 1980.
201. **Strakosch, C. R., Jefferys, D. B., and Keen, H.,** Blockage of chlorpropamide alcohol flush by aspirin, *Lancet,* 1, 394, 1980.
202. **Hansen, J. M. and Christensen, L. K.,** Drug interactions with oral sulfonylurea hypoglycemic drugs, *Drugs,* 13, 24, 1977.
203. **Hansten, P. D.,** *Drug Interactions,* 5th ed., Lea and Febiger, Philadelphia, 1985, chap. 4.
204. **Shin, A. F. and Shrewsbury, R. P.,** *Evaluations of Drug Interactions,* 3rd ed., C.V. Mosby Co., St. Louis, 1985, chap. 14.
205. **Brown, K. F. and Crooks, M. J.,** Displacement of tolbutamide, glibenclamide, and chlorpropamide from serum albumin by anionic drugs, *Biochem. Pharmacol.,* 25, 1175, 1976.

206. **Sherma, S. D., Vakil, B. J., Samuel, M. R., and Chadha, D. R.,** Comparison of pinbutolol and propanolol during insulin-induced hypoglycemic, *Curr. Ther. Res.,* 26, 252, 1979.

207. **Wade, A., Ed.,** *Martindale — The Extra Pharmacopoeia,* 27th ed., The Pharmaceutical Press, London, 1977, 797.

208. **Griffiths, M. C., Ed.,** *USAN and the USP Dictionary of Drug Names,* U.S. Pharmacopeial Convention, Rockville, Md., 1981.

209. **Windholz, M., Ed.,** *The Merck Index,* 9th ed., Merck and Co., Rahway, N.J., 1976.

210. **Kaistha, K. K.,** Selective assay procedure for chlorpropamide in the presence of its decomposition products, *J. Pharm. Sci.,* 58, 235, 1969.

211. **Bottari, F., Giannaccini, B., Nannipieri, E., and Saettone, M.,** Thermal Dissociation of Sulfonylureas. II. Dissociation of four N- and N'-substituted sulfonylureas in different media, *J. Pharm. Sci.,* 61, 602, 1972.

212. **Watanabe, C. K.,** Studies in the metabolic changes induced by administration of guanidine bases. I. Influence of injected guanidine hydrochloride upon blood sugar content, *J. Biol. Chem.,* 33, 253, 1918.

213. **Walker, R. S. and Linton, A. L.,** Phenethyldiguanide: a dangerous side effect, *Br. Med. J.,* 2, 1005, 1959.

214. **Anon.,** Phenformin: new labeling and possible removal from market, *FDA Drug Bull.,* 7, 6, 1977.

215. **Anon.,** HEW secretary suspends general marketing of phenformin, *FDA Drug Bull.,* 7, 14, 1977.

216. **Kreisberg, R. A.,** Lactic acidosis: interrelationships with diabetes mellitus and phenformin, in *Diabetes Mellitus,* Vol. 4, Fajans, S. S., Bennett, R. P. H., Freinkel, N., Kipnis, D., Lacy, P. E., and Winegrad, A. I., Eds., DHEW Publ. No. (NIH), 76-854, U.S. Government Printing Office, Washington, D.C., 1977, 142.

217. **Cohen, R. D. and Woods, F. H.,** Lactate metabolism, in *Clinical and Biochemical Aspects of Lactic Acidosis,* Blackwell Scientific, Oxford, 1976, chap. 2.

218. **Cohen, R. D. and Woods, F. H.,** The role of drug therapy in the pathogenesis of lactic acidosis, in *Clinical and Biochemical Aspects of Lactic Acidosis,* Blackwell Scientific, Oxford, 1976, chap. 7.

219. **Siitonen, O., Huttunen, J. K., Jarvinen, R., Palomaki, P., Aro, A., Juvonen, H., Korhonen, T., and Pitala, P.,** Effects of discontinuation of biguanide therapy on metabolic control in maturity-onset diabetes, *Lancet,* 1, 217, 1980.

220. **Shee, C. D.,** Stopping biguanide therapy, *Lancet,* 1, 426, 1980.

221. **Nunes-Correa, J., Pereira, E., Carreiras, F., and Correia, L. G.,** Stopping biguanide therapy, *Lancet,* 1, 427, 1980.

222. **Czyzyk, A., Lawecki, J., Sadowski, J., Ponikowska, L., and Szczepanik, Z.,** Effect of biguanides on intestinal absorption of glucose, *Diabetes,* 17, 492, 1968.

223. **Wicklmayr, M., Dietze, G., and Mehnert, H.,** Effect of phenformin on substrate metabolism of working muscle in maturity-onset diabetes, *Diabetologia,* 15, 99, 1978.

224. **Bratusch-Marrain, P. R., Korn, A., Waldhausl, W. K., Gasic, S., and Nowotny, P.,** Effect of buformin on splanchnic carbohydrate and substrate metabolism in healthy man, *Metabolism,* 30, 946, 1981.

225. **Dietze, G., Wicklmayr, M., Mehnert, H., Czempiel, H., and Henftling, H. G.,** Effect of phenformin on hepatic balances of glucogenic substrates in man, *Diabetologia,* 14, 243, 1978.

226. **Searle, G. L. and Gulli, R.,** The mechanism of the acute hypoglycemic action of phenformin (DBI), *Metabolism,* 29, 630, 1980.

227. **Nattrass, M., Todd, P. G., Hinks, L., Lloyd, B., and Alberti, K. G. M. M.,** Comparative effects of phenformin, metformin, and glibenclamide on metabolic rhythms in maturity-onset diabetics, *Diabetologia,* 13, 145, 1977.

228. **Davidoff, F.,** Guanidine derivatives in medicine, *N. Engl. J. Med.,* 289, 141, 1973.

229. **Waters, A. K., Morgan, D. B., and Wales, J. K.,** Blood lactate and pyruvate levels in diabetic patients treated with biguanides with and without sulfonylureas, *Diabetologia,* 14, 95, 1978.

230. **Bjorntorp, P., Carlstrom, S., Fagerberg, S. E., Hermann, L. S., Holm, A. G. L., Schersten, B., and Ostman, J.,** Influence of phenformin and metformin on exercise induced lactataemia in patients with diabetes mellitus, *Diabetologia,* 15, 95, 1978.

231. **Czyzyk, A., Lao, B., Bartosiewicz, W., Szczepanik, Z., and Orlowska, K.,** The effect of short term administration of antidiabetic biguanide derivatives on the blood lactate levels in healthy subjects, *Diabetologia,* 14, 89, 1978.

232. **Verdonck, L. F., Sangster, B., van Heijst, A. N. P., de Grott, G., and Maes, R. A. A.,** Buformin concentration in a case of fatal lactic acidosis, *Diabetologia,* 20, 45, 1981.

233. **Luft, D., Schnulling, R. M., and Eggstein, M.,** Lactic acidosis in biguanide-treated diabetics, *Diabetologia,* 14, 75, 1978.

234. **Conlay, L. A., Karam, J. H., Matin, S. B., and Loewenstein, J. E.,** Serum phenformin concentrations in patients with phenformin-associated lactic acidosis, *Diabetes,* 26, 628, 1977.

235. **Knatterud, G. L., Klimt, C. R., Osborne, R. K., Meinert, G. L., Martin, D. B., and Hawkins, B. S.,** A study of the effects of hypoglycemic agents on vascular complications in patients with adult-onset diabetes. V. Evaluation of phenformin therapy, *Diabetes,* 24(Suppl. 1), 65, 1975.

236. **Davidoff, F., Bertolini, D., and Haas, D.,** Enhancement of the mitochondrial Ca^{2+} uptake rate by phenethylbiguanide and other organic cations with hypoglycemic activity, *Diabetes,* 27, 757, 1978.

237. **Bohannon, N. V., Karam, J. H., Lorenzi, M., Gerich, J. E., Matin, S. B., and Forsham, P. H.,** Plasma glucagon suppression by phenformin in man, *Diabetologia,* 13, 503, 1977.

238. **Stout, R. W., Brunzell, J. D., Bierman, E. L., and Porte, D.,** Effect of phenformin on glucose-insulin relationships, *Diabetes,* 23, 624, 1974.

239. **Cohen, D., Pezzino, V., Vigneri, R., Avola, R., D'Agata, R., and Polosa, P.,** Phenformin increases insulin binding to human cultured breast cancer cells, *Diabetes,* 29, 329, 1980.

240. **Oates, N. S., Shah, R. R., Idle, J. R., and Smith, R. L.,** On the urinary disposition of phenformin and 4-hydroxy-phenformin and their rapid simultaneous measurement, *J. Pharm. Pharmacol.,* 32, 731, 1980.

241. **Unger, R. H.,** Diabetes and the alpha cell, *Diabetes,* 25, 136, 1976.

242. **Raskin, P.,** The role of somatostatin in managing diabetes, *Drug Therapy,* 8, 81, 1978.

243. **Sheppard, M., Shapiro, B., Pimstone, B., Kronheim, S., Berelowitz, M., and Gregory, M.,** Metabolic clearance and plasma half disappearance time of exogenous somatostatin in man, *J. Clin. Endocrinol. Metab.,* 48, 50, 1979.

244. **Efendic, S., Lins, P-E., and Luft, R.,** Somatostatin and insulin secretion, *Metabolism,* 27, 1275, 1978.

245. **Lins, P-E., Efendic, S., Meyers, C. A., Coy, D. H., Schally, A., and Luft, R.,** Selective effect of some somatostatin analogs on glucagon as opposed to insulin release in rats in vivo, *Metabolism,* 29, 728, 1980.

246. **Brown, M., Rivier, J., and Vale, W.,** Biological activity of somatostatin and somatostatin analogs on inhibition of arginine-induced insulin and glucagon release in the rat, *Endocrinology,* 98, 336, 1976.

247. **Vale, W., Rivier, J., Ling, N., and Brown, M.,** Biologic and immunologic activities and applications of somatostatin analogs, *Metabolism,* 27, 1391, 1978.

248. **Weir, G. C., Schwarz, J. A., and Mathe, C. J.,** Inhibition of glucagon and insulin secretion from the perfused rat pancreas by a β-cell selective somatostatin analog, *Metabolism,* 29, 68, 1980.

249. **Bloom, S. R., Adrian, T. E., Barnes, A. J., Long, R. G., Hanley, J., Mallinson, C. N., Rivier, J. E., and Brown, M. R.,** New specific long-acting somatostatin analogues in the treatment of pancreatic endocrine tumors, *Gut,* 19, 446, 1978.

250. **Skyler, J. S., Ed.,** Symp. Human Insulin Recombinant DNA Origin, *Diabetes Care,* 5 (Suppl. 2) 1, 1982.

251. **Karam, J. H. and Etzwiler, D. D., Eds.,** Int. Symp. Human Insulin, *Diabetes Care,* 6 (Suppl. 1), 1, 1983.

252. **Anon.,** *Facts and Comparisons,* Kastrup, E. K., Olin, B. R., and Hunsaker, L. M., Eds., Lippincott, 1985, 130b.

253. **Binder, C., Lauritzen, T., Faber, O., and Pramming, S.,** Insulin pharmacokinetics, *Diabetes Care,* 7, 188, 1984.

254. **Peterson, C. M., Ed.,** Symp. Optimal Insulin Delivery, *Diabetes Care,* 5 (Suppl. 1), 1, 1982.

255. **Anon.,** Labeling for oral hypoglycemic drugs of the sulfonylurea class, *Fed. Regist.,* 49, 14331, 1984.

256. **Anon.,** Symp. Current Res. Clinical Applications Second-Generation Sulfonylurea Glyburide, *Am. J. Med.,* 79, (3B), 1, 1985.

257. **Anon.,** Symp. New Perspectives in Noninsulin-Dependent Diabetes Mellitus and the Role of Glypizide in Its Treatment, *Am. J. Med.,* 75, (5B), 1, 1983.

258. **Asmal, A. C. and Marble, A.,** Oral hypoglycemic agents: an update, *Drugs,* 28, 62, 1984.

259. **Lockwood, D. H., Maloff, B. L., Nowak, S. M., and McCaleb, M. L.,** Extrapancreatic effects of sulfonylureas. Potentiation of insulin action through post-binding mechanisms, *Am. J. Med.,* 74, 102, 1983.

260. **Lockwood D. H., Gerich, J. E., and Goldfine, I., Eds.,** Symp. Effects Oral Hypoglycemic Agents Receptor Postreceptor Actions Insulin, *Diabetes Care,* 7 (Suppl. 1), 1, 1984.

261. **Kabadi, U. M.,** Adjuvant therapy with tolazamide and insulin improves metabolic control in type 1 diabetic mellitus, *Diabetic Care,* 8, 440, 1985.

262. **Rizza, R. A.,** Combined sulfonylurea and insulin therapy in insulin-dependent diabetes: research or clinical practice?, *Diabetes Care,* 8, 511, 1985.

HYPOTHALAMIC AND PITUITARY HORMONES

Leo E. Reichert, Jr., Thomas T. Andersen, James A. Dias, Paul W. Fletcher, and Patrick M. Sluss

INTRODUCTION

The pituitary gland, through its secretion of a variety of nonsteroid hormones, is considered the major physiologic regulator of bodily function. The secretion of the pituitary hormones is controlled by other hormones synthesized in and elaborated from the hypothalamus. Normal pituitary function is dependent upon an adequate vascular connection between the hypothalamus and the pituitary via the hypophysial portal blood vessels whose primary capillary bed lies in the median eminence of the brain. Hypothalamic hormones which stimulate release of the pituitary hormones are called "-liberins", such as corticoliberin which stimulates release of the adrenocorticotropic hormone from the pituitary gland. Hypothalamic hormones which inhibit release of pituitary hormones are called "-statins", such as somatostatin, which inhibits release of somatotropin (or growth hormone) from the anterior pituitary gland. The relationship between secretions of the hypothalamus, the pituitary gland, and target tissues of the pituitary hormones is a classic example of the servomechanism of hormone-release control. For example, corticoliberin stimulates secretion of adrenocorticotropic hormone which increases elaboration of cortisol from its target tissue, the adrenal gland. Cortisol, in turn, inhibits release of corticoliberin and adrenocorticotropic hormone, thus facilitating a return to steady state conditions. As a general principle, for pituitary hormones whose release is effected by products of their target tissue through negative feedback control, there exists a hypothalamic liberin only. However, for pituitary hormones for which there is no known specific target organ or target organ product, as with growth hormone (somatotropin), there exists a dual system of hypothalamic control — a liberin (somatoliberin) and a statin (somatostatin). In the case of the posterior pituitary hormones, there is no evidence for hypothalamic control of secretion. Hormones elaborated from the posterior pituitary gland are synthesized in the hypothalamus and transported to the posterior pituitary gland via axoplasmic flow through nonmyelinated nerve fibers. The release of posterior pituitary hormones is controlled by physiologic factors such as plasma osmolality or such neuroendocrine stimuli as that induced by suckling.

In the following sections, we will describe, for each of the recognized hormones of the pituitary gland and the hypothalamus, what is currently accepted in terms of their mechanism of action, structure-activity relationships, metabolism, uses and dosages, toxicity, physical chemical properties and approved nomenclature.

THE HYPOTHALAMIC HORMONES

GONADOTROPIN RELEASING HORMONE

Mechanism of Action

Evidence from several laboratories has suggested that gonadotropin releasing hormone (GnRH) action may be divided into three sequential steps: (1) interaction of GnRH with a specific plasma membrane receptor,[1] (2) mobilization of ionic calcium (Ca^{2+}),[2] and (3) expulsion of the contents of the gonadotropin secretory granule (either luteinizing hormone or follicle stimulating hormone) to the extracellular space.[3] At present the precise locus of action of Ca^{2+} is unknown. The question of whether cyclic nucleotides play a specific role

Table 1
ANALOGS OF GnRH; EXAMPLES OF DERIVATIVES RETAINING CONSIDERABLE BIOLOGICAL ACTIVITY

	Structural modification	Biological activity (GnRH = 100)
GnRH	PyroGlu–His–Trp–Ser–Tyr–Gly–Leu–Arg–Pro–GlyNH$_3$ 1 2 3 4 5 6 7 8 9 10,	100
Analogs		
	Formyl Ser[1]	53
	N-MePyr[1]	48
	3-(2-Naphthyl)-Ala[3]	52
	Pentamethyl Phe[3]	69
	Phe[5]	64
	D-Ala[6]	2830
	D-Leu[6]	2900
	N[6]-MeLeu[7]	102
	HomoArg[8]	22
	Pro[9]ethylamide	670
	Pro[9]propylamide	380

in the mechanism of luteinizing hormone (LH) and/or follicle stimulating hormone (FSH) release has remained enigmatic. It is apparent that fluctuations in cyclic nucleotide levels in response to GnRH can be detected under some experimental conditions;[4] however, it is equally clear that alterations in cyclic nucleotides can be uncoupled from stimulated LH release in other circumstances.[5] It should also be pointed out that GnRH releases both LH and FSH in vivo and in vitro. A specific peptide has not been isolated which will release only LH or FSH.

Structure-Activity Relationships

The structure of porcine GnRH was elucidated by Schally et al.[6] and is depicted in Table 1. GnRH is a decapeptide for which numerous methods of synthesis have been described. Five of the ten amino acids in the decapeptide are trifunctional and side reactions produced by these amino acids make synthesis and purification of synthetic GnRH difficult. It should also be noted that the first two amino acids and the carboxy terminal amino acid are identical to those in thyrotropin releasing hormone. Numerous analogs of GnRH have been prepared (see Table 1) and certain general structure-activity relationships can be inferred. PyroGlu[1] and His[2] seem to be crucial for biologic activity. Trp[3] may be substituted by pentamethyl Phe with retention of almost all of its biologic activity. Both Ser[4] and Tyr[5] seem to be of minor importance for the biological activity. The Gly[6]-Leu[7] bond appears to be crucial for stability in vivo. Substitution of Gly[6] either by free or protected D-amino acids leads to a significant increase in biological activity (Table 2). Leu[7] and Arg[8] are not essential for biological activity and may be replaced. However, if Pro[9] is replaced there is considerable loss of biological activity. The C-terminal glycinamide can be replaced by a number of aliphatic alkylamines with retention of activity. As seen in Table 1 replacement by ethylamide and propylamide leads to increased stability and prolonged biological activity due to the inability of brain enzymes to degrade this analog.

Metabolism

After intravenous injection of GnRH, the initial halflife in plasma is short (3 to 6 min), followed by a slower component (20 to 30 min). In experiments with radiolabeled GnRH a very long third component of more than 100 min is also observed.[7] Several metabolic

Table 2
CONTRIBUTION OF THE SIDE CHAIN IN POSITION TO BIOLOGICAL ACTIVITY OF GnRH

Residue	Name	Biological activity (GnRH = 1)
R = –H	GnRH(1-9)-nonapeptide-ethylamide	2·8
R = –CH$_3$	D-Ala^6	70·9
R = –CH$_2$–OH	D-Ser^6	65
R = –CH$_2$–O–C(CH$_3$)–CH$_3$ with CH$_3$	D-Ser(Bu^t)^6	172
	D-Leu^6	102
	D-Glu^6	28
	D-Glu(OBu^t)^6	44
	D-Lys^6	17·3
R = –CH$_2$–CH(CH$_3$)–H with CH$_3$	D-Lys(BOC)^6	38

R = –CH$_2$–CH$_2$–C(=O)(CH$_3$)–O–C–CH$_3$ with CH$_3$

R = –CH$_2$–CH$_2$–CH$_2$–CH$_2$–NH$_2$

R = –CH$_2$–CH$_2$–CH$_2$–CH$_2$–N(H)–C(=O)–O–C(CH$_3$)–CH$_3$ with CH$_3$

Note: D-amino acids strongly enhance biological activity (tested by superovulation in immature rats). Bu^t = *tert* butyl, bu^t = *tert* butyl-ether, BOC = *tert* butyloxycarbonyl.

pathways have been identified for the enzymatic breakdown of GnRH. Metabolic inactivation of GnRH occurs at the following sites as indicated by the vertical lines:

$$1 \qquad\qquad 5 \qquad\qquad 10$$
$$\text{PyroGlu|His|Trp-Ser-Tyr-Gly|Leu-Arg-Pro|GlyNH}_2$$

The main metabolites of GnRH are a hexapeptide GnRH$^{1-6}$ and a tetrapeptide GnRH. [7-10]

Uses and Dosage

Stimulatory analogs of GnRH with potent and long-acting activities have been developed for the purpose of simplifying GnRH treatment of infertility. However, GnRH and its agonistic derivatives have been found to exert paradoxical antifertility effects. It has been suggested that once daily intranasal spray application of 400 to 600 μg of the D-Ser(Bu^t)^6 derivative (see Table 2) is sufficient to inhibit ovulation.[8] GnRH is administered intravenously as a test of pituitary reserve and hypothalamic function and subcutaneously in the treatment of conditions associated with deficient gonadotropin secretion such as isolated gonadotropin deficiency, pituitary tumors, craniopharyngioma and anorexia nervosa.[9,10]

Toxicity

GnRH is active in all species studied to date, including nonmammalian species. In experimental animals such as the rat, the LD_{50} is 1.5 g/kg while the dose required for gonadotropin release is in the order of 2 μg/kg. However, secondary effects relative to release of FSH and LH suggest caution when GnRH is utilized in humans.

Physical-Chemical and Other Data

GnRH is soluble in water. Chymotrypsin, papain, subtilisin and thermolysin destroy the pituitary hormone releasing action of GnRH.

Chemical composition — $C_{55}H_{75}N_{17}O_{13}$ (mol wt = 1182.33).

Common names and abbreviations — Gonadoliberin, luteinizing hormone-releasing hormone, luliberin, folliberin, GnRH, LHRH, LRF, LH/FSH-RH.

THYROTROPIN RELEASING HORMONE

Mechanism of Action

The modern era of neuroendocrinology was ushered in just over a decade ago with the isolation and characterization from ovine and porcine hypothalamic tissue of a tripeptide which was designated thyrotropin-releasing hormone (TRH) by virtue of its capacity to stimulate the release of thyroid-stimulating hormone (TSH) from the mammalian anterior pituitary. TRH stimulates TSH release after binding to high-affinity receptors on the thyrotrope cell, activation of adenylate cyclase, and subsequent generation of cAMP.[11] The secretion of TSH is primarily regulated by negative feedback suppression of thyroid hormone $(T_3 + T_4)$ at the level of the pituitary gland, whereas TRH functions are the principal determinants of the "set point" of this interaction. Thyrotrope cell responsivity to TRH is also modulated by sex steroids, cortisol, and growth hormone. TRH is also a potent releasing hormone for prolactin.

Structure-Activity Relationships

A purified preparation of hypothalamic TSH-releasing factor was first obtained by Guillemin.[13] The structure of TRH of ovine[13] and porcine[12] origins were reported as follows: PyroGlu-His-ProNH$_2$. Numerous analogs of TRH have been prepared and studied, but few of them have significant biological activity. Substitution of the N-terminal amino acid usually leads to a marked decrease in activity. Only two analogs of higher activity than the parent molecule have been found: (N^γMeHis^2)-TRH with 8 times the activity and (L-β-[pyrazolyl-1]Ala^2)-TRH with 1.5 times the activity of native TRH. Some peptides have been described which are competitive antagonists of TRH. Cyclopentylcarbonyl-histidyl-pyrolidine inhibits TRH-induced TSH release at a 30-fold molar excess. Apparently this peptide binds to the pituitary TRH receptors rendering them refractory to TRH.

Metabolism

TRH is subject to rapid enzymatic breakdown in tissues[14] and body fluids.[15] It has also been shown that TRH is converted to a biologically active cyclized metabolite, histidyl-proline-diketopiperazine (His-Pro-DKP),[16] the formation of which is enhanced by TSH. His-Pro-DKP is metabolically active and is more effective than the parent tripeptide. These findings indicate that TRH in some instances may function as a prohormone for this metabolite, and that the effect of TSH on TRH metabolism provides a means by which the pituitary gland could exert a "feedback" on the hypothalamus to regulate its own function. The deaminated form of TRH is present in low concentrations in the brain and may be inactive. Studies with labeled TRH have indicated that it is rapidly cleared from the plasma and accumulated in liver, kidney, and pituitary gland. Labeled TRH has a plasma $t^{1/2}$ of 5 min and is rapidly excreted in the urine.[17]

Table 3
TOXICITY ENHANCEMENT BY TRH OF
DRUGS ACTING ON THE CENTRAL
NERVOUS SYSTEM[168]

Drug (i.p.)	Type	Fold increase in toxicity in presence of TRH
Chlorpromazine	Neuroleptic	38
Thioridazine	Neuroleptic	18
Haloperidol	Neuroleptic	2
Imipramine	Antidepressant	3
Amitriptyline	Antidepressant	7
Nomifensine	Antidepressant	4?
Amphetamine	Other	3
Caffeine	Other	2
Morphine	Other	2

Uses and Dosage

TRH is active by various routes, parenterally as well as nasally and orally. Nasal absorption is 5% and oral absorption 1% of the parenteral dose.[18,19] A therapeutic dose is 10 μg/kg in the human. TRH can be used as a test of pituitary TSH reserve to differentiate hypothalamic from pituitary dysfunction in patients with TSH deficiency.[20] TRH can be used to evaluate patients with inappropriate lactation and prolactinomas by monitoring serum prolactin response to its administration.[21] TRH does not stimulate growth hormone secretion in normal subjects, but stimulates release of growth hormone in 50% of the patients with acromegaly and thus can be of diagnostic help.[20] In addition, TRH stimulates ACTH secretion in some patients with Cushings' disease and Nelson's syndrome.[22]

Toxicity

TRH is relatively nontoxic in laboratory animals, with the LD_{50} being about 1.5 g/kg in the dog. The toxic consequences of TRH administration may be more substantial when used together with other drugs, such as neuroleptic, antidepressant, and stimulating drugs (Table 3). In these instances the LD_{50} of these drugs is significantly lowered.

Physical-Chemical and Other Data

TRH is partially soluble in chloroform or water, highly soluble in absolute methanol, and completely insoluble in pyridine.

Chemical composition — $C_{16}H_{22}N_6O_4$ (mol wt = 362.40).

Common names and abbreviations — Thyroliberin, TSH releasing hormone, TRH.

GROWTH HORMONE RELEASE-INHIBITING HORMONE

Growth hormone release-inhibiting hormone (somatostatin) action appears to involve the inhibition of the adenylate cyclase system. Thus, somatostatin added to rat pituitary inhibits the accumulation of cAMP during the first minutes of incubation.[23] The stimulatory effects of theophylline and dibutylryl-cAMP on growth hormone synthesis are antagonized by somatostatin in vitro.[24] This is associated with inhibition of the release of growth hormone and thyrotropin stimulating hormone. Other studies indicate that a dose-related increase in cGMP occurs in conjunction with the cAMP decrease.[25] The effects of somatostatin are shortlived requiring infusions or repeated injections. When infusions of somatostatin are stopped, however, there is a rebound with excess secretion of growth hormone, insulin, and gastrin.

Table 4
ANALOGS OF SOMATOSTATIN (GHRIH); SUMMARY OF BIOLOGICAL ACTIVITIES

Structure	Biological activity	
	In vivo	**In vitro**
┌─────── S ──────────── S ───────┐ H-Ala-Gly-Cys-Lys-Asn-Phe-Phe-Trp-Lys-Thr-Phe-Thr-Ser-Cys-OH (1 2 3 4 5 6 7 8 9 10 11 12 13 14)	100	100
AcGly²	—	65
Cys³	—	39
Desamino Cys³	—	60
( )	20	20
( )	15	15
( )	12	12
Thr¹	—	37
Ala²	135	190
D-Ala²	227	55
Ala⁵	112	130
Ala⁶	<10	1
Ala⁷	<10	3
Ala⁸	<10	<0.5
Nle⁹	0.5	—
DLys⁹	0.5	—
Ala¹⁰	<10	25
Ala¹¹	29	2
Ala¹²	22	4
Ala¹³	<10	6

Structure-Activity Relationships

The structure of somatostatin was elucidated by Brazeau et al.[26] and confirmed by Burgus et al.[27] by synthesis (Table 4). There has been some controversy about the relative biologic activity of linear somatostatin and cyclic somatostatin. Both forms are active in the dog in suppressing GH release. In humans the linear form is only slightly less active than the cyclic hormone on inhibition of insulin secretion.[28] Structure-activity relationships with the synthetic analogs of somatostatin (Table 4) indicate that the disulfide bridge (Cys³-Cys¹⁴) as well as the N-terminal dipeptide Ala¹-Gly² are not required for biological activity, whereas D-Ala² and D-Trp⁸ substitutions increase the biological activity two- to eightfold over the parent peptide. It appears that neither the size of the disulfide ring or the length of the peptide chain nor Lys⁴, Asn⁵, or Ser¹³ are critical for biological activity.

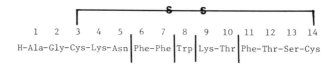

FIGURE 1. The primary structure of somatostatin. The vertical lines indicate sites of hydrolysis by brain peptides.

Table 5
LINEAR AMINO ACID SEQUENCE OF CRF

```
 1              5                  10                 15
H-Ser-Gln-Glu-Pro-Pro-Ile-Ser-Leu-Asp-Leu-Thr-Phe-His-Leu-Leu-Arg-
          20                 25                 30
Glu-Val-Leu-Glu-Met-Thr-Lys-Ala-Asp-Gln-Leu-Ala-Gln-Gln-Ala-His-
          35                 40
Ser-Asn-Arg-Lys-Leu-Leu-Asp-Ile-Ala-NH₂
```

Metabolism

After intravenous injection of somatostatin the plasma halflife is about 4 min.[29] In patients with liver disease this value is increased to 27 min as compared to 18 min in chronic renal failure. The metabolic inactivation of cyclic somatostatin by brain extracts starts with cleavage near Trp[8] and leads to preferential release of Phe[6], Phe[7], and Lys[9]. Linear somatostatin may have an additional cleavage site at Thr[10]-Phe[11]. The sites of breakdown are indicated by the vertical lines in Figure 1.

Uses and Dosages

At the present time synthetic somatostatin is being used in human and animal studies as an experimental tool to induce deficiency of certain hormones in order to assess their physiologic or pathologic importance.[30] For example, somatostatin has proven useful in establishing a physiologic role for glucagon in man and its importance in human diabetes mellitus.[31] When somatostatin is infused in man (100 to 500 μg/hr) glucose levels fall by 50% along with serum glucagon levels. In diabetics, somatostatin can decrease the insulin requirements by lowering blood glucose by 50%, and can prevent the development of diabetic ketoacidosis.

Toxicity

No serious adverse effects have been reported during administration of somatostatin to human subjects for as long as 3 days, although transient nausea, abdominal cramps, and, rarely, vomiting and diarrhea are observed. Prolonged treatment with somatostatin was toxic in baboons due to thrombocytopenia and reduced platelet aggregation.

Physical-Chemical and Other Data

Chemical composition — $C_{76}H_{104}N_{18}O_{19}S_2$ (mol wt = 1637.92).

Common names and abbreviations — Somatostatin, somatostatin release-inhibiting hormone, SRIH, GH-RIH.

CORTICOTROPIN RELEASING FACTOR

Mechanism of Action

Corticotropin Releasing Factor (CRF) (Table 5) regulates the release of corticotropin (ACTH) and stimulates ACTH synthesis.[32] ACTH release by CRF is Ca^{2+} and K^+ dependent and may involve the activation of adenylate cyclase.[33] The role of cAMP in CRF action is unclear, although 8-bromo-cAMP will elicit a response identical to CRF in isolated pituitary cells.[34]

Structure-Activity Relationships

Hypothalamic corticotropin releasing factor was the first neurohormone to be detected in hypothalamic and neurohypophysial tissue. Two types of CRF have been postulated and are referred to as alpha-CRF[35] and beta-CRF.[36] Beta-CRF is thought to be related, but not identical to lysine vasopressin and alpha-MSH. Recently, the purification, sequence analysis, and total synthesis of a 41 residue peptide that releases corticotropin in vitro has been reported[34] (Table 8). The COOH-terminal region in CRF (10-41) is 0.1% as potent as intact CRF, although CRF (4-41) is fully potent. CRF contains regions which are homologous with other known peptides, among them angiotensinogen, sauvagine, and urotensin I.

Metabolism

There are no reports on the metabolic fate or excretion of CRF.

Uses and Dosage

CRF is a relatively unknown entity, clinically. Experimental doses ranging from 30 to 3000 ng/kg are reported to elevate plasma ACTH 20-fold.[34]

Toxicity

Toxicity studies have not yet been accomplished with CRF due to the controversy over its structure.

Physical-Chemical and Other Data

Activity is destroyed by trypsin and thermolysin but unaffected by thioglycolate, pepsin, and chymotrypsin.

Common names — Corticotropin-releasing factor, corticoliberin, CRF.

THE ANTERIOR PITUITARY AND RELATED HORMONES

PROLACTIN

Mechanism of Action

The primary role of prolactin is considered to be the maintenance of lactation in humans, but it has several other actions as well.[37-39] During human pregnancy, prolactin is hyper-secreted by the pituitary and blood levels increase steadily until term. As a result of increased prolactin levels, together with the combined effects of estrogens and progesterone, development of the breast occurs, eventually forming milk in the acini.[40] Hydrocortisone and insulin have a permissive role in this process, and placental lactogen probably augments the effects of pituitary prolactin. At parturition, the removal of the placenta results in an abrupt decline in serum levels of estrogen and progesterone, and this decline initiates the onset of lactation. Lactation continues while estrogen levels are low and prolactin levels are high. Prolactin is essential for continued lactation in humans (but not in ruminants), and administration of drugs that inhibit prolactin secretion such as bromergocryptine causes lactation to cease. Although prolactin has well documented effects on parental behavior or salt retention in lower species such as birds or fish, respectively, no such effects have been thoroughly documented for humans.

At the cellular level, prolactin binds to the plasma membrane receptor with high affinity

Table 6
LINEAR AMINO ACID SEQUENCE OF HUMAN PITUITARY PROLACTIN

```
     1            5                10               15
NH₂-Leu-Pro-Ile-Cys-Pro-Gly-Gly-Ala-Ala-Arg-Cys-Gln-Val-Thr-Leu-Arg-Asp-Leu-Phe-
 20           25               30               35
Asp-Arg-Ala-Val-Val-Leu-Ser-His-Tyr-Ile-His-Asn-Leu-Ser-Ser-Glu-Met-Phe-Ser-Glu-
 40           45               50               55
Phe-Asp-Lys-Arg-Tyr-Thr-His-Gly-Arg-Gly-Phe-Ile-Thr-Lys-Ala-Ile-Asn-Ser-Cys-His-
 60           65               70               75
Thr-Ser-Ser-Leu-Ala-Thr-Pro-Glu-Asp-Lys-Glu-Gln-Ala-Gln-Gln-Met-Asn-Gln-Lys-Asp-
 80           85               90               95
Phe-Leu-Val-Ser-Ile-Leu-Ile-Leu-Arg-Ser-Trp-Asn-Glu-Pro-Leu-Tyr-His-Leu-Val-Thr-
100          105              110              115
Glu-Val-Arg-Gly-(Asx)-Gln-Glu-Ala-Pro-Glu-Ala-Ille-Leu-Ser-Lys-Ala-Val-Glu-Ile
120          125              130              135
Glu-Gln-Thr-Lys-Arg-Leu-Leu-Glu-Gly-Met-Glu-Leu-Ile-Val-Ser-Gln-Val-His-Pro-Glu-
140          145              150              155
Thr-Lys-Glu-Asp-Glu-Ile-Tyr-Pro-Val-Trp-Ser-Gly-Leu-Pro-Ser-Leu-Gln-Met-Ala-Asp-
160          165              170              175
Glu-Ser-Glu-Arg-Leu-Ser-Ala-Tyr-Tyr-Asn-Leu-Leu-His-Cys-Leu-Arg-Arg-Asp-Ser-His-
180          185              190              195        198
Lys-Ille-Asp-AsnTyr-Leu-Lys-Leu-Leu-Lys-Cys-Art-Ile-Ile-His-Asn-Asn-Asn-Cys-OH
```

although the means by which the message is transmitted to the protein synthesizing machinery is very poorly understood. There is no evidence that cAMP is the second messenger in prolactin physiology, but there is evidence that a stimulation of prostaglandin production precedes protein synthesis.[41] The result is a stimulation of the production of milk proteins (caseins and other proteins), lipids, and carbohydrates (notably lactose). The pentose pathway of glucose oxidation is stimulated as is the activity of pyruvate dehydrogenase. The synthesis of both components of lactose synthetase (α-lactalbumin and galactosyl transferase) is stimulated by prolactin. Electrolyte movement across the plasma membrane is regulated by prolactin through stimulation of the sodium-potassium ATPase activity.

Structure-Activity Relationships

The primary structure of human prolactin is given in Table 6. Many chemical and enzymatic modifications of prolactin have been made in an effort to define that portion of the molecule that interacts with its receptor, the so-called binding domain. Studies indicate that the lactogenic specificity of the hormone is in the amino terminal half of the molecule. (For the structurally similar growth hormones, the somatotrophic specificity resides in the carboxyl terminal half of the polypeptide chain.) However, researchers have as yet been unable to generate fragments (either by proteolysis or chemical cleavage) that contain biological activity.[42] Also, reduction of the disulfides leads to a loss of activity, as do numerous modifications of various amino acid residues. It was shown that four of the seven tyrosine residues could be modified without loss of activity, but further modification destroyed the binding or biological activity of the hormone.[43] It has also been reported that two of seven histidine residues are critical for interaction of prolactin with its receptor,[44] and the suggestion was made that the binding domain contains residues His[27], His[30], Tyr[28], and the tripeptide Leu[18], Phe[19], Asp[20].

Metabolism

Prolactin is synthesized by the anterior pituitary and its release into the blood is primarily under the control of a release inhibiting factor from the hypothalamus.[45] The prolactin-inhibitory factor, although not yet fully purified or chemically characterized, is released by the hypothalamus in response to dopaminergic inpulses. Dopamine may be a component of the prolactin inhibitory factor (or may be the factor). In addition, there is evidence that there are prolactin releasing factors, including (but not limited to) the thyrotropin-releasing hormone which has prolactin releasing activity.

Plasma prolactin levels for normal women range from 1 to 25 ng/mℓ with a mean of 8 ng/mℓ (3.5×10^{-9} mol/ℓ), while the range for normal men is 1 to 20 ng/mℓ with a mean of 4.7 ng/mℓ. Prolactin is episodically secreted and has a short (15 to 20 min) halflife in blood. The nocturnal rise in prolactin levels, like those of growth hormones, is due to the onset of sleep rather than to an intrinsic circadian rhythm.[45]

Several physiological situations give rise to increased prolactin release, notable among them being the stimulation of the breast and nipple during nursing.[41] Severe stress will lead to increased prolactin (and growth hormone) levels, and major surgery or the concomitant general anesthesia is often responsible for such an effect which is more prominent in women than in men. Estrogens, after several days of treatment, raise mean serum prolactin levels, probably due to an increased number of cells in the pituitary. Elevated estrogen levels probably account for the increased sensitivity of women compared to men for most or all situations leading to increased serum concentrations of prolactin.[45]

L-Dopa, probably after conversion to dopamine and actions at the hypothalamus, leads to a prompt (2 hr) decrease of serum prolactin which rebounds after another 2 to 3 hr. Of clinical interest are dopamine agonists such as the modified ergot derivative bromergocryptine (bromocriptine, CB-154) which have a longer duration of action than L-dopa and which directly affect the pituitary as well as the hypothalamus.[45]

Uses, Dosage, and Toxicity

Due to the availability of only small amounts of the human hormone, administration of physiologic or pharmacologic doses is not feasible for humans. Toxicity of prolactin may not be a serious problem if the human hormone becomes readily available except for the possible production of an immune response such as sometimes happens when insulin is given to diabetics, a caveat always to be considered.

Physical-Chemical and Other Data

Human prolactin is a protein hormone consisting of approximately 200 amino acid residues,[46] mol wt 22,800. Like all other mammalian prolactins, it has two tryptophan residues and three disulfide bonds,[46,47] including one which links the C-terminal residue to position 190. There is no covalently attached carbohydrate, and the isoelectric point is approximately 5.7. It is quite soluble at mildly alkaline pH, much less so near its pI. The amino acid sequence of human prolactin is known and is shown in Table 6. A great deal of physical-chemical data are available,[46] including its sedimentation coefficient ($s_{20,w}$ = 2.18), partial specific volume (0.732 cm³ g⁻¹), Stokes radius (24.9 Å), and frictional ratio (f/f$_o$ = 1.32).

Common names and abbreviations — Mammotropic H, mammotropin, lactotropic hormone, lactotropin, Prl, LTH, MTH

GROWTH HORMONE

Mechanism of Action

The mode of action of human growth hormone (GH, somatotropin) has not yet been fully elucidated, but it is known that it has both direct and indirect effects. In each instance, the hormone binds to a plasma membrane receptor, effecting intracellular changes secondarily. Direct effects include binding to diaphragm tissue, resulting in increased cAMP levels, and binding to erythrocytes, resulting in decreased glucose utilization. The indirect effects, which are of major importance, are mediated through production of secondary growth promoting peptides termed somatomedins (mol wt about 7000). Several different somatomedins have been demonstrated with slightly different physical and biological properties, including a sulfation factor (somatomedin A) and one with insulin-like activity (somatomedin C) which is not suppressible with antiinsulin antiserum. GH is an important anabolic hormone which leads to retention of nitrogen and potassium, a decrease in blood urea nitrogen, and an increase in serum phosphate. GH exhibits a marked species specificity in its action and only human GH is active in man.

Structure-Activity Relationships

A considerable amount of information is available concerning chemical modifications of specific residues in growth hormone, the intent of which is to define a portion of the molecule which is responsible for the biological activities of the hormone. In addition, many enzymatic cleavages have been made which indicate that the *entire* sequence is *not* needed for biological activity.[48] An exciting observation was made when it was shown that six residues could be removed from the middle of the hormone, leaving an active species of two polypeptides joined by a disulfide bond.[47] There is information that the active portion of somatotropin may include residues 96-133,[50,51] and studies such as these may lead to the production of chemically synthesized analogs which would be of use either an agonists or antagonists.

Metabolism

Human GH is synthesized by acidophilic cells of the anterior pituitary,[52] which contain approximately 8,500 μg of hormone and secrete about 500 μg/day. Plasma concentrations of somatotropin vary, but are approximately 1 to 5 ng/mℓ. There are various forms present in blood, referred to as "little", "big", and "large" GH, and these forms probably represent aggregates and/or prohormones. The halflife of little GH (monomeric) is 21 min, while that for big GH is 30 min.[52] The liver is the major site of clearance for most of the GH in man. Release of GH from the pituitary is regulated by the hypothalamus by means of a release inhibiting factor (somatostatin) and a putative somatotropin releasing factor (SRF), resulting in an episodic pattern of secretion. A nocturnal peak of GH release occurs 3 to 4 hr after the onset of sleep.

Uses and Dosages

Treatment with human growth hormone is effective in three of six types of dwarfs (types II, III, and IV, see Reference 52, Tables 4 to 10), and in patients with destructive pituitary or hypothalamic lesions leading to GH deficiency. Doses of 2 mg i.m. three times a week, increased to 4 mg i.m. three times a week if a growth rate of 6 cm/year is not obtained, were reported[53] to yield good results. Other doses of 2.5 mg twice weekly and 3.3 mg twice weekly were also effective.[54] Growth rates should approximate 9 cm/year for the first year and decrease by 1 cm/year for the second and third years. Treatment should begin as early as possible and continue until epiphyseal plate closure. In some cases, thyroid and adrenal replacement or oral anabolic agents may be indicated in conjunction with GH treatment.[55]

Toxicity

As with other protein hormones, the major toxicity problem is an immunological response to the exogenously administered GH. This can be mitigated by injecting monomeric growth hormone[56] rather than the cruder preparations which contain a significant proportion of aggregated hormone. Antibodies may develop in up to 50% of children treated with human GH.[57] However, children may respond to the monomeric GH preparation when they have become unresponsive to the more allergenic preparations.[58]

Physical-Chemical and Other Data

Human GH is a protein consisting of 191 amino acid residues, monomer mol wt 21,700 (Table 7). It has a propensity to aggregate to species of much higher molecular weight,

Table 7
LINEAR AMINO ACID SEQUENCE OF HUMAN GH

```
         1                    5                   10                   15
NH₂-Phe-Pro-Thr-Ile-Pro-Leu-Ser-Arg-Leu-Phe-Asp-Asn-Ala-Met-Leu-Arg-Ala-His-
     20                   25                   30                   35
Arg-Leu-His-Gln-Leu-Ala-Phe-Asp-Thr-Tyr-Gln-Glu-Phe-Glu-Glu-Ala-Tyr-Ile-Pro-
     40                   45                   50                   55
Lys-Glu-Gln-Lys-Tyr-Ser-Phe-Leu-Gln-Asn-Pro-Gln-Thr-Ser-Leu-Cys-Phe-Ser-Glu-
     60                   65                   70                   75
Ser-Ile-Pro-Thr-Pro-Ser-Asn-Arg-Glu-Glu-Thr-Gln-Gln-Lys-Ser-Asn-Leu-Gln-Leu-
     80                   85                   90
Leu-Arg-Ile-Ser-Leu-Leu-Leu-Ile-Gln-Ser-Trp-Leu-Glu-Pro-Val-Gln-Phe-Leu-Arg-
     95                  100                  105                  110
Ser-Val-Phe-Ala-Asn-Ser-Leu-Val-Tyr-Gly-Ala-Ser-Asn-Ser-Asp-Val-Tyr-Asp-Leu-
    115                  120                  125                  130
Leu-Lys-Asp-Leu-Glu-Glu-Gly-Ile-Glu-Thr-Leu-Met-Gly-Arg-Leu-Glu-Asp-Gly-Ser-
    135                  140                  145                  150
Pro-Arg-Thr-Gly-Gln-Ile-Phe-Lys-Gln-Thr-Tyr-Ser-Lys-Phe-Asp-Thr-Asn-Ser-His-
    155                  160                  165
Asn-Asp-Asp-Ala-Leu-Leu-Lys-Asn-Tyr-Gly-Leu-Leu-Tyr-Cys-Phe-Arg-Lys-Asp-Met-
    170                  175                  180                  185
Asp-Met-Asp-Lys-Val-Glu-Thr-Phe-Leu-Arg-Ile-Val-Gln-Cys-Arg-Ser-Val-Glu-Gly-
    190
Ser-Cys-Gly-Phe-COOH
```

often irreversibly. GH is devoid of covalently linked carbohydrate and contains two disulfide bonds which link positions 53 to 165 and 182 to 189. Like all known species of growth hormone, the human hormone contains a single tryptophan and a C-terminal phenylalanine. The N-terminus is also Phe, and the entire sequence is shown in Table 7. Its pI of 4.9 is lower than GH from other species, prolactins, or placental lactogens.

Common names and abbreviations — Growth hormone, somatotropin, STH, GH.

FOLLITROPIN

Mechanism of Action
Testis

FSH stimulates spermatogenesis and growth of the seminiferous tubules in testis of immature males. This action is mediated by a specific receptor for FSH which is present on the Sertoli cell. When FSH binds to its receptor, adenylate cyclase activity is stimulated[59] and cAMP levels increase. The activation of adenylate cyclase appears to involve the receptor mediated coupling of a guanyl nucleotide binding protein[60] with adenylate cyclase. The elevation of cAMP levels within Sertoli cells leads to the activation of an intracellular protein kinase which is in turn regulated by an FSH dependent protein kinase inhibitor.[61] Synthesis of the protein kinase inhibitor in addition to other Sertoli cell proteins is induced by FSH. Synthesis of Sertoli cell proteins may be influenced by the FSH induction of ornithine decarboxylase.[62] FSH also influences the secretion of androgen binding protein,[63] plasminogen activator,[64] inhibin,[65] and estrogen. The latter is synthesized from an androgen precursor supplied by the interstitial cells.[62,66] Regulation of FSH action appears to be related to an FSH induced loss of its own receptors,[67] synthesis of protein kinase inhibitor, and decline in phosphodiesterase activity. FSH affects Sertoli cell microfilament formation (actin and myosin) resulting in alteration of cell shape.[68] Such a microfilament assembly/disassembly cycle may be an essential part of spermatogonia movement towards the tubule lumen and spermatid expulsion.

Table 8
PRIMARY AMINO ACID SEQUENCE OF THE α-SUBUNIT OF HUMAN FOLLITROPIN

```
  1                                10
Ala-Pro-Asp-Val-Gln-Asp-Cys-Pro-Glu-Cys-Thr-Leu-Gln-Glu-Asn-Pro-Phe-Phe-
      20                               30
Ser-Gln-Pro-Gly-Ala-Pro-Ile-Leu-Gln-Cys-Met-Gly-Cys-Cys-Phe-Ser-Arg-Ala-
          40                               50            *
Tyr-Pro-Thr-Pro-Leu-Arg-Ser-Lys-Lys-Thr-Met-Leu-Val-Gln-Lys-Asn(CHO)-Val-
              60                               70
Thr-Ser-Glx-Ser-Thr-Cys-Cys-Val-Ala-Lys-Ser-Tyr-Asn-Arg-Val-Thr-Val-
                                  80
Met-Phe-Lys-Val-Glx-Asn(CHO)-His-Thr-Ala-Cys-His-Cys-Ser-Thr-Cys-Tyr-Tyr-
              90
His-Lys-Ser-COOH
```

Note: CHO* denotes the presence of an oligosaccharide moiety.

Ovary

The target cells for FSH in the female are the granulosa cells of the ovary. Ovaian follicles stimulated by FSH will grow and develop multiple layers of granulosa cells and form a follicular space called an antrum. Full development of the follicle also requires luteinizing hormone (LH).[69] FSH appears to act in rats by regulating the number of follicles destined to ovulate by rescuing small (200 to 400 μm) follicles from atresia.[70] Secretion of follicular fluid, the mitotic proliferation of granulosa cells, and the transformation of the surrounding stroma into a layer of theca cells are also actions regulated by FSH. Ovarian FSH receptors are localized on the granulosa cell membrane. The interaction (binding) of FSH with its ovarian receptor activates adenylate cyclase and elevates cAMP levels within the cells. Granulosa cell receptors for LH are increased by FSH[71] demonstrating further a synergistic role of FSH and LH in the ovary. The majority of estrogen produced appears to be derived from the granulosa cell and estrogen is a mitogen[72] for granulosa cell proliferation. Granulosa cell production of estrogen involves the stimulation of aromatase activity[73] induced by FSH and requires aromatizable androgen (Δ^4-androstenedione or testosterone) which is presumably produced by thecal cells.[74] FSH stimulates progesterone synthesis in granulosa cells, in vitro, but the presence of androgen is required.[75] Granulosa cell plasminogen activator is synthesized in response to FSH[76] and ornithine decarboxylase activity also appears to be induced by FSH.[77] FSH induces a rise in membrane microviscosity of granulosa cells[78] and the depletion of norepinephrine from Graafian follicles.[79] The latter effect of FSH may play a role in the formation and/or function of the corpus luteum.

Structure-Activity Relationships

FSH is composed of an α-subunit which is common to LH, thyroid stimulating hormone (TSH), and human chorionic gonadotropin (hCG), and a hormone-specific β-subunit. Neither subunit alone has significant in vitro or in vivo biological activity.[80] The amino acid sequence of the α-subunit of human[81] FSH has been determined (Table 8). The amino acid sequence of the β-subunit of human FSH has been proposed (Table 9).[82] The α-subunit has two points of N-glycosidic linked carbohydrate attachment on asparagine residues 56 and 82. The β-subunit has one at asparagine residue 7. Biological activity of FSH is markedly decreased after enzymic deglycosylation.[83] Periodate oxidation destroys carbohydrate moieties with a loss of biological activity in vivo. Sialic acid residues are not essential for retention of full biological activity in vivo or in vitro as shown after desialylation by careful oxidation and reduction[84] or by neuraminidase treatment.[85] Attempts to derivatize the tryptophan residue of intact FSH with 2-hydroxy-5-nitrobenzyl bromide (HNBB) were without effect on activity but caused a loss in activity when the β-subunit alone was treated prior to recombination

Table 9
LINEAR AMINO ACID SEQUENCE OF THE β-SUBUNIT OF HUMAN FOLLITROPIN

```
1                   7      *        10
Asn-Ser-Cys-Glu-Leu-Thr-Asn(CHO)-Ile-Thr-Ile-Ala-Ile-Glu-Lys-Glu-Glu-Cys-Arg-
   20                                      30
Phe-Cys-Leu-Thr-Ile-Asn(CHO)-Thr-Thr-Trp-Cys-Ala-Gly-Tyr-Cys-Tyr-Thr-Arg-Asp-
        40                                 50
Leu-Val-Tyr-Lys-Asn-Pro-Ala-Arg-Lys-Asx-Ile-Gln-Lys-Thr-Cys-Thr-Phe-Lys-Glu-
          60                                 70
Leu-Val-Tyr-Glu-Thr-Val-Arg-Val-Pro-Gly-Cys-Ala-His-His-Ala-Asp-Ser-Leu-Tyr-
          80                                 90
Thr-Tyr-Pro-Val-Ala-Thr-Gln-Cys-His-Cys-Gly-Lys-Cys-Asp-Ser-Asp-Ser-Thr-Asp-
          100                                  110
Cys-Thr-Val-Arg-Gly-Leu-Gly-Pro-Ser-Tyr-Cys-Ser-Phe-Gly-Glu-Met-Lys-Gln-Tyr-

Pro-Thr-Ala-Leu-Ser-Tyr
```

Note: CHO* denotes an oligosaccharide moiety.

with α-subunits.[86] This suggests that the tryptophan is in a region of subunit-subunit interaction and this proposal has been supported by circular dichroism studies of N-bromosuccinimide oxidized FSH.[87] The ε-amine groups of the α- and β-subunits are essential for biological activity.[88] There are five disulfide linkages in the α-subunit and six in the β-subunit, although their exact positions are not yet well established.[119]

Metabolism

The metabolism of FSH involves the usual pathways of blood clearance including the liver and urine. Gonadotropin present in the urine of postmenopausal women is biologically active. The halflife of FSH in the human is characterized by a rapid initial (α) phase of disappearance followed by a more prolonged secondary (β) phase. Estimates of the α-phase $t\,^1/_2$ for FSH in humans vary from 30 min to 4 hr, and for the β-phase $t\,^1/_2$ has been estimated to vary from 50 to 70 hr.[90]

Uses and Dosage

Purified gonadotropin from the urine of postmenopausal women (Pergonal, Serono, Inc.) is used clinically and is commercially available. Pergonal contains equal unit doses of FSH and LH activity; however, chorionic gonadotropin must be administered to induce ovulation. The recommended initial dose is 75 IU i.m. daily for 9 to 12 days, followed by the 10,000 IU of chorionic gonadotropin on the last day. The FSH is used in conjuction with hCG to induce ovulation in women. Occasionally ovulation may occur before treatment with hCG. Some infertile men with hypopituitarism have been successfully treated with gonadotropins.

Toxicity

Complications include excessive ovarian enlargement and multiple births. Ovarian hyperstimulation after hCG may lead to pain in the abdomen and bleeding into the peritoneal cavity. No direct toxic effects are known but extreme caution in its use is warranted until more definitive studies have been completed.

Physical-Chemical and Other Data

An acidic glycoprotein, human FSH has a reported isoelectric point of 5.5 and an average mol wt estimate of 33,500. The sedimentation coefficient of FSH has been estimated to be approximately 2.8 $S_{20,w}$. These individual determinations have been summarized in Table 10. FSH is very soluble in water, physiological saline, or 50% alcohol.

Table 10
SOME PHYSICAL CHARACTERISTICS OF
PITUITARY FSH FROM VARIOUS SPECIES

Species	Mol wt	Sedimentation coefficient $s_{20,w}$ (Svedbergs)	Isoelectric point (pI)	Ref.
Human pituitary	25,000	4.63	5.6	91
	35,000	2.9	3.4—5.55	92
Ovine pituitary	32,095	3.5	4.4	93
Bovine pituitary	37,000	—		94
Equine pituitary	33,200	—	—	95

Common names and abbreviations — Follitropin, follicle stimulating hormone, FSH.

LUTROPIN/CHORIOGONADOTROPIN

Mechanism of Action

Testis

The target cell for LH in the testis is the Leydig cell. The biological properties of hCG appear to be identical with those of LH and the two glycoproteins are thought to bind to the same receptor sites in the testis. LH has two major effects on Leydig cells: (1) it acts to promote and maintain the differentiation of Leydig cells prior to puberty and (2) maintains a basal level of testosterone production. One bioassay for LH is based on the weight increase of the ventral prostate following LH administration.[96] This bioassay demonstrates an indirect effect of LH via testosterone. The mechanism of action of LH on Leydig cells begins with the binding of LH to its receptor. Leydig cells acquire LH receptor at approximately the same time that they develop smooth endoplasmic reticulum and the capacity to synthesize steroids. The binding of LH to its receptor activates adenylate cyclase and causes the formation of cAMP and the activation of protein kinase.[97] Leydig cells exhibit a rapid rise in oxygen uptake following addition of LH. The significance of this "respiratory burst" is not clear. The events which are sequal to LH binding undoubtedly play a role in enhancing steroidogenesis. It appears that *de novo* mRNA synthesis is not a prerequisite to LH enhanced testosterone biosynthesis.[98] Apparently LH also induces phosphorylation of several cytosolic proteins through a cAMP mechanism.[99] The consequences of this effect remain to be elucidated but are probably similar to those seen in the ovarian system (below).

Ovary

The target tissues for LH and hCG in the ovary include the granulosa cells of the developing (preovulatory) follicle and the highly differentiated luteal cells of the corpus luteum. The biochemical properties of LH and hCG action on these cells appear to be identical. The corpus luteum is formed subsequent to ovulation. Bioassays for LH using the female rat as a model have used hormone induced ovarian hyperemia and the depletion of ascorbic acid from the ovary.[100] The action of LH on the ovarian cells requires the presence of receptors for LH. These receptors have been localized on the thecal and interstitial cells of the rat ovary and on granulosa cells and on luteal cells. It should be noted that only granulosa cells in follicles which are preovulatory have LH receptors. This concept has been supported by

Table 11

LINEAR AMINO ACID SEQUENCE OF THE β-SUBUNIT OF HUMAN LH

```
                                  10
Ser-Arg-Glu-Pro-Leu-Arg-Pro-Trp-Cys-His-Pro-Ile-Asn-Ala-Ile-Leu-Ala-Val-
    20                                        30            *
Glu-Lys-Glu-Gly-Cys-Pro-Val-Cys-Ile-Thr-Val-Asn-(CHO)-Thr-Thr-Ile-Cys-Ala-
              40                                     50
Gly-Tyr-Cys-Pro-Thr-Met-Arg-Met-Leu-Leu-Glx-Ala-Val-Leu-Pro-Pro-Val-Pro-
                        60                                      70
Gln-Pro-Val-Cys-Thr-Thr-Arg-Asx-Val-Arg-Phe-Glx-Ser-Ile-Arg-Leu-Pro-Gly-
                                  80
Cys-Pro-Arg-Gly-Val-Asp-Pro-Val-Val-Ser-Phe-Pro-Val-Ala-Leu-Ser-Cys-Arg-
    90                                        100
Cys-Gly-Pro-Cys-Arg-Arg-Ser-Thr-Ser-Asp-Cys-Gly-Gly-Pro-Lys-Asx-His-Pro-
          110
Leu-Thr-Cys-Asx-Glx-Asx-Ser-Lys-Gly-COOH
```

Note: CHO* denotes an oligosaccharide moiety.

the observation of development-dependent responsiveness of granulosa cells to LH.[101] The appearance of LH receptors on granulosa cells is most likely related to cell differentiation. The luteinization process of granulosa cells is accelerated by LH as is the sequence of events that leads to ovulation. A mechanism for LH induced ovulation has been suggested which involves the production of plasminogen activator by granulosa cells presumably resulting in follicle rupture due to tissue breakdown.[102] Cellular levels of cAMP are elevated following LH stimulation as a consequence of adenylate cyclase activation in both granulosa and luteal cells. Granulosa cells from small to medium sized follicles respond to FSH but not LH, and cAMP levels in cells from preovulatory follicles are elevated by either LH or FSH treatment.[103] This is in keeping with the concept of "development dependent" responsiveness of granulosa cells to LH. cAMP has been implicated in nearly all of the actions of LH including its effects on luteal cell progesterone synthesis. cAMP activates protein kinase and results in the phosphorylation of cytosolic proteins, events which lead to steroidogenesis in follicular and luteal cells.[104] Progesterone biosynthesis in the luteal cell is stimulated by LH while thecal cells respond to LH by the production of androgen which appears to be the substrate for FSH-induced estrogen production by granulosa cells.

Structure-Activity Relationships

Luteinizing hormone and hCG are composed of two protein subunits with branched carbohydrate side chains. Amino acid sequences for the β-subunit of each hormone have been proposed[105,106] (Tables 11 and 12). The sequence of the α-subunit is similar to that of FSH (Table 8). Some of the carbohydrate side chains terminate with sialic acid. Human chorionic gonadotropin contains 12%, and LH contains 1% sialic acid on a weight basis, whereas, hCG has 30% and LH has 16% total carbohydrate on a weight basis. Some sulfation of carbohydrate has been demonstrated for LH.[107] Sialic acid removal from hCG results in a loss of biological activity in vivo with only a slight change of activity in vitro.[108] The former effect is largely due to a decrease in the plasma halflife ($t \, ^1/_2$) of the desialylated hCG. Treatment of LH with neuraminidase does not markedly affect its activity.[109] There are 30 additional amino acid residues in the carboxyl terminal extension of the β-subunit of hCG relative to hLH. This segment is rich in proline and serine residues, the latter of which are attachment points for O-glysocidically linked carbohydrate.[110] Structures of the N-glycosidically linked carbohydrate in hCG have been proposed[110] as well as the N-glycosidically linked carbohydrate in LH.[111] Partial deglycosylation of LH results in a slight loss of LH receptor binding activity,[112] but prevents cAMP accumulation, steroidogenesis,[113] and ovulation.[114] Selective deglycosylation of α- and β-subunits of LH suggests that the α-subunit

Table 12
LINEAR AMINO ACID SEQUENCE OF THE β-SUBUNIT OF HUMAN CHORIONIC GONADOTROPIN

```
                              10                        *
Ser-Lys-Glu-Pro-Leu-Arg-Pro-Arg-Cys-Arg-Pro-Ile-Asn(CHO)-Ala-Thr-Leu-
              20                              30
Ala-Val-Glu-Lys-Glu-Gly-Cys-Pro-Val-Cys-Ile-Thr-Val-Asn(CHO)-Thr-Thr-
                      40
Ile-Cys-Ala-Gly-Tyr-Cys-Pro-Thr-Met-Thr-Arg-Val-Leu-Gln-Gly-Val-Leu-
      50                              60
Pro-Ala-Leu-Pro-Gln-Val-Val-Cys-Asn-Tyr-Arg-Asp-Val-Arg-Phe-Glu-Ser-
              70                              80
Ile-Arg-Leu-Pro-Gly-Cys-Pro-Arg-Gly-Val-Asn-Pro-Val-Val-Ser-Tyr-Ala-
                      90                              100
Val-Ala-Leu-Ser-Cys-Gln-Cys-Ala-Leu-Cys-Arg-Arg-Ser-Thr-Thr-Asp-Cys-
                              110
Gly-Gly-Pro-Lys-Asp-His-Pro-Leu-Thr-Cys-Asp-Asp-Pro-Arg-Phe-Gln-Asp-
      120                                      130
Ser-Ser-Ser-Ser(CHO)-Lys-Ala-Pro-Pro-Pro-Ser(CHO)-Leu-Pro-Ser-Pro-Ser
                              140
(CHO)-Arg-Leu-Pro-Gly-Pro-Ser(CHO)-Asp-Thr-Pro-Ile-Pro-Gln-CONH₂
```

Note: CHO* denotes an oligosaccharide moiety.

carbohydrate may be essential for biological activity.[115] Similar results have been reported with hCG. Chemical modification of the amino groups of lysine residues of LH causes a loss of biological activity.[116] Disulfide bond assignment in α-[117] and β-[118] subunits of LH and hCG have been difficult due to disulfide bond interchange during the process of cleavage. With this in mind, it has been suggested that one should regard current assignments of disulfide bonds in these hormones with some caution.[119] Finally, it should be recognized that hCG has some FSH-like activity. This activity is not due to contamination with FSH but is a consequence of the structural homology between the two molecules.[120]

Metabolism

The metabolism of human LH has been studied in humans. A biphasic halflife is evident. The initial (α) phase of LH disappearance from the circulation has been approximated to range from 20 to 80 min.[121] The secondary (β) phase of disappearance has been estimated to range from 2 to 4 hr. In contrast, hCG has a much longer halflife than hLH with an α-phase of 8.9 hr and a β-phase of clearance of 37.2 hr. This difference is considered a consequence of the relative sialic acid content of the two hormones. The presence of sialic acid reduces the rate of hepatic uptake and metabolism of sialoproteins in general, thus prolonging their plasma survival time.

Uses and Dosage

Chorionic gonadotropin purified from urine of pregnant women is available for clinical use as the commercial preparations Glukor (Hyre Pharmaceuticals), Follutein (Squibb), and A.P.L. (Ayerst). Its uses include the treatment of cryptorchism not associated with anatomic obstruction and the treatment of male hypogonadism secondary to pituitary failure. Human chorionic gonadotropin is used to induce ovulation in anovulatory infertile women whose anovulation is not due to ovarian failure. Administration is usually by intramuscular injection. The dosage regime is variable and depends upon such factors such as age, weight, and physician's experience. Due to its very short halflife and limited availability, LH has been used primarily for selected research projects rather than routine clinical applications.

Toxicity

Complications are possible such as ovarian enlargement and ascites with or without pain

Table 13
SOME PHYSICAL PROPERTIES OF LH AND
hCG

Species	Sedimentation coefficient $s_{20,w}$ (Svedbergs)	Isoelectric point (pI)	Mol wt	Ref.
Human LH	—	6.2—6.95	—	122
hCG	—	2.89	48,000	123
Ovine LH	2.3—2.68	7.3	30,000	124
Bovine LH	2.63	—	33,000	124
Porcine LH	2.46	—	30,000	124

and/or pleural effusion. Rupture of ovarian cysts with bleeding into the peritoneum may occur. Other complications include multiple births, thromboembolism, and precocious puberty and water retention. Caution is advised in use of hCG or LH for clinical problems.

Physical-Chemical and Other Data

Highly purified human LH is a white powder which is soluble in water. Chymotrypsin destroys the gonadotropin action of LH but not FSH. LH has an approximate mol wt of 30,000 and an isoelectric point of approximately 7.4. Human chorionic gonadotropin is precipitated as long thin needles in 60% alcohol. It is soluble in water, glycerol, and glycols; insoluble in anhydrous organic solvents; and it is precipitated by acetone or molybdic and phosphotungstic acids. It has an approximate mol wt of 46,000 and an isoelectric point of 2.9. Table 13 summarizes some of the known physical properties of hLH and hCG.

Common names and abbreviations — Lutropin, luteinizing hormone, interstitial cell stimulating hormone, LH, ICSH/human chorionic gonadotropin, choriogonadotropin, hCG, and CG.

THYROTROPIN

Mechanism of Action

Thyrotropin (TSH) increases colloid formation by the secretory epithelium of the thyroid gland and increases its iodine uptake. TSH controls the rate of formation and release of thyroid hormones and also stimulates the conversion of glycerophosphate to phosphatidic acid in thyroid tissue.[125] TSH secretion is regulated by thyroid hormone (negative feedback), and in the absence of thyroid hormone pituitary tumors may form. Biological assay of TSH utilizes as endpoints physiological responses to the hormone such as iodine depletion of stored iodine[126] and phosphorous uptake.[127]

Binding of TSH to its receptor represents the initial stage of its mechanism of action.[128] The next stage involves the activation of adenylate cyclase and the accumulation of cAMP.[129] Ornithine decarboxylase activity as well as protein kinase activity of thyroid cells is also increased by TSH.[130]

Structure-Activity Relationships

The amino acid sequence of human TSH has been proposed.[122] The carbohydrate content of TSH is about 16%. Acid labile sulfate appears as a component of the α-subunit of TSH. Significant amounts of sialic acid are not found in TSH. The COOH terminal dipeptide of TSH is implicated as a possible receptor recognition site.[131] The α- and β-subunits of TSH can be crosslinked with retention of up to 100% of original activity suggesting that the subunits do not have to dissociate to elicit a biological effect.[132] TSH is inactivated by

Table 14

LINEAR AMINO ACID SEQUENCE OF THE β-SUBUNIT OF HUMAN TSH

```
                          10
Phe-Cys-Ile-Pro-Thr-Glx-Tyr-Met-Thr-His-Val-Glu-Arg-Arg-Glx-Cys-Ala-Tyr-
      20                    *                       30
Cys-Leu-Thr-Ile-Asn(CHO)-Thr-Thr-Ile-Cys-Ala-Gly-Tyr-Cys-Met-Thr-Arg-Asx-
              40                                  50
Ile-Asx-Gly-Lys-Leu-Phe-Leu-Pro-Lys-Tyr-Ala-Leu-Ser-Gln-Asx-Val-Cys-Thr-
                          60                                  70
Tyr-Arg-Asp-Phe-Ile-Tyr-Arg-Thr-Val-Glx-Ile-Pro-Gly-Cys-Pro-Leu-His-Val-
                              80
Ala-Pro-Tyr-Phe-Ser-Tyr-Pro-Val-Ala-Leu-Ser-Cys-Lys-Cys-Gly-Lys-Cys-Asx-
      90                              100
Thr-Asx-Tyr-Ser-Asp-Cys-Ile-His-Glu-Ala-Ile-Lys-Thr-Asx-Tyr-Cys-Thr-Lys-
              110
Pro-Glx-Lys-Ser-Tyr-COOH
```

Note: CHO* denotes an oligosaccharide moiety.

oxidizing agents such as potassium permanganate and elemental iodine. The primary structure of the β-subunit of human TSH is given in Table 14. The primary structure of the α-subunit is similar to that of human FSH (Table 8).

Metabolism

The halflife of TSH in normal humans has been reported to be 54 min, 35 min in euthyroid, 27 min in hyperthyroid, and 98 min in hypothyroid patients.[133]

Uses and Dosage

TSH is commercially available as Thytropar (Armour) which is a partially purified bovine anterior pituitary TSH. It is not used as a therapeutic agent but rather, (1) to diagnose thyroid disorders such as subclinical hypothyroidism or low thyroid reserve, (2) to differentiate between hypopituitarism and primary myxedema, (3) to assess thyroid status while receiving thyroid medication, and (4) to differentiate primary and secondary hypothyroidism. Dosage is usually 10 IU in 2 mℓ of saline (i.m. or s.c.). In view of the many effects related to its stimulation of thyroid hormone release, caution should be exercised when TSH is utilized for human studies or therapy.

Toxicity

Prolonged usage of TSH may cause generation of antibodies to TSH rendering treatment ineffective.[134] Menstrual irregularities, nausea, vomiting, urticaria, transitory hypotension, tachycardia, atrial fibrillation, fever, headache, thyroid swelling, and postinjection flare have been reported. Adrenal cortical suppression may occur.

Physical-Chemical and Other Data

TSH is a glycoprotein possessing two nonidentical subunits whose mol wt is estimated to be 26,000 to 30,000. The estimated sedimentation coefficient is 2.6S. It is soluble throughout a wide range of pHs and dissolves readily in saline. The β-subunit has one glycoprotein moiety. Sialic acid has been found only in human TSH. A summary of some known physical properties of TSH is presented in Table 15.

Common names and abbreviations — Thyrotropin, thyroid stimulating hormone, and TSH.

PREGNANT MARE SERUM GONADOTROPIN

Mechanism of Action

Pregnant Mare Serum Gonadotropin (PMSG) is present in the serum of horses between

Table 15
SOME PHYSICAL
PROPERTIES OF
THYROTROPIN

Sedimentation coefficient $S_{w,20}$ (Svedbergs)	Mol wt	Ref.
2.5—2.9	—	135
2.82	26,000—31,000	136
2.4—3.0	33,000	137

days 40 and 130 of pregnancy. Specialized trophoblast cells of the embryo invade the maternal endometrium by day 36 of gestation, and develop into small uterine growths known as endometrial cups. This hormone (PMSG) secreted by the endometrial cups possesses both LH and FSH activities in other species. Evidence of this is provided by bioassay for PMSG which uses rat ovarian weight gain as an endpoint.[138] In the rat, PMSG induces uterine as well as follicular growth, interstitial tissue stimulation, and some luteinization, and in addition to maintaining the corpora lutea of pregnancy, PMSG stimulates the formation of secondary corpora lutea. PMSG competes with FSH and LH for their receptors in gonadal tissue, thus the initial event of PMSG action in the gonads involves a receptor binding step.[139,140] As with the other glycoprotein hormones, this binding interaction leads to the activation of adenylate cyclase, elevation of cAMP levels,[141] and stimulation of enzyme pathways leading to the synthesis and the secretion of the steroid hormones.[142]

Structure-Activity Relationships

As with the other glycoprotein hormones discussed above, PMSG possesses two subunits which by themselves have little activity. The high carbohydrate content (45%) of PMSG is critical to its in vivo biological activity. Different glycosylated forms of PMSG exist in mare serum.[146] Desialylation of PMSG diminishes its potency in vivo.[144] Iodination of the α-subunit of PMSG prior to combination with its β-subunit results in a loss of FSH activity when tested in the rat.[139] The fact that PMSG does not stimulate follicular growth in the mare indicates that it has only an LH-like function in the mare similar to the LH-like function of hCG in the human.

If the α-subunit of PMSG is recombined with the β-subunit of ovine FSH, the potency of hybrid FSH is greater than native ovine FSH. However, the β-subunit of PMSG does not recombine readily with either ovine LH α or hCG α-subunits. Modification of the histidine residues of PMSG resulted in a loss of biological but not immunological activity.[143]

Metabolism

The halflife of PMSG in the horse is about 6 days and in the sheep it is 21 hr.[145] The long halflife is attributed to its high sialic acid and carbohydrate content. Relatively little PMSG is found in the urine of pregnant mares.

Uses and Dosage

Gonadotropin from pregnant mares' serum has not been routinely used clinically, and reliable information on dosage regimes or information of toxicity is not available.

Toxicity
Physical-Chemical and Other Data

The amino acid sequence of the α- and β-subunits of PMSG has not been proposed. The carbohydrate content of PMSG may vary, but is approximately 45% with about 10% sialic acid.[146] The mol wt of PMSG is about 64,000.[147] Estimates of sedimentation coefficients range from 2.5S to 3.5S.[148] The isoelectric point of equine chorionic gonadotropin (eCG) is low (pI = 1.8) presumably due to the high sialic acid content of the carbohydrate.[148] It is soluble in water, alcohol, glycerol, and glycol and is stable in neutral or alkaline solutions.

Common names and abbreviations — Pregnant mare serum gonadotropin, equine chorionic gonadotropin, PMSG, and eCG.

ADRENOCORTICOTROPIN AND PRO-OPIOMELANOCORTIN (POMC) PEPTIDES

Mechanism of Action

As with other protein and peptide hormones, peptides of this group of related hormones produce their biological effects by binding to specific receptors present on the plasma membranes of target tissues. Detailed information on the mechanism of action is available for adrenocorticotropin (ACTH) and the opioid peptides (endorphins and enkephalins).

ACTH maintains the adrenal cortex of hypophysectomized mammals, causes depletion of cholesterol, lipids, and ascorbic acid in the adrenals, and stimulates the biosynthesis and release of adrenal cortical steroids (glucocorticoids, mineralcorticoids and androgens).[149-151] ACTH stimulates adrenal cortical function by binding to receptors for ACTH which results in activation of adenylate cyclase. Intracellular cAMP is thereby increased and functions as a hormonal second messenger leading to induction of adrenal steroidogenesis. ACTH at high concentrations also results in skin pigmentation (Addison's disease) and the release of fatty acids from adipose tissue.[149]

The opioid peptides are unusual in that the characterization of their receptors led to the prediction of the existence of previously unknown hormones.[152] Opioid peptide stimulation is as diverse as the biological actions of opiates.[152-155] These include the induction of analgesia, production of a physiological dependence, respiratory depression, decreased diastolic blood pressure and heart rate, release of prolactin and GH, constipation, decreased intestinal motility, and a wide range of behavioral effects. Additionally, β-endorphin has been shown to alter LH secretion[156] and may play a role in the physiological response to stress. The mechanism of these actions involves binding of opioid peptides to receptors which are widely distributed in the body, followed by the activation of adenylate cyclase, and increased cAMP production in target cells. Binding to receptors is sensitive to cations (especially Mg^{2+} and Na^+) and the activation of adenylate cyclase is modulated by guanyl nucleotides.[152]

β-Lipotropin stimulates fat mobilization in rabbit adipose tissue but is weakly active in the rat and inactive in the mouse. Intact β-lipotropin has no opiate-like activity even though the complete sequences of the endorphins and enkephalins are contained in this peptide. Little information is available on the mechanism of action of this hormone.

Melanocyte-stimulating hormone (MSH) stimulates pigmentation in the skin by causing movement and redistribution of melanin granules in the melanocyte.[149] Sensitive bioassays for MSH have been developed using reptilian and fish tissue.[149] The physiological significance of MSH has been reviewed.[157] The mechanism of action involves binding to specific receptors for MSH located on the plasma membrane followed by functional alterations in the cytoskeleton of the cell, an action which presumably involves fluctuations in intracellular calcium levels.

Structure-Activity Relationships

ACTH and MSH were the first of these hormones to be isolated, purified, and sequenced. Procedures for synthesizing ACTH and MSH rapidly followed. The details of the discovery, isolation, purification, and synthesis of ACTH and MSH have been reviewed in detail.[149]

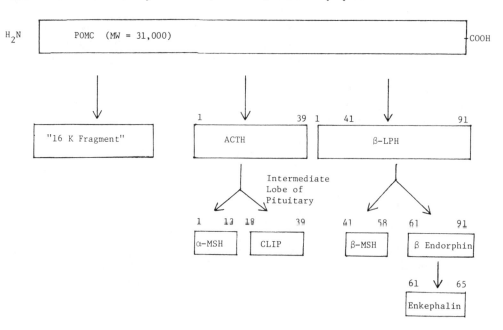

FIGURE 2.   Derivation of POMC peptide hormones.

More recently, β-LPH was isolated, purified, and sequenced.[158] Subsequently, it was observed that these hormones as well as the opioid peptides were structurally related and it is now clear that they are all products of the same precursor protein, POMC.[158-160] The generation of these peptide hormones from post-translational processing of POMC is shown in Figure 2. The actual hormones produced depend on the location of the secretory cells. For example, ACTH is secreted from anterior pituitary cells but it is further degraded to α-MSH and corticotropin-like intermediate lobe peptides (CLIP) in intermediate lobe pituitary cells. In addition to the peptides shown in Figure 2, γ-endorphin (61-77), α-endorphin (61-76), γ-MSH (12 amino acid peptides from the 16 K fragment), and γ-LPH (1-58) have been isolated from pituitary glands. The amino acid sequence is known for each of these hormones and synthetic analogs are available. Thus, a great deal of information concerning structure-function relationships have been accumulated and reviewed in detail.[149,155,161-164]

The structures of the major products of POMC processing are shown in Figure 3. Interestingly, β-MSH from various species shows considerable variability (Figure 3) while the structure of α-MSH is conserved. Ovine, porcine, and bovine ACTH each differ from human ACTH at positions 25, 31, and 33. However, the 1-24 amino acid fragment of ACTH retains full biological activity. α-MSH, β-MSH, and ACTH all contain a common sequence (His-Phe-Arg-Tyr) which is required for biological activity. Additionally, there is a great deal of homology in amino acids 1 to 13 among these three hormones. This is the basis for the ability of ACTH to increase skin pigmentation at high doses. The potency and duration of action of synthetic ACTH preparations can be increased by various amino acid substitutions, however, no clinical advantages have been reported.[151] The analgesic and behavioral modifying properties of the endorphins and enkaphalins and the identification of POMC peptides in the CNS suggest that these hormones may become clinically significant in the near future.

Metabolism

ACTH is not active when given orally since it is rapidly destroyed by gastrointestinal proteases. Its plasma halflife is about 15 min.[151] ACTH appears to be degraded in the tissues since no biologically active material can be detected in the urine;[151] however, the degradation

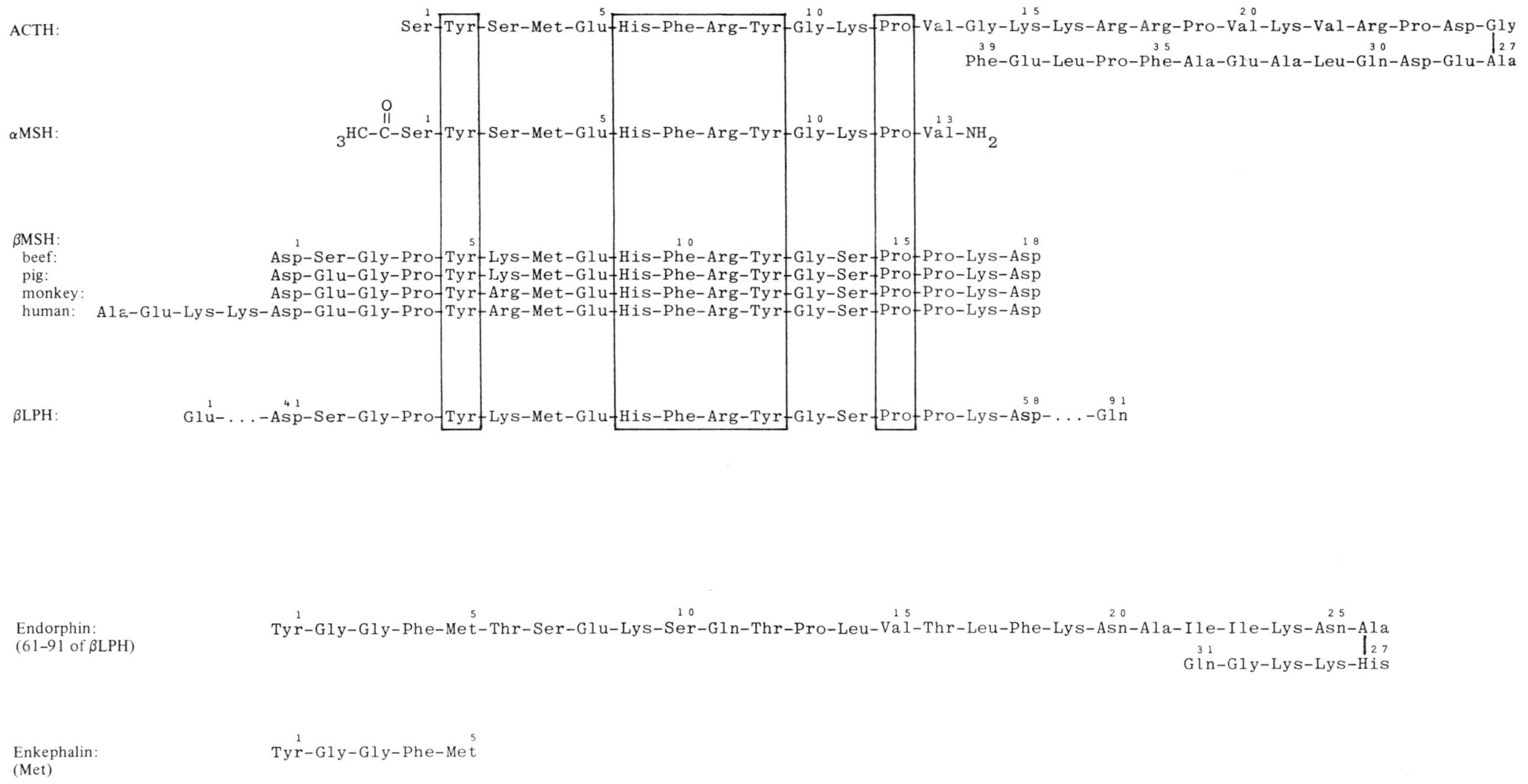

ACTH:

    Ser-Tyr-Ser-Met-Glu-His-Phe-Arg-Tyr-Gly-Lys-Pro-Val-Gly-Lys-Lys-Arg-Arg-Pro-Val-Lys-Val-Arg-Pro-Asp-Gly
    Phe-Glu-Leu-Pro-Phe-Ala-Glu-Ala-Leu-Gln-Asp-Glu-Ala

αMSH:

    O
    ‖
    $_3$HC-C-Ser-Tyr-Ser-Met-Glu-His-Phe-Arg-Tyr-Gly-Lys-Pro-Val-NH$_2$

βMSH:

    beef: Asp-Ser-Gly-Pro-Tyr-Lys-Met-Glu-His-Phe-Arg-Tyr-Gly-Ser-Pro-Pro-Lys-Asp
    pig: Asp-Glu-Gly-Pro-Tyr-Lys-Met-Glu-His-Phe-Arg-Tyr-Gly-Ser-Pro-Pro-Lys-Asp
    monkey: Asp-Glu-Gly-Pro-Tyr-Arg-Met-Glu-His-Phe-Arg-Tyr-Gly-Ser-Pro-Pro-Lys-Asp
    human: Ala-Glu-Lys-Lys-Asp-Glu-Gly-Pro-Tyr-Arg-Met-Glu-His-Phe-Arg-Tyr-Gly-Ser-Pro-Pro-Lys-Asp

βLPH:

    Glu-...-Asp-Ser-Gly-Pro-Tyr-Lys-Met-Glu-His-Phe-Arg-Tyr-Gly-Ser-Pro-Pro-Lys-Asp-...-Gln

Endorphin:
(61—91 of βLPH)

    Tyr-Gly-Gly-Phe-Met-Thr-Ser-Glu-Lys-Ser-Gln-Thr-Pro-Leu-Val-Thr-Leu-Phe-Lys-Asn-Ala-Ile-Ile-Lys-Asn-Ala
    Gln-Gly-Lys-Lys-His

Enkephalin:
(Met)

    Tyr-Gly-Gly-Phe-Met

FIGURE 3.   Primary structures of the major POMC-derived peptides.

and excretion of ACTH require further study. Endogenous ACTH is secreted in a pulsatile fashion with fastigia occurring at about 3 hr intervals. The amplitude of the secretory peaks shows a circadian rhythm reaching a maximum shortly before walking and a nadir shortly before the onset of sleep.[165]

Uses and Dosages

ACTH is used primarily for diagnostic testing of adrenal function.[151,166] Diagnostically, 10 to 25 IU of ACTH in 500 mℓ of 5% glucose are administered intravenously over an 8-hr period.[151,166] Therapeutically, ACTH is used for the control of chronic inflammatory disease, due to its stimulation of glucocorticoids, and treatment of adrenocortical insufficiency. When used chronically, ACTH has been administered intramuscularly in doses below 40 IU per day and requires gradual dose reduction when treatment is terminated. Dosages are individualized after establishing adrenal responsiveness. ACTH given as a single dose in the morning has the advantage of producing intermittent inhibition of endogenous ACTH in contrast to the continuous suppression of the hypothalamopituitary axis due to glucocorticoid therapy. Additionally, treatment with ACTH causes increased levels of glucocorticoids, mineralcorticoids, and androgens; this differs significantly from the treatment of many of these clinical conditions with corticoids.[151]

Toxicity

The toxic effects of ACTH result from the stimulation of adrenal steroids or from hypersensitivity reactions.[151] ACTH therapy is contraindicated in patients with osteoporosis, scleroderma, systemic fungal infections, ocular herpes simplex, recent surgery, a history of or presence of peptic ulcer, congestive heart failure, hypertension, or sensitivity to proteins of porcine origin. Prolonged treatment with ACTH has been associated with subcapsular cataracts and glaucoma, decreased resistance to infection, and an inability to localize infection. Although the incidence is rare, some individuals are capable of producing antibodies to synthetic ACTH and allergic reactions and anaphylaxis have been reported.[167] Following the abrupt termination of ACTH therapy, relative adrenocortical insufficiency has been reported.[167]

Physical-Chemical and Other Data

Adenocorticotropic hormone is also referred to as adrenocorticotrophic hormone or corticotropin and is abbreviated as ACTH. It is marketed as, among others, Acethropan, Acortan, Acorto, Acthar, Acton, Actonar, Adrenomone, Alfatrofin, Cibacthen, Corstiline, Cortiphyson, Cortophin, Isactid, Reacthin, Solacthyl, and Tubex. Additionally, synthetic ACTH which contains only the first 24 amino acids of ACTH is available as tetracosactide (generic). α-ACTH is distinguished from the acid or pepsin degraded product, β-ACTH.

ACTH is available for intravenous or intramuscular injection and some preparations contain zinc hydroxide or gelatin to slow the rate of absorption. ACTH is a white powder which is freely soluble in water. Pure ACTH has a potency of 150 to 200 USP units per milligram.

POSTERIOR PITUITARY HORMONES

INTRODUCTION

Vasopressin and oxytocin are polypeptide hormones synthesized in the hypothalamus from a larger prohormone, then split by proteolytic cleavage. They remain bound (noncovalently) to carrier proteins, called neurophysins, during transport down the nonmyelinated nerve fibers of the pituitary stalk to the posterior pituitary where they are stored in secretory

Table 16
THE STRUCTURE OF VASOPRESSIN AND OXYTOCIN

Vasopressin (Arg vasopressin: mol wt = 1085)

```
       ┌────── S ────── S ──────┐
       │                        │
 Cys-Tyr-Phe-Gln-Asn-Cys-Pro-Arg-Gly-NH₂

   1    2   3   4   5   6   7   8   9
```

Oxytocin (mol wt = 1007)

```
       ┌────── S ────── S ──────┐
       │                        │
 Cys-Tyr-Ile-Gln-Asn-Cys-Pro-Leu-Gly-NH₂

   1    2   3   4   5   6   7   8   9
```

granules. Both hormones have been extracted and purified from posterior pituitary glands. Their structures have been described and methods of synthesis developed. Thus, there are many analogs of these hormones available and much of the structural basis of their biological actions have been elucidated. Recently, a peptide of mol wt 4000 has been isolated from the posterior pituitary. It has been suggested that this "hormone", coherin, stimulates coordinate contractions of the intestine, and is thought to be distinct from oxytocin and vasopressin. Consideration of coherin must await future developments.

VASOPRESSIN

Mechanism of Action

Receptors for vasopressin have been shown in arterial vessel walls, distal tubules of the renal medulla, and in the hypothalamus.[168] Vasopressin binding to receptor stimulates adenylate cyclase activity and cAMP production which in turn activates luminal membrane-bound protein kinase. These events ultimately result in the alteration of membrane permeability (antidiuretic effect) or arterial vessel diameter (pressor effect). The action of vasopressin (primarily an antidiuretic) is modulated by Ca^{2+}, Mg^{2+}, prostaglandins, and α-adrenergic blocking agents,[168,169] probably at the level of binding to receptor and adenylate cyclase activation.

Structure-Activity Relationships

The structure of arginine vasopressin (AVP), shown in Table 16, was described in 1953 and confirmed by synthesis in 1956. AVP has been isolated from human, beef, chicken, horse, and sheep pituitaries. A similar hormone (lysine vasopressin) having Lys^8 rather than Arg^8 has been isolated from pig pituitaries.[175] Vasopressin stimulates the uptake of water by the distal convoluted tubules and collecting ducts of the kidney resulting in the formation of more concentrated urine (antidiuresis). Vasopressin also has vasopressor activity resulting in hypertension, decreased cardiac output, decreased coronary blood flow, and decreased oxygen saturation in cardiac venous blood.[169] Phe^3 and Arg^8 are required for vasopressin activity, which is assayed by the rat pressor assay and the rat antidiuretic assay. Antidiuretic and pressor activities of vasopressin can be separated by selective substitution at various positions during synthesis. Substitutions at positions 1, 2, 4, and 8, especially with 1-

Table 17
USE OF VASOPRESSIN IN THE TREATMENT OF
DIABETES INSIPIDUS

Hormone	Dosage and route	Duration of effect (hr)
Aqueous vasopressin	5—10 IU s.c.	3—6
Vasopressin tannate (Pitressin) in oil	5 IU i.m.	24—72
Lypressin	10—20 IU intranasal	3—8
DDAVP	10—20 μg intranasal	12—24

desamino compounds, cause increased antidiuretic activity. Substitutions at position 4 which increase lipophilicity (e.g., Val^4) decrease pressor activity as well as increasing antidiuretic activity of the hormone. 1-Desamino (Val^4, D-Arg^8) vasopressin (DDAVP) is the most potent antidiuretic hormone available and has almost no pressor activity. Substitutions at positions 3 and 8 (e.g., Orn^8 and Ile^3) result in enhanced pressor activity of the hormone. Vasopressin (Phe^2, Ile^3, Orn^8), for example, has a pressor:antidiuretic ratio of 220. The pharmacology of synthetic analogs of vasopressin has been reviewed[168,171,172] and a catalog of more than 200 analogs is available.[173]

Vasopressin appears to potentiate adenocorticotropin (ACTH) release by corticotropin releasing factor (CRF).[174,175] It has been suggested that vasopressin is involved in overcoming corticoid feedback inhibition of ACTH secretion during certain stress states.[176]

Metabolism

The concentration[170] of vasopressin in plasma is 10^{-11} to 10^{-12} M. There is no evidence for significant binding of vasopressin to serum proteins.[168,169] Vasopressin is cleared from serum in a biphasic fashion (early phase $1/2 = 1$ to 2 min). Vasopressin is excreted in free form in the urine (6 to 30% of exogenous doses) and inactivated by the liver and kidneys. The ability of isolated organs to enzymatically degrade vasopressin indicates that the spleen, pancreas, small intestine, and CNS (hypothalamus and cortex) as well as liver and kidney, are capable of inactivating the hormone. The substitution of compounds into synthetic vasopressins can alter the duration of the effect of the hormone. DDAVP, for example, has a longer effective duration than AVP.[169]

Uses and Dosage

Clinically, vasopressin is used primarily as an antidiuretic in the treatment of diabetes insipidus.[169,177] Vasopressin is also used as a hemostatic (pressor activity), especially for gastrointestinal hemorrhage, since it effectively reduces portal blood flow. Synthetic analogs are drugs of choice due to the separation of antidiuretic and pressor activities in these compounds. Table 17 summarizes some common uses of vasopressin in the treatment of diabetes insipidus.

Toxicity

The primary effect of vasopressin in the human is due to its antidiuretic activity. Vasopressor effects are seen at pharmacological doses, e.g., doses used to produce hemostatic effects. Coronary, intestinal and peripheral ischemia, local gangrene, and bradycardia have been reported following treatment with high doses of vasopressin.[178] Pulmonary abnormalities, local irritation of the nasal mucosa, and induction of asthmatic attacks have been associated with the use of snuff powders containing vasopressin or analogs for the treatment of diabetes insipidus.[168] The use of nonsynthetic vasopressin has been associated with antibody formation to vasopressin (bovine and porcine), antibody formation to growth hormone (an impurity), and allergic reactions.[178] Prolonged administration of any form of vasopressin with antidiuretic activity will result in water intoxication unless water intake is carefully managed.

Physical-Chemical and Other Data

Vasopressin is water soluble. Pure ADH has a mol wt = 1085 (Arg-ADH) and an activity of 400 IU/mg.[178]

Vasopressin (IUPAC/IUB) is also referred to as antidiuretic hormone, adiuretin, and β-hypophamine or abbreviated as VP or ADH. It is marketed as, among others, Leiovomone, Pitressin, Tonephin, and Vasophysin.

Common names and abbreviations — Antidiuretic H and ADH.

OXYTOCIN

Mechanism of Action

Oxytocin receptors have been reported to be present in kidney, uterus, mammary gland, and hypothalamus. The hormonal action of oxytocin, like vasopressin, involves activation of adenylate cyclase and requires Ca^{2+} and Mg^{2+}. Prostaglandins appear to interact with oxytocin in effecting uterine contractibility.[168] Additionaly, uterotonic effects of oxytocin are enhanced by estrogens.[169]

Structure-Activity Relationships

The structure of oxytocin, shown in Table 16, was reported in 1953 and confirmed by synthesis in 1956. In contrast to vasopressin, oxytocins purified from beef and pig pituitaries have identical amino acid sequences. While differing from vasopressin by only two amino acids, oxytocin has very little antidiuretic activity. Oxytocin causes milk ejection and increased uterine contraction; actions which are used as the basis for the bioassay of oxytocin activity in the rat. Oxytocin is probably involved with the initiation of parturition although women with posterior pituitary failure or diabetes insipidus can deliver normally.[169]

The ring structure (amino acids 1-6) of oxytocin is important to its biological action. The ring structure of oxytocin (tocinamide) alone retains uterotonic activity. However, the disulfide bridge is not essential to biological activity of the molecule and can be replaced by carbon or selenium. Furthermore, removal of the N-terminal amino group enhances oxytocin activity. Thus, desamino-1-carbo-oxytocin and desamino-1-seleno-oxytocin are several times as potent as the natural hormone. Milk ejection activity of the hormone can be selectively enhanced by amino acid (e.g., Val, Asn) substitutions at position 4. Substitutions of amino acids at positions 1, 2, or 4 have enabled the production of partial agonists or inhibitors of oxytocin. Relationships between conformational changes of oxytocin and its biological action have been considered in detail.[179] The pharmacology of synthetic analogs of oxytocin has been reviewed[168,171,172] and a catalog of analogs is available.[171]

Metabolism

The metabolism of oxytocin is very similar to that of vasopressin.[168] Steady state clearance is more rapid and biological halflife is shorter for oxytocin during periods of lactation in rats. Additionally, the mammary gland contributes to the degradation of oxytocin but not vasopressin.

Uses and Dosage

Clinical conditions associated with altered concentrations of oxytocin have not been described. Oxytocin is used in the human as a regulator of uterine activity for assisting labor and augmenting abortion induction. In animals, oxytocin is also used to stimulate milk let-down. Synthetic analogs are preferred for therapeutic purposes since they are generally free of impurities and are available with increased and specific (milk ejection vs. uterotonic) potencies.

Toxicity

Natural oxytocin has antidiuretic activity (about 1% that of vasopressin) which can result in water intoxication in both mother and fetus when pharmacologic doses of oxytocin are administered in conjunction with electrolyte free fluids. Oxytocin increases the risk of uterine rupture.[178] Adverse effects following oxytocin administration for the induction of labor include cervical lacerations, depression of respiration, jaundice in the newborn,[180] and an increased risk of neonatal asphyxia following maternal toxemia.[178] Vomiting and placental retention have been reported following oxytocin and intra-amniotic urea administration for the induction of abortion.

Physical-Chemical and Other Data

Oxytocin is a water soluble material prepared by synthesis or isolated from posterior pituitary glands. Pure oxytocin has a mol wt = 1007 and an activity of 450 to 500 USP units per milligram. Oxytocin (IUPAC/IUB) is also referred to as ocytocin and α-hypophamine and is abbreviated as OT or OXT. It is marketed as, among others, Endopituitrina, Pitocin, Syntocinon, Nobitocin S, Orasthin, Oxystin, Partocon, Synpitan, Piton-S, and Uteracon.

REFERENCES

1. **Marshall, J. C., Shakespear, R. A., and Odell, W. D.,** Pituitary plasma membrane luteinizing hormone releasing hormone binding: evidence for the presence of specific binding sites in other tissues, *J. Endocrinol.*, 67, 38, 1975.
2. **Conn, P. M., Kilpatrick, D., and Kirshner, N.,** Ionoporetic Ca^{2+} mobilization in rat gonadotropes and bovine adrenomedullary cells, *Cell Calcium*, 1, 129, 1980.
3. **Conn, P. M., Rogers, D. C., and Sandhu, F. S.,** Alteration of the intracellular calcium level stimulates gonadotropin release from cultured rat anterior pituitary cells, *Endocrinology*, 105, 1122, 1979.
4. **Borgeat, P., Chavancy, G., Dupont, A., Labrie, F., Arimura, A., and Schally, A. V.,** Stimulation of adenosine 3′,5′-cyclic monophosphate accumulation in anterior pituitary gland *in vitro* by synthetic luteinizing hormone releasing hormone, *Proc. Natl. Acad. Sci. U.S.A.*, 69, 2677, 1972.
5. **Sen, K. K. and Menon, K. M. J.,** Dissociation of cyclic AMP accumulation from that of luteinizing hormone (LH) release in response to gonadotropin releasing hormone (GnRH) and cholera enterotoxin, *Biochem. Biophys. Res. Commun.*, 87, 221, 1979.
6. **Schally, A. V., Arimura, A., Baba, Y., Nair, R. M. G., Matsuo, H., Redding, T. W., Debeljuk, L., and White, W. F.,** Isolation and properties of the FSH and LH-releasing hormone, *Biochem. Biophys. Res. Commun.*, 43, 393, 1971.
7. **Redding, T. W., Kastin, A. J., Gonzalez-Barcena, D., Coy, D. H., Coy, E. J., Schalch, D. S., and Schally, A. V.,** The half-life, metabolism and excretion of tritated luteinizing hormone-releasing hormone (LH-RH) in man, *J. Clin. Endocrinol. Metab.*, 37, 626, 1973.
8. **Bergquist, C., Nillius, S. J., and Wide, L.,** Inhibition of ovulation in women by intranasal treatment with a luteinizing hormone-releasing hormone agonist, *Contraception*, 19, 497, 1979.
9. **Mortimer, C. H., Besser, G. M., and McNeilly, A. S.,** Gonadotropin releasing hormone therapy in the induction of puberty, potency, spermatogenesis and ovulation in patients with hypothalamic-pituitary-gonadal dysfunction, in *Hypothalamic Hormones*, Proceedings of the Serono Symposium, Motta, M., Crosignani, P. G., and Martini, L., Eds., Academic Press, New York, 1975, 325.
10. **Nillius, S. J., Fries, H., and Wide, L.,** Successful induction of follicular maturation and ovulation by prolonged treatment with LH-releasing hormone therapy in women with anorexia nervosa, *Am. J. Obstet. Gynecol.*, 122, 921, 1975.

11. **Hershman, J. M.,** Clinical application of thyrotropin-releasing hormone, *N. Engl. J. Med.,* 290, 886, 1974.

12. **Schally, A. V.,** Aspects of hypothalamic regulation of the pituitary gland: its implications for the control of reproductive processes, *Science,* 202, 18, 1978.

13. **Guillemin, R.,** Peptides in the brain: the new endocrinology of the neuron, *Science,* 202, 390, 1978.

14. **Griffiths, E. C., White, N., and Jeffcoate, S. L.,** Age-dependent in the inactivation of thyrotropin-releasing hormone by different areas of rat brain, *Neurosci. Lett.,* 13, 57, 1979.

15. **Jackson, I. M. D., Papapetrou, P. D., and Reichlin, S.,** Metabolic clearance of thyrotropin-releasing hormone in the rat in hyperthyroid states: comparison with serum degradation *in vitro, Endocrinology,* 104, 1292, 1979.

16. **Peterkofsky, A. and Battaini, A.,** The biological activities of the neuropeptide histidyl-proline diketo-piperazine, *Neuropeptides,* 1, 105, 1980.

17. **Bassiri, R. M. and Utiger, R. D.,** Metabolism and excretion of exogenous thyrotropin releasing hormone in humans, *J. Clin. Invest.,* 52, 1616, 1973.

18. **Redding, T. W. and Schally, A. V.,** A study on the mode of administration of thyrotropin releasing hormone (TRH) in mice, *Neuroendocrinology,* 6, 329, 1970.

19. **Gordon, J. H., Bollinger, J., and Reichlin, S.,** Plasma thyrotropin responses to thyrotropin-releasing hormone after injection into the third ventricle, systemic circulation, median eminence and anterior pituitary, *Endocrinology,* 91, 696, 1972.

20. **Jackson, I. M. D.,** Diagnostic tests for the evaluation of pituitary tumors, in *The Pituitary Adenoma,* Post, K. D., Jackson, I. M. D., and Reichlin, S., Eds., Plenum Press, New York, 1980, 219.

21. **Kleinberg, D. L., Noel, G. L., and Frantz, A. G.,** Galactorrhea: a study of 235 cases, including 48 with pituitary tumors, *N. Engl. J. Med.,* 296, 589, 1977.

22. **Krieger, D. T. and Condon, E. M.,** Cyproheptadine treatment of Nelson's syndrome: restoration of plasma ACTH circadian periodicity and reversal of response to TRF, *J. Clin. Endocrinol. Metab.,* 46, 349, 1978.

23. **Borgeat, P., Labrie, P., and Drouin, J.,** Inhibition of adenosine 3′,5′-cyclic monophosphate accumulation in anterior pituitary gland *in vitro* by growth hormone release inhibiting hormone, *Biochem. Biophys. Res. Commun.,* 56, 1052, 1974.

24. **Vale, W., Brazeau, P., and Grant, G.,** Premières observations sur le mode d'action de la somatostatin, un facteur hypothalamique qui inhibe la sécrétion de l'hormone de croissance, *C.R. Acad. Sci. Paris,* 275, 2913, 1972.

25. **Kaneko, T., Oka, H., and Munemura, M.,** Stimulation of guanosine 3′,5′-cyclic monophosphate accumulation in rat anterior pituitary gland in vitro by synthetic somatostatin, *Biochem. Biophys. Res. Commun.,* 61, 53, 1974.

26. **Brazeau, P., Vale, W., Burgus, N., Ling, M., Butcher, M., Rivier, J., and Guillemin, R.,** Hypothalamic polypeptide that inhibits the secretion of immunoreactive pituitary growth hormone, *Science,* 179, 77, 1973.

27. **Burgus, R., Ling, N., Butcher, M., and Guillemin, R.,** Primary structure of somatostatin, a hypothalamic peptide that inhibits the secretion of pituitary growth hormone, *Proc. Natl. Acad. Sci. U.S.A.,* 70, 684, 1973.

28. **Leblanc, H. and Yen, S.,** Comparison of cyclic and linear forms of somatostatin in the inhibition of growth hormone, insulin and glucagon secretion, *J. Clin. Endocrinol. Metab.,* 40, 906, 1975.

29. **Pimstone, B., Berelowitz, M., and Konheim, S.,** Somatostatin, *S. Afr. Med. J.,* 50, 1471, 1976.

30. **Gerich, J. E.,** Somatostatin modulation of glucagon secretion and its importance in human glucose homeostatis, *Metabolism,* 27, 1283, 1978.

31. **Gerich, J. E.,** Somatostatin and diabetes, *Am. J. Med.,* 70, 619, 1981.

32. **Buckingham, J. C. and Hodges, J. R.,** The use of corticotropin production by adenohypophysial tissue *in vitro* for the detection and estimation of potential corticotropin releasing factors, *J. Endocrinol.,* 72, 187, 1977.

33. **Labrie, F., Borgeat, P., Ferland, L., Lemay, A., Dupont, A., Lemaire, S., Peletier, G., Barden, N., Drouin, J., DeLean, A., Belanger, A., and Jolicoeur, P.,** Mechanism of action and modulation of activity of hypothalamic hypophysiotropic hormones, in *Hypothalamic Hormones,* Motta, M., Crosignani, P. G., and Martini, L., Eds., Academic Press, New York, 1979.

34. **Vale, W., Spiess, J., Rivier, C., and Rivier, J.,** Characterization of a 41-residue ovine hypothalamic peptide that stimulates secretion of corticotropin and β-endorphin, *Science,* 213, 394, 1981.

35. **Schally, A. V., Lipscomb, H. S., and Guillemin, R.,** Isolation and amino acid sequence of α_2-corticotropin-releasing factor (α_2-CRF) from hog pituitary glands, *Endocrinology,* 71, 164, 1962.

36. **Schally, A. V. and Guillemin, R.,** Isolation and chemical characterization of a β-CRF from posterior pituitary glands, *Proc. Soc. Exp. Biol. Med.,* 112, 1014, 1963.

37. **Riddle, O.,** Prolactin invertebrate function and organization, *J. Natl. Cancer Inst.,* 31, 1039, 1963.

38. **Nicoll, C. S. and Bern, H. A.,** Prolactin, in *Ciba Foundation Symposium on Lactogenic Hormones,* Wolstenholme, G. E. W. and Knight, J., Eds., Churchill Livingstone, London, 1972, 299.

39. **Frantz, A. G.,** Prolactin and its functions, in *Peptide Hormones,* Parsons, J. A., Ed., University Park Press, Baltimore, 199, 1975.
40. **McNeilly, A. S.,** Lactation and the physiology of prolactin secretion, *Postgrad. Med. J.,* 51, 231, 1975.
41. **Horrobin, D. F.,** *Prolactin 1975,* Eden Press, Montreal, 1975, chap. 4—10.
42. **Wong, T. M., Cheng, C. H. K., and Li, C. H.,** Radioimmunoreactivity and receptor-binding activity of the recombined molecule obtained by complementation of two fibrinolysin fragments of ovine prolactin, *Proc. Natl. Acad. Sci. U.S.A.,* 78, 88, 1981.
43. **Andersen, T. T., Zamierowski, M. M., and Ebner, K. E.,** Effect of nitration on prolactin activities, *Arch. Biochem. Biophys.,* 192, 112, 1979.
44. **Andersen, T. T. and Ebner, K. E.,** Reaction of histidines of prolactin with ethoxyformic anhydride, a binding site modification, *J. Biol. Chem.,* 254, 10995, 1979.
45. **Clemons, J. A. and Meites, J.,** Comparative mammalian studies of the control of prolactin secretion, in *Lactogenic Hormones, Fetal Nutrition, and Lactation,* Josinovich, J. B., Reynolds, M., and Cobo, E., Eds., John Wiley & Sons, New York, 1974, 111.
46. **Bewley, T. A. and Li, C. H.,** Studies of pituitary lactogenic hormone physicochemical characterization of porcine prolactin, *Arch. Biochem. Biophys.,* 167, 80, 1975.
47. **Wallis, M.,** The primary structure of bovine prolactin, *FEBS Lett.,* 44, 205, 1974.
48. **Kostyo, J. L.,** The search for the active core of pituitary growth hormone, *Metabolism,* 23, 885, 1974.
49. **Li, C. H., Hayadshida, T., Doneen, B. A., and Rao, A. J.,** Human somatotropin: biological characterization of the recombinant molecule, *Proc. Natl. Acad. Sci. U.S.A.,* 73, 3463, 1976.
50. **Graf, L. and Li, C. H.,** Isolation and properties of two biologically active fragments from limited tryptic hydrolysis of bovine and ovine pituitary growth hormone, *Biochemistry,* 13, 5408, 1974.
51. **Yamasaki, N., Shimanaka, J., and Sonenberg, M.,** Studies on the common active site of growth hormone; revision of the amino acid sequence of an active fragment of bovine growth hormone, *J. Biol. Chem.,* 250, 2510, 1975.
52. **Dillon, R. S.,** Hormones and disorders of the anterior pituitary and the hypothalamus, in *Handbook of Endocrinology,* 2nd ed., Lea and Febiger, Philadelphia, 1980, 213.
53. **Soyka, L. F., Bode, H. H., Crawford, J. D., and Flynn, F. J.,** Effectiveness of long-term human growth hormone therapy for short stature in children with growth hormone deficiency, *J. Clin. Endocrinol. Metab.,* 30, 1, 1970.
54. **Zuppinger, K., Joss, E., and Locher, A.,** Treatment of pituitary growth retardation, *Praxis,* 64, 1101, 1975.
55. **Guyda, H., Friesen, H., and Bailey, J. D.,** Medical Research Council of Canada therapeutic trial of human growth hormone, *Can. Med. Assoc. J.,* 112, 1301, 1975.
56. **Moore, W. V. and Jin, D.,** The role of aggregated hGH in therapy of hGH deficient children, *Endocrinology (Suppl.),* 100, 210, 1977.
57. **Uthne, K.,** Human somatomedins, purification and some studies on their biologic actions, *Acta Endocrinol. (Suppl.),* 73, 175, 1973.
58. **Underwood, L. E., Voina, S. J., and Van Wyk, J. J.,** Restoration of growth by human growth hormone (ROOS) in hypopituitary dwarfs immunized by other growth hormone preparations: clinical and immunologic studies, *J. Clin. Endocrinol. Metab.,* 38, 288, 1974.
59. **Jahnsen, T., Purvis, K., Birnbaumer, L., and Hansson, V.,** FSH and LH/hCG responsive adenyl cyclases in adult rat testes: methodology and assay conditions, *Int. J. Androl.,* 3, 396, 1980.
60. **Limbird, L. E.,** Activation and attenuation of adenylate cyclase, *Biochem. J.,* 195, 1, 1981.
61. **Tash, J. S., Welsh, M. J., and Means, A. R.,** Regulation of protein kinase inhibitor by follicle stimulating hormone in Sertoli cells *in vitro, Endocrinology,* 108, 427, 1981.
62. **Francis, G. L., Triche, T. J., Brown, T. J., Brown, H. C., and Bercu, B. B.,** *In vitro* gonadotropin stimulation of bovine Sertoli cell ornithine decarboxylase activity, *J. Androl.,* 2, 312, 1981.
63. **Louis, B. G. and Fritz, I. B.,** Follicle stimulating hormone and testosterone independently increase the production of androgen-binding protein by Sertoli cells in culture, *Endocrinology,* 104, 454, 1979.
64. **Lacroix, M., Smith, F. E., and Fritz, I. B.,** Secretion of plasminogen activator by Sertoli cell-enriched cultures, *Mol. Cell. Endocrinol.,* 9, 227, 1977.
65. **Steinberger, A. and Steinberger, E.,** Secretion of an FSH-inhibiting factor by cultured Sertoli cells, *Endocrinology,* 99, 918, 1976.
66. **Dorrington, J. H. and Armstrong, D. T.,** Effects of FSH on gonadal functions, *Rec. Progr. Hormone Res.,* 35, 301, 1979.
67. **O'Shaughnessy, P. J. and Brown, P. S.,** Reduction in FSH receptors in the rat testis by injection of homologous hormone, *Mol. Cell. Endocrinol.,* 12, 9, 1978.
68. **Davis, J. C., Himmelstein, A., Bordy, M., and Desjardins, C.,** Follicle stimulating hormone induced adenosine 3',5' monophosphate mediated movement of immature rat Sertoli cells in primary culture, *Endocrinology,* 105, 1419, 1979.

69. **Steelman, S. L. and Pohley, F. M.,** Assay of the follicle stimulating hormone based on the augmentation with human chorionic gonadotropin, *Endocrinology,* 53, 604, 1953.

70. **Hirshfield, A. N. and Midgley, A. R., Jr.,** The role of FSH in the selection of large ovarian follicles in the rat, *Biol. Reprod.,* 19, 606, 1978.

71. **May, J. V., McCarty, K., Jr., Reichert, L. E., Jr., and Schomberg, D. W.,** Follicle stimulating hormone-mediated induction of functional luteinizing hormone/human chorionic gonadotropin receptors during monolayer culture of porcine granulosa cells, *Endocrinology,* 107, 1041, 1980.

72. **Hillier, S. G., Reichert, L. E., Jr., and Van Hall, E. V.,** Control of preovulatory follicular estrogen biosynthesis in the human ovary, *J. Clin. Endocrinol. Metab.,* 52, 847, 1981.

73. **Gore-Langton, R. E. and Dorrington, J. H.,** FSH induction of aromatose in cultured rat granulosa cells measured by a radiometric assay, *Mol. Cell. Endocrinol.,* 22, 135, 1981.

74. **Tsang, B., Armstrong, D. T., and Whitefield, J. F.,** Steroid biosynthesis by isolated human ovarian follicular cells *in vitro, J. Clin. Endocrinol. Metab.,* 51, 1407, 1980.

75. **Nimrod, A.,** Studies on the synergistic effect of androgen on the stimulation of progestin secretion by FSH in cultured rat granulosa cells: progesterone metabolism and the effect of androgens, *Mol. Cell. Endocrinol.,* 8, 189, 1977.

76. **Beers, W. H. and Strickland, S.,** A cell culture assay for follicle stimulating hormone, *J. Biol. Chem.,* 253, 3877, 1978.

77. **Osterman, J. and Hammond, J. M.,** FSH and LH stimulation of ornithine decarboxylase activity: studies with porcine granulosa cells *in vitro, Endocrinology,* 101, 1335, 1977.

78. **Strulovici, B., Lindner, H. R., Shinitzky, M., and Zor, U.,** Elevation of apparent membrane viscosity in ovarian granulosa cells by follicle stimulating hormone, *Biochim. Biophys. Acta,* 640, 159, 1981.

79. **Ben-Jonathan, N., Bran, R. H., Reich, L. R., Bahr, J. M., and Tsafriri, A.,** Norepinephrine in Graafian follicles is depleted by follicle stimulating hormone, *Endocrinology,* 110, 457, 1982.

80. **Reichert, L. E., Jr., Trowbridge, C. G., Bhalla, V. K., and Lawson, G. M., Jr.,** The kinetics of formation and biological activity of native and hybrid molecules of human follicle stimulating hormone, *J. Biol. Chem.,* 249, 6472, 1974.

81. **Rathnam, P. and Saxena, B. B.,** Primary amino acid sequence of follicle stimulating hormone from human pituitary glands, *J. Biol. Chem.,* 205, 6735, 1975.

82. **Saxena, B. B. and Rathnam, P.,** Amino acid sequence of the β-subunit of follicle-stimulating hormone from pituitary glands, *J. Biol. Chem.,* 251, 993, 1976.

83. **Saxena, B. B.,** Gonadotropin receptors, in *Methods in Receptor Research,* Part I, Bleeker, M., Ed., Marcel Dekker, New York, 1976, 354.

84. **Reichert, L. E., Jr.,** Human FSH: purification properties and some structure function relationships, in *Gonadotropins,* Saxena, B. B., Belling, C. G., and Gandy, Eds., John Wiley & Sons, New York, 1972, 107.

85. **Finne, E.,** Inactivation of endogenous FSH by neuraminidase from *vibrio cholerae, Endokrinologia,* 72, 365, 1978.

86. **Rathnam, P. and Saxena, B. B.,** Studies on the modification of tryptophan, methionine, tyrosine and arginine residues of human follicle stimulating hormone and its subunits, *Biochim. Biophys. Acta,* 576, 81, 1979.

87. **Giudice, L. C., Pierce, J. G., Cheng, K. W., Whitley, R., and Ryan, R. J.,** Circular dichroism of mammalian follitripins and the effects of treatment with N-bromosuccinimide, *Biochem. Biophys. Res. Commun.,* 81, 725, 1978.

88. **Sairam, M. R.,** Studies on pituitary follitropin. III. Functional role of the amino groups in subunit and receptor interactions of the ovine hormone, *Arch. Biochem. Biophys.,* 194, 79, 1979.

89. **Fujiki, Y., Rathnam, P., and Saxena, B. B.,** Studies on the disulfide bonds in human pituitary follicle stimulating hormone, *Biochim. Biophys. Acta,* 624, 428, 1980.

90. **Kjeld, J. M., Harsoulis, P., Kuku, S. F., Marshall, J. C., Kaufman, B., and Fraser, T. R.,** Infusions of hFSH and hLH in normal men, *Acta Endocrinol.,* 81, 225, 1976.

91. **Papkoff, H., Mahlmann, L. J., and Li, C. H.,** Some chemical and physical properties of human pituitary follicle stimulating hormone, *Biochemistry,* 6, 3976, 1976.

92. **Reichert, L. E., Jr., Kathan, R. H., and Ryan, R. J.,** Studies on the composition and properties of immunochemical grade human pituitary follicle stimulatory hormone (FSH): comparison with luteinizing hormone (LH), *Endocrinology,* 82, 109, 168.

93. **Cahill, C. L., Shetlor, M. R., Payne, R. W., Endicott, B., and Li, Y. T.,** Isolation and characterization of ovine follicle stimulating hormone, *Biochim. Biophys. Acta,* 154, 40, 1968.

94. **Grimek, H. J., Gorski, J., and Wentworth, B. C.,** Purification and characterization of bovine follicle stimulating hormone: comparison with ovine follicle stimulating hormone, *Endocrinology,* 104, 145, 1979.

95. **Braselton, W. E., Jr. and McShan, W. H.,** Purification and properties of follicle stimulating and luteinizing hormones from horse pituitary glands, *Arch. Biochem. Biophys.,* 139, 45, 1970.

96. **Greep, R. O., Van Dyke, H. G., and Chow, B. F.,** Use of the anterior lobe of the prostate gland in the assay of metakentrin, *Proc. Soc. Exp. Biol. Med.,* 46, 644, 1941.

97. **Dufau, M. L., Tsuruhara, T., Horner, K. A., Podesta, E., and Catt, K. J.,** Intermediate role of adenosine 3′,5′-cyclic monophosphate and protein kinase during gonadotropin-induced steroidogenesis in testicular interstitial cells, *Proc. Natl. Acad. Sci. U.S.A.,* 74, 3419, 1977.

98. **Cooke, B. A., Janszen, F. H. A., and van Driel, M. J. A.,** Inhibition of Leydig cell steroidogenesis: effect of actinomycin D before and after preincubation of Leydig cells *in vitro, Int. J. Androl. (Suppl.),* 2, 240, 1978.

99. **Dufau, M. L., Sorrell, S. H., and Catt, K. J.,** Gonadotropin-induced phosphorylation endogenous proteins in the Leydig cell, *FEBS Lett.,* 131, 229, 1981.

100. **Parlow, A. F. and Reichert, L. E., Jr.,** Biological assay of luteinizing hormone (LH, ICSH) by the ovarian hyperemia method of Ellis: an evaluation, *Endocrinology,* 72, 955, 1963.

101. **Zeleznik, A. J., Keyes, P. L., Menon, K. M. J., Midgley, A. R., Jr., and Reichert, L. E., Jr.,** Development-dependent response of ovarian follicles to FSH and hCG, *Am. J. Physiol.,* 233, 229, 1977.

102. **Beers, W. H., Strickland, S., and Reich, E.,** Ovarian plasminogen activator: relationship to ovulation and hormonal regulation, *Cell,* 6, 387, 1975.

103. **Hamberger, L., Nordenstrom, K., Rosberg, S., and Sjorgen, A.,** Acute influence of LH and FSH on cAMP formation in isolated granulosa cells of rat, *Acta Endocrinol.,* 88, 567, 1978.

104. **Hunzicker-Dunn, M. and Jungmann, R. A.,** Rabbit ovarian protein kinases. II. Effect of an ovulatory dose of human chorionic gonadotropin or luteinizing hormone on the multiplicity of follicular and luteal protein kinases, *Endocrinology,* 103, 431, 1978.

105. **Papkoff, H., Sairam, M. R., and Li, C. H.,** Amino acid sequence of the subunits of ovine pituitary interstitial cell-stimulating hormone, *J. Am. Chem. Soc.,* 93, 1531, 1971.

106. **Morgan, F. J., Birken, S., and Canfield, R. E.,** Amino acid sequence of human chorionic gonadotropin, *J. Biol. Chem.,* 250, 5247, 1975.

107. **Hortin, G., Natowicz, M., Pierce, J., Baenziger, J., Parsons, T., and Boime, I.,** Metabolic labelling of lutropin with [^{35}S] sulfate, *Proc. Natl. Acad. Sci. U.S.A.,* 78, 7466, 1981.

108. **Brand, E. C., Odink, J., and Van Hall, E. V.,** Discrepancy between the effects of desialylation of human chorionic gonadotropin on *in vitro* ovarian biological activity and on receptor binding, *Acta Endocrinol.,* 95, 75, 1980.

109. **Papkoff, H. and Li, C. H.,** Studies on the chemistry of interstitial cell-stimulating hormone, in *Gonadotropins and Ovarian Development,* Butt, W. R., Crooke, A. C., and Rife, M., Eds., Churchill Livingston, Edinborough, 1970, 138.

110. **Kessler, M. J., Reddy, M. S., Shah, R. H., and Bahl, O. P.,** Structures of N-glycosidic carbohydrate units of human chorionic gonadotropin, *J. Biol. Chem.,* 254, 7901, 1979.

111. **Bahl, O. P., Reddy, M. S., and Bedi, G. S.,** A novel carbohydrate structure in bovine and ovine luteinizing hormones, *Biochem. Biophys. Res. Commun.,* 96, 1192, 1980.

112. **Sairam, M. R. and Schiller, P. W.,** Receptor binding, biological and immunological properties of chemically deglycosylated pituitary lutropin, *Arch. Biochem. Biophys.,* 197, 294, 1979.

113. **Sairam, M. R. and Fleshner, P.,** Inhibition of hormone induced cAMP production and steroidogenesis in interstitial cells by deglycosylated lutropin, *Mol. Cell. Endocrinol.,* 22, 41, 1981.

114. **Sairam, M. R.,** Inhibition of LH-induced ovulation in the rat by a hormonal antagonist, *Contraception,* 21, 651, 1980.

115. **Sairam, M. R.,** Deglycosylation of ovine pituitary lutropin subunits: effects on subunit interaction and hormone activity, *Arch. Biochem. Biophys.,* 204, 199, 1980.

116. **Tertrin-Clary, C., Roy, M., and De la Llosa, P.,** Nitroguanidyl-lutropin, a derivative which inhibits the stimulation of ovarian adenylate cyclase by lutropin, *FEBS Lett.,* 118, 77, 1980.

117. **Mise, T. and Bahl, O. P.,** Assignment of disulfide bonds in the α-subunit of human chorionic gonadotropin, *J. Biol. Chem.,* 255, 8516, 1980.

118. **Mise, T. and Bahl, O. P.,** Assignment of disulfide bonds in the β-subunit of human chorionic gonadotropin, *J. Biol. Chem.,* 256, 6587, 1981.

119. **Pierce, J. G. and Parsons, T. F.,** Glycoprotein hormones: structure and function, *Ann. Rev. Biochem.,* 50, 465, 1981.

120. **Taliadouros, G. S., Amr, S., Louvet, J.-P., Birken, S., Canfield, R. E., and Nisula, B. C.,** Biological and immunological characterization of crude commercial human chorianogonadotropin, *J. Clin. Endocrinol. Metab.,* 54, 1002, 1982.

121. **Pepperell, R. J., DeKretser, D. M., and Burger, H. G.,** Studies on the metabolic clearance rate and production rate of human lutenizing hormone and on the initial half-time of its subunits in man, *J. Clin. Invest.,* 56, 118, 1975.

122. **Sairam, M. R. and Li, C. H.,** Human pituitary thyrotropin: the primary structure of the α and β subunits, *Can. J. Biochem.,* 55, 755, 1977.

123. **Bahl, O. P.,** Human chorionic gonadotropin. I. Purification and physico chemical properties, *J. Biol. Chem.,* 244, 567, 1969.

124. **Ward, D. N., Adams-Mayne, M., Ray, N., Balke, B. E., Coffey, J., and Showalter, M.,** Comparative studies of luteinizing hormone from beef, pork, and sheep pituitaries. I. Purification and physical properties, *Gen. Comp. Endocrinol.,* 8, 44, 1967.

125. **Florsheim, W. H., Williams, A. D., and Schonbaum, E.,** On the mechanism of the McKenzie Bioassay, *Endocrinology,* 87, 881, 1970.

126. **McKenzie, J. M.,** The bioassay of thyrotropin in serum, *Endocrinology,* 63, 372, 1958.

127. **Greenspan, F. S., Kriss, J. P., Moses, L. E., and Lew, W.,** An improved bioassay method for thyrotropic hormone using thyroid uptake of radiophosphorous, *Endocrinology,* 58, 767, 1956.

128. **Tate, R. L., Schwartz, H. I., Holmes, T. M., Kohn, L. D., and Winand, R. J.,** Thyrotropin receptors in thyroid plasma membranes, *J. Biol. Chem.,* 250, 6509, 1975.

129. **Zor, A., Kaneko, T., Lowe, I. P., Bloom, G., and Field, J. B.,** Effect of thyroid stimulating hormone and prostaglandins on thyroid adenyl cyclase activation and cyclic adenosine 3',5',-monophosphate, *J. Biol. Chem.,* 259, 244, 1984.

130. **Friedman, Y., Hladis, P., Babiarz-Crowell, D., and Burke, G.,** Effects of cholera toxin on thyroid cyclic AMP-dependent protein kinase and ornithine decarboxylase activities, *Endocrinol. Res. Commun.,* 6, 71, 1979.

131. **Cheng, K. W., Glazer, A. N., and Pierce, J. G.,** The effects of modification of the COOH terminal regions of bovine thyrotropin and its subunits, *J. Biol. Chem.,* 246, 7930, 1973.

132. **Parsons, T. R. and Pierce, J. G.,** Biologically active covalently crosslinked glycoprotein hormones and the effects of modification of the COOH-terminal region of their α-subunits, *J. Biol. Chem.,* 254, 6010, 1979.

133. **Bakke, J., Lawrence, N., and Roy, S.,** Disappearance rate of exogenous thyroid stimulating hormone (TSH) in man, *J. Clin. Metab.,* 22, 352, 1962.

134. **Hays, M., Solomon, D. H., and Werner, S. C.,** The effect of purified bovine thyroid stimulating hormone in man. II. Loss of effectiveness with prolonged administration, *J. Clin. Endocrinol. Metab.,* 21, 1475, 1961.

135. **Pierce, J. G. and Nyc, J. F.,** A method for the preparation of high potency concentrates of thyrotropic hormone, *J. Biol. Chem.,* 222, 777, 1956.

136. **Fontaine, Y. A. and Condliffe, P. G.,** Density gradient centrifugation of bovine thyroid-stimulating hormone, *Biochemistry,* 2, 290, 1963.

137. **Jacobson, G., Roos, P., and Wide, L.,** Human pituitary thyrotropin: characterization of five glycoproteins with thyrotropin activity, *Biochim. Biophys. Acta,* 490, 403, 1977.

138. **Cole, H. H. and Erway, J.,** 48 Hour assay test for equine gonadotropin with results expressed in international units, *Endocrinology,* 29, 514, 1941.

139. **Moore, W. T. and Ward, D. N.,** Pregnant mare serum gonadotropin: an *in vitro* biological characterization of the lutropin-follitropin dual activity, *J. Biol. Chem.,* 255, 6930, 1980.

140. **Licht, P., Bona Gallo, A., Aggarwal, B. B., Farmer, S. W., Castelino, J. B., and Papkoff, H.,** Biological and binding activities of equine pituitary gonadotropins and pregnant mare serum gonadotropin, *J. Endocrinol.,* 83, 311, 1979.

141. **Farmer, S. W. and Papkoff, H.,** Pregnant mare serum gonadotropin and follicle stimulating hormone stimulation of cyclic AMP production in rat seminiferous tubule cells, *J. Endocrinol.,* 76, 391, 1978.

142. **Suzuki, K., Kawakura, K., and Tamoski, B.,** Effect of pregnant mares serum gonadotropin on the activities of Δ⁴-5α reductase, aromatase, and other enzymes in the ovaries of immature rats, *Endocrinology,* 102, 1595, 1978.

143. **Aggarwal, B. B. and Papkoff, H.,** Effects of histidine modification on the biological and immunological activities of equine chorionic gonadotropin, *Arch. Biochem. Biophys.,* 202, 121, 1980.

144. **Schams, D. and Papkoff, H.,** Chemical and immunochemical studies on pregnant mare serum gonadotropin, *Biochim. Biophys. Acta,* 263, 139, 1972.

145. **McIntosh, J. E. A., Moor, R. M., and Allen, W. R.,** Pregnant mare serum gonadotropins: rate of clearance from the circulation of sheep, *J. Reprod. Fertil.,* 44, 95, 1975.

146. **Agarwal, B. B., Farmer, S. W., Papkoff, H., and Seidel, G. E.,** Biochemical properties of equine chorionic gonadotropin from two different pools of pregnant mare sera, *Biol. Reprod.,* 23, 570, 1980.

147. **Moore, W. T. and Ward, D. N.,** Pregnant mare serum gonadotropin. Rapid chromatographic procedures for the purification of intact hormone and isolation of subunits, *J. Biol. Chem.,* 255, 6923, 1980.

148. **Combarnous, Y., Salesse, R., and Garnier, J.,** Physiochemical properties of pregnant mare serum gonadotropin, *Biochim. Biophys. Acta,* 667, 267, 1981.

149. **Hofman, K.,** Relations between chemical structure and function of adrenocorticotropin and melanocyte-stimulating hormone, in *Handbook of Physiology,* Vol. 4, Section 7, Greep, R. O. and Astwood, E. B., Eds., American Physiological Society, Washington, D.C., 1974, chap. 22.

150. **Dillon, R. S.**, *Handbook of Endocrinology*, Lea & Febiger, Philadelphia, 1980, chap. 5.
151. **Haynes, R. D., Jr. and Larner, J.**, Adrenocorticotropic hormone; adrenocortical steroids and their synthetic analogs; inhibitors of adrenocortical steroid biosynthesis, in *The Pharmacological Basis of Therapeutics*, Goodman, L. S. and Gilman, A., Eds., MacMillan, New York, 1975, 1472.
152. **Synder, S. H. and Childers, S. R.**, Opiate receptors and opioid peptides, *Ann. Rev. Neurosci.*, 2, 35, 1979.
153. **Terenius, L.**, Endogenous peptides and analgesia, *Ann. Rev. Pharmacol.*, 18, 189, 1978.
154. **Miller, R. J. and Cuatrecasas, P.**, Enkephalins and endorphins, *Vitamins Hormones*, 36, 297, 1978.
155. **Morley, J. S.**, Structure-activity relationships of enkephalin-like peptides, *Ann. Rev. Pharmacol. Toxicol.*, 20, 81, 1980.
156. **Parvizi, N. and Ellendorff, F.**, β-Endorphin alters luteinizing hormone secretion via the amygdala but not the hypothalamus, *Nature (London)*, 286, 812, 1980.
157. **Howe, A.**, The mammalian pars intermedia: a review of its structure and function, *J. Endocrinol.*, 59, 385, 1973.
158. **Cretien, M., Benjannet, S., Seidah, N. G., and Lis, M.**, Beta-lipotropin, endorphins and enkephalins, in *Clinical Neuroendocrinology: A Pathophysiological Approach*, Tolis, G., Ed., Raven Press, New York, 1979, 147.
159. **Lerner, A. B.**, The intermediate lobe of the pituitary gland, in *Peptides of the Pars Intermedia*, Evered, D. and Lawrenson, G., Eds., Ciba Foundation Symposium 81, Pitman Medical Ltd., London, 1981, 3.
160. **Crine, P., Gossard, F., Seidah, N. G., Gianoulakis, C., Lis, M., and Cretien, M.**, Biosynthesis of β-endorphin in the rat pars intermedia, in *Synthesis and Release of Adenohypophyseal Hormones*, Jutisz, M. and McKerns, K. W., Eds., Plenum Press, New York, 1980, 263.
161. **Eberle, A. N.**, Structure and chemistry of the peptide hormones of the intermediate lobe, in *Peptides of the Pars Intermedia*, Evered, D. and Lawrenson, G., Eds., Ciba Foundation Symposium 81, Pitman Medical Ltd., London, 1981, 13.
162. **Blake, J., Tseng, L. F., Chang, W. C., and Li, C. H.**, The synthesis and opiate activity of human β-endorphin analogs, *Int. J. Peptide Prot. Res.*, 11, 323, 1978.
163. **Walter, J. M., Sandman, C. A., Berntson, G. G., McGivern, R. F., Coy, O. H., and Kastin, A. J.**, Endorphin analogs with potent and long-lasting analgesic effects, *Pharmacol. Biochem. Behav.*, 7, 543, 1977.
164. **Morgan, B. A.**, Enkephalins and endorphins, in *Amino-Acids, Peptides and Proteins*, Sheppard, R. C., Ed., Special Periodical Rep. 9, Chemical Society, London, 1978, 481.
165. **Conroy, R. T. W. L. and Mills, N. J.**, *Human Circadian Rhythms*, Churchill Livingston, London, 1970.
166. **Goth, A.**, *Medical Pharmacology*, C. V. Mosby, St. Louis, 1976, chap. 38.
167. **von Eickstedt, K. W.**, Corticotrophins and corticosteroids, in *Meyler's Side Effects of Drugs*, Dukes, M. N. G., Ed., Excerpta Medica, Amsterdam, 1980.
168. **Sandow, J. and Konig, W.**, Chemistry of the hypothalamic hormones, in *The Endocrine Hypothalamus*, Jeffcoate, S. L. and Hutchinson, J. S. M., Eds., Academic Press, New York, 1978, 149.
169. **Dillon, R. S.**, *Handbook of Endocrinology*, Lea and Febiger, Philadelphia, 1980, chap. 5.
170. **Schroder, E. and Lubke, K.**, *The Peptides*, Vol. 2, Academic Press, New York, 1966, 336.
171. **Rudinger, J., Pliska, V., and Krejci, I.**, Oxytocin analogs in the analysis of some phases of hormone action, *Rec. Progr. Hormone Res.*, 28, 166, 1972.
172. **Sawyer, W. H. and Manning, M.**, Synthetic analogs of oxytocin and the vasopressins, *Ann. Rev. Pharmacol.*, 13, 5, 1973.
173. **Fasman, G. D. and Sober, H. A., Eds.**, *Handbook of Biochemistry and Molecular Biology*, Vol. 3, 3rd ed., CRC Press, Boca Raton, Fla., 1976.
174. **Yates, F. E., Russell, S. M., Dallman, M. F., Hedge, G. A., McCann, S. M., and Dhariwal, A. P. S.**, Potentiation by vasopressin of corticotropin release induced by corticotropin-releasing factor, *Endocrinology*, 88, 3, 1971.
175. **Buckingham, J. L. and Hodges, J. R.**, The use of corticotropin production by adenohypophyseal tissue *in vitro* for the detection and estimation of potential corticotropin releasing factors, *J. Endocrinol.*, 72, 187, 1977.
176. **Jones, M. T.**, Control of corticotropin (ACTH) secretion, in *The Endocrine Hypothalamus*, Jeffcoate, S. L. and Hutchinson, J. S. M., Eds., Academic Press, New York, 1978, 389.
177. *Physicians Desk Reference*, 36th ed., Baker, C. E., Jr., Publ., Medical Economics Co., Oradell, N.J., 1982.
178. **von Eickstedt, K. W.**, Miscellaneous hormones, in *Meyler's Side Effects of Drugs*, Dukes, M. N. G., Ed., Excerpta Medica, Amsterdam, 1980, 720.
179. **Walter, R., Schwartz, J. L., Darnell, J. H., and Urry, D. S.**, Relation of the conformation of oxytocin to the biology of neurologic hormones, *Proc. Natl. Acad. Sci. U.S.A.*, 58, 1355, 1971.
180. **Oski, F. A.**, Oxytocin and neonatal hyperbilirubinemia, *Am. J. Dis. Child.*, 129, 1139, 1975.

RADIOPAQUES

David D. Shaw

INTRODUCTION

Radiopaque compounds, commonly referred to as contrast media, are drugs which allow for the internal opacification of blood vessels, body cavities, and organ systems and accordingly are classified as diagnostic aids. Due to the presence of organically bound iodine atoms on the contrast molecule, usually one to three, the penetration of an X-ray electron beam through the body is attenuated when the electrons strike an iodine atom. Due to its high electron absorption coefficient, coupled with its ease of incorporation covalently into a wide variety of organic compounds, iodine has remained the most widely used component in contrast media since its initial use in the early 1920s as NaI.[1,2] Aside from barium sulfate which must be used orally, all contrast media approved for human use are iodinated compounds.

The historical development of media used in diagnostic radiology has been comprehensively surveyed by Grainger,[3] Miller and Skucas,[4] and Killen.[5] The interested reader is referred to these publications for more detailed information on the evolution of existing contrast media.

The sole function of a contrast medium is to impede the beam of electrons generated by the X-ray machine passing through the body, and as such are diagnostic agents in contradistinction to therapeutic drugs which exert defined pharmacologic actions. Because contrast media may be given in extremely high doses, it is of paramount importance that these agents exhibit as little physiological and biochemical effects as possible. Thus, the continued development of newer contrast media over the preceding 30 years has centered primarily on chemical modifications which decrease their systemic toxicity.[6-9] The clinical uses of contrast media fall into three broad categories of applications: (1) oral and rectal administration for visualization of the gastrointestinal tract and hepatobiliary system; (2) intravenous and intraarterial administration for opacification of the vascular system, and (3) intrathecal or subarachnoid injection for delineation of the spinal cord. Certain radiopaque compounds are restricted to one application area (e.g., barium sulfate for oral or rectal use only) while several may be used in all three areas (e.g., newer nonionic media).

With the exception of barium sulfate already mentioned, all contrast media approved for human use are triiodinated derivatives of benzoic acid. Since these agents are diagnostic rather than therapeutic, their efficacy (radiopacity) is determined solely by the amount of iodine which is bound to the parent molecule, and thus its content in solution. Contrast media may vary in concentration from 10 to 80% w/v. Because of this it will be more appropriate to organize this chapter differently from others presented in this volume since these agents do not strictly exhibit a mechanism of action, any structure-activity relationships, or in vivo metabolism (metabolic conversion). Since toxicity and patient tolerance have been the overriding factors in the development of contrast media, these will serve as the major focus with attendant factors noted as needed.

This review will focus mainly on the most commonly accepted agents which have been approved by the U.S. Food and Drug Administration, but where appropriate will also include generically equivalent and/or newer agents which are in use outside the U.S., and agents which are still in experimental stages of development both in the U.S. and abroad. The use of barium sulfate for gastrointestinal visualization and oil based media, which have largely been replaced, are outside the scope of this review, and thus, the interested reader is referred to other references.[10-13] Thus, the remaining radiopaques to be discussed here are all water soluble, iodinated organic compounds which may be used essentially in all human application areas.

IONIC MONOMERIC

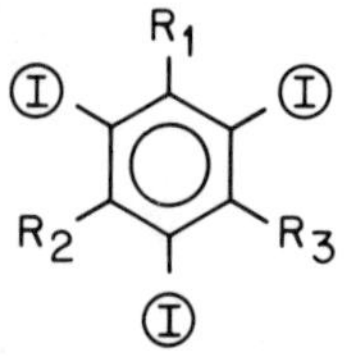

	R_1	R_2	R_3
DIATRIZOATE	$-COO^-$	$-NHCOCH_3$	$-NHCOCH_3$
IOTHALAMATE	$-COO^-$	$-NHCOCH_3$	$-CONHCH_3$
METRIZOATE	$-COO^-$	$-NCOCH_3$ $\quad$ CH_3	$-NHCOCH_3$
IODAMIDE	$-COO^-$	$-NHCOCH_3$	$-CH_2NHCOCH_3$
IOGLICATE	$-COO^-$	$-NHCOCH_3$	$-CONHCH_2CONHCH_3$
IOXITHALAMATE	$-COO^-$	$-NHCOCH_3$	$-CONHCH_2CH_2OH$
IOPANOATE	$-CH_2CH-COO^-$ $\quad$ CH_2CH_3	$-H$	$-NH_2$
IPODATE	$-CH_2CH_2COO^-$	$-H$	$-N=CHN(CH_3)_2$
IOCETAMATE	$-NCH_2CHCOO^-$ $\quad$ $COCH_3$ CH_3	$-H$	$-NH_2$
TYROPANOATE	$-CH_2CHCOO^-$ $\quad$ CH_2CH_3	$-H$	$-NHCOCH_2CH_2CH_3$

FIGURE 1. Chemical structures of representative ionic monomeric contrast media.

CHEMISTRY

The chemical development and evolution of contrast media has resulted in four major classes of compounds: ionic monomers, ionic dimers, nonionic monomers, and nonionic dimers. The generic names, chemical structures, empirical formulas, molecular weights, route of application, trade names, and manufacturers are given in Figures 1 to 4 and Tables 1 to 4 for representative compounds in each class.

IONIC MONOMERIC COMPOUNDS

Ionic monomers represent the most widely used contrast media today, and the synthesis, in the early 1950s of diatrizoic acid led to the wide variety of derivatives currently available. In order to increase the solubility of the pure acid form for vascular injection, numerous cations were tried[14] and eventually sodium[15] and N-methylglucamine (meglumine)[16] were found to be the most acceptable. Because sodium salts have a higher toxicity but lower

IONIC DIMERIC

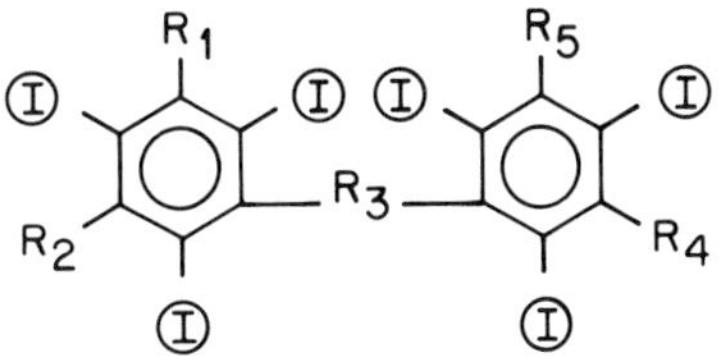

	R_1	R_2	R_3	R_4	R_5
IOXAGLATE	$-COO^-$	$-CONHCH_2CH_2OH$	$-NHCOCH_2NHOC-$	$-NCOCH_3$ CH_3	$-CONHCH_3$
IODOXAMATE	$-COO^-$	$-H$	$-NHCO(CH_2CH_2O)_4CH_2CH_2COHN-$	$-H$	$-COO^-$
IODIPAMIDE	$-COO^-$	$-H$	$-NHCO(CH_2)_4COHN-$	$-H$	$-COO^-$
IOSEFAMATE	$-COO^-$	$-CONHCH_3$	$-NHCO(CH_2)_8COHN-$	$-CONHCH_3$	$-COO^-$
IOSULAMIDE	$-COO^-$	$-NCOCH_3$ CH_2CH_3	$-NHCOCH_2CH_2-SO_2-CH_2CH_2COHN-$	$-NCOCH_3$ CH_2CH_3	$-COO^-$

FIGURE 2. Chemical structures of representative ionic dimeric contrast media.

NONIONIC MONOMERIC

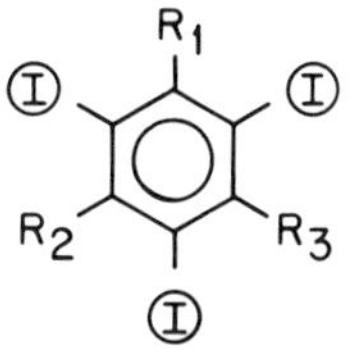

	R_1	R_2	R_3
METRIZAMIDE	$-CONH-2DEOXY-D-GLUCOSE$	$-NCOCH_3$ CH_3	$-NHCOCH_3$
IOPAMIDOL	$-CONHCHCH_2OH$ CH_2OH	$-NHCOCHOHCH_3$	$-CONHCHCH_2OH$ CH_2OH
IOGLUNIDE	$-NHCO(CHOH)_4CH_2OH$	$-NCOCH_3$ CH_3	$-CONHCH_2CH_2OH$
IOHEXOL	$-CONHCH_2CHOHCH_2OH$	$-NCOCH_3$ $CH_2CHOHCH_2OH$	$-CONHCH_2CHOHCH_2OH$
IOPROMIDE	$-CONHCH_2CHOH$ CH_3 CH_2OH	$-NHCOCH_2OCH_3$	$-CONHCH_2CHOHCH_2OH$
IOGULAMIDE	$CO-CO-(CHOH)_3-CH_2OH$ $-NH$	$-CONHCH_2CHOHCH_2OH$	$-CONHCH_2CHOHCH_2OH$

FIGURE 3. Chemical structures of representative nonionic monomeric contrast media.

NONIONIC DIMERIC

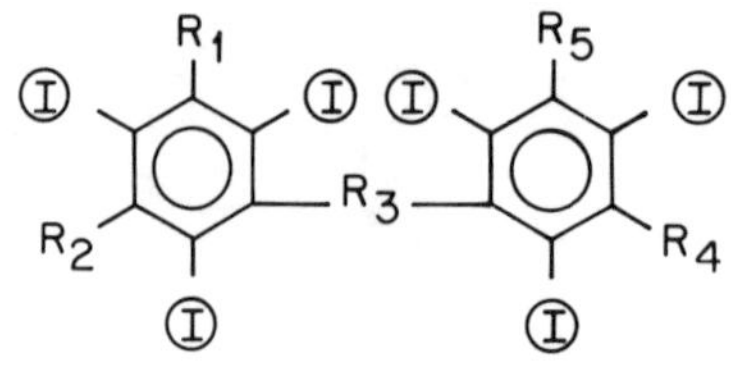

	R₁	R₂	R₃	R₄	R₅
IOTROL	-CONHCHCH₂OH / CHOHCH₂OH	-CONHCHCHOHCH₂OH / CH₂OH	-NCOCH₂CON- / CH₃ CH₃	-CONHCHCHOHCH₂OH / CH₂OH	-CONHCHCH₂OH / CHOHCH₂OH
IODECOL	-CONHCH / CH₂OH / CH₂OH	-CONHCH / CH₂OH / CH₂OH	-NCOCH₂CON- / CH₂OH CH₂OH	-CONHCH / CH₂OH / CH₂OH	-CONHCH / CH₂OH / CH₂OH
IOTASUL	-CONCH₂CHOHCH₂OH / CH₃	-CONCH₂CHOHCH₂OH / CH₃	-NHCOCH₂CH₂-S-CH₂CH₂COHN-	-CONCH₂CHOHCH₂OH / CH₃	-CONCH₂CHOHCH₂OH / CH₃

FIGURE 4. Chemical structures of representative nonionic dimeric contrast media.

Table 1
CHEMICAL COMPOSITION OF REPRESENTATIVE IONIC MONOMERS

Generic name	Molecular formula	Mol wt[a]	Iodine (%)	Cations	Route of administration	Tradename (manufacturer)
Diatrizoic acid	$C_{11}H_9I_3N_2O_4$	613.92	62.1	Sodium Meglumine Sodium and Meglumine	Oral Intravascular (arterial and venous)	Renograftin® (Squibb) Hypaque® (Winthrop) Angiovist® (Schering AG)
Iothalamic acid	$C_{11}H_9I_3N_2O_4$	613.92	62.1	Sodium Meglumine	Oral Intravascular (arterial and venous)	Conray® (Mallinckrodt)
Metrizoic acid	$C_{12}H_{11}I_3N_2O_4$	627.03	60.8	Sodium Calcium Magnesium Meglumine	Oral Intravascular (arterial and venous)	Isopaque® (Nyegaard)
Iodamic acid	$C_{12}H_{11}I_3N_2O_4$	627.94	60.7	Meglumine	Oral Intravascular (arterial and venous)	Uromiro® (Bracco) Renovue® (Squibb)
Ioglicic acid	$C_{13}H_{12}I_3N_3O_5$	670.97	56.8	Sodium Meglumine Sodium and meglumine	Oral Intravascular (arterial and venous)	Rayvist® (Schering AG)
Ioxithalamic acid	$C_{12}H_{11}I_3N_2O_5$	643.94	59.2	Sodium Meglumine Sodium and Meglumine	Oral Intravascular (arterial and venous)	Telebrix® (Guebet)
Iopanoic acid	$C_{11}H_{12}I_3NO_2$	570.93	66.7	Sodium	Oral	Telepaque® (Winthrop)
Ipodic acid	$C_{12}H_{13}I_3N_2O_2$	597.04	63.8	Sodium	Oral	Oragrafin® (Squibb)
Iocetamic acid	$C_{12}H_{13}I_3N_2O_3$	613.96	62.1	—	Oral	Cholobrine® (Mallinckrodt)
Tyropanoic acid	$C_{15}H_{17}I_3NO_3$	640.11	59.5	Sodium	Oral	Bilopaque® (Winthrop)

[a] Acid form.

Table 2
CHEMICAL COMPOSITION OF REPRESENTATIVE IONIC DIMERS

Generic name	Molecular formula	Mol wt[a]	Iodine (%)	Cations	Route of administration	Tradename (manufacturer)
Ioxaglic acid	$C_{24}H_{21}I_6N_5O_8$	1268.89	60.0	Sodium Meglumine Sodium and meglumine	Oral Intravascular (arterial and venous)	Hexabrix® (Guerbet) Hexabrix® (Mallinckrodt)
Iodipamide	$C_{20}H_{14}I_6N_2O_6$	1139.77	66.8	Sodium Meglumine	Intravascular (venous)	Cholografin® (Squibb)
Iodoxamic acid	$C_{26}H_{26}I_6N_2O_{10}$	1287.93	59.2	Meglumine	Intravascular (venous)	Cholovue® (Squibb) Endobile® (Bracco)
Iosefamic acid	$C_{28}H_{28}I_6N_4O_8$	1309.98	58.2	Meglumine	Intravascular (venous)	— (Mallinckrodt)
Iosulamide	$C_{28}H_{28}I_6N_4O_{10}S$	1569.25	48.6	Meglumine	Intravascular (venous)	— (Winthrop)

[a] Acid form.

viscosity than meglumine salts,[17,18] combination formulations were developed.[19-21] The comparative toxicity of several ionic monomers is shown in Table 5. Generally, the toxicities of these compounds are similar except for those in which the 5 position of the benzene ring is unsubstituted (e.g., iopanoate, tyropanoate). These compounds are highly protein bound (80 to 100%)[22-24] and are excreted primarily through the hepatobiliary systems as glucuronide conjugates[25,26] which make them preferred agents for cholecystography[27-29] and cholangiography[30-32] (Table 6). Unfortunately, most of these agents can only be given orally due to their low water solubility and higher systemic toxicity.[33]

Of the ionic media which are injectable, all are highly water soluble and have a low binding to plasma proteins.[34,35] As such these compounds are rapidly excreted through the kidneys[36-38] and are preferred for vascular procedures (Table 7).

IONIC DIMERIC COMPOUNDS

With the exception of ioxaglate which is intended for vascular use, the compounds in this class are primarily used for visualization of the hepatobiliary system via intravenous injection. The protein binding of these compounds is greater than with fully substituted ionic media and is thus preferentially excreted into the bile. As one would expect, based on their chemical structures, those compounds which are fully substituted on the ring are also eliminated to a greater extent through the kidneys (e.g., ioxaglate, iosefamate, iosulamide). A correlation exists between the protein binding and toxicity of these compounds (and for ionic monomers as well) and is presented in Tables 6 and 7.

NONIONIC MONOMERIC COMPOUNDS

In order to decrease toxicity and improve tolerance, Almen[39] in 1969 suggested that compounds which did not dissociate in solution be synthesized. This approach minimized two problems associated with ionic media. First, the osmolality of the solution was essentially decreased by one half, and second, toxic ions like sodium could be eliminated. Metrizamide (Amipaque®) was the culmination of this research effort, but due to its physical-chemical properties is not autoclavable in solution and must be reconstituted from a lyophilized form immediately prior to use.[40] However, the basic principles were established for the future approach to contrast media, namely nonionic compounds.

Table 3
CHEMICAL COMPOSITION OF REPRESENTATIVE NONIONIC MONOMERS

Generic name	Molecular formula	Mol wt	Iodine (%)	Cations	Route of administration	Tradename (manufacturer)
Metrizamide	$C_{18}H_{22}I_3N_3O_8$	789.10	48.2	—	Oral Intravascular (arterial and venous) Intrathecal subarachnoid	Amipaque® (Nyegaard) Amipaque® (Winthrop)
Iopamidol	$C_{17}H_{22}I_3N_8O_8$	777.09	49.0	—	Oral Intravascular (arterial and venous) Intrathecal subarachnoid	Niopam® (Bracco) Solutrast® (Bracco) Isovue® (Squibb)
Ioglunide	$C_{18}H_{24}I_3N_3O_9$	807.12	47.2	—	Oral Intravascular (arterial and venous) Intrathecal subarachnoid	— (Guebet)
Iohexol	$C_{19}H_{26}I_3N_3O_9$	821.14	46.4	—	Oral Intravascular (arterial and venous) Intrathecal subarachnoid	Omnipaque® (Nyegaard) Omnipaque® (Winthrop)
Iopromide	$C_{18}H_{29}I_3N_3O_8$	791.12	48.2	—	Oral Intravascular (arterial and venous) Intrathecal subarachnoid	— (Schering AG)
Iogulamide	$C_{20}H_{26}I_3N_3O_{12}$	881.15	43.2	—	Oral Intravascular (arterial and venous) Intrathecal subarachnoid	— (Mallinckrodt)

In the past several years a variety of highly water soluble, nonionic media have been synthesized[41-45] and tested.[46-48] Compared to ionic compounds, both monomers and dimers, these are significantly less toxic (Table 8) and have more favorable physical-chemical properties (Table 9) which have made them acceptable for all radiographic procedures, including, especially, injection into the subarachnoid space.[49] All the agents in this class are of very similar structure (Figure 3), and properties (Tables 7 and 8). As can be seen, all contain polyhydric groups which confer the extremely high water solubility (over 100% w/v) of these compounds.[50] Although the viscosity of nonionic monomers is higher than that of ionic monomers at equi-iodine concentration (Table 9), no practical problems have arisen in their clinical usage.

NONIONIC DIMERIC COMPOUNDS

With the realization that nonionic monomers were a significant advance over ionic ones, current research has focused on developing compounds which would have all the excellent

Table 4
CHEMICAL COMPOSITION OF REPRESENTATIVE NONIONIC DIMERS

Generic name	Molecular formula	Mol wt	Iodine (%)	Cations	Route of administration	Tradename (manufacturer)
Iotrol	$C_{37}H_{48}I_6N_6O_{18}$	1626.24	46.9	—	Oral Intravascular (arterial and venous) Intrathecal subarachnoid	— (Schering AG)
Iodecol	$C_{35}H_{44}I_6N_6O_{16}$	1566.19	48.7	—	Oral Intravascular (arterial and venous) Intrathecal subarachnoid	— (Schering AG)
Iotasul	$C_{38}H_{50}I_6N_6O_{14}S$	1608.33	47.4	—	Oral Intravascular (arterial and venous)	— (Schering AG)

Table 5
COMPARATIVE TOXICITY OF SELECTED IONIC RADIOPAQUE COMPOUNDS IN THE MALE MOUSE

	Iodine concentration (mg/mℓ)	Route	LD_{50} (g/kg)	Ref.
Ionic monomers				
Diatrizoate, sodium	300	IV[a]	14.0	94
Diatrizoate, meglumine	300	IV	11.1	95
Iothalamate, sodium	400	IV	13.3	96
Iothalamate, meglumine	282	IV	12.0—14.0	96
Metrizoate, sodium + meglumine + calcium	370	IV	12.8—15.8	97,98
Metrizoate, calcium + meglumine	280	IV	13.4	97,98
Iopanoate, sodium	150	0[b]	2.9	99
	150	IV	0.3	99
Tyropanoate, sodium	144	0	4.0—7.8	100
	144	IV	0.7	100
Ionic dimers				
Ioxaglate, sodium + meglumine	320	IV	17.5—22.3	101
Iodipamide, meglumine	260	IV	2.4—2.9	102
Iosulamide, meglumine	259	IV	10.4—14.1	102, 103

[a] IV = intravenous.
[b] O = oral.

Table 6

**PHYSIOLOGIC-PHARMACOLOGIC PROPERTIES OF
CHOLECYSTOCHOLANGIOGRAPHY CONTRAST AGENTS**

Generic (trade) name	Recommended dose	Route administered	Route eliminated	Relative protein binding	Relative water solubility	Time to maximal Gallbladder opacification
Iopanoate (Telepaque®)	3.0 g	Oral	Hepatobiliary	High	Very low	14—19 hr
Ipodate (Oragrafin®)	3.0—6.0 g	Oral	Hepatobiliary	High	Low	10—12 hr
Iocetamate (Cholobrine®)	3.0—4.5 g	Oral	Hepatobiliary	High	Low	10—15 hr
Tyropanoate (Bilopaque®)	3.0 g	Oral	Hepatobiliary	High	Low	4—10 hr
Iodipamide (Cholografin®)	5.1 g	Intravenous	Hepatobiliary and renal	High	Low	15—30 min
Iodoxamate (Cholovue®)	Unknown	Intravenous	Hepatobiliary	High	Low	15—30 min
Isofemate (—)	Not established	Intravenous	Hepatobiliary and renal	Moderate to high	Moderate	10—20 min
Iosulamide (—)	Not established	Intravenous	Hepatobiliary and renal	Moderate to high	Moderate	10—20 min

Table 7

**PHYSIOLOGIC-PHARMACOLOGIC PROPERTIES OF ANGIOUROGRAPHIC
CONTRAST AGENTS**

Generic name	Recommended dose (g)	Route administered	Route eliminated	Relative protein binding	Relative water solubility	Time to maximum organ opacification
Urographic Diatrizoate Iothalamate Metrizoate Ioxaglate Iohexol Iopamidol	≤60	Intravenous	Renal	All low	All high	5—20 min
Angiographic Same as urographic	≤87.5	Intraarterial	Renal	All low	All high	Sec
Myelographic Metrizamide Iopamidol Iohexol	≤3.0	Subarachnoid	Renal	All very low	All very high	1—3 min

properties of the former but would have properties which would make them iso-osmotic to body fluids at acceptable iodine concentrations required for imaging. The compounds listed in Table 8, and shown in Figure 4, are currently in initial human investigation. Thus far, these have shown promise clinically. The major drawback to these is their higher viscosity which may make them impractical for rapid hand or power injection.

BIOLOGICAL EFFECTS (PHARMACOLOGY/PHYSIOLOGY)

As stated earlier, contrast media do not possess specific activities, and in fact their design

Table 8
COMPARATIVE TOXICITY OF SELECTED NONIONIC RADIOPAQUE COMPOUNDS IN THE MALE MOUSE

	Iodine concentration (mg/mℓ)	Route	LD$_{50}$ (g/kg)	Ref.
Nonionic monomers				
Metrizamide	300	Intravenous	28.2—38.3	104, 105
	370	Intravenous	27.9—36.0	104, 105
Iopamidol	300	Intravenous	30.2—35.9	106
	370	Intravenous	33.5	106
Iohexol	300	Intravenous	52.0	101, 105, 106
	370	Intravenous	46.1—52.4	101, 105
Iopromide	300	Intravenous	28.6—39.2	106
Nonionic dimers				
Iotrol	300	Intravenous	>50	107
Iodecol	300	Intravenous	>50	107

Table 9
PHYSICAL-CHEMICAL PROPERTIES OF REPRESENTATIVE RADIOPAQUE COMPOUNDS

	Iodine concentration (mg/mℓ)	Osmolality (mOsm/kg H$_2$O)	Viscosity (mPa at 37°C)
Ionic monomers			
Diatrizoate, sodium	300	1450	2.5
Diatrizoate, sodium + meglumine	370	1950	8.4
Diatrizoate, meglumine			
Iothalamate, sodium	400	2230	4.7
Iothalamate, meglumine	282	1440	3.8
Metrizoate, meglumine + calcium + sodium + magnesium	440	2660	10.9
Metrizoate, meglumine + sodium + calcium	370	2150	8.4
Metrizoate, meglumine + calcium	280	1440	4.0
Ionic dimers			
Ioxaglate, sodium + meglumine	320	580	7.5
Ioxaglate, sodium	320	580	4.0
Nonionic monomers			
Metrizamide	370	580	16.0
	280	430	5.0
Iopamidol	370	800	9.5
	280	570	3.8
Iohexol	370	980	13.5
	300	690	4.1
Nonionic dimers			
Iotrol	300	360	—
Iodecol	300	280	—

has been such that they possess the most minimal effect on the body's systems as possible. However, certain consequences from the administration of contrast media are well known, and in most instances these can be related to the route, speed, or concentration of administration,[51,52] as well as the particular physical-chemical[53,54] and chemotoxic properties[55,56] of the different formulations.

With the exception of nonionic dimers, all contrast media are markedly hyperosmotic to blood and cerebrospinal fluid and this may, in part, be responsible for hypervolemia,[57] electrolyte disturbances,[58] vasodilation,[59] pulmonary hypertension,[60] breakdown of the blood brain barrier,[61] myocardial depression and bradycardia,[62,63] diuresis,[64,65] pain,[66] and endothelial injury[67] which have been reported after contrast medium exposure.

Alternatively, all contrast media possess inherent chemotoxic properties which may be more accurately correlated to their effects on enzyme[68] and cellular systems,[69] such as complement activation,[70] lysozyme inhibition,[71] protein binding,[72] and histamine liberation.[73] Regardless of whether it is the physical-chemical or chemotoxic properties, or both, of the newer nonionic contrast media, these agents cause far fewer and less severe perturbations than ionic media.

Intravascularly administered contrast media are rapidly distributed throughout the extracellular compartment[74,75] and the primary route of excretion is primarily determined by the agents' affinity for serum proteins, notably albumin.[76-78] Typically, the distribution and excretion of ionic[79-81] and nonionic[82,83] media can be described by either a two-[80] or three-[83] compartment system. This difference may be more methodologic than real as the newer techniques of high powered liquid chromatography (HPLC) in quantifying concentrations are several times more sensitive.[84] Regardless, urinary excretion of diatrizoates, iothalamates, metrizoates, and all nonionics occurs through glomerular filtration[85] and is close to 100% within 24 hr. Those agents which are protein bound and thus handled through the hepato biliary system are removed at a rate 4 to 5 times slower.[86,87]

Orally administered media (iopanoate, tyropanoate, ipodate) are dependent upon bile salts for their absorption in the small intestine,[88,89] but as their water solubility increases this dependency decreases.[90] These agents are transported into the hepatobiliary system bound to plasma albumin, metabolized to glucuronide conjugates, and actively excreted into the hepatic ducts and gall bladder. The time from administration to maximal gall bladder concentration may vary from 3 to 20 hr and depends on solubility characteristics and transfer functions from intestine to plasma. Table 9 presents the more important characteristics of these orally administered contrast media. Intravenously administered agents (iodipamide, iosefamate, iosulamide) used for hepatobiliary opacification are considerably more water soluble[91] and reach maximal biliary concentrations sooner.[92]

INDICATIONS AND DOSAGES

The major procedural indication areas and recommended maximum single exposure dosage of selected contrast media are presented in Tables 6 and 7. The volume of contrast medium administered will depend not only on the concentration of the solution used, but also on the route and mode of administration, the size of the patient (or systems to be visualized), and the physiological (or pathological) state of the patient. Single exposure dosage should not exceed 87.5 g of iodine as recommended by the American College of Radiology. Administration of contrast media to infants and children must be closely monitored as the immaturity of the kidney will significantly delay total excretion.[93,94] Used within the framework of good clinical practice and understanding of basic physiological principles, contrast media are extraordinarily safe drugs. With the introduction and addition of newer and safer nonionic media to the radiologist's already large armementarium, a significant step in patient safety has been realized.

AUTHOR'S NOTE

Due to the numerous number of radiopaque substances which are available throughout the world today, it has been possible to mention only a selected number of these. A more complete, although not entirely comprehensive listing of compounds is found in Appendix 1 along with the CAS registry number of each. If additional, or more in-depth technical information is desired, especially on the newer agents which may not be listed in the USAN (U.S. Adopted Names, 1984), the reader may contact the research departments of the major pharmaceutical companies listed in Appendix 2.

Finally, any errors which remain are solely the responsibility of the author, and hopefully are minimal.

ACKNOWLEDGMENT

I wish to express my sincere appreciation to Mrs. Wendy Hankle for her expert typing and collating of this manuscript and to Mrs. Colleen Hassett for proofreading it.

Appendix 1

USAN: generic name	CAS number	USAN: generic name	CAS number
Acetrizoate, sodium	129-63-5	Iophendylate	1320-11-2
Acetrizoic acid	85-36-9	Iophenoxic acid	96-84-4
Barium sulfate	7727-43-7	Ioprocemic acid	1456-52-6
Diatrizoate, meglumine	131-49-7	Iopromide	73334-07-3
Diatrizoate, sodium	737-31-5	Iopronic acid	37723-78-7
Diatrizoic acid		Iopydol	5579-92-0
(amidotrizoic acid)	117-96-4	Iopydone	5579-93-1
Ethiodized oil	8808-53-5	Iosefamic acid	5591-33-3
Iobenzamic acid	3115-59-7	Ioseric acid	51876-99-4
Iobutoic acid	13445-12-0	Iosulamide, meglumine	6284-40-8
Iocarmate meglumine	54605-45-7	Iosumetic acid	37863-70-0
Iocarmic acid	10397-75-8	Iotasul	71767-13-0
Iocetamic acid	16034-77-8	Iotetric acid	60019-19-4
Iodamide	4440-58-4	Iothalamate, meglumine	13087-53-1
Iomide, meglumine	6284-40-8	Iothalamate, sodium	1225-20-3
Iodecol	81045-33-2	Iothalamic acid	2276-90-6
Iodipamide, meglumine	3521-84-4	Iotrol	79770-24-4
Iodipamide, sodium	24360-85-8	Iotroxic acid	51022-74-3
Iodipamide	606-17-7	Ioxaglate, meglumine	59018-13-2
Iodized oil	8001-49-9	Ioxaglate, sodium	67992058-9
Iodopyracet	—	Ioxaglic acid	59017-64-0
Iodoxamate, meglumine	51764-33-1	Iozomic acid	31598-07-9
Iodoxamic acid	31127-82-9	Ipodate, sodium	1221-56-3
Ioglicic acid	49755-67-1	Ipodic acid	5587-89-3
Ioglucol	63941-73-1	Methiodal, sodium	126-31-8
Ioglucomide	63941-74-2	Metrizamide	31112-62-6
Ioglunide	56562-79-9	Metrizoate, sodium	7225-61-8
Ioglycamic acid	2618-25-1	Metrizoic acid	1949-45-7
Iogulamide	75751-89-2	Methiodal	143-47-5
Iohexol	66108-95-0	Tyropanoate, sodium	7246-21-1
Iopamidol	60166-93-9	Tyropanoic acid	27293-82-9
Iopanoic acid	96-83-3		

Appendix 2

Bracco Industria Chemica
20134 Milano
Italy

E. R. Squibb and Sons
Diagnostic Division
P.O. Box 191
New Brunswick, N.J. 08903

Laboratoire Guerbet
16-24 rue Jean Chaptal
93609 Aulnay-Sous-Bois
Cedex
France

Lafayette Pharmacal Inc.
Diagnostic Products Division
P.O. Box 4499
Lafayette, Indiana 47904

Mallinckrodt
Diagnostic Products Division
675 McDonnell Boulevard
St. Louis, Mo. 63134

Nyegaard and Company, A/S
Postbox 4220 Torshov
Oslo 4
Norway

Schering AG
Mullerstrasse 170-172
D-1000 Berlin 65
West Germany

Winthrop-Breon Laboratories
90 Park Avenue
New York, N.Y. 10016

REFERENCES

1. **Osborne, E. D., Sutherland, C. G., Scholl, A. J., and Roundtree, L. G.,** Roentgenography of the urinary tract during excretion of sodium iodide, *JAMA*, 80, 368, 1923.
2. **Berberich, J. and Hirsch, S.,** Die Rontgenographische darstellung der Arterien und venen am lebenden Menschen, *Klin. Wochenschr.*, 2, 2226, 1923.
3. **Grainger, R. G.,** Intravascular contrast media — the past, the present and the future, *Br. J. Radiol.*, 55, 1, 1982.
4. **Miller, R. E. and Skucas, J.,** *Radiographic Contrast Agents*, University Park Press, Baltimore, 1977.
5. **Killen, D. A.,** Angiographic contrast media: a historical resume, *Surgery*, 73, 333, 1973.
6. **Hoppe, J. O., Larsen, A. A., and Coulston, F.,** Observations on the toxicity of a new urographic contrast medium, sodium 3,5-diacetamido-2,4,6-triiodobenzoate and related compounds, *J. Pharm. Exp. Ther.*, 116, 394, 1956.
7. **Hoppe, J. O.,** Some pharmacological aspects of radioopaque compounds, *Ann. N.Y. Acad. Sci.*, 78, 727, 1959.
8. **Langecker, H., Harwart, A., and Junkmann, K.,** 3,5-Diacetylamino-2,4,6-triiodbenzoesaure als Rontgenkontrastmittel, *Arch. Exp. Pathol. Pharmakol.*, 222, 584, 1954.
9. **Almen, T.,** Contrast agent design. Some aspects on the synthesis of water-soluble contrast agents of low osmolality, *J. Theor. Biol.*, 24, 216, 1969.
10. **Miller, R. E. and Skucas, J.,** Barium Sulfate, in *Radiographic Contrast Agents*, Miller, R. E. and Skucas, J., Eds., University Park Press, Baltimore, 1977, 9.
11. **Miller, R. E. and Skucas, J.,** Barium sulfate, in *Radiographic Contrast Agents*, Miller, R. E. and Skucas, J., Eds., University Park Press, Baltimore, 1977, 85.
12. **House, A. J. S.,** Iodinated bronchographic agents, in *Radiographic Contrast Agents*, Miller, R. E. and Skucas, J., Eds., University Park Press, Baltimore, 1977, 389.
13. **Batnitzky, S.,** Positive contrast myelography, water-insoluble iodinated organic agents, in *Radiographic Contrast Agents*, Miller, R. E. and Skucas, J., Eds., University Park Press, Baltimore, 1977, 429.
14. **Archer, S.,** Chemical aspects of radiopaque agents, *Ann. N.Y. Acad. Sci.*, 78, 720, 1959.
15. **Wallingford, V. H.,** General aspects of contrast media research, *Ann. N.Y. Acad. Sci.*, 78, 707, 1959.
16. **Steinwall, O.,** An improved technique for testing the effect of contrast media and other substances on the blood-brain barrier, *Acta Radiol.*, 49, 281, 1958.

17. **Fischer, H. W. and Cornell, S. H.,** The toxicity of sodium and methylglucamine salts of diatrizoate, iothalamate, and metrizoate: an experimental study of their circulating effects following intracarotid injection, *Radiology*, 85, 1013, 1965.

18. **Cornell, S. H. and Fischer, H. W.,** Comparison of mixtures of metrizoate and iothalamate salts with their methylglucamine solutions by the carotid injection technique, *Invest. Radiol.*, 2, 41, 1967.

19. **Hoppe, J. O., Duprey, L. P., Borisenok, W. A., and Bird, J. G.,** Selective radiopacity in cardiovascular angiography, *Angiology*, 18, 257, 1967.

20. **Fischer, H. W.,** Introduction to angiographic contrast agents, in *Radiographic Contrast Agents*, Miller, R. E. and Skucas, J., Eds., University Park Press, Baltimore, 1977, 329.

21. **Gootman, N., Rudolph, A. M., and Buckley, N. M.,** Effects of angiographic contrast media on cardiac function, *Am. J. Cardiol.*, 25, 59, 1970.

22. **Mudge, G. H., Stibitz, G. R., Robinson, M. S., and Gemborys, M. W.,** Competition for binding to multiple sites of human serum albumin for cholecystographic agents and sulfobromophthalein, *Drug Metab. Dispos.*, 6, 440, 1978.

23. **Lang, J. H. and Lasser, E. C.,** Binding of roentgenographic contrast media to serum albumin, *Invest. Radiol.*, 2, 396, 1967.

24. **Sokoloff, J., Berk, R. N., Lang, J. H., and Lasser, E. C.,** The role of Y and Z hepatic proteins in the excretion of radiographic contrast materials, *Radiology*, 106, 519, 1973.

25. **McChesney, E. W. and Hoppe, J. O.,** Observations on the metabolism and excretion of the glucuronide of iopanoic acid by the cat, *Arch. Int. Pharmacodyn. Ther.*, 99, 127, 1954.

26. **Barnhart, J. L., Berk, R. N., Janes, J. O., and Witt, B. L.,** Isolation, hepatic distribution, and intestinal absorption of the glucuronide metabolite of iopanoic acid, *Invest. Radiol.*, 15, S109, 1980.

27. **Loeb, P. M., Berk, R. N., and Janes, J. O.,** The effect of fasting on gallbladder opacification during oral cholecystography: a controlled study in normal volunteers, *Radiology*, 126, 395, 1978.

28. **Berk, R. N. and Loeb, P. M.,** Pharmacology and physiology of the biliary radiographic contrast materials, *Semin. Roentgenol.*, 11, 147, 1976.

29. **Russell, J. G. and Frederick, P. R.,** Clinical comparisons of tyropanoate sodium, ipodate sodium and iopanoic acid, *Radiology*, 112, 519, 1974.

30. **Marshall, T. R. and Ling, J. T.,** Present status of intravenous cholangiography, *Curr. Med. Dig.*, 30, 33, 1963.

31. **McNutly, J. G.,** Drip infusion cholecystocholangiography, *Radiology*, 90, 570, 1968.

32. **Feldman, M. I. and Keshane, M.,** Slow infusion intravenous cholangiography, *Radiology*, 87, 355, 1966.

33. **Taketa, R. M., Berk, R. N., Lang, J. H., Lasser, E. C., and Dunn, C. R.,** The effect of pH on the intestinal absorption of Telepaque, *Am. J. Roentgenol.*, 114, 767, 1972.

34. **Lasser, E. C., Farr, R. S., Fujimagri, T., and Tripp, W. N.,** The significance of protein binding of contrast media in roentgen diagnosis, *Am. J. Roentgenol.*, 87, 338, 1962.

35. **Olsson, O.,** Excretion of sodium metrizoate through the liver during urography, *Acta Radiol. Diag.*, 11, 85, 1971.

36. **Dawson, J. B., McChesney, E. W., and Teller, F. F.,** Excretion of metrizoate in man, *Acta Radiol. Scand.*, 7, 502, 1968.

37. **Cattell, W. R.,** Excretory pathways for contrast media, *Invest. Radiol.*, 5, 473, 1970.

38. **Becker, J. A. and Berdon, W. E.,** Blood clearances of contrast material in patients with impaired renal function, *Radiology*, 93, 1301, 1969.

39. **Almen, T.,** Contrast agent design. Some aspects of the synthesis of water soluble contrast agents of low osmolality, *J. Theor. Biol.*, 24, 215, 1969.

40. **Holtermann, H.,** personal communication.

41. **Pitre, D. and Felder, E.,** Development, chemistry and physical properties of iopamidol and its analogues, *Invest. Radiol.*, 15, S301, 1980.

42. **Haavaldsen, J.,** Iohexol: introduction, *Acta Radiol. Scand.*, Suppl. 362, 9, 1980.

43. **Speck, U., Mutzel, W., Mannesmann, G., Pfeiffer, H., and Siefert, M.,** Pharmacology of nonionic dimers, *Invest. Radiol.*, 15, 317, 1980.

44. **Hoey, G. B., Hopkins, R. M., Smith, K. R., and Wiegert, P. E.,** Synthesis and biological testing of nonionic iodinated X-ray contrast media, *Invest. Radiol.*, 15, S289, 1980.

45. **Amiel, M., Gressard, A., Janin, A., and Touboul, P.,** Comparison chez l'homme au cours de la coronarographie selective des effets electro-physiologiques d'un sel de l'acide diatrizoique et d'un sel de l'acide ioxaglique, *Ann. Radiol.*, 22, 461, 1979.

46. **Gonsette, R. E.,** Animal experiments and chemical experiences in cerebral angiography with a new contrast agent (ioxaglic acid) with a low hyperosmolality, *Ann. Radiol.*, 21, 271, 1978.

47. **Aakhus, T. O., Sommerfelt, S. C., Stormorken, H., and Dahlstrom, K. D.,** Tolerance and excretion of iohexol after intravenous injection in healthy volunteers, *Acta Radiol. Scand.*, Suppl. 362, 131, 1980.

48. **Hammer, B. and Lackner, W.,** Iopamidol, a new nonionic hydrosoluble contrast medium for neuroradiology, *Neuroradiology*, 19, 119, 1980.

49. **Almen, T.,** Experience from 10 years of development of water-soluble nonionic contrast media, *Invest. Radiol.,* 15, S283, 1980.

50. **Jacobsen, T.,** The preclinical development of iohexol (Omnipaque), *Farmakoterapi,* 38, 45, 1982.

51. **Chahine, R. A. and Raizner, A. E.,** The mechanism of hypotension following angiography, *Invest. Radiol.,* 11, 472, 1976.

52. **Fischer, H. W.,** Hemodynamic reactions to angiographic media — a survey and commentary, *Radiology,* 91, 66, 1968.

53. **Wolf, G., Gerlings, E. D., and Wilson, W. J.,** Depression of myocardial contractility induced by hypertonic coronary injections in the isolated, perfused dog heart, *Radiology,* 107, 655, 1973.

54. **Popio, K. A., Koss, A. M., Oravec, J. M., and Ingram, J. T.,** Identification and description of separate mechanisms for two components of Renografin toxicity, *Circulation,* 58, 520, 1978.

55. **Sovak, M., Ranganathan, R., Lang, J. H., and Lasser, E. C.,** Concepts in design of improved intravascular contrast agents, *Ann. Radiol.,* 21, 283, 1978.

56. **Rapoport, S. I. and Levitan, H.,** Neurotoxicity of X-ray contrast media, *Am. J. Roentgenol.,* 122, 156, 1974.

57. **Hammermeister, K. E. and Warbasse, J. R.,** Immediate hemodynamic effects of cardiac angiography in man, *Am. J. Cardiol.,* 31, 307, 1973.

58. **Kutt, H., Milhorat, T. H., and McDowell, F.,** The effect of iodinized contrast media upon blood proteins, electrolytes and red cells, *Neurology,* 13, 492, 1963.

59. **Lindgren, P.,** Hemodynamic responses to contrast media, *Invest. Radiol.,* 5, 424, 1970.

60. **Friesinger, G., Schaffer, J., Criley, M., Gaertner, R., and Ross, J.,** Hemodynamic consequences of the injection of radiopaque material, *Circulation,* 31, 370, 1965.

61. **Jeppson, P. G. and Olin, T.,** Neurotoxicity of roentgen contrast media. Study of the blood-brain barrier in the rabbit following selective injection into the internal carotid artery, *Acta Radiol. Diag.,* 10, 17, 1970.

62. **Fischer, H. W. and Thomson, K. R.,** Contrast media in coronary arteriography: a review, *Invest. Radiol.,* 13, 450, 1978.

63. **Higgins, C. B.,** Effects of contrast media on the conducting system of the heart, *Radiology,* 124, 599, 1977.

64. **McLennon, B. L. and Becker, J. A.,** Excretory urography: choice of contrast material, *Clin. Radiol.,* 100, 591, 1971.

65. **Saxton, H. M.,** Review article: urography, *Br. J. Radiol.,* 42, 321, 1969.

66. **Holder, J. C. and Dalrymple, G. V.,** Pain and aortofemoral arteriography: the importance of chemical structure and osmolality of contrast agents, *Invest. Radiol.,* 16, 508, 1981.

67. **Ritchie, W. G. M., Lynch, P. R., and Stewart, G. J.,** The effect of contrast media on normal and inflamed canine veins, *Invest. Radiol.,* 9, 444, 1974.

68. **Schultz, B.,** Serine proteases as mediators of radiographic contrast media toxicity, *Invest. Radiol.,* 15, S18, 1980.

69. **Lasser, E. C., Lang, J. H., Hamblin, A. E., Lyon, S. G., and Howard, M.,** Activation systems in contrast idiosyncrasy, *Invest. Radiol.,* 15, S2, 1980.

70. **Lasser, E. C., Lang, J. H., Lyon, S. G., and Hamblin, A. E.,** Complement and contrast material reactors, *J. Allergy Clin. Immunol.,* 64, 105, 1979.

71. **Lasser, E. C., Lang, J. H., Lyon, S. G., and Hamblin, A. E.,** Complement and contrast material reactors, *J. Allergy Clin. Immunol.,* 64, 105, 1979.

72. **Lasser, E. C. and Lang, J. H.,** Contrast-protein interactions, *Invest. Radiol.,* 5, 446, 1970.

73. **Lasser, E. C., Walters, A. J., Reuter, S. R., and Lang, J. H.,** Histamine release by contrast media, *Radiology,* 100, 683, 1970.

74. **Cattell, W. R.,** Excretory pathways for contrast media, *Invest. Radiol.,* 5, 473, 1970.

75. **Dawson, J. B., McChesney, E. W., and Teller, F. F.,** Excretion of metrizoate in man, *Acta Radiol. Diag.,* 7, 502, 1968.

76. **Olsson, O.,** Excretion of sodium metrizoate through the liver during urography, *Acta Radiol. Diag.,* 11, 85, 1971.

77. **Lasser, E. C.,** Pharmacodynamics of biliary contrast media, *Radiol. Clin. N. Am.,* 4, 511, 1966.

78. **Muller, W. E.,** The binding of intravenous and oral biliary contrast agents to human and bovine serum albumin, *Naunyn-Schmiedebergs Arch. Pharm.,* 302, 227, 1978.

79. **McChesney, E. W. and Hoppe, J. O.,** Studies on the tissue distribution and excretion of sodium diatrizoate in laboratory animals, *Am. J. Roentgenol.,* 78, 137, 1957.

80. **Newhouse, J. H.,** Fluid compartment distribution of intravenous iothalamate in the dog, *Invest. Radiol.,* 12, 364, 1977.

81. **Blaufox, M. D., Sanderson, D. R., Tauxe, W. N., Wakim, K. G., Orvis, A. L., and Owen, C. A.,** Plasmatic diatrizoate-^{131}I disappearance and glomerular filtration in the dog, *Am. J. Physiol.,* 204, 536, 1963.

82. **Golman, K.,** Excretion of metrizamide. I. Comparison with diatrizoate and iothalamate after intravenous administration in rabbits, *Acta Radiol.,* Suppl. 335, 253, 1973.

83. **Mutzel, W., Speck, U., and Weinmann, H. J.,** Pharmacokinetics of iopromide in rat and dog in contrast media, in *Urography, Angiography and Computerized Tomography,* Taenzer, V. and Zeitler, E., Eds., Thieme-Stratton, New York, 1983, 85.

84. **Edelson, J.,** personal communication.

85. **Donaldson, I. M. L.,** Comparison of the renal clearances of inulin and radioactive diatrizoate (Hypaque) as measures of the glomerular filtration rate in man, *Clin. Sci.,* 35, 513, 1968.

86. **Moss, A. A., Lin, S. K., and Riegelman, S.,** Pharmacokinetics of iopanoate and iodoxamate in Rhesus monkeys, *Invest. Radiol.,* 15, S132, 1980.

87. **Moss, A. A., Lin, S. K., Margules, E. R., Motson, R. W., and Riegelman, S.,** Pharmacokinetics of iopanoic acid in the Rhesus monkey: biliary excretion, plasma protein binding and biotransformation, *Invest. Radiol.,* 14, 171, 1979.

88. **Loeb, P. M., Barnhart, J. L., and Berk, R. N.,** The dependence of the biliary excretion of iopanoic acid on bile salts, *Gastroenterology,* 74, 174, 1978.

89. **Amberg, J. R., Thompson, W. M., Goldberger, L., Williamson, S., Alexander, R., and Bates, M.,** Factors in the intestinal absorption of oral cholecystopaques, *Invest. Radiol.,* 15, S136, 1980.

90. **Moss, A. A., Amberg, J. R., and Jones, R. S.,** Relationship of bile salts and bile flow to biliary excretion of iopanoic acid, *Invest. Radiol.,* 7, 11, 1972.

91. **Koehler, R. E., Stanley, R. J., and Evens, R. G.,** Iosefamate meglumine: an iodinated contrast agent for hepatic computed tomography scanning, *Radiology,* 132, 115, 1979.

92. **Nelson, J. A., White, G. L., and Nakashima, E. N.,** Iosulamide: human tolerance study of a new intravenous cholangiographic drug, *Invest. Radiol.,* 15, 511, 1980.

93. **Krovetz, L. J., Grumbar, P. A., Hardin, S., Morgan, A. V., and Schiebler, G. L.,** Complications following use of four angiocardiographic contrast media in infants and children, *Invest. Radiol.,* 4, 13, 1969.

94. **Krovetz, L. J., Shanklin, D. R., and Schiebler, G. L.,** Serious and fatal complications of catheterization and angiocardiography in infants and children, *Am. Heart J.,* 76, 39, 1968.

95. **Duprey, L. P. and Drobeck, H. P.,** Acute IV toxicity study comparing Hypaque-76 and Renografin-76 in the mouse, Report in the Files of the Sterling-Winthrop Research Institute, Rensselaer, New York.

96. **Aspelin, P. and Almen, T.,** Studies on the acute toxicity of ionic and non-ionic contrast media following rapid intravenous injection. An experimental study in mice, *Invest. Radiol.,* 11, 309, 1976.

97. **Salvesen, S., Nilsen, P. L., and Holtermann, H.,** Effects of calcium and magnesium ions on the toxicity of isopaque sodium, *Acta Radiol.,* Suppl. 270, 17, 1967.

98. **Drobeck, H. P. and Duprey, L. P.,** Acute intravenous toxicity of Isopaque 370 in the mouse, rat and rabbit, Report in the Files of the Sterling-Winthrop Research Institute, Rensselaer, New York, 1970.

99. **Drobeck, H. P. and Duprey, L. P.,** Acute oral toxicity (LD_{50}) in mice of two Bilopaque granulations (comparison with commercial Bilopaque), Report in the Files of the Sterling-Winthrop Research Institute, Rensselaer, New York.

100. **Duprey, L. P.,** Acute intravenous toxicity of five cholecystographic agents, Report in the Files of the Sterling-Winthrop Research Institute, Rensselaer, New York.

101. **Piller, R. N. and Duprey, L. P.,** Intravenous ALD_{50} of Win 39424 (iohexol) and Hexabrix, Report in the Files of the Sterling-Winthrop Research Institute, Rensselaer, New York, 1980.

102. **Rosenberg, F. J., Ackerman, J. H., and Nickel, A. R.,** Iosulamide, a new intravenous cholangiocholecystographic medium, *Invest. Radiol.,* 15, S142, 1980.

103. **Duprey, L. P. and Drobeck, H. P.,** Acute intravenous toxicity of win 31122 (iosulamide) lyophil in the mouse, Report in the Files of the Sterling-Winthrop Research Institute, Rensselaer, New York, 1979.

104. **Salvesen, S.,** Acute toxicity tests of metrizamide, *Acta Radiol.,* Suppl. 335, 5, 1973.

105. **Salvesen, S.,** Acute intravenous toxicity of iohexol in the mouse and in the rat, *Acta Radiol.,* Suppl. 362, 73, 1980.

106. **Mutzel, W. and Speck, U.,** Tolerance and biochemical pharmacology of iopromide, in *Contrast Media in Urography, Angiography and Computerized Tomography,* Taenzer, V. and Zeitler, E., Eds., Thieme-Stratton, New York, 1983, 11.

107. **Speck, U.,** personal communication.

THE VITAMINS

Richard A. Ferrari

VITAMINS AS A CLASS OF BIOLOGICALLY ACTIVE COMPOUNDS

A vitamin is an organic chemical compound that is required in very small amounts for the maintenance of health and for the preservation of life in the nutrition of animals and many microorganisms. Vitamins do not provide energy nor are they part of the structural elements of the body, but act as cofactors or other regulators of metabolism. They are present naturally in the diet of animals or the media of microorganisms and in some cases may be synthesized by intestinal bacteria, but are not normally accumulated within the body to any appreciable extent. A critically low intake of a vitamin will produce a particular set of clinically recognizable deficiency symptoms which can be corrected or reversed by the administration of that vitamin.

Casimir Funk, a Polish biochemist, gave the name "vitamine" to a substance that cured scurvy, beriberi, and pellagra.[1] While he was unable to determine its structure, he thought that it was an organic base or amine vital to life.

The major experimental thrust on the vitamins began in the early 1900s and culminated in the isolation of vitamin B_{12} in 1948.[2] However, early writings on the prevention of scurvy in the 1700s[3] by the inclusion of citrus fruit in the diet of seafarers antedated more modern investigations by some 200 years. The science of nutrition may be regarded as the father of biochemistry in that many of the water soluble vitamins were found to be cofactors in enzymatic reactions which were then assembled into metabolic pathways. During the investigative period, many vitamins were discovered, rediscovered, or discarded as invalid. This is exemplified by a numerical listing of the B complex vitamins (Table 1).[4-7] Great strides have been made recently in elucidating the molecular biology of the fat soluble vitamins after years of incomprehension.

VITAMIN A

Discovery and Nutritional Background

Independent investigations by McCollum and Davis,[8] and Osborne and Mendel[9] in 1913 provided evidence that a substance in butter fat and egg yolk when added to an otherwise adequate purified diet allowed young rats to grow normally. Olive oil and certain other vegetable oils did not contain this essential nutrient. However, McCollum and Davis[10] found that when saponified butter fat was extracted with a mixture of olive oil (lacking this substance) and ether, the olive oil remaining after the evaporation of the ether was now able to support growth in rats. They later named the lipid extractable substance, fat-soluble A.

Steenbock and Gross[11] in 1919 discovered that yellow colored vegetables such as carrots and sweet potatoes contained fat-soluble A whereas white vegetables such as potatoes and parsnips or red colored vegetables such as beets lacked this nutrient. This substance, named vitamin A, was thought to be associated with the yellow pigment, carotene, associated with these vegetables. This was only partly correct, because when pork liver, which was devoid of carotene and other yellow pigments, was added to pigment-free rations of white leghorn chicks, they grew normally and laid a normal number of eggs.[12] However, the yolks from these eggs lacked their usual yellow color. These and similar feeding experiments proved that vitamin A present in animal tissues was not synonymous with certain carotenoid pigments found in plant tissues.

The relationship between carotenes and vitamin A was established by Moore in 1929.[13] Purified carotene was fed to young rats made deficient in vitamin A. The livers of these

Table 1
THE B VITAMINS: PAST AND PRESENT

B	Mixture of B vitamins; original designation for "water soluble B"
B_1	Thiamin
B_2	Riboflavin
B_3	Older designation for pantothenic acid and later abandoned
B_4	A mixture which cured paralysis in rats and chicks, later abandoned
B_5	Properties similar to niacin, later abandoned
B_6	Pyridoxin
B_7	A mixture required for nutrition of pigeons, later abandoned
B_8	Identified as adenylic acid, later abandoned
B_9	Not used
B_{10}	Growth factor and feathering in chicks, later abandoned
B_{11}	Same as B_{10}, probably a mixture of B_{12} and folic acid
B_{12}	Cyanocobalamine
B_{13}	Identified as α-lipoic acid or orotic acid, designation later abandoned
B_{14}	Probably a metabolite of xanthopterin, unconfirmed
B_{15}	Pangamic acid, a pseudovitamin
B_{16}	Unknown
B_{17}	Laetrile, a pseudovitamin

rats contained vitamin A in nearly colorless form. Moore, therefore, proved that carotene was a precursor or provitamin of the vitamin A found in rat liver. This experiment explained how the chicks on a vitamin A-free ration grew normally and hatched eggs when supplemented with pork liver.

Isolation, Structure, and Chemical Synthesis

Steenbock's association of vitamin A and carotene and Moore's proof that carotene was pro-vitamin A led to the isolation of vitamin A (retinol) from saponified fish liver oil by Karrer and co-workers[14] in 1931. Having established the structure of β-carotene the year before, Karrer wrote the structure of vitamin A as being the 20 carbon alcohol derived from one half of the β-carotene molecule (see Figure 1). Physical properties of retinol are given in Table 2.

Two laboratories reported the chemical synthesis of retinol a year apart. Fuson and Christ[15] condensed β-cyclocitral with dimethyl acrolein to form an aldehyde which they reduced to vitamin A alcohol. Kuhn and Morris[16] condensed β-ionylidene acetaldehyde with β-methyl crotonaldehyde in the presence of piperidine to give the aldehyde which they reduced to retinol.

Deficiency

Vitamin A deficiency in young experimental animals is fairly easy to show.[17] Epithelial tissue of the skin lining the alimentary canal and in glandular ducts shows abnormally severe keratinization and metaplastic changes. Characteristic changes in eyes, xerophthalmia, take place. The conjunctiva of the inner eyelid and the outer coating of the cornea become dry, scaly or opaque resulting in blindness. Cells within the kidney medulla keratinize and renal calculi may form. Cornification of the lining of glandular ducts causes blockage and eventual loss of function. Respiratory tract infections occur. Bone growth fails to take place because of defective chondroitin sulfate synthesis. A deficiency of 3'-phosphoadenosine 5'-phosphosulfate which is required for sulfation of mucopolysaccharides may be the cause. In addition, lysosomal sulfatase may hasten chondroitin sulfate degradation. Poor bone development in the cranium and increased cerebrospinal fluid pressure lead to damage of the central nervous system.

In humans, an early sign of vitamin A deficiency is night blindness. This type of blindness

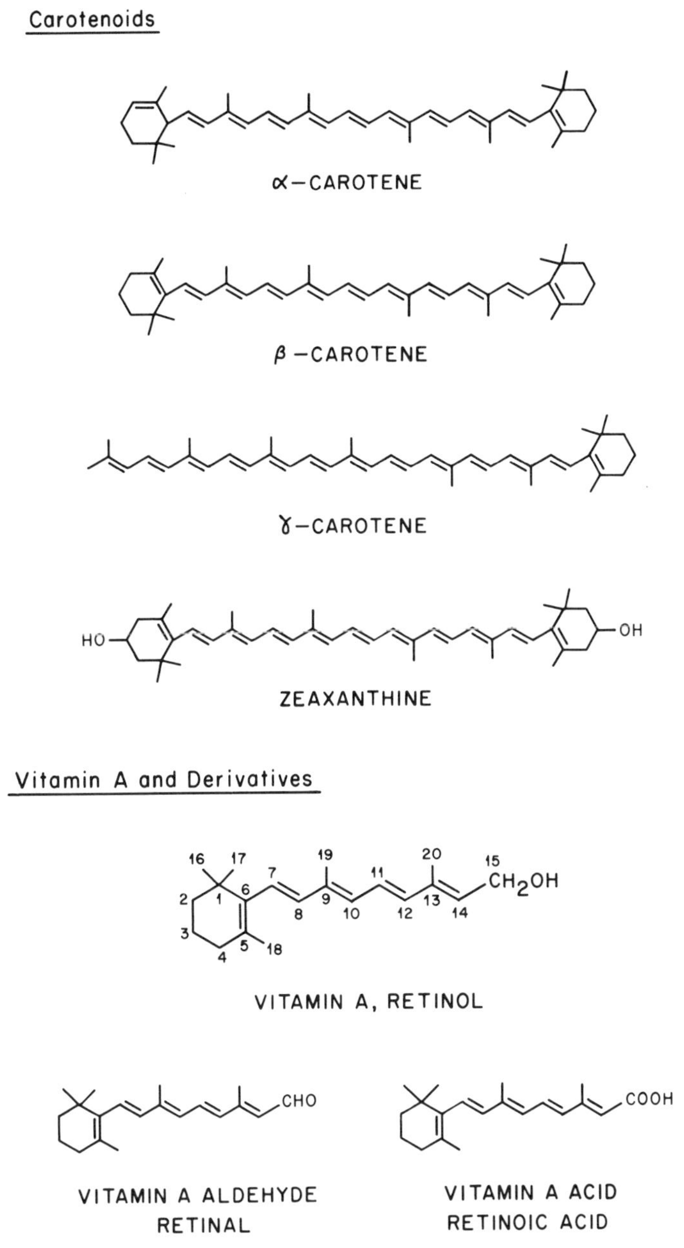

Carotenoids

α–CAROTENE

β–CAROTENE

ɣ–CAROTENE

ZEAXANTHINE

Vitamin A and Derivatives

VITAMIN A, RETINOL

VITAMIN A ALDEHYDE
RETINAL

VITAMIN A ACID
RETINOIC ACID

FIGURE 1. Carotenoids and vitamin A derivatives.

is not related to the hyperkeratotic xerophthalmia mentioned before, because the deficiency is in the visual pigment rhodopsin. Humans also may develop a hyperkeratotic infiltration of the pilosebaceous canal and sweat ducts with a layer of stratum corneum several times as thick as is normal.[18]

Reproduction in the males and females is impaired by vitamin A deficiency, due again to its effect in epithelial tissue. The germinal epithelium of the testes fails to develop or degenerates if already formed, resulting in arrested spermatogenesis. In the female, the vaginal epithelium becomes hyperkeratotic but, more importantly, the placenta fails to develop normally giving rise to stillborn or weak offspring.[19]

Table 2
PHYSICAL PROPERTIES OF THE VITAMINS

Vitamin	Solubility[186]	pK_a[187]	Mp[186]	Stability[32,186]
Vitamin A (retinol)	Insoluble in water Soluble in EtOH, ether, and oils	—	62—64°C	Unstable UV light, alkali and O_2; fairly stable to heat
Vitamin D_2 (calciferol)	Insoluble in water Soluble in organic solvents	—	84—85°C	Less stable at acid pH
Vitamin E (α-tocopherol)	Insoluble in water Soluble in fats and oils	—	2.5—3.5°C	Oxidized in air and light, rapidly by iron and silver salts
Vitamin K_1	Insoluble in water Soluble in benzene, and petroleum ether	—	An oil	Dec. light and alkali
Thiamin HCl	1 g/mℓ water	4.8 9.0	248°C dec.	Dec. aqueous soln.>pH5.5 or heat
Riboflavin	1 g/3000—15,000 mℓ H_2O; soluble in alkaline pH, slightly soluble in EtOH	10.2	278—288°C dec.	Dec. light and in alkaline soln.
Nicotinic Acid	1 g/60 mℓ H_2O Soluble in hot H_2O Insoluble in ether	4.85	236.6°C	Incompatible $NaNO_2$ Stable to heat, light, acid, or base
Nicotinamide	1 g/mℓ H_2O Soluble in ether	0.5 3.35	128—131°C	Fairly stable as above
Pyridoxine	1 g Hydrochloride/4.5 mℓ H_2O Insoluble in ether	5.0 8.96	160°C	Fairly stable in acid Soln. dec. in light
Folic Acid	Insoluble in cold H_2O Soluble in hot H_2O Insoluble in ether	8.26[188]	250°C dec.	Fairly stable in dil. acid and base; unstable to light and heat at acidic pH
Vitamin B_{12}	1 g/80 mℓ H_2O Soluble in EtOH Insoluble in ether	—	>300°C	Stable pH 4.5-5
Pantothenic Acid	Soluble in H_2O Mod. soluble in ether Insoluble in $CHCl_3$	4.4[189]	An oil	Unstable in acids, bases and heat
Biotin	1 g/4500 mℓ H_2O Soluble in MeOH, EtOH	—	232—233°C	Stable to heat and air
Ascorbic Acid	1 g/3 mℓ H_2O Soluble in EtOH Insoluble in ether	4.17 11.57	190—192°C	Oxidizes in air and light; more stable acid pH; unstable with copper and iron

Vitamin A deficiency in adults is less common because the liver acts as a store for the vitamin that may serve for a matter of years. Also, pure vitamin A deficiency is unlikely in a person consuming an inadequate diet. Multiple deficiencies would be expected.

Dietary Sources

Approximately 65% of the vitamin A in western diets is derived from carotenoids present in green leafy vegetables and fruits.[17] Vegetables particularly high in carotenoids are sweet potatoes, carrots, broccoli, spinach, swiss chard, winter squash, raw pepper, collards, turnips and other greens, and canned vegetable soups. Apricots, raw peaches, canned plums, and pumpkin are good fruit sources. Vitamin A content in the following meats, dairy products, and fish are high: chicken and beef liver including liverwurst, butter and cheese, crabmeat, swordfish and whitefish.[20]

The availability of vitamin A and the carotenoids is limited in individuals with malabsorption states such as steatorrhea. In underdeveloped countries in particular, absorption may be curtailed by the lack of dietary lipid which acts as a solvent for this fat soluble vitamin. Emulsification aids in absorption.

The vitamin A content of diets was previously expressed in international units. At present, recommended dietary allowances are expressed in terms of retinol equivalents. One retinol equivalent (R.E.) is 1 μg of retinol or 6 μg of β-carotene and 1 R.E. is 3.33 IU of vitamin A activity from retinol or 10 IU of activity from β-carotene.[21] The recommended dietary allowances range from 400 R.E. in children to 1000 R.E. in adult males.

Due to man's inefficient absorption of provitamin forms from the diet, about one third is considered to be utilized, giving figures which are lower than the analyzed amounts of the carotenoids. One must also take into account the vitamin A conversion factors for the carotenes and the xanthophylls. While retinol is fairly unstable (Table 2), β-carotene is more resistant to deterioration during food processing and storage.[22]

Structure-Activity Relationships

The structure of vitamin A or retinol, and two biologically active (but not equivalent) congeners are given in Figure 1. Retinol is considered to be the true vitamin. The aldehyde and acid forms are metabolic transformation products.[17] All three are classified as "retinoids". As was mentioned before, β-carotene from plant sources may serve as a precursor of vitamin A by being cleaved in half to form two molecules of retinol. Alpha- and gamma-carotenes give only one molecule of retinol since the opposite end of the molecule is dissimilar to the β-ionine ring of retinol. Vitamin A, as it occurs naturally, is in the all *trans* configuration.

Retinal (the aldehyde form) and retinol are readily interconvertible enzymatically. Retinoic acid is formed by an irreversible oxidation of the aldehyde and is on the pathway of excretion of vitamin A. However, retinoic acid can partially replace vitamin A in that it promotes bone growth and the growth of soft tissues.[17] It is able to sustain sperm production but not the maturation of embryos. Retinal functions as a precursor of 11-*cis* retinal which is a constituent of the visual pigment.[23] Retinol, the vitamin, is effective in all respects, namely, in growth promotion, differentiation and maintenance of epithelial tissue, reproductive processes, and in vision via retinal.

Biological and Therapeutic Effects of Retinoids

In 1926, the association of vitamin A deficiency and the development of neoplasms was made.[24] Further observations that vitamin A deficient diets led to precancerous cell changes that were corrected by vitamin A supplementation led ultimately to the examination of the various forms of the vitamin (Figure 1) and synthetic analogs for antineoplastic activity. More than 1500 retinoids have been synthesized and, of these, many have been studied extensively in the laboratory and the clinic.

Tretinoin

All *trans* retinoic acid (tretinoin) has been used successfully in the treatment of acne by accelerating the formation of loose keratinized cells within the pilosebaceous canal resulting in the expulsion of existing comedones. The acne condition worsened during the first 6 weeks of treatment due to skin irritation prior to improvement of the condition.[25] Tretinoin has also been used topically in other hyperkeratotic states, such as lamellar ichthyosis.[26] Topical retinoic acid treatment followed by topical glucocorticoid application was beneficial in the treatment of psoriasis.[27] The limiting factor in treating these hyperkeratotic skin conditions was irritation by tretinoin necessitating reducing the concentration or frequency of application.

13-cis Retinoic Acid

13-*cis* retinoic acid, called isotretinoin, has also been successfully used in the treatment of nodulocystic acne when given orally to patients.[28] The sebaceous glands were reduced in size and sebum secretion was markedly decreased. Unlike tretinoin, isotretinoin was ineffective in psoriasis. Isotretinoin was also found useful in the treatment of other skin diseases characterized by disordered epidermal cell growth and differentiation such as lamellar ichthyosis, epidermolytic hyperkeratosis (both diseases characterized by excessive scaly skin production), and Darier's disease (papules developing into scaly encrustations).[29]

Isotretinoin has been found to have antineoplastic activity without the cytotoxicity associated with classical chemotherapeutic agents.[30] For example, isotretinoin inhibited the clonal growth of two human myeloid leukemia cell lines.[31] This property was shared with tretinoin, but the *cis* form is less toxic to the liver.[24]

Etretinate

This wholly synthetic vitamin A analog has an aromatic ring. Etretinate given orally produced a good to excellent response in 43% of 751 patients with psoriasis.[29] Since this disease responds initially to most treatments and long term remissions are difficult to obtain, clinical testing in many long term trials will be necessary to be convincing. It is interesting, in terms of specificity, that etretinate had no effect in acne patients.[29]

Vitamin A Antagonists

The toxic reactions to sodium benzoate, bromobenzene, or citral in rats were reversed by large amounts of vitamin A.[32] The mechanisms of the toxic effects were not known.

Mechanism of Action

The involvement of vitamin A aldehyde (retinal) in the visual process developed from the work of Wald and co-workers.[3] All *trans*-retinol stored in the liver is isomerized to the 11-*cis* form. Retinol is transported from the liver to the visual pigment receptor, opsin, in the eye bound to a protein called retinol-binding protein of the plasma. This binding protein can also transport the *cis*- or *trans*-isomers of retinal. The 11-*cis* form of retinol and retinal are interconvertible in the retina by retinal reductase using either NAD or NADP as cofactors with the equilibrium in favor of the alcohol. The combination of 11-*cis* retinal with the membrane bound glycoprotein opsin at the ϵ-amino group of an exposed lysine residue to form the visual pigment rhodopsin is an energy-yielding, spontaneous reaction and results in a conformational change of the protein.[17] *Trans*-retinal cannot form this bond. A photon entering the eye causes dissociation of rhodopsin through a series of transformations that can be observed spectrophotometrically by slowing down the reaction at very cold temperatures. The product *trans*-retinal can be reisomerized and used again or it can be reduced to retinol and re-enter the cycle.

Some of the above steps are still unclear, but studies within the past 2 years[23] have shown that there are two other light catalyzed reactions. These are the phosphorylation of rhodopsin and activation of the enzyme cGMP phosphodiesterase. It has also been found that photolysis of rhodopsin leads to the closing of sodium channels in the membrane of the rod cell together with an increased expulsion of calcium ions to the extracellular space. The involvement of the phosphodiesterase is attractive, because activation of this enzyme occurs within 125 msec of light excitation of rhodopsin and the event is amplified by the concomitant disappearance of 50,000 molecules of cGMP. The reaction sequences and which one is primary or secondary have yet to be established.

Cone vision differs from rod vision, given above, by the presence of at least three different pigments in separate structures to account for the detection of color. Pigments with absorption maxima in the blue (430 nm), green (540 nm), and red (575 nm) regions have been found.[17]

11-*cis* Retinal appears to function in each type of cone, but the type of protein in the opsin may be different. In hereditary color blindness, one or another of the types of opsins may be missing. The red and green opsins appear to be linked to the X chromosome.[17]

One of the major functions of vitamin A is in maintaining the integrity of epithelial tissue. It has been shown in the past 10 years, that vitamin A regulates the glycosylation of epithelial proteins. Vitamin A regulated the incorporation of glucosamine into glycoproteins in the cornea and conjunctiva of the eye.[33] In another epithelial system, the incorporation of mannose into membrane glycoproteins was mediated by mannosylretinylphosphate. This carrier of mannose residues was synthesized from guanosine diphosphate mannose and retinylphosphate by an enzyme in rat liver microsomes.[34]

A review by Zile and Cullum[35] presents current models of vitamin A action in the areas of growth, differentiation, reproduction, vision, and membrane structure and function. Investigators are looking for a molecular basis of action for retinoids in these phenomena. In particular, they are interested in cellular retinoid receptors, isomerization reactions in pathways other than vision, electron transfer reactions along the conjugated double bond chain of retinoids, and the modification of gene expression by binding to nucleoproteins. With respect to the latter, there is epidemiological evidence that maintenance of sufficient (but not excessive) vitamin A stores protects against lung cancer in smokers.[35]

Biosynthesis

Beta-carotene biosynthesis parallels that for sterols initially. Mevalonate is phosphorylated by ATP in green plants to form mevalonate-5-phosphate, mevalonate-5-pyrophosphate and isopentenyl pyrophosphate and then isomerization to dimethylallyl pyrophosphate takes place. This product is the precursor for the formation of carotenes and sterols. Dimethylallyl pyrophosphate condenses with isopentenyl pyrophosphate to form geranyl pyrophosphate. At this point the pathways for sterol and carotinoid biosynthesis diverge. Geranyl pyrophosphate is converted to farnesyl pyrophosphate for sterol synthesis, but in carotenoid biosynthesis two molecules of geranyl pyrophosphate condense to form geranyl geranyl pyrophosphate which condenses with itself enzymatically to form phytoene. Phytoene is desaturated stepwise to form lycopene which cyclizes on one end to form α-carotene and then on the other end to give β-carotene (Figure 1).[36]

Pharmacokinetics

The major site for the conversion of carotenoids to vitamin A is in the intestinal tract by the enzyme 15,15'-dioxygenase which requires iron and NADH or NADPH.[17] Vitamin A then passes through the intestinal wall and is transported to the liver dissolved in the lipids of the chylomicrons.[37] Vitamin A is stored in the liver as retinyl palmitate, mainly, and mobilized by being hydrolyzed and bound to a specific retinol binding protein (RBP).[38] The vitamin A-RBP complex then combines with prealbumin in the plasma for transport in the circulatory system to specific receptor sites in target tissues where the complex is broken down and vitamin A enters the cell perhaps to be phosphorylated and glycosylated to perform its metabolic role.[37] The RBP is released, re-enters the circulation where it exhibits less affinity for prealbumin than before, and binds to more vitamin A in the liver. The structure of RBP has been described.[37] Vitamin A toxicity was suggested to occur when the vitamin A circulates in a form not bound to RBP and interacts with cells in a different manner.[38]

The degradation of spent vitamin A occurs via retinoic acid produced by oxidation of the terminal alcohol group probably in the tissues on which it acts. Sixty percent or more of the metabolites appear in the bile and only 12% of these is the β-glucuronide. The remainder appear to be polar metabolites not yet identified.[39] 5,6-Epoxyretinoic acid, and an intermediate in one of the metabolic pathways 13-*cis*-4-oxoretinoic acid have been identified.[40] 13-*cis* Retinoic acid appears to be metabolized much like the all-*trans* form but the proportion of metabolites was different.[41] Many of the metabolites have yet to be identified.

Toxicity

Vitamin A and β-carotene have the potential of becoming overused to the extent that vitamin C is today. The antineoplastic activity of vitamin A was alluded to earlier under the heading Biological and Therapeutic Effects of Retinoids. They have been shown to antagonize the effects of carcinogens on cells or to reverse their neoplastic activity, to act as inhibitors of tumor growth, and to act as adjuvants in stimulating host cell mediated immunity.[42] Since vitamin A is involved in epithelial cell differentiation, its influence on epidermal disorders is paramount. Toxic doses of vitamin A, 1 million IU, were given for short periods of time, 5 to 14 days, to patients with pityriasis rubra pilaris[43] or with Darier's disease.[44] The hyperkeratotic and keratodermatous lesions in pityriasis rubra pilaris peeled leaving smooth, normal underlying skin. The patients with Darier's disease also experienced some desquamation of the limbs and trunk as part of the treatment.

β-Carotene has also been suggested for cancer prevention and treatment.[45] It was thought that this substance would be much less toxic than vitamin A when ingested in quantities up to 350 mg/day for a 70 kg person.

Hypervitaminosis A following a meal of polar bear or seal liver by Arctic explorers is the most dramatic illustration of acute toxic effects of this vitamin. The symptoms of acute toxicity are headaches, stomach ache, nausea, and dizziness.[46] The majority of cases are from chronic ingestion of the vitamin or its precursors. The list of symptoms includes dryness of the skin, rashes, fissures of the skin, and generalized desquamation. High intake of β-carotene resulted in yellow to orange colored skin.[46] High vitamin A intake also caused liver damage, neurological damage including increased intracranial pressure and hydrocephalus in children, thyroid suppression, muscle stiffness, mental changes, teratogenic effects in experimental animals, and pain in the bones and joints.[47]

One report[48] advocated the administration of a β-cyclodextrin analog after retinoic acid treatment in order to reduce the toxic effects of this retinoid. Concurrent administration, however, increased toxicity.

Vitamin A and the other fat soluble vitamins are stored by the body, especially in the liver and depot body fat. The carotenoids are stored in the fat especially.[49]

VITAMIN D

History and Nutritional Background

According to McCollum,[3] the beneficial effect of sunlight on bone development was recorded by the Greek historian Herodotus (484 to 425 B.C.), who examined the skulls of Persians and Egyptians slain on a battlefield many years before. The skulls of the Persians were very thin whereas the Egyptian skulls were thicker. Some Egyptians in the region said that this was caused by the Persians wearing turbans whereas the Egyptians went bareheaded, exposing themselves to sunlight. Francis Glisson in 1650 wrote of the bone deformities characteristic in England at that time called rickets. He said the name came from the archaic English word *wrikken,* which meant bent or twisted.[3]

Schuette may have been the first one to use cod liver oil therapeutically for rickets in 1824, but its success rate was variable and not well accepted. It was almost 100 years later that the antirachitic factor in cod liver oil was discovered.

Mellanby in the 1920s conducted feeding experiments with puppies employing diets containing the three accessory nutrients known at that time, vitamin A, water soluble B which cured beriberi, and vitamin C, the antiscorbutic substance. Mellanby thought that rickets was caused by a toxic component in cereals he called "toxamine" which prevented the proper deposition of calcium and phosphorus in bone.[3] Experiments with butterfat and cod liver oil by McCollum and co-workers provided evidence that there was another fat soluble factor in cod liver oil besides vitamin A and that this substance was the one responsible for the prevention of rickets in young animals. Both butterfat and cod liver oil prevented xerophthalmia in growing rats but only cod liver oil prevented rickets. When oxygen was passed through these heated oils, the vitamin A value was destroyed but the antirachitic activity was stable. McCollum named this new substance vitamin D since it was the fourth accessory nutrient found.[3]

Isolation, Structures, and Chemical Synthesis

Pure vitamin D was first isolated in 1930 by Askew and co-workers[50] from irradiated ergosterol by fractional distillation and crystallization. The isolation procedure for the D vitamins from natural sources or irradiated sterol mixtures is a multistep process involving saponification, chromatographic removal of vitamin A, concentration and elution by adsorption chromatography, esterification and fractional crystallization of the esters followed by hydrolysis of the ester to obtain the pure vitamin.[5]

The structural formulas of some of the more important forms of the D vitamins and their precursors are given in Figure 2. Ergosterol is a plant sterol. Calciferol is made by irradiating ergosterol with UV light. This form of the vitamin is commonly used for dietary supplementation. The physical properties of calciferol are given in Table 2.

The total synthesis of vitamin D_3 has been accomplished by two laboratories; each process entails over 20 steps.[5]

Deficiency

Rickets is an abnormality of bone growth. The formation of the bone matrix continues, but the zone of calcification is poorly defined and the deposition of calcium and phosphate especially at the epiphyses to comprise a mineralized, fully rigid structure fails to take place.[51,52] The long bones of the legs display curvature due to the weight placed on them and later harden in this configuration. Osteomalacia is the vitamin D deficiency disease in adults. Bone is a metabolically active tissue undergoing renewal and repair constantly. In the absence of vitamin D and calcium, the bones lose calcium in order to maintain normal plasma levels and to prevent tetany.[51] Therefore, vitamin D appears to be necessary for absorption of calcium from the intestinal tract, for calcification of growing or regenerating bones with parathyroid hormone, and for the maintenance of plasma calcium levels.[51]

Dietary Sources

Dietary sources of previtamin D and vitamin D are secondary in importance to the formation of this vitamin by UV irradiation of the skin surface. It is believed that exposure of the skin to sunlight in the summer months greatly reduces the dependence on a dietary source for this vitamin.[21]

Foods rich in vitamin D are fish liver oils, liver, and eggs. Vitamin D has the narrowest distribution of any vitamin. Daily requirements are for 5 to 10 µg of vitamin D_3, or its equivalent. Since vitamin D is sensitive to oxygen and light, food storage and processing should take this into account.[22]

Structure-Activity Relationships

Structures of the different active forms of the vitamin and previtamins are found in Figure 2. The fully active form, 1,25-dihydroxy vitamin D, can be made from either vitamin D_3 or 25-hydroxy-D_3 in people with normal liver and kidney function. The activity of the synthetic compound alfacalcidol (Figure 3) is one half that of $1,25(OH)_2D_3$, because it is not quantitatively converted.[51]

1α-Hydroxy vitamin D_2 and the D_3 analogs are equally active in intestinal transport of calcium and in bone mineralization, but 1α(OH)-D_2 has only one fifth the calcium mobilization properties as alfacalcidol which would be desirable in osteoporosis patients where

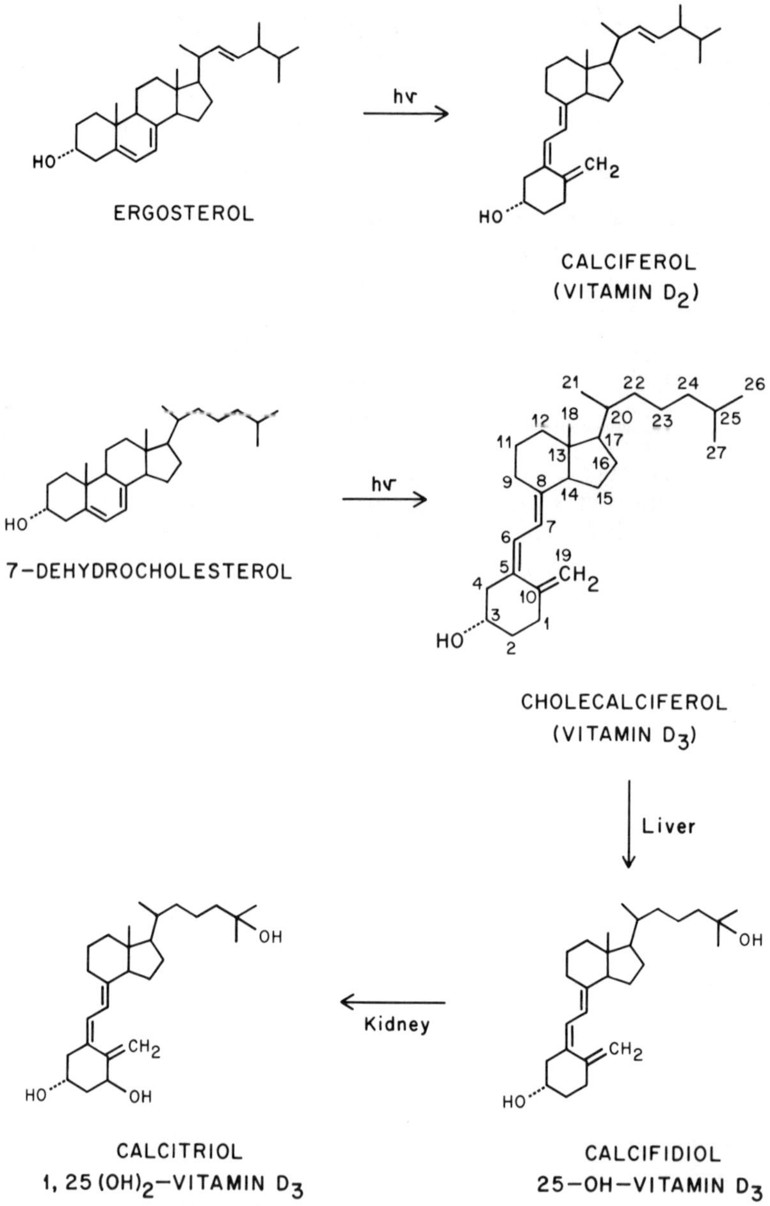

FIGURE 2.   Structural formulas of vitamin D and biosynthetic pathway.

mobilization of bone would be a handicap.[51] Dihydrotachysterol is about three times as potent as vitamin D_2 and of shorter duration of action.[53]

Certain fluoro analogs of vitamin D_3 have been tested and found to have potent biological activity in inducing a calcium binding protein in tissue culture. The compound 24,24-difluoro-1,25(OH)$_2$ vitamin D3 (Figure 3) is about four times as potent as 1,25(OH)$_2$D$_3$ and is the most potent compound found yet in this test system.[54] It is also at least as potent as 1,25(OH)$_2$D$_3$ in stimulating calcium absorption in the intestine and in calcium mobilization from bone.

Vitamin Antagonists

Two compounds synthesized as antagonists of the 25-hydroxylase enzyme in liver proved

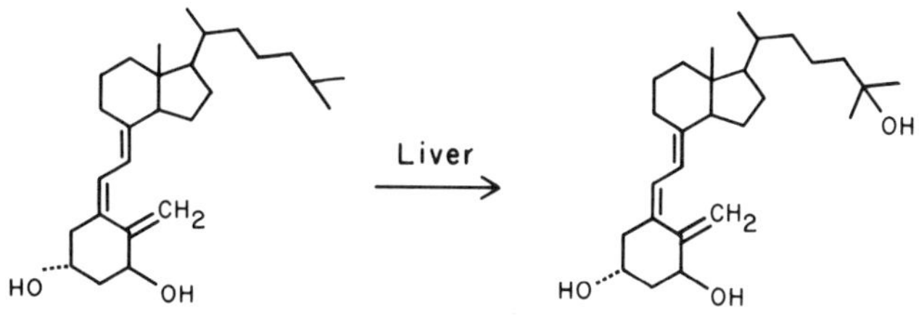

1α (OH) Vitamin D_3
(Alfacalcidol)

1,25 $(OH)_2$–Vitamin D_3

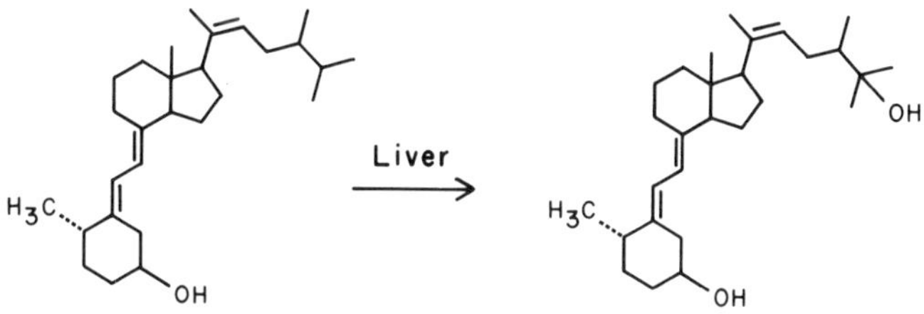

Dihydrotachysterol

25 (OH) Dihydrotachysterol

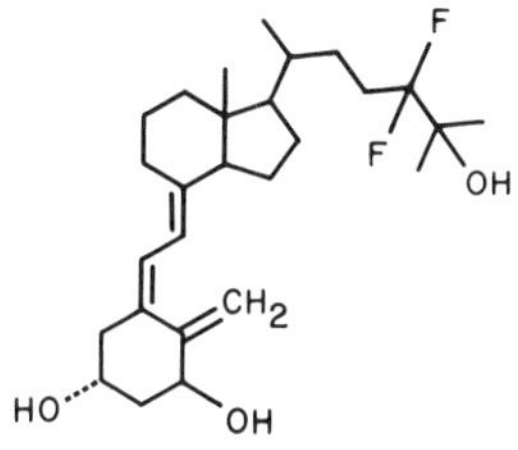

24,24–F_2–1α,25$(OH)_2$–
Vitamin D_3

FIGURE 3. Synthetic analogs of the D vitamins.

to be physiological antagonists of vitamin D_3. 25-Azavitamin D_3 and 19-hydroxy-(10S)-19-dihydrovitamin D_3 (Figure 4) were effective antagonists with potential use in hypercalcemic patients.[51]

Mechanism of Action

Vitamin D is transformed by the liver and kidney to the active form 1,25-$(OH)_2$-D_3 which is transported to distant sites where it acts. In this context, vitamin D is a hormone in the classic sense. In target tissues 1,25-$(OH)_2$-D_3 binds to a high affinity receptor. The affinity of this receptor for the different analogs of vitamin D parallels their biological activities.[55] Also, there is a lag period between feeding vitamin D and biological effect, e.g., uptake of calcium by the intestine, indicating that metabolic transformations are necessary prior to initiating intracellular events.[56,57] It has been shown that oral vitamin D is absorbed from the rat intestine into the lymph and 90% is associated with chylomicrons. When lymph mixes with blood, the vitamin D is transferred to an α-globulin.[58] The target tissues for this

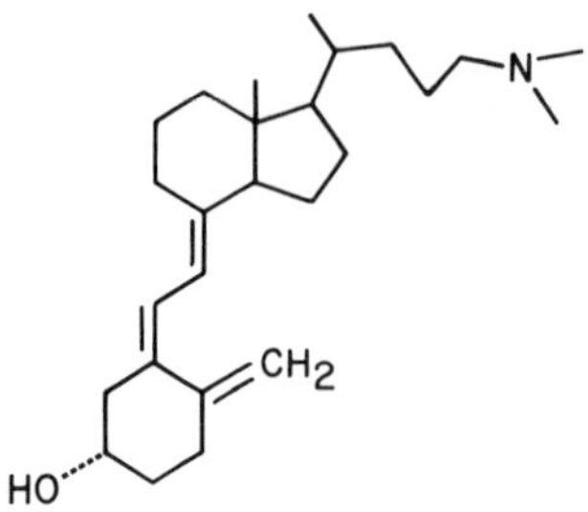

25-Aza Vitamin D$_3$ 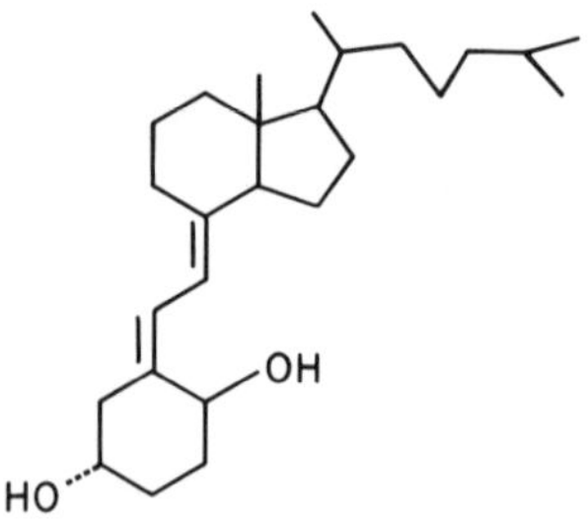   19(OH)-(10S)-19-Dihydro Vitamin D$_3$

FIGURE 4.   Other vitamin D analogs.

vitamin so far identified are intestinal villi, osteoblasts of bone, parathyroid gland, glandular cells of the stomach, certain cells of the pituitary, epidermis of the skin, renal tubules, cells in the pancreas,[51] placenta,[59] and chick embryo chorioallantoic membrane.[55]

The hormone receptor complex in the target tissue is transferred from the cytosol to the nuclear compartment where the expected hormone-mediated events take place, namely the synthesis of a protein which binds calcium.[51] Inhibitors of *de novo* protein and RNA synthesis block calcium transport.[57,60] Other investigators contend that calcium binding protein itself is not responsible for calcium transport but that it induces an alteration in brush border membrane structure to increase its fluidity, thereby allowing calcium to pass through the membrane.[61] The mechanism of calcium transport is being actively pursued and has yet to be resolved.

Vitamin D also regulates phosphate absorption and transport. Under conditions of low blood phosphate levels, 1,25-$(OH)_2D_3$ concentration in blood is increased.[51] Therefore, vitamin D regulates the utilization of both minerals that give bone its rigidity.

Biosynthesis of the D Vitamins

Cholesterol biosynthesis[17] from acetyl coenzyme A in liver and skin takes place by the condensation and cyclization of six mevalonic acid units to form squalene and then lanosterol. At this point, the pathway splits. One branch leads to desmosterol and the other to 7-dehydrocholesterol immediately prior to formation of cholesterol. 7-Dehydrocholesterol in skin is the immediate precursor of cholecalciferol (vitamin D$_3$). The precursor may also be made by the dehydrogenation of cholesterol in the intestine. Upon exposure to UV light from the sun, the B ring is split yielding vitamin D$_3$. Ergosterol synthesized by yeast and certain other plants has an additional methyl group at C-24 derived from *S*-adenosylmethionine. UV irradiation of ergosterol produces vitamin D$_2$ (Figure 2).

Vitamins D$_2$ and D$_3$ are further metabolized by identical pathways. The above vitamins are hydroxylated in the 25 position (Figure 2) by a microsomal, flavoprotein mixed function oxidase and cytochrome P-450.[51] This reaction takes place in the liver. The 25-OH vitamin D then circulates to the kidney where it is 1α-hydroxylated in mitochondria by an enzyme requiring NADPH, ferredoxin, and cytochrome P-450. Calcitriol is the most potent member of the D vitamin family.

Certain synthetic analogs of vitamin D also have biological activity after being converted to active forms in the body. Alfacalcidol and dihydrotachysterol are ultimately metabolized into more active compounds by the liver (Figure 3).[51,53,62]

Pharmacokinetics

It was noted earlier that most of the vitamin D requirements may be normally met by exposure of endogenous 7-dehydrocholesterol in the skin to sunlight. Absorption of dietary vitamin dissolved in dietary fat is taken into the lymphatic system from the intestine in the chylomicron fraction.[58] When the lymph mixes with blood, vitamin D is transferred to the α-globulin fraction for transport. 25-OH vitamin D_3 and 24,25-OH_2 vitamin D_3 has greater affinity for this binding protein than vitamin D_3 or 1α,25-$(OH)_2$vitamin D_3.[58] The major circulating form of the vitamin was found to be 25-OH vitamin D_3.[51]

Further metabolism of 1,25$(OH)_2$ vitamin D_3 to 1,24,25$(OH)_3$ vitamin D_3 and then to the 24-carboxy derivative is known, but whether or not these represent the final excretion products is still under investigation. Present evidence indicates that the major route of excretion of the vitamin is via the bile with minor amounts present in the urine.[51]

Toxicity

One review on vitamin toxicity stated that vitamin D was probably the most toxic of the vitamins when used in excess and that cases of overuse exceed vitamin D deficiency.[63] Hypervitaminosis D results in hypercalcemia, greater renal tubular absorption of calcium, and increased demineralization of bone. This decalcification leaves the individual with greater risk of stress fractures. These effects were reported to be due to calcidiol rather than calcitriol.[64] If vitamin D is used to treat osteoporosis, care should be taken not to aggravate the condition by this seemingly anomalous behavior of the vitamin.

The toxicity of vitamin D is due mainly to the deposition of calcium in soft tissue such as renal tubules, blood vessels, the heart, pancreas, lungs, and gastric mucosa. Death, when it occurs, arises from renal failure.[60] Symptoms of hypervitaminosis D include hypertension, nausea, loss of appetite, and weakness. This fat soluble vitamin is stored in adipose tissue in mammals and in the liver of fish. Treatment for vitamin D overdosing includes corticosteroids as well as decreased calcium and vitamin D intake.[63]

VITAMIN E

Discovery and Nutritional Background

Prior to 1923, four vitamins were known to exist. They were vitamins A, B, C, and D. During this period, experimentation with semipurified rations took place. Diets that were adequate for growth and maintenance and which contained sources of these four vitamins were found to be deficient in terms of reproduction. Sterility, fetal death followed by resorption of the fetus, stillbirth or premature delivery, and failure of the newborn to survive were observed. Cows fed only wheat or oats failed to deliver live young. Rats fed cow's milk supplemented with iron appeared to be normal in terms of growth, but were often sterile. Matill and co-workers ascribed the problem to a substance required for reproductive development that was missing in milk.[3] This substance was named "Factor X".

In 1923, Evans and Scott found that supplementing rat feed with fresh lettuce, wheat germ, or alfalfa cured this deficiency. They systematically ruled out the involvement of vitamins A, B, C, and D. At the same time Sure found that adding velvet bean pods, polished rice, rolled oats, and yellow corn to the ration corrected reproductive failure. He named this "substance X" vitamin E, the fertility vitamin, as being the next micronutrient described for proper nutrition of animals.[5] The name tocopherol was derived from the Greek words "tokos", childbirth, and "phero", to bear.

Isolation, Structures, and Chemical Synthesis

In 1931, Olcott and Matill found an antioxidant fraction of lettuce oil that was able to serve as a potent source of vitamin E. In 1936, Evans and co-workers fractionated wheat germ oil and found an equally effective source of this vitamin which was called α-tocopherol.[3] The physical properties are given in Table 2.

Fernholtz in 1938 heated and oxidized α-tocopherol to fragments which enabled him to propose a structure for vitamin E (Figure 5). A year later, Karrer who deduced the structure

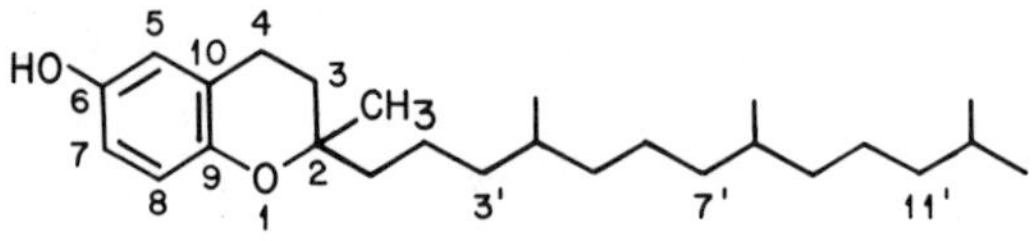

Tocol

α − Tocopherol	5, 7, 8 − Trimethyltocol
β − Tocopherol	5, 8 − Dimethyltocol
γ − Tocopherol	7, 8 − Dimethyltocol
δ − Tocopherol	8 − Methyltocol
ζ − Tocopherol	5, 7, 8 − Trimethyltocol−3′,7′,11′−trienol
ε − Tocopherol	5, 8 − Dimethyltocol−3′,7′, 11′−trienol
η − Tocopherol	7, 8 − Dimethyltocol−3′, 7′, 11′−trienol
8 − Methyl − tocopherol	8 − Methyltocol−3′, 7′, 11′− trienol

FIGURE 5.   Naturally occurring tocopherols.

of vitamin A, successfully synthesized α-tocopherol and proved that it had the biological properties of vitamin E.[3] Trimethylhydroquinone was condensed with phytyl bromide in the presence of anhydrous zinc chloride. The product was only half as active biologically as the natural product. Consequently, the diasterioisomers made by reacting with 3-bromo-(+)-camphorsulfonyl chloride were separated, one of which had the expected biological potency.[5]

Eight naturally occurring tocopherols were found.[65] Each is named here as a derivative of tocol, a synthetic compound, consisting of a chromane ring structure and a phytol side chain (Figure 5).

Deficiency

Evans and Bishop in 1922[3] found that the rat fetus was normal up to the 8th day of gestation at which point a deformed liver and abnormalities in heart and blood vessels began to emerge. Death by oxygen deprivation occurred near the 13th day. They were able to distinguish these anatomical findings as being unique to vitamin E deficiency.

Other deficiency symptoms were paralysis of the hind limbs of rats, rabbits, and guinea pigs born of mothers given a ration which was supplemented with just enough vitamin E to allow survival of the offspring. Creatinuria developed and histological examination of the affected muscle tissue revealed pigmented ceroid spots and degeneration like that seen in muscular dystrophy. Administration of vitamin E supplements cured this condition. Muscular dystrophy in humans was not cured by administering vitamin E.[66] Therefore, vitamin E deficiency in animals is not an animal model for human muscular dystrophy.

Many of the deficiency symptoms seem to be related to the antioxidant activity of the tocopherols. Incorporating highly unsaturated fats or rancid fats in the ration of experimental animals caused the symptoms of vitamin E deficiency: loss of hair, skin lesions, anorexia, emaciation, intestinal hemorrhages, muscle and nerve lesions, and exudative diathesis in chicks. Giving vitamin E supplements at the same time as the oxidized or polyunsaturated lipids did not prevent the symptoms, because the vitamin E was destroyed on contact with the lipids. However, if the vitamin E was given the day before and the day after feeding these lipids, protection against the deficiency occurred.

It used to be said that there was no known nutritional requirement for vitamin E in humans and that deficiency symptoms could only be demonstrated in animals. This was largely true because the fat soluble vitamin stores in the liver and adipose tissue provided sufficient reserves of the vitamin for long periods. Also, since vitamin E was broadly distributed in normal diets, there was little chance of avoiding this vitamin. However, cases of vitamin E deficiency disease in children have appeared in which there was chronic liver disease, malabsorption syndrome,[67] or in which low birth weight children were fed formulas with a low ratio of vitamin E to polyunsaturated lipids.[68]

Six children with cholestatic liver disease with vitamin E malabsorption developed muscular weakness and neurologic damage over a period of several years. Oral supplements of vitamin E did not produce normal circulating levels of this vitamin. Low birth weight children on formulas low in vitamin E developed anemia, reticulocytosis, thrombocytosis, decreased red blood cell survival time, and edema. Oral vitamin E therapy reversed these deficiency signs in part but not completely, because of poor intestinal absorption of the vitamin. As a result of these observations and those of others in patients in special predicaments, the human requirement for vitamin E has been documented. A firm value for the recommended allowance in normal individuals, however, is difficult to establish.

Dietary Sources

The tocopherols are widely distributed in nature. Good sources are vegetable oils, whole grain cereals and cereal products, eggs, butter, liver, and legumes. The most concentrated natural source is wheat germ oil. Fish liver oils do not contain tocopherols. Conventional cooking techniques do not destroy an appreciable amount of α-tocopherol. However, cooking in copper vessels or high temperature processing in vegetable oil should be avoided.[22]

The recommended dietary allowance for vitamin E is 8 to 10 mg of α-tocopherol equivalents for women and men, respectively. Dietary intake of this vitamin is dependent upon the level of polyunsaturated fats ingested and other factors such as concomitant large dosages of other vitamins. Alpha-tocopherol units are equivalent to milligrams of d-α-tocopherol acetate and 1 mg of this form of the vitamin equals 1 international unit (I.U.), an earlier designation of units of activity.[21] The synthetic and natural forms of vitamin E are equivalent when expressed in terms of the unesterified d-isomer.

Structure-Activity Relationships

There are three sites of stereoisomerism in the tocopherols, position 2 on the chromane ring and positions 4' and 8' on the phytyl chain.[69] Changes in configuration on the side chain did not change biological activity very much, but a change from the d to l configuration at ring carbon atom number 2 did. The d isomer was the naturally occurring one. d-α-Tocopherol had the greatest activity in preventing resorption and in maintaining gestation or in preventing hemolysis in vivo. The activity fell off in the following order: d-α>d-β>d-ζ>d-γ>d-ϵ>d-η>d-δ tocopherol with relative potencies of 135, 54, 29, 11, 5, 3, and 1, respectively.[69]

Biological activity was recorded for α-tocopherolquinone[70] and α-tocopherolhydroquinone.[71] These compounds were able to re-establish fertility in rats on a vitamin E deficient diet at a dose of 5 mg orally and 5 mg i.p. per rat during gestation.

Smith et al.[72] synthesized α-tocopheramine in 1942 and reported that it had biological activity comparable to α-tocopherol in the gestation-resorption test. This synthetic compound differs from α-tocopherol in having an amino group substituted for the hydroxyl on position 6 of the chromane ring (Figure 6). Schwieter and co-workers[73] synthesized α-tocopheramine and 15 analogs of it and showed that two had biological activity in preventing hemolysis. These were d,l-N-methyl-β-tocopheramine and d,l-N-methyl-γ-tocopheramine (Figure 6). Bieri and Prival[74] further characterized these compounds and found them to be equal in potency to d,l-α-tocopherol in preventing exudative diathesis in chicks. Blood levels in rats

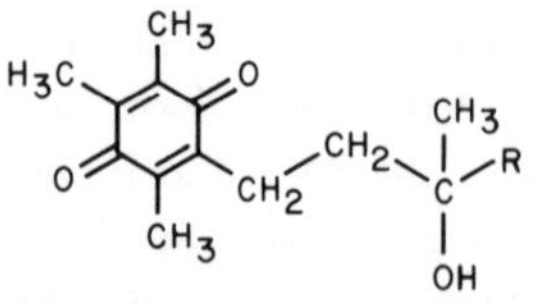

α-Tocopherylquinone

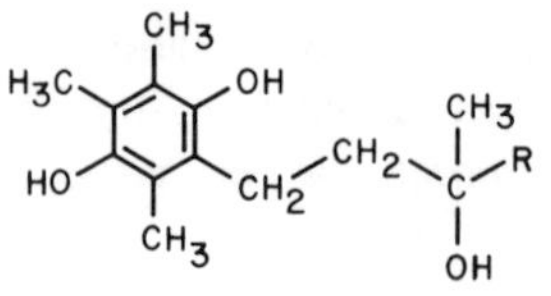

α-Tocopherylhydroquinone

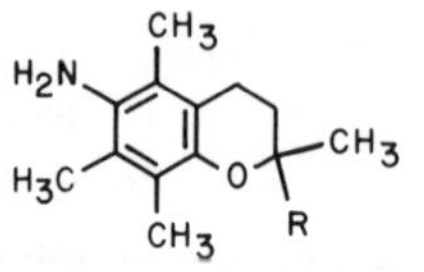

α-Tocopheramine

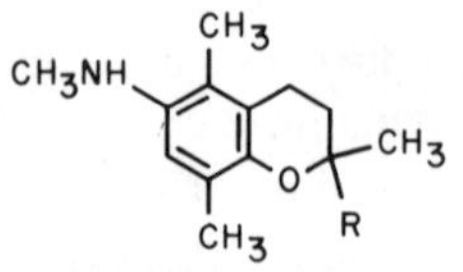

N-Methyl-β-Tocopheramine

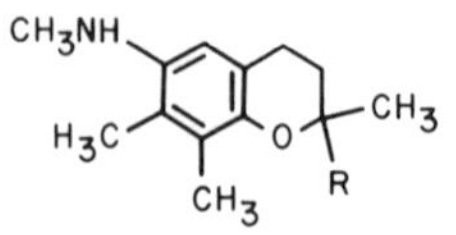

N-Methyl-γ-Tocopheramine

R = 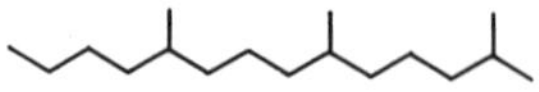

FIGURE 6. Analogs of tocopherol.

given equal doses of *N*-methyl-β and *N*-methyl-γ-tocopheramine were one half that of α-tocopherol, but they were stored in liver at twice the concentration of the natural vitamin. Analysis of liver fractions showed the same distribution as for α-tocopherol and, moreover, neither compound had been converted to its corresponding tocopherol. Wasserman and Taylor[68] concluded that the tocopherols must have three methyl groups either all on the ring or two on the ring and one on the amino group for optimal activity.

Vitamin Antagonists

Whether or not α-tocopheroquinone mentioned in the previous section is an antagonist of α-tocopherol is questionable. The biologically effective dose and the toxic dose possibly causing this antagonism may be close. Other antagonists listed are oxidizing agents. Since one mechanism of action of the tocopherols (see below) is as an antioxidant, this activity is nonspecific.

Mechanism of Action

The cellular function of tocopherols has not been firmly established, but various modes of action have been recorded. The mode of action with the greatest amount of evidence is that vitamin E and selenium act in adipose tissue, in plasma lipoproteins, and in the membranes of mitochondria and cell membranes, including those of erythrocytes, as antioxidants to maintain their integrity against assaults by peroxidized polyunsaturated fatty acids and other peroxides generated during metabolism. The yellow-brown ceroid pigment found in certain human organs is probably polymerized peroxides of fatty acids. In experimental animals these pigment deposits can be prevented from forming by adequate levels of vitamin E or other antioxidants or by reducing the intake of unsaturated fats. The requirement for α-tocopherol is directly proportional to the dietary level of polyunsaturated fat. Consequently, people who alter their diet in favor of polyunsaturated fats in order to prevent coronary artery disease require more than the minimal amount of vitamin E.[66]

The types of diseases prevented by vitamin E, selenium, antioxidants, or a combination of these agents have been listed by Scott.[75] Vitamin E cannot be replaced by any other agent in prevention of male sterility in a number of animal species nor for prevention of nutritional muscular dystrophy. Therefore, the role of vitamin E is distinct and not just due to antioxidant activity per se. Other mechanisms of action suggested, such as possible involvement in enzymatic reactions, have not been proven as yet.

Biosynthesis of the Tocopherols

The tocopherols are synthesized in green plants, algae, and some fungi. In photosynthetic plants, the most widespread form is α-tocopherol and it is localized mainly in the chloroplasts.[76] The pathways were studied using etiolated seedlings — seedlings grown in the dark — since they are very active metabolically and readily absorb various radioactive precursors. precursors.

Biosynthesis of the aromatic ring may take place via shikimic acid and is deduced from the pathway found in *Escherichia coli*. The participation of homogentisic acid has been established but from that step forward to γ-tocotrienol is still uncertain.[76] The condensation of isoprene units to form the side chain and chromenol ring formation by cyclization of the quinone is under investigation.

Pharmacokinetics

Vitamin E is absorbed in the intestinal tract by passive diffusion.[77] The rate of absorption is linear with concentration. Since this vitamin is insoluble in aqueous media, lipids need to be present for proper solubilization and transport through the lumen of the intestine. Fatty acids and bile acids form micelles with vitamin E. Absorption of the vitamin is enhanced by short and medium chain fatty acids and decreased by long chain polyunsaturated fatty acids. The polyunsaturated fatty acids are better solvents for the tocopherols and therefore are partitioned in favor of the micelle rather than toward the absorptive surfaces of the intestinal cell membranes. The tocopherols enter the blood stream via the lymphatics and are associated with lipoprotein fractions particularly rich in lipids. The tocopherols reach peak concentrations in tissues by 4 to 8 hr after ingestion. The tissue concentration is proportional to the log of the tocopherol concentration in blood. As was mentioned before, adipose tissue is an important store of this fat-soluble vitamin and excessive fat deposits in the body may compete with tissues that require vitamin E.[78] Two metabolites of α-tocopherol have been identified in human urine after hydrolysis of their conjugates. They are 2-(3-hydroxy-3-methyl-5-carboxypentyl)-3,5,6-trimethylbenzoquinone and its γ-lactone.[79]

Toxicity

Supplementation with vitamin E is a common practice based on the presumed benefits to be derived, namely, the prevention of ischemic heart disease, peripheral atherosclerosis, thrombophlebitis, the vascular complications of diabetes, leg cramps, sterility, and aging in general due to free-radical bombardment of vital organs.[80] Again, vitamin E is an essential, fat-soluble vitamin in small amounts, but carries the *a priori* risk of toxicity in huge amounts since it can be stored in fat depots throughout the body.

Toxic effects recorded as a consequence of megadoses of vitamin E are thrombophlebitis (which it is supposed to prevent), pulmonary embolism, hypertension, visual impairment and interference in blood coagulation due to its antagonisms of vitamins A and K, gynecomastia due to its estrogen-like activity and various, nonspecific complaints such as fatigue, headache, dizziness, nausea, and muscular weakness.[80]

Megavitamin usage is considered to be 100 to 300 mg of d-α-tocopheryl acetate compared with its nutritional requirement of 8 to 10 mg. It is fortunate that the vitamin E supplement of commerce is all-rac-α-tocopheryl acetate which is a mixture of isomers.[80]

VITAMIN K

Discovery and Nutritional Background

The discovery of vitamin K is credited to Henrik Dam during the time he was a student in 1929 at the University of Copenhagen. His assignment was to determine how chickens synthesized cholesterol. He added various sources of lipids to a fat-free experimental ration and produced, in one such combination, hemorrhagic lesions in the skin and muscles resembling scurvy. Adding lemon juice did not cure this condition. This new deficiency state was produced by the absence of a fat-soluble factor necessary for blood coagulation which he named vitamin K for "Koagulation".[3]

Isolation, Structures, and Chemical Synthesis

During the course of isolating the antihemorrhagic factor from natural sources, investigators found that two different chemical agents were biologically effective. One form of the vitamin from plant sources was isolated from alfalfa by Karrer and co-workers[81] and by Doisy's laboratory[82] in 1939. The procedure employed extraction, chromatography, adsorption of impurities, and isolation of the pure oil or crystallization at low temperatures. Another form of vitamin K was extracted, purified, and crystallized starting with fermented fish meal by Doisy's group.[83] Henrik Dam and Edward Doisy shared in the 1943 Nobel prize in physiology and medicine for the discovery of vitamin K and for its synthesis, respectively.

Determination of the structures of the K vitamins (Figure 7) was accomplished by degradation and comparison of the fragments with known compounds and with synthetic analogs.[5] Oxidation of vitamin K_1 with chromic acid gave phthalic acid and traces of 2-methyl-1,4-naphthoquinone-3-acetate.[84] The side chain was found to contain one double bond because the number of moles of hydrogen consumed was one more than that required to reduce the naphthoquinone portion. From work on other fat soluble vitamins, the side chain was found to consist of a phytyl substituent like that on α-tocopherol published 1 year earlier. The structure of vitamin K_2 from fish meal was done in much the same manner. The side chain was thought to be a difarnesyl group based on ozonolysis,[5] but the complete structure was not accepted until synthesis of the complete vitamin had been accomplished.

Synthesis of vitamin K_1 was done by condensing phytyl bromide with the sodium salt of 2-methyl-1,4-naphthoquinone in 1939 by Doisy's laboratory.[85] Menadione was synthesized by oxidation of 2-methylnaphthalene.[5] Therefore, in the space of time between 1929 and 1939, the K vitamins were discovered, isolated and synthesized. Physical properties of K_1, as representative, are given in Table 2.

Vitamin K Deficiency

Vitamin K deficiency results in reduced blood coagulation. Any reduction in biliary circulation to the small intestine results in poor absorption of this fat soluble vitamin. Transfer of vitamin K across the placental membrane is not very efficient. Consequently, the newborn may be temporarily low in this antihemorrhagic factor. When the normal bacterial flora of the intestinal tract is established after birth, this reduction in vitamin K is remedied. In the adult, this deficiency is rare because sources of this vitamin are widespread.

Dietary Sources

Sources of vitamin K_1 are distributed among the green leafy vegetables, meats, and dairy products. In addition, bacterial synthesis in the intestinal tract supplies approximately one

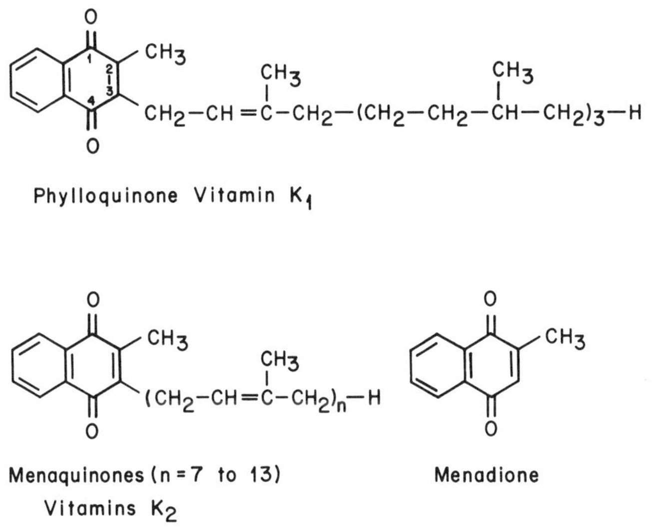

FIGURE 7. Structures of the K vitamins.

half of the daily requirement. The additional intake in the diet has been estimated to be 70 to 140 μg in adult men and 100 to 200 μg in women.[21] Vitamin K and niacin are the most stable vitamins in terms of resistance to destruction during food storage and processing.[22]

Structure-Activity Relationships

Fieser, et al.[86] reported on the antihemorrhagic activity of 79 compounds synthesized or selected on the basis of similarity to the basic 1,4-naphthoquinone structure. On a molar basis, vitamin K_2 was about 82% as active as K_1, which in this biological test was nearly equivalent. The same near molar equivalency exists for menadione vs. the natural vitamins (Figure 7). A double bond in the β position of the side chain enhanced potency, but further unsaturation did not have much effect on biological activity. A side chain length of 20 to 30 carbon atoms gave optimum activity and a branched chain was more effective than a straight chain. Removal of the methyl group on position 2 of the naphthalene ring gave 1/65 of the orginal activity, but elongation of this group to 2 carbons or more abolished activity. Likewise, alkylation on any other position resulted in inactivity. Introduction of a hydroxyl group also reduced or abolished activity.

Vitamin Antagonists

The most important antagonists of vitamin K are the anticoagulants dicumarol and warfarin. Arora and Mathur[87] reported structure-activity relationships of 35 derivatives of coumarin. The 7,8-dimethoxy analog of dicumarol was more active than dicumarol (Figure 8) as was calophyllolide. Tromexan, used in the treatment of thromboembolisms, was less active than dicumarol. In general, other substituents on coumarin resulted in compounds with poorer anticoagulant properties.

Mechanism of Action

A short time after the involvement of vitamin K in blood coagulation was demonstrated, the requirement of the vitamin in the formation of prothrombin was found. Subsequently, vitamin K was shown to be required for the synthesis of three more factors involved in coagulation, Factor VII, Factor IX, and Factor X. The intrinsic coagulation pathway occurs in the circulatory system following the deposition of platelets on the surface of blood vessels. The triggering mechanism is thought to be surface contact. The extrinsic system is initiated

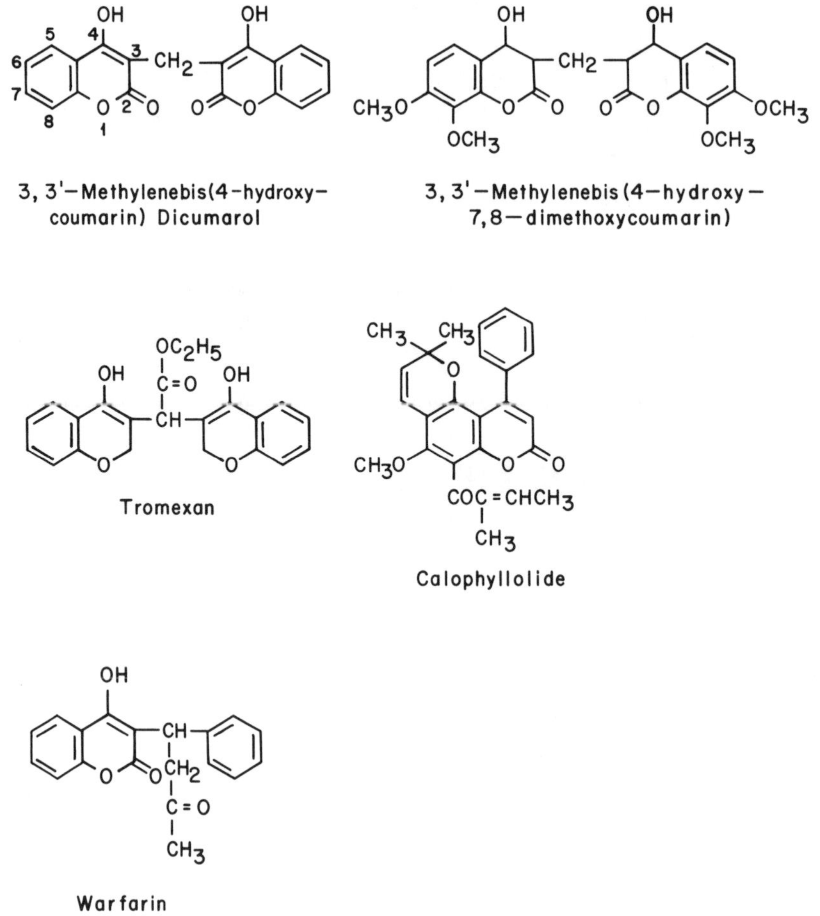

3,3'—Methylenebis(4-hydroxy—
coumarin) Dicumarol

3,3'—Methylenebis(4—hydroxy—
7,8—dimethoxycoumarin)

Tromexan

Calophyllolide

Warfarin

FIGURE 8.   Vitamin K antagonists.

by tissue injury activating Factor VII and others which merge with the intrinsic pathway in a cascade of reactions leading to the formation of a solid fibrin clot.[88] The early activation steps take place in phospholipid membranes and many are dependent on Ca^{2+} ions.[89] The inactive precursors, or zymogens, are transformed into their active forms by proteolytic enzymes which in turn act on other zymogens. The action of the serine proteinase thrombin on fibrinogen to produce the insoluble fibrin clot takes place outside of the lipoprotein matrix.

Vitamin K added in vitro to the coagulation system did not increase prothrombin formation. The vitamin was required for a synthetic process that was lacking in the deficient animal. The site of action of vitamin K was found to be the carboxylation of glutamic acid to yield a new amino acid, γ-carboxyglutamic acid (Figure 9) in ten positions on the prothrombin polypeptide chain.[89,90] In vitamin K deficiency an abnormal and inactive prothrombin was made in the liver. Gamma-carboxyglutamic acid residues were also discovered in osteocalcin, a protein found in mineralized bone tissue.

Three forms of vitamin K are involved in its role as a coenzyme for rat liver or ox liver microsomes in vitro (Figure 9).[90,91] The 2,3-epoxide, a major metabolite of the vitamin, is converted to the quinone by a sulfhydryl enzyme not yet identified in a reaction that is sensitive to the coumarin-type anticoagulants. Dithiothreitol (DTT) substitutes for this sulfhydryl reductant in vitro. The further reduction of the quinone to the hydroquinone compound

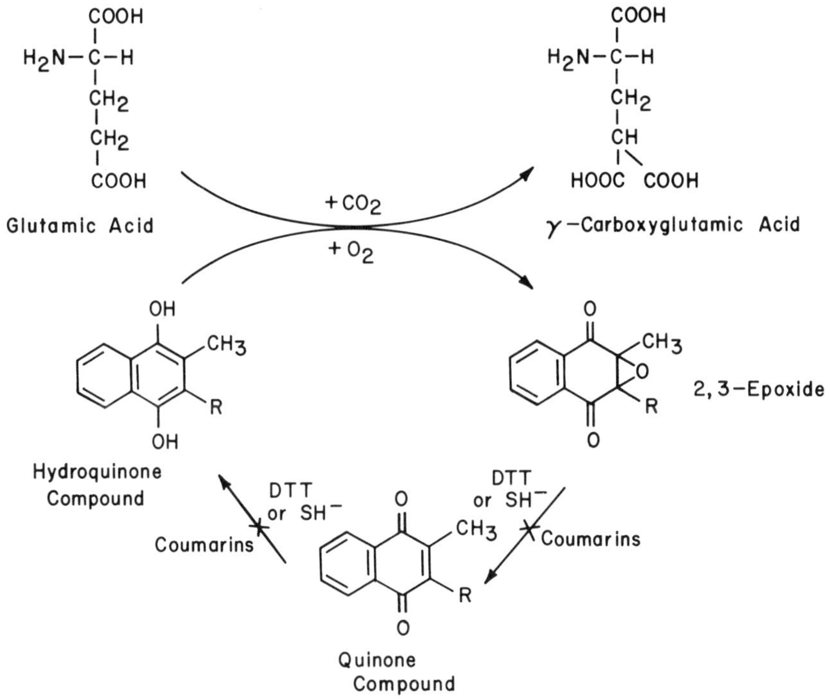

FIGURE 9.   Synthesis of γ-carboxyglutamate residues on prothrombin.

is also sensitive to these anticoagulants. The hydroquinone form of the vitamin appears to be the coenzyme species responsible for oxidative carboxylation of glutamic acid.

Biosynthesis of Vitamin K

The phylloquinones (K_1) are synthesized in plants and the menaquinones (K_2) are made by bacteria and certain fungi.[76] All seven carbon atoms of shikimic acid are incorporated into the simplest naphthoquinones, lawsone (2-hydroxy-1,4-naphthoquinone) or juglone (5-hydroxy-1,4-naphthoquinone) in plants. Dansette and Azerad[92] proposed that a succinic semialdehyde-thiamin pyrophosphate anion reacted with chorismate to give O-succinylbenzoate which then condensed to yield 1,4-dihydroxy-2-naphthoic acid. This was decarboxylated to give 1,4-naphthoquinol. The 2-methyl group was added by S-adenosylmethionine. The intermediate then went on to give methaquinone or naphthoquinones. The pathway for the formation of the polyprenyl side chain probably took place by the route used for steroid synthesis.[76] A polyprenylpyrophosphate group may be attached to the ring by electrophilic aromatic substitution, although the pathways are unproven.

Pharmacokinetics

When 1′,2′-phylloquinone was administered orally to human subjects, 54 to 60% of a 1-mg dose was recovered in the feces. Almost all of this was lipid soluble. About 15 to 23% was unchanged vitamin K_1. Absorption from the intestine was 40 to 46%. When vitamin K_1 was given intravenously, 34 to 38% was recovered in the feces. This meant that there was excretion into the intestine via the bile.[93] The mechanism of absorption of vitamin K_1 differed from that for K_2. Vitamin K_1 absorption was saturable as measured both in vivo and in vitro and required energy for its transport across the intestinal wall. In contrast, vitamin K_2 absorption was not saturable and took place passively.[77]

It was found that lymph was the major route of transport of intestinally absorbed vitamin

K_1 in rat and man.[93] The vitamin was carried in mixed micelles of fatty acids and bile salt. Most of the absorption occurred in the small intestine with lesser amounts in the colon.

An intravenous injection of vitamin K_1 in man produced two exponential plasma clearance curves, one with a t 1/2 of 24 min and a second with a t 1/2 of 104 min.[93] In a study employing rats, the liver took up the major portion of vitamin K_1 from blood. Phylloquinone was rapidly metabolized by human subjects to three polar compounds with shortened side chains. These were excreted predominantly in the urine as glucuronides.

Toxicity

Animal toxicity experiments with various natural and synthetic forms of vitamin K demonstrated that menadione had an oral LD_{50} in mice of 500 mg/kg whereas the natural compound, vitamin K_1, gave no deaths at 25 g/kg.[63] Both compounds are lipid soluble.

Newborn humans were reported to experience hemolytic anemia which was sometimes fatal upon vitamin K overtreatment. Adverse circulatory effects in adults given vitamin K or one of its synthetic analogs intravenously have been reported.[63]

THIAMIN

Discovery and Nutritional Background

C. Eijkman,[3] a military physician in the Dutch Indies during the late 1800s, made an important discovery regarding the prevalent disease beriberi. He was carrying out nutritional experiments with chickens which he fed scraps from the kitchen of the military hospital where he worked. These leavings consisted mainly of cooked, polished rice which was a staple of the diet on the wards. The chickens developed a paralysis. A newly appointed administrator of the hospital refused to allow Eijkman to use these leftovers. Instead he had to feed the chickens whole unpolished rice upon which the chickens recovered from their paralysis. Eijkman made the connection between paralysis in his chickens and the symptoms of neuritis in patients suffering from beriberi. However, he came to the erroneous conclusion that the rice grain contained a neurotoxic substance which was neutralized by a substance in the bran. The correct cause of beriberi was made by Grijns,[3] who in 1901 concluded that rice bran contained a nutrient that was lacking in polished rice.

Funk in 1912 and 1913 prepared a crude extract of rice polishings and of yeast[94] which cured polyneuritis in pigeons. The properties of this crude material were similar to organic bases which led him to name this substance "vitamine", an amine vital to life.[1] Later, Funk found that polyneuritis in pigeons developed more readily on a diet high in carbohydrate. This led to the belief by other investigators that there was an aberration in carbohydrate metabolism in cases of beriberi. In a historic paper, McCollum and Kennedy[95] made the distinction between "fat soluble A" and "water soluble B" which were the only two vitamins thought to exist in 1916. The vitamin that cured polyneuritis was later named vitamin B_1.

Isolation, Structure, and Chemical Synthesis

Williams and associates[96] isolated thiamin hydrochloride from rice bran by adsorbing the vitamin on fuller's earth and eluting it with quinine sulfate. The yield was very small — 5 g/ton of rice bran. They were, however, able to obtain enough of the material for a structure determination.[97]

In 1936, Williams and Cline[98] synthesized the pyrimidine portion of thiamin and condensed it with the thiazole portion made previously by Buchman[99] to give the first complete chemical synthesis of thiamin. Formylacetate reacted with ethoxyethyl ether to give ethyl-β-ethoxy-α-formylpropionate which condensed with acetamidine to form a substituted pyrimidine. The 4-hydroxy group was converted in two steps to an amino and then to a dibromo derivative. Synthesis of the thiazole portion of thiamin began with ethyl acetoacetate and ethylene oxide which gave a lactone which was chlorinated and then cleaved and decarboxylated to give 3-acetyl-3-chloropropanol. The latter was condensed with thioformamide to yield the thiazole moiety. The thiazole portion and the substituted pyrimidine fragment were heated together to give thiamin bromide hydrobromide which was converted to the chloride form with silver chloride. This procedure led to a commercial synthesis of thiamin which made this vitamin widely available. The physical properties are given in Table 2.

Thiamin Deficiency

The deficiency syndrome in fowl has been described as polyneuritis. The head of the bird is reflected back over the neck. There is muscular weakness, ataxic gait, tachycardia, cardiac failure, and cardiac necrosis. In adult humans there are generally two types of beriberi, the so-called dry type and the wet type.[100] The dry or chronic type of beriberi is characterized by peripheral neuropathy such as loss of deep tendon reflexes and abnormal sensitivity of the skin and a prickly feeling. This is accompanied by muscular pain and weakness, fatigue, mental confusion, and inability to work. In more severe cases, edema in the wet form of beriberi caused by cardiac failure may occur. Tachycardia may result from even slight exertion. Anorexia and digestive complaints may also be present. A very severe form of beriberi was noted in infants between the first and fourth months of age.[100] In some, an apparently healthy infant nursed by a thiamin-deficient mother may suddenly succumb to cardiac failure. In others, neurological signs such as silent crying may occur. Recovery is rapid when a thiamin supplement is given.

The foregoing forms of beriberi are rare in western countries. In the Orient, where the diet consists of large amounts of polished rice, and poverty coexists, beriberi may be seen. A disease of the western world caused by thiamin deficiency is called Wernicke-Korsakoff's Syndrome.[101] This disease is seen most often in alcoholics with poor nutritional status in which alcohol and carbohydrates comprise the main source of calories. It is characterized by mental confusion, poor recall, and ataxia. Diagnosis of this disease and beriberi may be made by measuring the erythrocyte transketolase activity with and without thiamin addition to an in vitro test system. The status of pyridoxine and vitamin B_{12} should be assessed in patients with Wernicke-Korsakoff's syndrome or other peripheral neuropathies, because a combination of deficiencies may be present. Treatment is afforded by intravenous drip or intramuscular injection of thiamin followed by a balanced diet supplemented with oral thiamin.

Dietary Sources

Flour sold in stores today is enriched with 2.0 to 2.5 mg of thiamin per pound as well as with riboflavin, niacin, and iron according to minimum and maximum levels set by U.S. government standards.[20] Thiamin is widely distributed in foodstuffs, but is particularly high in yeast. Other sources richer in thiamin than most are pork, nuts, and the germ part of cereal grains, such as wheat germ.[20]

Thiamin and ascorbic acid are the vitamins most sensitive to destruction during food storage and cooking.[22] Thiamin is more stable than thiamin pyrophosphate which is approximately 50% of the total. Thiamin is degraded in neutral or basic environments such as in chocolate cake of pH 8 whereas it is much better preserved in white bread of pH 5.8[22] (see Table 2). Thiamin is a water soluble vitamin. Therefore, losses in cooking water occur.

The recommended dietary allowance of thiamin ranges between 0.3 mg for infants and 1.5 mg for adolescents and adults. A small increment (0.4 to 0.5 mg) is suggested in the case of pregnancy and lactation.

Structure-Activity Relationships

Thiamin acts as a coenzyme in carbohydrate metabolism, a topic to be covered in the

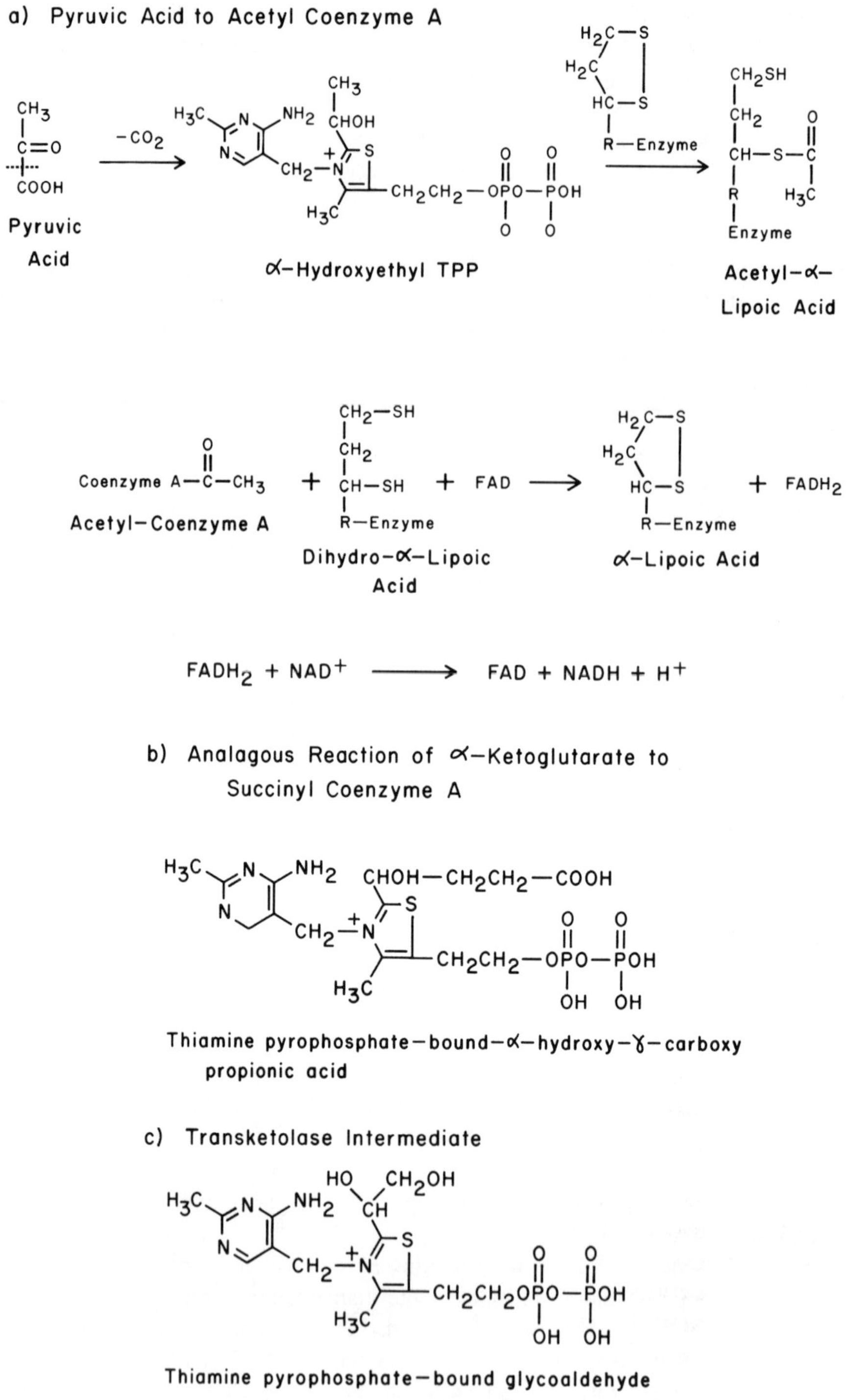
a) Pyruvic Acid to Acetyl Coenzyme A
Pyruvic Acid
−CO2
α−Hydroxyethyl TPP
R—Enzyme
Acetyl−α−Lipoic Acid
Enzyme
Coenzyme A—C—CH3
Acetyl−Coenzyme A
R—Enzyme
Dihydro−α−Lipoic Acid
FAD
FADH2
α−Lipoic Acid
FADH2 + NAD+ → FAD + NADH + H+
b) Analagous Reaction of α−Ketoglutarate to Succinyl Coenzyme A
Thiamine pyrophosphate−bound−α−hydroxy−γ−carboxy propionic acid
c) Transketolase Intermediate
Thiamine pyrophosphate−bound glycoaldehyde

FIGURE 10. Biochemical reactions involving thiamin pyrophosphate.

section on Mechanism of Action. The active form of the vitamin is thiamin pyrophosphate (Figure 10) and this is the most prevalent form in body tissues. In rat brain,[102] thiamin triphosphate was the next most plentiful form followed by thiamin monophosphate and then thiamin.

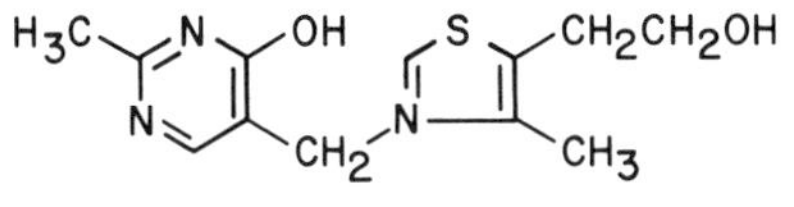

Oxythiamin

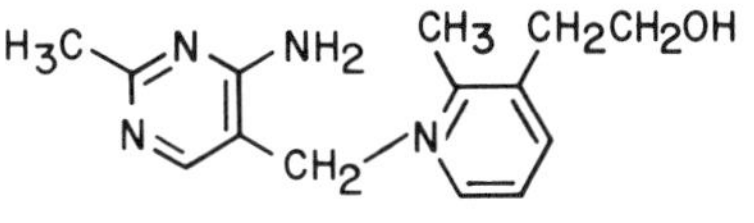

Neopyrithiamin

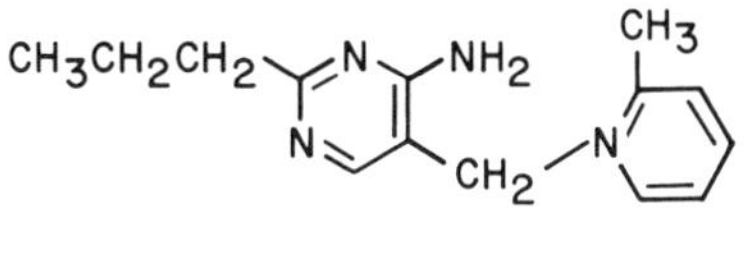

Amprolium

FIGURE 11.   Thiamin antagonists.

Thiamin Antagonists

Three important thiamin antagonists have been studied: oxythiamin, neopyrithiamin, and amprolium (Figure 11). The agent named pyrithiamin was found to be a mixture of compounds whose structures have not been defined.[103] Oxythiamin has a hydroxyl substituent in place of the amino group at position 4 of the pyrimidine moiety. Oxythiamine is a substrate for the thiamin activating enzyme thiamin phosphokinase. Oxythiamin diphosphate competes for thiamin diphosphate in its role as a coenzyme.[103] It decreases food consumption, weight gain, and growth in experimental animals and causes cardiac hypertrophy and bradycardia but no polyneuritis.

A second compound, neopyrithiamin has a pyridine ring substituted for the thiazole moiety and acts differently from oxythiamin. Neopyrithiamin inhibits thiamin phosphokinase preventing thiamin from being converted to its active form. It causes polyneuritis as well as weight loss and changes in cardiac function.[103]

The third antagonist, amprolium,[104] has been used for treatment of coccidiosis in poultry. This agent cannot take part in thiamin pyrophosphate-catalyzed reactions, because it lacks the hydroxyethyl group which is the site of phosphorylation. In addition, it is an inhibitor of this enzyme. Amprolium, blocks thiamin absorption from the intestinal tract, a process that is mediated by the phosphokinase and that correlates well with the known active transport of the vitamin.

Another type of thiamin antagonism came to light through observations in animal husbandry. Silver foxes fed raw fish developed a disease named Chastek paralysis, named for the farmer who first noticed this problem.[32] An allied disease called fern poisoning of cattle was observed in Oregon.[19] Both disorders were cured by adding additional thiamin to the ration. The cause of these neurological symptoms was the presence of the enzyme thiaminase I which occurs in certain bacteria in the gastrointestinal tract of freshwater fish and shellfish and in bracken ferns.[105] Thiaminase I cleaves the vitamin into pyrimidine and thiazole fragments.

Mechanism of Action

Thiamin pyrophosphate (TPP), the active form of vitamin B_1, was originally named cocarboxylase because it was found to be a cofactor which assisted in the oxidative decarboxylation of α-keto acids. Today, TPP is known to function as a carrier of an α-hydroxyethyl group in the pyruvate dehydrogenase enzyme complex, as a carrier of the α-hydroxy-γcarboxypropyl group in the conversion of α-ketoglutarate to succinyl coenzyme A and to carry active glycoaldehyde in the enzyme transketolase (Figure 10).[17]

The first of these enzymes converts pyruvate to acetyl coenzyme A. This step represents the branch point between the cytoplasmic reactions of glycolysis and the oxidative, energy producing reactions in the citric acid cycle housed in the mitochondria. The first step is the reaction between pyruvate and TPP within the matrix of the mitochondria. Thiamin bearing the α-hydroxyethyl group, is bound to pyruvic dehydrogenase. This group is then passed along to α-lipoic acid bound to an adjacent enzyme, lipoyl transacetylase. In the process of opening the disulfide bond of α-lipoic acid to form the reduced disulfide of this second coenzyme, the substrate is oxidized to acetate, still bound to α-lipoic acid. Coenzyme A from a dissociable enzyme in the mitochondria accepts the acetyl group to form acetyl coenzyme A. To regenerate the enzyme complex in a form ready to react with another pyruvate, α-lipoic acid is reoxidized by dihydrolipoyl dehydrogenase. The hydrogens are passed on to an enzyme-bound molecule of flavin adenine dinucleotide (FAD) which then reduces 1 mol of nicotinamide adenine dinucleotide (NAD+) which in turn enters the electron transport system to generate adenosine triphosphate (ATP). The overall reaction utilizes five coenzymes: thiamin, riboflavin (FAD), niacin (NAD+), α-lipoic acid, and pantothenic acid (coenzyme A). The entire process is essentially irreversible and is orchestrated by five enzymes to produce potential energy in the form of ATP and acetyl coenzyme A which enters the citric acid cycle for more energy production or synthetic reactions for the formation of fatty acids and steroids.[17]

A second enzymatic reaction involving TPP is one in which α-ketoglutaric acid is transformed into succinyl coenzyme A in the citric acid cycle. The reaction mechanism is very similar to the conversion of pyruvate to acetyl coenzyme A. A four-carbon unit from α-ketoglutarate attached to TPP is transferred to α-lipoic acid. The four-carbon fragment is oxidized to succinate during the reduction of α-lipoic acid and coenzyme A accepts the succinate to form succinyl coenzyme A.[17] This also is an irreversible reaction sequence.

The transketolase reaction has been used to monitor thiamin levels in humans suspected of suffering from a vitamin B_1 deficiency.[100] This reaction takes place in the hexose monophosphate shunt and is responsible for the formation of NADPH (reduced nicotinamide adenine dinucleotide phosphate) and for the synthesis of pentoses which are constituents of nucleotides. Transketolase catalyzes the reversible transfer of the two-carbon unit glycoaldehyde from xylulose-5-phosphate to ribose-5-phosphate to give sedoheptulose-7-phosphate and glyceraldehyde-3-phosphate.[17] The glycoaldehyde moiety is attached to TPP during the transfer reaction.

Biosynthesis of Thiamin

Studies on the biosynthesis of this vitamin have relied heavily on the incorporation of isotopically labeled precursors into the pyrimidine and thiazole portions. It was found that intermediates in the biosynthesis of pyrimidines were not involved in the synthesis of the pyrimidine moiety of thiamin.[106] Instead, 5-aminoimidazole ribonucleotide, an intermediate in purine biosynthesis, branched off to form 4-amino-5-hydroxymethyl-2-methyl pyrimidine,[107] which was then incorporated into thiamin. The source of the carbons differed in the bacterial and yeast synthetic pathways. Neither the methyl nor the sulfur portion of methionine appeared to be involved despite earlier evidences to the contrary. Methionine was found to be a coprecipitated impurity in the isolated intermediate.

Pharmacokinetics

It was mentioned before that the thiamin antagonist amprolium and neopyrithiamin inhibited the enzyme thiamin pyrophosphokinase and that this inhibition blocked absorption of thiamin from the gastrointestinal tract.[104] This indicates that thiamin is phosphorylated during an active transport process. Although free thiamin has been detected in the cytosol of rat brain, the major portion in membrane fractions of mitochondria occurred as the diphosphate ester with lesser amounts of the mono- and triphosphates.[102]

A large number of metabolites of thiamin have been found and the structures of six of them have been determined. They are 2-methyl-4-amino-5-pyrimidine carboxylic acid, 4-methylthiazole-5-acetic acid, 2-methyl-4-amino-5-hydroxymethylpyrimidine, 5-(2-hydrox-yethyl)-4-methylthiazole, 3-(2'-methyl-4'-amino-5'-pyrimidylmethyl)-4-methylthiazole-5-acetic acid, and 2-methyl-4-amino-5-formylaminomethylpyrimidine.[108] The enzyme thia-minase in the bacteria of the gastrointestinal tract may hydrolyze thiamin into pyrimidine and thiazole fragments which may be reabsorbed and further metabolized. The six metabolites named above were isolated from urine of rats or man.

Toxicity

Toxicity due to massive oral intake of thiamin has not been found, but deleterious effects have been reported when this vitamin was given parenterally in large amounts. When more than 400 mg were administered parenterally, there was a transient increase in mental alertness followed by lethargy and sleepiness, nausea, anorexia, and acute hypotension.[63] Allergy to thiamin has been reported. Pharmaceutical workers handling this vitamin occasionally con-tracted contact dermatitis or eczema.[109] Fatal anaphylactic shock to injection of thiamin has been reported in seven sensitized individuals.[63]

RIBOFLAVIN

Discovery and Nutritional Background

Hauge and Carrick[110] discovered that brewers' yeast from one source allowed good growth in rats but failed to prevent neuritis in young chickens. Corn, on the other hand, was rich in the antineuritic substance but poor in the growth promoting factor. They concluded that the two micronutrients were not identical. Using another line of evidence, Smith and Hendrick[3] autoclaved yeast from a source different from that used by Hauge and Carrick and found that the antineuritic substance was destroyed by heat and that the growth promoting substance survived this treatment. These two experiments indicated that there were two distinct vitamins responsible for curing the two different deficiency syndromes. The antineuritic substance was later named vitamin B_1 and the growth promoting vitamin was named vitamin B_2 since it was the second of the B vitamins to be discovered.

There remained one obstacle to the clear-cut delineation of this vitamin. In 1926, Gold-berger and Lillie[3] produced a syndrome in rats that they believed resembled pellagra in dogs. The syndrome included the tongue lesions of pellagra; therefore, they named the curative substance vitamin P-P for pellagra-preventive factor. Later the deficiency disease was shown not to be analogous to black tongue in dogs but could be cured by the heated yeast extract of Smith and Hendrick.

Isolation, Structure, and Chemical Synthesis

Salmon, Guerrant, and Hays[111] separated a B-P factor which prevented polyneuritis in pigeons from P-P factor, which was the so-called anti-pellagra factor in rats, on fuller's earth. P-P factor was adsorbed at pH 0.08 and B-P factor between pH 3 and 5.5 thereby separating the two B vitamins. Kuhn et al.[112] isolated "ovoflavin" from egg whites. Thirty kilograms of dried egg albumin yielded 30 mg of three times recrystallized ovoflavin. The riboflavin pigment Kuhn and co-workers isolated corresponded to the yellow pigment ob-served by Warburg and Christian and which was associated with their preparation of an oxidative enzyme later named "old yellow enzyme".[3]

The structure of riboflavin was deduced by photolysis of the compound in alkaline solution

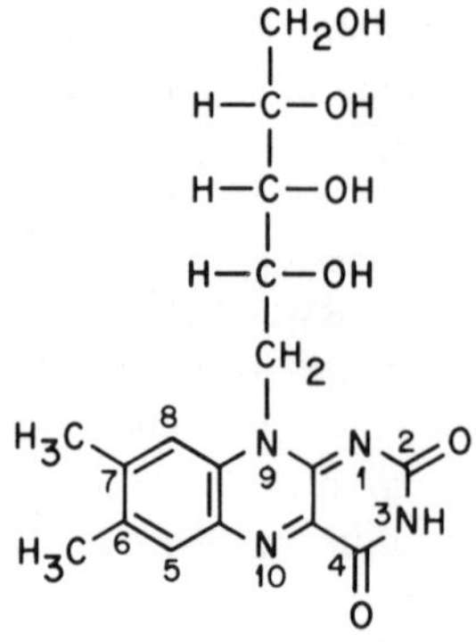

Riboflavin

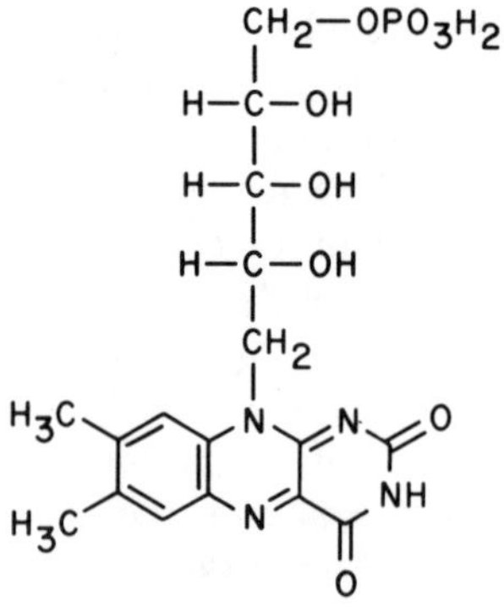

FMN, Flavin Mononucleotide

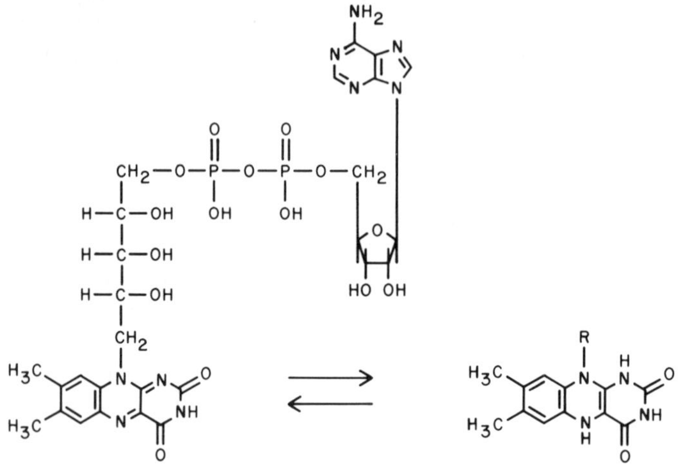

FAD, Flavin Adenine Dinucleotide (Oxidized Form)

FAD (Reduced Form)

FIGURE 12. Riboflavin and its co-enzyme forms.

to yield lumiflavin which had a methyl group in place of ribose in position 9 (Figure 12).[5] Lumiflavin was degraded further in alkali to give a bicyclic keto acid and urea. This keto acid was cleaved to 4-amino-1, 2-dimethyl-5-methylaminobenzene with heat under alkaline conditions. This compound was condensed with alloxan to give lumiflavin, confirming the structure. The side chain was shown to be ribose by tetra-acetylation and by formation of the di-isopropylidine derivative with acetone.[5]

In 1935, two groups successfully synthesized riboflavin. Karrer and co-workers[113,114] synthesized riboflavin, 6,7-dimethyl-9-(1′-*D*-ribityl) isoalloxazine, in six steps starting with *O*-nitroxylidine. Kuhn and associates[115] employed nitroxylidine also as a starting material but condensed this with ribose directly to give an imino sugar intermediate which was catalytically reduced to 1,2-dimethyl-4-amino-5-ribitylaminobenzene (I). Condensation of (I) with alloxan was a common step in the two methods. Some physical properties of riboflavin are given in Table 2.

Deficiency Symptoms

The primary deficiency symptom associated with riboflavin is growth retardation in experimental animals. Rats exhibit, in addition, alopecia, eczema, conjunctivitis, corneal opacities, and irreversible sterility. Riboflavin deficient females may deliver abnormal offspring if they are fertile at all.[116] Humans suffer from cheilosis which is cracks at the corners of the mouth, seborrhea of the nasolabial folds, shark-like appearance of the skin and glossitis, and a magenta colored tongue.[18] However, some of the above changes such as those of the skin resemble niacin or iron deficiencies and are not unique.[17] It should be emphasized that poor nutrition usually results in a multiplicity of vitamin, mineral, protein, or caloric deficiencies. Therefore, treatment may be general vitamin supplementation, especially of the water-soluble vitamins which are not stored to the extent that the fat-soluble vitamins are.

Dietary Sources

Riboflavin is widely distributed.[20] Good dietary sources of riboflavin are yeast, milk, egg whites, liver, heart, kidney, and green leafy vegetables. The recommended dietary allowance is between 0.4 to 0.6 mg for infants and 1.3 to 1.7 mg for adults. Riboflavin is included in the standard of identity for enriched flour. Riboflavin is more stable than thiamin to food cooking and storage but is degraded in alkaline solution and by light (see Table 2). It is preserved in cooked meats but being water soluble, some may be lost in the drippings.[22]

Structure-Activity Relationships

Riboflavin occurs in tissues as free ribityl-5'-phosphate and is combined with 5'-adenylic acid. These are the coenzyme forms of the vitamin and are called FMN for flavin mononucleotide (erroneously) and FAD for flavin adenine dinucleotide (correctly). The structures are given in Figure 12.

Flavin coenzymes are attached very strongly to the apoenzymes which they subserve. Dissociation constants range between 10^{-8} to 10^{-9} which is considerably less than for the niacin coenzymes.[17] Riboflavin phosphate was attached to the "old yellow enzyme" at the imino group at position 3 (Figure 12) and by the phosphate attached to ribitol. The point of attachment of flavin to enzyme varies with the particular enzyme. Limited alterations could be made in the substituents at positions 6 and 7 without decreasing the affinity of the coenzyme for the apoenzyme.[117]

A large number of analogs of riboflavin have been prepared and tested for biological activity.[118] Replacement of the D,1'-ribityl group on position 9 by other 5 carbon pentose alcohols resulted in inactive compounds except for L,1'-arabityl or D,1'-xylityl substituents which gave less activity than riboflavin. Glycoside-bonded pentoses resulted in total loss of biological activity. A 3-methyl substituent abolished activity. The methyl groups at positions 6 and 7 may be replaced either singly or together by ethyl groups without total loss of activity, but unsubstitution at these positions (two hydrogens) resulted in a toxic compound.[119] A complete discussion of biological potency of the many analogs of riboflavin may be found in the references cited.[117-119]

Vitamin Antagonists

Many structural analogs of riboflavin have been synthesized and tested for biological activity either in the nutrition of the B_2-deficient rat or for growth of microorganisms. Dichloroflavin, the first inhibitory analog of riboflavin to be reported, blocks the growth of *Staphylococcus aureus* and *Streptobacterium plantarum,* but not yeast or *Lactobacillus casei.* The inhibition is reversed by adding riboflavin to the growth medium.[118] Diethyl riboflavin was found to substitute completely for the growth of *L. casei* and *Bacillus lactis acidi.* Diethyl riboflavin supported growth of rats at low dose levels but decreased survival in conjunction with rapid weight gains at high doses.[117] Isoriboflavin blocked growth of rats supplemented with 10 μg of riboflavin per day but 40 μg/day of riboflavin prevented this inhibitory effect. Isoriboflavin was without effect on growth of *L. casei*.[118,119] D-Arabino-flavin retarded growth of rats receiving either low (10 μg/day) or high (300 μg/day) riboflavin supplements. It also inhibited growth of a lactic acid producing bacteria. L-Arabinoflavin, as was mentioned earlier, appeared to substitute somewhat for riboflavin in rats. Galactoflavin blocked growth in rats on a diet supplemented with 10 or 40 μg riboflavin per day. Gal-actoflavin stimulated growth of *L. casei* at low levels but inhibited at high levels.[117] Lum-ichrome and lumiflavin were reported to be inhibitory toward the growth of microorganisms. Both inhibited *Neurospora* and lumiflavin, at high concentrations, inhibited *L. casei*.[118]

The antimalarials atabrine, quinine, and some related compounds inhibited growth of *L. casei*. Atabrine inhibited the flavin enzymes D-amino acid oxidase and cytochrome reduc-tase.[118] While some antimalarials are riboflavin antagonists, others such as paludrine are not, indicating an imperfect correlation with respect to mode of action of these medicinal agents.[119]

Al-Hassan and coauthors[120] described a large number of inhibitors of the enzyme riboflavin synthase which condenses two molecules of lumazine to riboflavin. Substrate analogs such as pyrido [2,3-d] pyrimidines and transition state analogs were presented. The purpose of the synthetic work was to elicit compounds which would be effective in a parasite but not in the host.

Mechanism of Action

Riboflavin acts at the cellular level in electron transport and during oxidation-reduction reactions of intermediary metabolism. Many of the flavoproteins are oxidases which reduce oxygen to H_2O_2. L-Amino acid oxidase of liver uses two FAD molecules per unit of enzyme whereas the same enzyme in the kidney uses two FMN molecules.[17] The peroxides formed are cleaved by catalase or peroxidase. Enzymes such as dihydro-orotic dehydrogenase and cytochrome P-450 reductase use both FAD and FMN as cofactors in hydrogen transfer.[17] Protein-bound flavins may be partially reduced to free radical red or blue semiquinones which have characteristic spectra. The flavin may accept either one or two protons at a time.

Reducing equivalents accepted by flavoproteins are transferred directly to oxygen, to the electron-transferring flavoprotein or to ubiquinone in the electron chain of oxidative phos-phorylation. Reduced nicotinamide adenine dinucleotide (NADH) transfers electrons to FMN and then to ubiquinone. In the oxidation of succinate to fumarate in the citric acid cycle, succinic dehydrogenase containing bound FAD accepts two hydrogens which are then passed on to ubiquinone without NAD+ being involved as an intermediate. FAD is covalently linked to a histidine residue of the enzyme at the 7 position of riboflavin (Figure 12).[17]

Biosynthesis of Riboflavin

All green plants and many species of bacteria, yeast, and fungi synthesize riboflavin. Guanosine triphosphate (GTP) is the precursor of riboflavin.[106] All carbon atoms of GTP are incorporated into this vitamin except C-8 which is given off as formate. The carbon atoms of the ribityl unit are also derived from GTP. Regulation of riboflavin biosynthesis may occur by the effect of an intermediate in the pathway on the first enzyme in the sequence, GTP cyclohydrolase II.[106]

FMN, riboflavin-5'-phosphate, and FAD may be made in animals by the enzymes fla-vokinase utilizing ATP and by flavin nucleotide pyrophosphorylase and ATP, respectively.[17]

Pharmacokinetics

Absorption of riboflavin by man and rats from the intestinal tract occurs by a saturable process but the mechanism is presently unknown. Maximum levels in the blood occur 1/2 to 2 hr after ingestion. Dietary riboflavin is presented in the form of riboflavin phosphate and FAD which must be converted to free riboflavin for intestinal absorption. The release of the vitamin from riboflavin-5'-phosphate is accomplished by FMN phosphatase located in brush border membranes of intestinal mucosa. FAD pyrophosphatase performs the same function and its location is the same as for the phosphatase. Inhibition of uptake of riboflavin-^{14}C by riboflavin formed by hydrolysis of FMN and FAD speaks to the saturable process.[121]

Riboflavin-binding protein, a transport protein, has been found in the serum, egg whites, and yolks of laying hens and other birds and serves as a means of ensuring that little riboflavin is lost during development of the embryo.[122] This transport protein was analyzed and found to bind riboflavin above pH 4.5 and to release the vitamin at a more acid pH.[123] It is a complex glycoprotein containing N-acetylglucosamine, sialic acids containing N-acetylneuraminic acid, fucose, and galactose. The process of release of the riboflavin to the cell by the riboflavin-binding protein is unknown. Binding to plasma proteins in mammals is not a major consideration.[124]

An appreciable amount of the riboflavin in mammalian tissues is excreted unchanged. The larger the amount of riboflavin ingested and the faster the absorption rate, the more unchanged vitamin is excreted. Slower absorption and utilization results in more vitamin B_2 being metabolized. Halflives for excretion are 1.2 hr in man and 0.4 hr in the rat. The nature of the metabolites in mammals is unknown but intestinal bacteria degrade riboflavin to lumichrome and other unidentified metabolites none of which are conjugates. Riboflavin is excreted mainly in the urine in most species (50 to 90%). Secretion into the intestinal tract via the bile has been demonstrated in the rat and man.[124]

Toxicity

The low toxicity reported for riboflavin is probably caused by its limited intestinal absorption and its low solubility in aqueous media, about 190 mg/ℓ.[63] The LD_{50} for riboflavin in the rat was 560 g/kg i.p.[116] The corresponding value for mice was 340 g/kg i.p. which translates into 5000 times a therapeutic dose of riboflavin.[116]

NIACIN

Discovery and Nutritional Background

Niacin is the generally recognized name for this B vitamin which consists of nicotinic acid and its amide. The deficiency disease related to the lack of niacin in the diet is pellagra which was reported in 1735 by Gaspar Casal, a physician to King Philip V of Spain.[17] In 1786, Goethe wrote that the Italians developed a brown pigmented skin upon exposure to the sun and he postulated that this sickness was due to their diet of corn.[3]

In 1914, Voegtlin proved that pellagra was a dietary deficiency disease by testing two diets on human pellegra patients. The diet containing milk, meat, and eggs cured their symptoms whereas the one containing cereal grains and small amounts of ham and milk was ineffective.[3]

Spencer in 1916 linked canine "black tongue" disease and pellagra in man.[3] At about the same time, Goldberger was commissioned by the U.S. Public Health Service to investigate the cause of pellagra. Using inmates at the Rankin Farm of the Mississippi State Penitentiary, he and his co-workers concluded that this disease was caused by an amino acid deficiency, a mineral deficiency, or the lack of some unknown vitamin. He was able to rule out an infectious agent by testing sputum and feces of pellagra patients.[125]

Somewhat later, Elvehjem and co-workers discovered that the pellagra preventative factor was different from the vitamin that cured beriberi. Sebrell and colleagues isolated a filtrate from rice bran that cured black tongue in dogs. Also, they found that better results were obtained by the addition of riboflavin. In 1937, Elvehjem and associates found that black tongue was cured by nicotinic acid obtained from a liver extract. This substance when given to humans cured pellagra in a short time and the remaining skin lesions were alleviated by the administration of riboflavin. They also found that tryptophan could reduce the amount of nicotinic acid needed to cure pellagra and that this amino acid was a precursor of niacin.[125]

It is interesting to note that pellagra did not become a disease entity until the introduction of cultivated corn in Europe and America. Since corn was an inexpensive foodstuff, it was used in place of higher quality protein from meat and eggs. Investigators believed that something in corn increased the dietary requirement for niacin.[3,125]

Isolation, Structure, and Chemical Synthesis

The active substance, a filtrate factor from liver or yeast, was found by Fouts, Sebrell, Elvehjem, and their associates[5] to consist of nicotinic acid, a substance which had been prepared from nicotine by nitric acid oxidation in 1867 by Huber. The placement of the carboxyl group on the pyridine ring was established as being at the 3-position by showing that the products of thermal decarboxylation of both pyridine-2,3- and -3,4-dicarboxylic acids produced a common product, nicotinic acid.[5] Some physical properties of nicotinic acid and nicotinamide are given in Table 2. Niacin is one of the more stable vitamins.

Deficiency Symptoms

The symptoms of pellagra described by Horwitt[126] are characterized by dermatitis, diarrhea, and dementia. Early signs are weakness, lethargy, poor appetite, and indigestion. Skin lesions of more severe pellagra occur on the face, hands, feet, and on those parts of the body subject to trauma. Sunlight exacerbates the condition. Alimentary tract disorders of diarrhea, vomiting, anorexia, and sore mouth occur. The neuronal lesions appear to be central in location. Myelin degeneration and changes in cortical neurons may be responsible for the irritability, loss of memory, headaches, and in advanced cases, psychoses.

Dietary Sources of Niacin

Thiamin, riboflavin, and niacin as well as iron come under the U.S. Federal Standards for enrichment of flour, cornmeal, rice, and macaroni products. The purpose of this legislation was to ensure that people at the poverty level who subsist on relatively inexpensive cereal products (compared with meat, fish, and eggs) would not lack for proper intake of these essential nutrients.

The table of Recommended Dietary Allowances lists "niacin equivalent" requirements as being between 6 to 8 mg for infants to 19 mg for late teenagers.[21] One niacin equivalent is equal to 1 mg of niacin as the free acid or amide or 60 mg of tryptophan. This amino acid is a presursor of niacin but it is also required for protein synthesis in the amount of about 500 mg per day. Therefore, the total daily intake of tryptophan must be at least 560 mg.

Niacin is stable to heat, light, acid, and alkali. Loss occurs if the water used in cooking vegetables or the meat drippings is discarded. Trigonelline (*N*-methyl-nicotinic acid) is inactive as a niacin substitute, but it is present in the seeds of many plants including coffee. Roasting coffee liberates nicotinic acid so that it may serve as a source of niacin.[20]

Good sources of niacin are meat, poultry, fish, and cereal grains. Dairy products and eggs are rich in tryptophan but not of the preformed vitamin.

Structure-Activity Relationships

The two active forms of niacin are nicotinic acid and its amide. Structures are given in a later section.

Vitamin Antagonists

3-Pyridinesulfonamide is a competitive inhibitor of nicotinic acid in some species of bacteria. 3-Pyridinesulfonic acid inhibition is reversible by nicotinic acid after incubating bacterial cultures for 1 day or longer. Rat growth was retarded slightly by this analog but mice were unaffected by it. It failed to enhance the appearance of pellagra in dogs fed a niacin deficient ration. Acetylpyridine (pyridine-3-methylketone) was more effective as an antagonist of niacin in animals than in bacterial cultures. Acetylpyridine caused the onset of symptoms of pellagra in dogs, mice, and rabbits. Nicotinic acid or tryptophan in the diet prevented onset of the deficiency. 6-Aminonicotinic acid interferred with p-aminobenzoic acid in some bacterial strains and this inhibition was overcome by adding niacin to the growth medium.[5]

It was mentioned earlier that pellagra developed more easily on a deficient diet containing corn. Attempts have been made to isolate the inhibitory substance without success.

Mechanism of Action

Nicotinic acid amide functions as a constituent of the two coenzymes nicotinamide adenine dinucleotide (NAD) and nicotinamide adenine dinucleotide phosphate (NADP) (Figure 13). Like the riboflavin coenzymes, niacin coenzymes carry out oxidation-reduction reactions. NAD and some flavoproteins are sometimes reduced at the substrate level. In other cases, NAD is reduced, passing on hydrogens to FMN in the electron transport scheme for the production of ATP. There are over 250 different dehydrogenases utilizing niacin as a cofactor. It is no wonder that lack of this vitamin and tryptophan in the diet results in such diverse and severe deficiency symptoms.

Some dehydrogenases operate efficiently with either NAD or NADP, others have an absolute requirement for one or the other and still other enzymes use one in preference but operate less efficiently with the other. The end result of oxidation-reduction equilibria in cells is that NAD is mostly in the oxidized form and NADP is mostly in its reduced form. Another generalization is that the enzymes that employ NAD are usually ones that generate energy for the cell via oxidative phosphorylation and enzymes that use NADP are biosynthetic ones.[17] An example of the latter is NADP-requiring glucose-6-phosphate dehydrogenase which is the first enzyme in the hexose monophosphate shunt that is responsible for the synthesis of pentoses required by nucleotides for the formation of RNA and DNA. There are also transhydrogenases that exchange reducing equivalents between NAD in one compartment of a cell and NADP in another compartment.

NAD performs functions unrelated to oxidation or reduction. The enzyme DNA ligase uses NAD or ATP for the synthesis of 3'-5'-phosphodiester linkages during DNA replication or repair. The pyrophosphate bond of NAD is split with the release of nicotinamide mononucleotide.

Hydrogen transfer to NAD + or NADP + to form the reduced coenzyme takes place in a stereospecific manner by enzymes (Figure 13). The pyridine ring is planar with one hydrogen on carbon 4. The second hydrogen is added to this position during reduction and can project outward from the plane of the ring or back, away from the observer. The outward projection is called the 4-pro-R side (A type of reduction) or inward called the 4-pro-S side or B type of reduction. The reaction takes place on one side or the other depending upon the specific enzyme performing the reduction. Yeast alcohol dehydrogenase or heart lactic dehydrogenase are A type reductases, whereas glucose dehydrogenase of liver or glucose-6-phosphate dehydrogenase from yeast add the hydride ion to the B side of the ring.[17] One hydrogen reduces the niacin coenzyme and the second is released to the medium as a proton.

Biosynthesis of Niacin

The metabolic route from tryptophan to NAD[17] is illustrated in Figure 13. The first reaction is carried out by tryptophan-2,3-dioxygenase in liver and requires copper and heme as cofactors. N-Formylkynurenine is cleaved to kynurenine by kynurenine formylase and then is oxidized to 3-hydroxykynurenine by kynurenine-3-hydroxylase which uses NADPH and

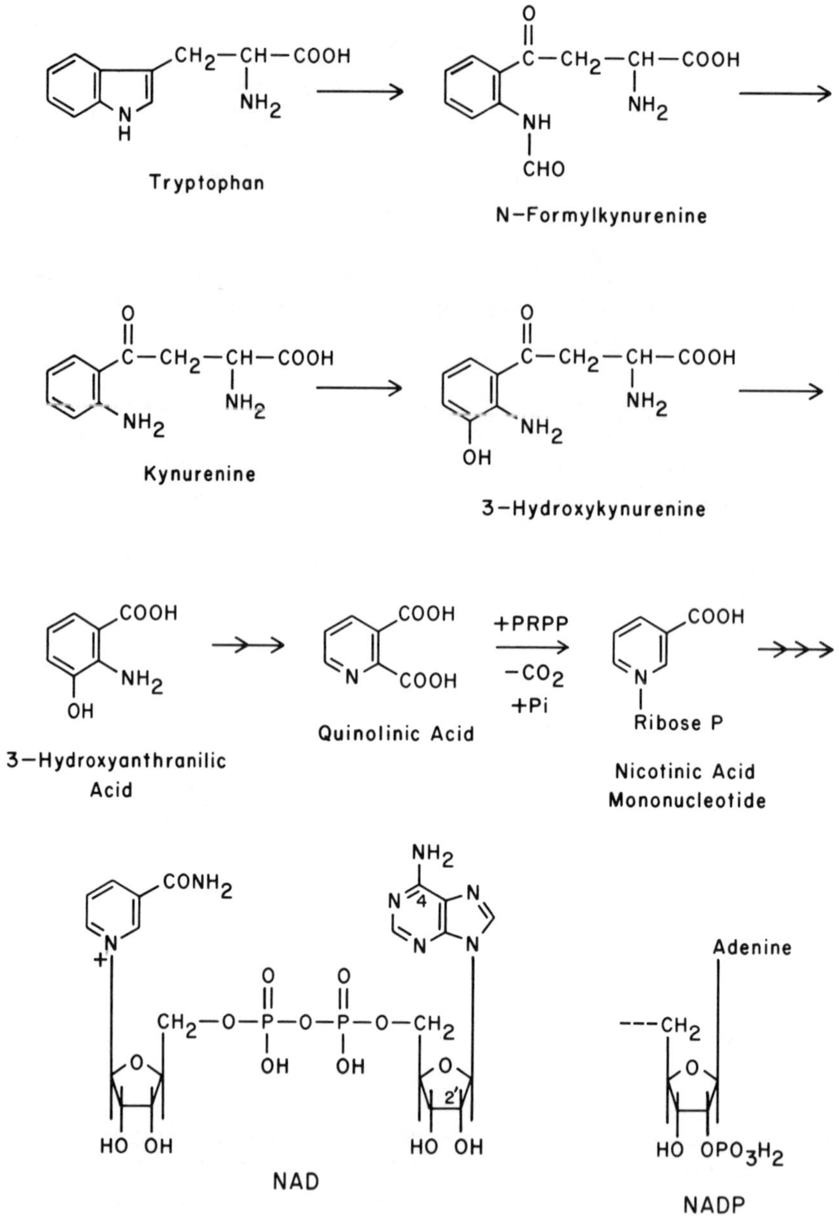

FIGURE 13.   Biosynthesis of NAD.

oxygen in the reaction. Kynureninase with pyridoxal phosphate converts 3-hydroxykynurenine to 3-hydroxyanthranilic acid which is then cleaved to 2-amino-3-carboxymuconic semialdehyde by 3-hydroxyanthranilate oxygenase in liver or kidney. This intermediate undergoes rearrangement and is cyclized to give quinolinic acid. Quinolinic acid combines with 5-phosphoribosyl-1-pyrophosphate (PRPP) with loss of a carboxyl group to give nicotinic acid mononucleotide by a reaction carried out by quinolinate transphosphoribosylase. Also, dietary nicotinic acid can be converted to nicotinic acid mononucleotide using PRPP. Deamino NAD is formed by condensation with ATP and the release of inorganic pyrophosphate. The amino group on the carboxyl of nicotinic acid is added by NAD synthetase which requires ATP and an amino group from glutamine, NADP is phosphorylated by NAD kinase and ATP using NAD as the substrate.

Pharmacokinetics

Intestinal transport of nicotinic acid appears to be by diffusion.[127] Absorption of amino acids occurs mainly in the small intestine and takes place by an active transport process dependent upon the chemical class into which it falls. Neutral amino acids compete with each other for a common carrier as do acidic and basic amino acids. Tryptophan is one of the aromatic basic amino acids essential for man and must be absorbed preformed in the diet.

NAD and NADP are metabolized by tissues to nicotinamide and adenosine diphosphate ribose. The nicotinamide moiety is methylated in the liver to N'-methylnicotinamide by S-adenosylmethionine enzymatically. This is the principal metabolite of niacin found in the urine.[17] Other metabolites of nicotinamide have been identified in the urine of animals and man, namely the 2- and 6-pyridones of N'-methylnicotinamide, nicotinuric acid, and others.[32]

Toxicity

Large amounts (3 to 6 g/day) of nicotinic acid, relative to the nutritional requirement of 10 to 20 mg, have been administered to humans in order to reduce blood levels of cholesterol and triglycerides as an antiatherosclerotic agent.[126] Side effects include flushing due to peripheral vasodilatation, pruritis, and gastric irritation.[63]

VITAMIN B_6, PYRIDOXINE

Discovery and Nutritional Background

By employing purified diets, the cause of "rat pellagra" was investigated in 1934 and found not to be due to a deficiency of thiamin, riboflavin, or niacin. Gyorgy[3] concluded from his studies that a new alkali-stable substance was the required micronutrient. He studied the properties of this new factor: its electronegativity, solubility, and reactivity toward certain derivatizing agents and found that it was a basic compound lacking a primary amino group but containing an hydroxyl substituent. This compound was distinguished from Factor II, which later was identified as pantothenic acid. Biotin, which had been isolated and crystallized by this time, was not effective in curing these skin symptoms called "pellagra" or acrodynia in rats. By 1936, the cause of these deficiency symptoms had been narrowed down to the substance Gyorgy named vitamin B_6.[3]

Isolation, Structure, and Chemical Synthesis

Lepkovsky, Keresztesy, and Gyorgy and their respective co-workers were able to isolate and crystallize the vitamin in 1938. The structure of B_6 was determined in 1939 by Stiller et al. by degradation. In the same year, Harris and Folkers synthesized pyridoxine which is 4,5-di(hydroxymethyl)-3-hydroxy-2-methylpyridine (Figure 14) in six steps beginning with the condensation of ethoxyacetylacetone and cyanoacetamide.[5] Physical properties of pyridoxine are given in Table 2.

Deficiency Symptoms

The discriminative deficiency symptom in rats is acrodynia which is a scaly dermatitis with loss of hair about the ears, nose, chin, and chest.[128] Pyridoxine deficiency also results in muscle weakness, fatty liver, convulsions, nerve degeneration, adrenal enlargement, reproductive failure, and increased excretion of xanthurenic acid, urea, and oxalic acid. Xanthurenic acid is a tryptophan metabolite which accumulates when kynureninase, the enzyme which converts 3-hydroxykynurenine to 3-hydroxyanthranilic acid in the biosynthesis of niacin, is blocked due to lack of its cofactor pyridoxal phosphate.

In man, pyridoxine deficiency takes some time to develop and the deficiency syndrome is poorly defined. A seborrheic dermatitis around the eyes, nose, and mouth developed in

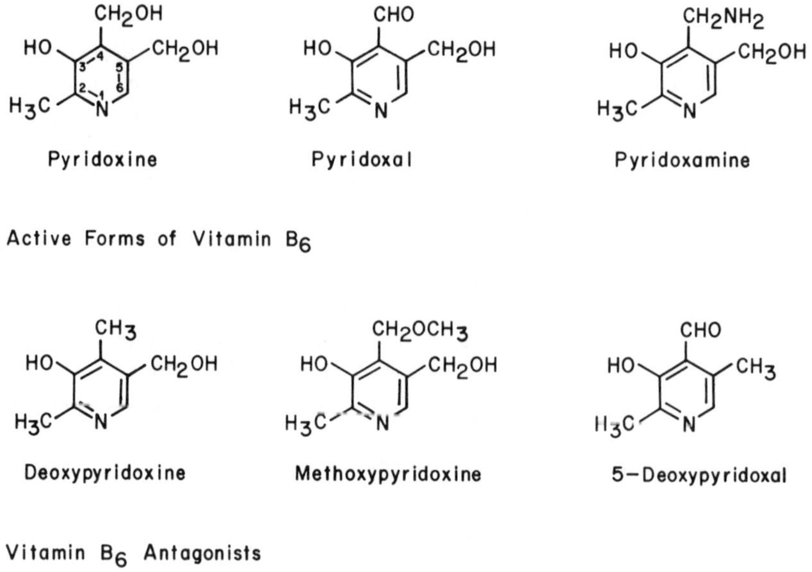

Active Forms of Vitamin B₆

Vitamin B₆ Antagonists

FIGURE 14.   Forms of vitamin B_6 and B_6 antagonists.

human subjects fed a pyridoxine deficient diet together with a pyridoxine antimetabolite deoxypyridoxine. These volunteer subjects also developed a cheilosis at the corners of the mouth like that seen with riboflavin deficiency and glossitis and a reddening of the tongue and mouth, similar to niacin deficiency. Giving riboflavin or niacin did not clear up these symptoms, but a pyridoxine supplement cured the condition within 2 to 3 days.[18] The resemblance of the dermatitis of essential fatty acid deficiency to that in pyridoxine deficiency may be due to the requirement of pyridoxine for the enzymatic conversion of linolenic to arachidonic acid. The enlarged adrenals of pyridoxine deficiency may result from the involvement of this vitamin in adrenalcortical function.[18] Convulsions in the newborn may also occur with mothers on a pyridoxine-restricted diet.

Dietary Sources of Vitamin B₆

Good sources of the B_6 vitamins are fish, poultry, and meat.[21] Vitamin B_6 is not a single chemical entity but comprises pyridoxine, pyridoxamine, and pyridoxal, all of which are biologically equivalent. Pyridoxine predominates in vegetable sources whereas pyridoxal and pyridoxamine occur in animal tissues. Information on the utilization of these forms of the vitamin is inaccurate because of insufficient data.

The recommended dietary allowances of vitamin B_6 range from 0.3 to 2.2 mg as maintenance levels in infants and adults, respectively. The amount of vitamin B_6 required also is proportional to protein intake. The B_6 content of food may be decreased 20% by cooking[21] and it is destroyed by light at a pH of 6 and above.

Structure-Activity Relationships

Vitamin B_6 includes pyridoxal and pyridoxamine derived from animal sources and pyridoxine from plant sources. The active co-enzymes are pyridoxal-5-phosphate and pyridoxamine-5-phosphate. The latter can function only in transaminase reactions (Figure 14).

Vitamin B₆ Antagonists

Many structural analogs of pyridoxine have been synthesized. Three of the most important antagonists are illustrated in Figure 14. The effective antagonists are substituted either in position 4 or 5.[129]

Deoxypyridoxine (substituted on the 4 position) has been studied the most. Reducing pyridoxine in the diet accelerated the appearance of deficiency syndrome with this antagonist. Giving B_6 supplements cured the deficiency. During the initial stage of B_6 deficiency, the liver had a normal content of the B_6 vitamins and the activity of the enzymes was not decreased unless the deficiency was allowed to progress. Deoxypyridoxine appeared to be phosphorylated in the same manner as pyridoxal. Both phosphate esters were found to compete for binding to B_6-requiring enzymes. But, as in the case of acute deficiency states, if the enzyme already had pyridoxal phosphate bound to it, the deoxypyridoxine would not displace it.[129]

Isonicotinic acid hydrazide is an antagonist of the pyridoxal phosphate-requiring enzyme tryptophanase but not of decarboxylase which also requires the same co-enzyme. Also, isoniazid is effective against the tuberculosis bacillus but the addition of vitamin B_6 to the culture did not reverse the effect of isoniazid.[129] Therefore, the action of isoniazid is that of an irreversible antagonist of pyridoxal or of its phosphate.

The pyrimidine fragment of thiamin, 4-amino-5-hydroxymethyl-2-methylpyrimidine, called toxopyrimidine was phosporylated with phosphorous oxychloride. This phospho-pyrimidine was a competitive antagonist of pyridoxal phosphate for the enzyme tyrosine decarboxylase in cultures of *Streptococcus faecalis*.[130]

Mechanism of Action

Pyridoxine takes part in the metabolism of amino acids. The active co-enzyme forms are the 5-phosphates of pyridoxal and pyridoxamine in the case of transamination reactions but only pyridoxal-5-phosphate with respect to other transformations. The co-enzyme is synthesized in liver, brain, and kidney by ATP and pyridoxal kinase.

Pyridoxal phosphate takes part in the following reactions:

1. Transaminases
2. Decarboxylases
3. Desulfhydrases
4. Dehydratases
5. Glycogen phosphorylase
6. Amino acid synthesis
7. Serine hydroxymethyltransferase
8. Niacin biosynthesis

Transaminase reactions involved the interchange of an α-amino group and an α-keto group to form a new amino acid and the corresponding α-keto acid. Aminotransferases are known for all amino acids except threonine and lysine.[17] Glutamic acid is usually involved as one of the reactants and glutamic-aspartate and glutamic-alanine aminotransferases are particularly important since excess protein in the diet is used for energy production by way of generation of pyruvic acid and α-ketoglutaric acid for entry into the citric acid cycle. In man, the eight essential amino acids are not formed by transamination from corresponding α-ketoacids.

The mechanism of the transaminase reaction is illustrated in Figure 15. Enzyme-bound pyridoxal phosphate reacts at the 4 position with an α-amino acid to form a Schiff base with the aldehyde group. The pyridoxal phosphate ends up as pyridoxamine phosphate and the α-amino acid becomes an α-keto acid. Pyridoxal phosphate is regenerated by the back reaction in which a second α-keto acid accepts the amino group from pyridoxamine phosphate to make a new amino acid.[17]

Amino acid decarboxylases are widespread in nature. All decarboxylases except for that acting on histidine require pyridoxal phosphate.[17] Carbon dioxide is evolved from an amino acid attached as a Schiff base intermediate in a reaction similar to the transaminase reaction.

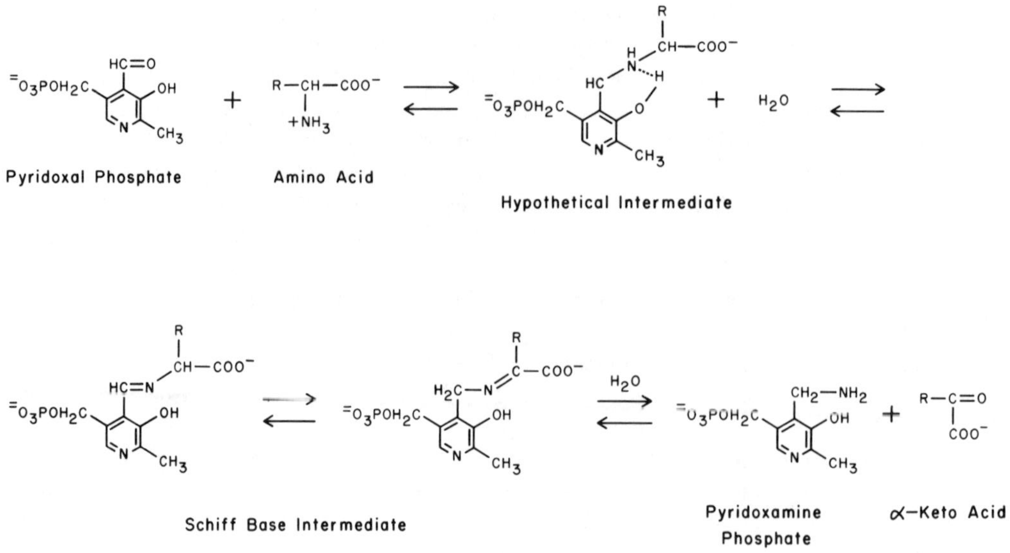

FIGURE 15.   Mechanism of the transaminase reaction.

Desulfhydrases, such as cysteine desulfhydrases in bacteria, liberate ammonia, H_2S, and pyruvic acid from cysteine.[17] Pyridoxal phosphate serves as a cofactor.

Related to desulfhydrases is a pyridoxal phosphate-requiring enzyme called serine dehydratase that dehydrates serine to a dehydroalanine intermediate followed by its deamination to pyruvic acid.[17]

Glycogen phosphorylase has pyridoxal phosphate linked covalently to the ε-amino group of a lysine residue of the enzyme. Removal of this cofactor whose function is unknown results in an inactive enzyme.[17]

Amino acid synthases, such as threonine synthase, utilizes O-phosphohomoserine bound to pyridoxal phosphate in Schiff's base linkage where the elimination of the phosphate residue and a shift of double bonds result in moving the hydroxyl group from the terminal position to one β to the carboxyl group to form threonine. The threonine then dissociates from the pyridoxal phosphate-enzyme complex.[17] Synthesis of protoporphyrin, a precursor of hemoglobin, is carried out by the pyridoxal phosphate requiring enzyme δ-aminolevulinate synthase.

Serine hydroxymethyltransferase, another pyridoxal phosphate-requiring enzyme, condenses acetaldehyde and glycine to make threonine by an alternate route. This enzyme also transfers the β-carbon of serine to tetrahydrofolate to form glycine and generates a formyl group for synthetic pathways utilizing N^5, N^{10}-methylenetetrahydrofolate.[17]

Deficiency of pyridoxine also results in the excretion of xanthurenic acid, a side product in the biosynthesis of niacin. Thus, the conversion of tryptophan to niacin is interrupted by a pyridoxine deficiency. The enzyme requiring pyridoxal phosphate, kynureninase, is blocked from forming 3-hydroxyanthranilic acid (see Figure 13).[17]

Biosynthesis

Hill et al.,[131] using radiolabeled precursors, showed that pyridoxine was synthesized from three glycerol molecules. One as a 2-carbon unit was obtained from pyruvate at the oxidation level of acetaldehyde and the other two glycerols were incorporated intact at the level of glyceraldehyde-3-phosphate.

Pharmacokinetics

Absorption of pyridoxine from the lumen of the small intestine occurs rapidly and appears to be by simple diffusion.[127] Pyridoxal phosphate is also absorbed, partly after hydrolysis by alkaline phosphatase in the intestinal wall and partly intact by a saturable process that was inhibited by L-phenylalanine and pyridoxamine phosphate but not by pyridoxamine.[132]

Vitamin B_6 compounds in the cytosol are transported into the mitochondria in the phosphorylated state at a linear rate. Pyridoxal and pyridoxamine are phosphorylated in the cytosol by pyridoxal kinase before transport. About 20% of the vitamin B_6 compounds are in the mitochondria where many reactions employing B_6 enzymes take place. Mixing of endogenous and exogenous pyridoxal phosphate is less homogenous in the mitochondria where they are bound to matrix proteins than in the cytosol. Hydrolysis of pyridoxal phosphate by the hydrolase may take place in the intermembrane space of mitochondria and on the plasma membrane where alkaline phosphatase is also located. It is probable that dephosphorylation of pyridoxal and pyridoxamine phosphates may take place mainly by alkaline phosphatase.[133]

4-Pyridoxic acid comprises the major metabolite of the B_6 co-enzymes excreted in the urine. This compound is pyridoxine oxidized to the corresponding carboxylic acid at position 4. Other metabolites are pyridoxal, pyridoxamine and their 5-phosphates and a small amount of pyridoxine.

Toxicity
Large amounts of vitamin B_6 were given to pregnant women for treatment of nausea without ill effects on the mother or offspring.[63] This vitamin appears to be relatively nontoxic.

FOLIC ACID

Discovery and Nutritional Background
The chronicle of the discovery of folic acid began in 1931 when Wills described an autolyzed yeast fraction which cured macrocytic anemia. This material was named Will's Factor.[5] From this time on into the 1940s, various factors were put forward as new vitamins or growth factors. These include vitamin M, Factor U, Vitamin Bc, Norit Eluate Factor, and Citrovorum Factor. The confusion occurred because folic acid was not a single compound but a family of pteroylglutamic acids which were active to varying degrees in biological systems which utilized one or more of them for growth in the case of bacteria or for the cure of anemia and gastrointestinal disorders in animals.

Vitamin M was so named because a factor in yeast or liver extracts cured a nutritional macrocytic anemia in monkeys.[118] Factor U was identified as a growth factor for chicks maintained on a purified ration.[5] Vitamin Bc was the name given to a substance which prevented macrocytic anemia in chicks and was found in yeast and in a liver fraction.[5] Norit Eluate Factor, also called *Lactobacillus casei* factor, was a micronutrient from liver extract adsorbed on Norit and eluted with 0.5 N ammonium hydroxide. This substance was reported to be necessary for growth of this microorganism.[5] Citrovorum Factor was required for the growth of cultures of *Leuconostoc citrovorum*.

p-Aminobenzoic acid has been listed as a vitamin. It is now recognized that *p*-aminobenzoic is part of the folic acid structure and functions as such. Some bacteria require *p*-aminobenzoic acid for synthesis of the complete folic acid molecule.[32]

Isolation, Structure, and Chemical Synthesis
Angier and co-workers reported the isolation, degradation, and synthesis of the liver *Lactobacillus casei* factor in a preliminary note in 1945. Pfiffner and associates[134] isolated and characterized the chick antianemia factor from hog liver, horse liver, and yeast and found that it was identical to Angier's *L. casei* factor in 1947. Pfiffner started with 1000 lb

Table 3
THE NATURAL OCCURRENCE OF FOLATES AND
OTHER PTERINS

Name	Occurrence
Folic acid, pteroyl-L-glutamic acid	Yeast, autolyzed liver, spinach
Pteroyldiglutamic acid	Propionibacteria
Pteroylhexaglutamic acid (vitamin Bc conjugated)	Yeast
N5-Formyltetrahydrofolic acid (citrovorum factor, synthetic leucovorin, folinic acid SF)	Liver
N10-Formyltetrahydrofolic acid	Liver mitochondria, red blood cells, plants
5-Methyltetrahydrofolic acid (pre-folic acid)	Liver, plants
Rhizopterin; N10-formylpteroic acid	*Rhizopus nigricans* butterfly wings
Xanthopterin	Insects, amphibia
Biopterin and tetrahydrobiopterin	Insects, amphibia, humans

of hog liver and successfully adsorbed and eluted the vitamin from Amberlite IR-4, Superfiltrol, and Norit. After butanol extraction and barium-zinc precipitation, the vitamin was crystallized at acid pH to yield about 7 mg of product.

The synthesis of pteroylglutamic acid was reported in detail by Walker et al. (including Angier), in 1948.[135] Equimolar amounts of 2,4,5-triamino-6-hydroxypyrimidine and *p*-aminobenzoylglutamic acid were dissolved in water and reacted with α,β-dibromopropionaldehyde to give a 30 to 50% yield of crude pteroylglutamic acid. The crude material was neutralized, filtered, and crystallized at pH 3. Physical properties of folic acid are given in Table 2.

Deficiency Symptoms

Folic acid deficiency is characterized by megaloblastic anemia. Symptoms include weakness, tiredness, shortness of breath, sore tongue, diarrhea, neurological impairment, anorexia, headache, and palpitations.[136] Megaloblastic anemia occurs frequently in women during the third trimester of pregnancy in regions where poor diet includes marginal folic acid content.[32] Folic acid and vitamin B_{12} are interrelated in terms of deficiency syndrome, hematopoiesis and metabolic roles.[137]

Dietary Sources

Plants and some bacteria are the only organisms able to synthesize folic acid. Monogastric animals, lacking ruminant microorganisms and certain bacteria such as *Lactobacillus casei* used to assay folic acid, require a source of the vitamin.[21] Folic acid is widely distributed. Good food sources are liver, leafy vegetables, and some fruit.[138] The recommended dietary allowance for folic acid and its conjugates is 100 to 400 μg/day for adults and 30 to 45 μg/day for infants. Some heat destruction occurs during food processing. This becomes pronounced if left on a steam table.[22] Like many vitamins, folic acid is light sensitive (see Table 2).

Structure-Activity Relationships

Folic acid refers to pteroylglutamic acid, but it also encompasses a group of related vitamins found with varying numbers of glutamic acid residues and a limited number of other substituents. Naturally occurring folic acid derivatives and other pterins are listed in Table 3 together with other names given to them at one time and their natural sources.[139]

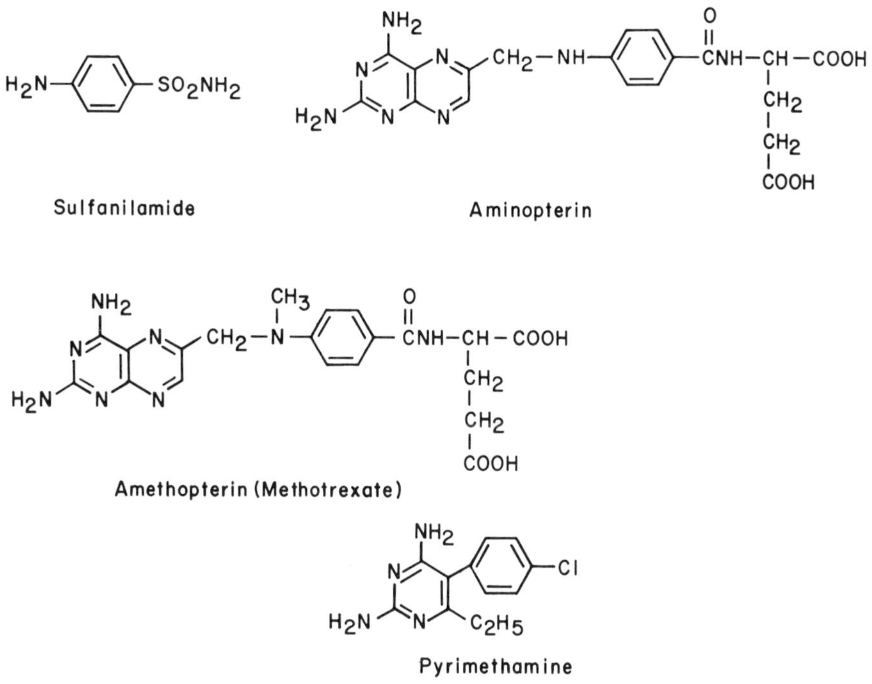

FIGURE 16. Folic acid antagonists.

Folic Acid Antagonists

A very large number of folic acid antagonists have been synthesized and many of them (Figure 16) have therapeutic activity. Since microorganisms synthesize their own folic acid analogs and humans must assimilate them preformed, any inhibitor that specifically inhibits folic acid biosynthesis would ultimately kill the bacteria. Sulfonamides[140] are structural analogs of p-aminobenzoic acid. Therefore, folate biosynthesis at the p-aminobenzoic acid incorporation step would be blocked.

The reduction of dihydrofolate to tetrahydrofolate by dihydrofolate reductase is inhibited by aminopterin (4-aminopteroylglutamic acid) and amethopterin (4-amino-10-methylpter-oylglutamic acid, methotrexate).[140] The reduced cofactor is required for purine nucleotide biosynthesis and, hence, cell division. Rapidly growing tumor cells are more susceptible than normal cells to these antagonists. Since folic acid deficiency produces leucopenia as well as anemia in humans, methotrexate was found to cause remissions in patients with leukemia.

Pyrimethamine,[141] an antimalarial compound, is one of a large class of 2,4-diaminopyr-imidine folic acid antimetabolites synthesized. Different types of chemical substitution yield-ing folic acid antagonists include pyrimidine, purine, and pteridine analogs, alterations in the pterin ring, different amino acids substituting for glutamic acid, alkylated — and therefore blocked — pteroylglutamic acids, different substituents on the pterin ring, and sulfonyl rather than carboxyl groups between the p-aminobenzene moiety and the glutamic acid substituents.[142]

Mechanism of Action

The folic acid group of vitamins act as co-enzymes in 1-carbon transfer reactions in the biosynthesis of many essential metabolic intermediates. Folic acid is successively reduced to dihydrofolate and then to its co-enzymatically active form tetrahydrofolate (THF) by folic acid reductase and dihydrofolate reductase, each requiring NADPH (Figure 17).[17]

The enzyme serine transhydroxymethylase requires pyridoxal phosphate as a cofactor and

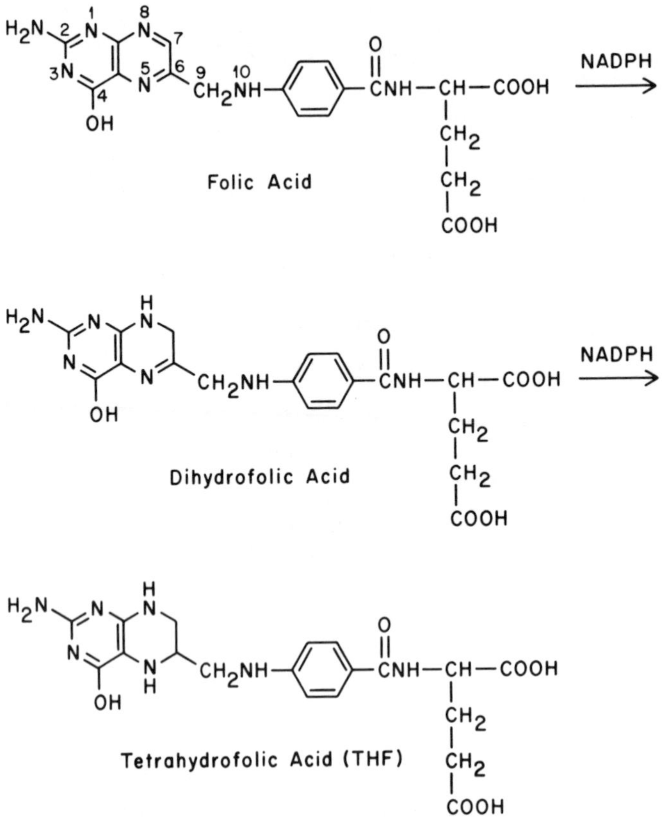

FIGURE 17.   Formation of tetrahydrofolic acid.

transfers the β-carbon of serine to THF to yield glycine and N^5, N^{10}-methylene-THF (Figure 18).[17] The amino group of serine may be held in the form of a Schiff base characteristic of pyridoxal phosphate enzymes, as was discussed under Vitamin B_6. N^5, N^{10}-methylene THF is oxidized by N^5, N^{10}-methylene-THF dehydrogenase and NADP to N^5, N^{10}-methenyl THF which is hydrolyzed by N^5, N^{10}-methenyl cyclohydrolase to N^{10}-formyl THF. N^{10}-Formyl THF can be synthesized directly from formic acid, THF, and ATP by yet another enzyme called formyl THF synthetase.[17]

Another form of THF used in 1-carbon transfers is N^5-methyl THF which is formed by reduction of N^5, N^{10}-methylene THF and NADH by N^5, N^{10}-methylene THF reductase.[17] The methyl groups on the N^5 position can be used to methylate homocysteine to give methionine in microorganisms and betaine to give choline.

Thus, folic acid in the reduced form can act as a carrier of one carbon units at three oxidation states, methyl, hydroxymethyl, and formate.[139]

THF can also accept a formimino group from formiminoglutamic acid, an intermediate in histidine degradation, to yield N^5-formimino THF. This requires the enzyme formiminoglutamate formimino transferase. The formimino group is then deaminated by N^5-formimino THF cyclodeaminase to give N^5, N^{10}-methenyl THF.[139] These reactions are summarized in Figure 18.

N^5, N^{10}-methylene THF participates in nucleic acid metabolism. The enzyme thymidylate synthetase and this 1-carbon carrier transforms deoxyuridine 5′-phosphate to thymidine 5′-phosphate and dihydrofolate. THF is then regenerated by dihydrofolate reductase and NADPH. *De novo* biosynthesis of the purine nucleus is accomplished with the aid of THF as a supplier of formate residues comprising purine carbons 2 and 8.[17]

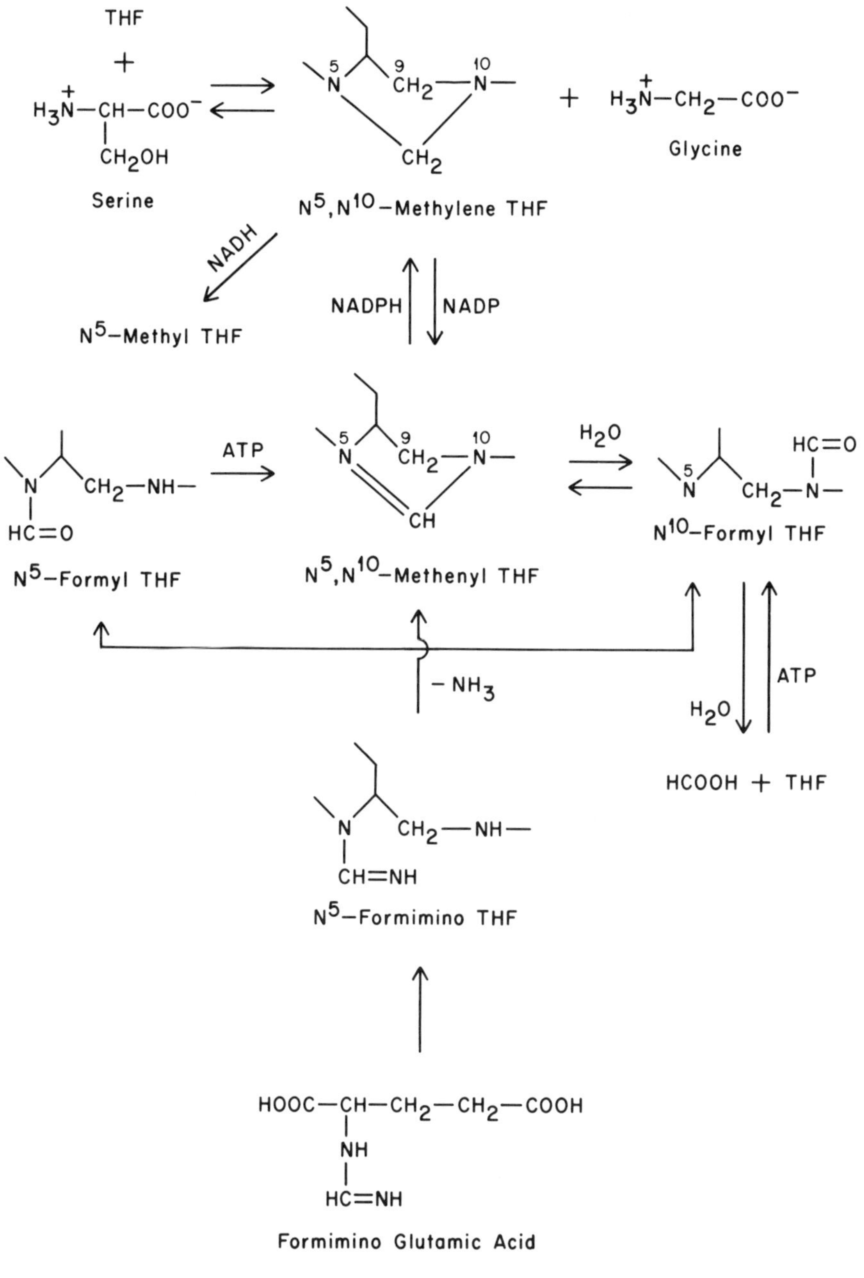

FIGURE 18. 1-Carbon transfer reactions involving tetrahydrofolate.

Folate, THF, and its methylated analogs are required in the cytosol and mitochondria of the cell, but they cannot pass through the mitochondrial membrane. Serine and glycine are permeable to this membrane and serve as a shuttle for 1-carbon units between these cellular compartments.[17]

Biosynthesis of Folic Acid

Guanosine triphosphate is the precursor of the pterin ring. The first three reactions appear to be catalyzed by a single enzyme from *Escherichia coli*. Dihydroneopterin triphosphate is the end product of this reaction sequence catalyzed by GTP cyclohydrolase. When two of the three intermediates were added to an in vitro system they were converted to this product. Further along in the sequence of reactions, *p*-aminobenzoate is added to the pterin nucleus to give dihydropterin. The enzyme can also add *p*-aminobenzoylglutamate or a sulfonamide to produce dihydrofolic acid or an inactive coenzyme. Thus, sulfonamides appear to compete with *p*-aminobenzoate for synthesis of folic acid. After the addition of one glutamate residue, others can be attached by other enzymes.[106]

Pharmacokinetics

Folic acid occurs in the diet as glutamate polypeptides of various chain lengths. In order to be absorbed all but one must be removed by an enzyme called conjugase.[136] The liberated folic acid is then absorbed through the intestine at an optimal pH of 6 by both a saturable process and a nonsaturable one at low and high folate concentrations, respectively. Experiments with isolated brush border membrane vesicles demonstrated that the folic acid analogs methotrexate and 5-methyl THF competed with folic acid for uptake.[143] Current information indicates that folate is transported in the blood in the free form, bound loosely to serum proteins and bound tightly to a protein carrier.[136] Less is bound in the high affinity state than by the other two modes. The form of folate most prevalent in the circulatory system is the N^5-methyl THF. N^5-methyl THF is transported against a concentration gradient to bone marrow cells, red blood cells, liver, cerebrospinal fluid, and kidney cells. Folate is stored to the extent of 5 to 10 mg in the liver in the form of polyglutamates. Release of folic acid from the liver requires cleavage of these glutamate residues.

About 100 μg of folate, daily, enters the enterohepatic circulation as biologically active compounds. These aid in maintaining normal serum levels of folic acid.[136]

Excretion in the urine and bile of both biologically active and inactive forms of folic acid takes place. There is tubular reabsorption of folic acid which is in competition with folic acid analogs such as aminopterin and amethopterin.[139] Reabsorption through the cell membranes of renal tubules is by a metabolically active process. The principal breakdown product of folic acid in the urine is acetamidobenzoylglutamic acid which indicates that folic acid is cleaved between the 9 and 10 positions and that the *p*-aminobenzoylglutamic acid portion is acetylated probably by the liver before excretion.

Toxicity

Studies in rats and in human epileptics have suggested that folic acid in intravenous doses of 45 and 14 mg, respectively, caused seizures.[136] This is about 100 times the recommended dietary allowance for this vitamin. Undoubtedly, the toxicity of folic acid would be lower in normal subjects given the vitamin by the oral route.

VITAMIN B$_{12}$

Discovery and Nutritional Background

Vitamin B$_{12}$ was the last of the legitimate vitamins to be characterized. The description of pernicious anemia reached back into the mid nineteenth century. A nutritional deficiency was suspected, because the disease was characterized by partial degeneration of the gastric mucosa. The link between vitamin B$_{12}$, or what was later named B$_{12}$, and pernicious anemia was slow to develop for several reasons. Folic acid and B$_{12}$ deficiencies result in macrocytic anemias which are functionally similar. Thus, the initial search for one vitamin sometimes led in the direction of the other. Secondly, B$_{12}$ deficiency more often developed due to the lack of a glycoprotein responsible for its transport across the intestinal walls into the blood stream than to lack of the vitamin itself in the diet. This limiting agent responsible for B$_{12}$ absorption was called "intrinsic factor".[136] Thirdly, assay for vitamin B$_{12}$ activity was initially done using humans suffering from pernicious anemia. There was no animal model

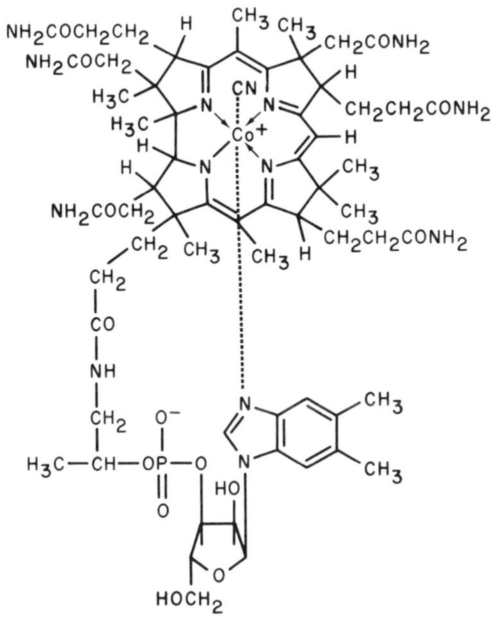

FIGURE 19.   Vitamin B_{12}.

of this deficiency disease.[5] Lastly, human stores of vitamin B_{12} are sufficient for 3 to 6 years before symptoms of a deficiency state make their appearance.[136]

A parallel series of investigations into a so-called "animal protein factor" were conducted in 1946 and 1947 by Rubin and Bird[144] among others. Hens on a diet of corn and soybean meal laid eggs that failed to hatch well. The addition of a small amount of cow manure to the ration improved hatchability. An acid precipitate of water extract of cow manure, known as an animal protein factor, was later shown to be identical to vitamin B_{12} upon its isolation in 1948.

In 1926, Minot and Murphy[145] announced that adding large amounts of liver to the diets of patients with anemias cured their condition and restored the red blood cell count to normal. Minot, Murphy, and their colleague Whipple were awarded the Nobel Prize in 1934 in physiology and medicine for this major advance in therapeutics. However, it remained until 1948 for the active principle in liver to be identified as vitamin B_{12}.

Isolation, Structure, and Chemical Synthesis

In 1948, two laboratories reported the isolation and crystallization of vitamin B_{12}.[5] Rickes et al. isolated red, crystalline, cyanocobalamine which was found to be efficacious in humans with pernicious anemia and also as a growth factor for *Lactobacillus lactis* Dorner. This microorganism, it was found, could replace humans for biological assay of B_{12} activity. The second group to isolate vitamin B_{12} was Lester-Smith and Parker in England. The fractionation steps from liver to acetone precipitate of the purified material were accomplished by chromatography and solvent extraction.[5]

Determination of the structure of vitamin B_{12} was another matter. The molecule was very complex and required 7 years of analysis of fragments and X-ray crystallographic evidence to arrive at the final structure, which is given in Figure 19.[5] Another Nobel Prize was awarded for work on vitamin B_{12} in 1964, this time for the X-ray crystallographic identification of the molecular structure by Hodgkin and her associates.

Vitamin B_{12} consists of two main structural portions. The most prominent feature is the planar corrin ring which is made up of four pyrrol rings bridged on three sides by methylene groups and on the fourth side by a direct linkage. The six double bonds are conjugated and form a resonant system. A central cobalt atom is in a coordination complex with the four nitrogens in the corrin ring. The outer portions of the ring are substituted by methyl, acetamide, or propionamide groups in the same sequence found in uro-porphyrin III.[2] Also contained in the coordination complex is an unusual nucleotide, 5,6-dimethylbenzimidazole, in α-glycosidic linkage with ribose-3-phosphate. The usual nucleotide linkage between sugar and base is in the β configuration. The other end of the phosphate group is esterified to 1-amino-2-propanol. The nitrogen of the latter is connected to a propionic acid substituent on one ring by an amide bond. The benzimidazole ring is nearly perpendicular to the corrin ring.

Vitamin B_{12} is the cyano coordination compound of the above structure known as "cobalamine" by convention. Other cobalamines are known and will be discussed under Structure-Activity Relationships. The presence of the cyano group does not imply that this is the form in which the vitamin exists in the body. It is, however, a stable form of B_{12} and lends a very rich, red color to the coordination complex.

Synthesis of vitamin B_{12} was accomplished in 1973, 25 years after its isolation, by a team led by Woodward at Harvard and Eschenmoser in Zurich.[146] The coordinated efforts of 99 chemists from 19 countries were required to accomplish the 60-step synthesis of cyano-cobalamine in the space of 11 years. Some physical properties of this vitamin are given in Table 2.

Deficiency Symptoms

Dietary deficiency of vitamin B_{12} results only rarely and that is caused by strict adherence to a vegetarian diet that excludes all animal products. The more prevalent form of B_{12} deficiency is due to a lack of intrinsic factor which permits absorption of the vitamin from the gastrointestinal tract.

Pernicious anemia is the deficiency state caused by lack of absorption of vitamin B_{12}. It is characterized by megaloblastic bone marrow, a macrocytic anemia usually a permanent defect in production of intrinsic factor normally present in gastric juice, low rate of hydrochloric acid production in the stomach, atrophy of the gastric mucosa and, late in the disease, neurological degeneration, especially in the spinal cord.[101,147]

Dietary Sources

Microorganisms are responsible for the production of all of the vitamin B_{12} required by higher animals and many simpler forms of life.[148] As you might recall, cow manure is a very rich source of animal protein factor which was later identified as vitamin B_{12}. The vitamin produced by microorganisms is stored in animal tissues. Thus, meat and meat products, fish, poultry, eggs, and milk are good sources of the vitamin. Vegetable products are devoid of vitamin B_{12} unless they are contaminated by bacteria.[136] Clams and oysters which filter large quantities of plankton-laden seawater are good sources. Stability to food processing at pH 4 to 5 is good, but destruction by light takes place.[22]

The NRC requirements for vitamin B_{12} range from 0.5 μg per day in infants to 3 μg in adults. The infant levels were obtained from the average B_{12} content in human milk.

Structure-Activity Relationships

Vitamin B_{12} is the cyano derivative of cobalamine and was the form of the vitamin first isolated from liver.[136] Cyanocobalamin is the pharmaceutical preparation of the vitamin and is the most stable chemically. Other groups can replace the cyano group in the cobalt coordination complex. Examples are hydroxyl as in vitamin $B_{12}a$, water as in vitamin $B_{12}b$, or nitro as in vitamin $B_{12}c$. A large number of analogs have been synthesized[2] many of which have B_{12} activity.

Vitamin B_{12} exists as a coenzyme like most other B vitamins. Two coenzyme forms have

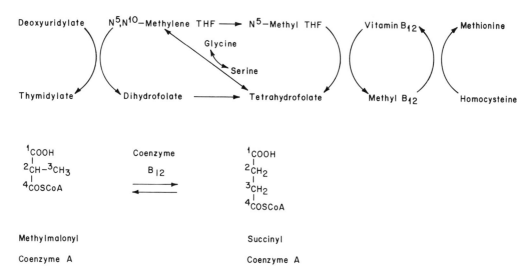

FIGURE 20. Co-enzyme reactions of vitamin B_{12}.

been isolated. Methylcobalamin and 5'-deoxyadenosylcobalamin are cobalt coordination complexes replacing the cyano group. In addition, B_{12} is probably linked to a peptide in its storage and active forms.[136]

Vitamin B_{12} Antagonists

A number of antimetabolites of vitamin B_{12} were sought by replacement of the nucleotide group, hydrolysis of the amide bonds, halogenation, preparation of lactams, lactones, and other derivatives.[2] While they sometimes were effective against certain microorganisms, they were almost always ineffective in higher species. It was hoped that a B_{12} antimetabolite might be effective against a blood disorder such as leukemia in a manner similar to the folic acid antagonists. That hope has not been realized as yet.

A recent paper[149] describes succinylacetone pyrrole, a B_{12} biosynthesis inhibitor. It is a competitive inhibitor of α-aminolevulinic acid dehydratase, the enzyme responsible for synthesis of porphobilinogen. This is of consequence only in microorganisms, because animals require preformed B_{12}.

Mechanism of Action

Megaloblastic changes in the bone marrow are due to an interruption in DNA synthesis whereby cells enlarge but do not divide. Folic acid and vitamin B_{12} are both required for a rate limiting step in DNA synthesis, the methylation of deoxyuridylate to thymidylate.[137] The methyl donor is N^5,N^{10}-methylenetetrahydrofolate (see Figure 18), which is made from tetrahydrofolate (THF). The major form of folate in blood and tissues is N^5-methyl THF. In order to transform N^5-methyl THF to THF, an enzyme with vitamin B_{12} as the cofactor is required. The methyl group is handed off to B_{12} to give methyl B_{12} which, in turn passes the methyl group to homocysteine to form methionine (Figure 20). In the process, THF is generated for resynthesis of N^5,N^{10}-methylene THF. Vitamin B_{12} deficiency is known to reduce this conversion and N^5-methyl THF accumulates. The latter is "trapped" or not converted to the N^5,N^{10}-methylene THF, because the back reaction (Figure 18) is not re versible in man.[150,151] This requirement for folic acid and vitamin B_{12} may aid in explaining the megaloblastic anemia common to the deficiency of either of these vitamins.

Vitamin B_{12} functions as a coenzyme in one other enzymatic reaction in man, the iso-merization of methylmalonyl coenzyme A to succinyl coenzyme A.[17] This pathway deals with the metabolism of propionyl CoA obtained from odd-numbered fatty acids, and from the metabolism of isoleucine and valine. In this reaction the entire thioester group migrates. The excretion of elevated amounts of methylmalonic acid is considered diagnostic of vitamin B_{12} deficiency.[137]

Biosynthesis

The corrin nucleus of vitamin B_{12} is assembled in a manner similar to porphyrins.[2] Delta-aminolevulinic acid combines to form the ringed structure and the methyl groups on the periphery are derived from S-adenosylmethionine.[17] The 5,6-dimethylbenzimidazole portion of the molecule is derived from 6,7-dimethyl-8-ribityllumazine (DMRL), an intermediate in riboflavin biosynthesis. The riboside is obtained from nicotinamide mononucleotide in an exchange reaction.[152] The final step is the assembly of cobalamin on 70S ribosomes with the loss of a phosphate group to give the coenzyme form of vitamin B_{12}. It is interesting to note the participation of riboflavin and niacin in the biosynthesis of vitamin B_{12} by microorganisms.

Pharmacokinetics

The absorption and transport of vitamin B_{12} has been studied extensively. Intrinsic factor is a glycoprotein that is made in the acid-secreting parietal cells of the stomach.[148] There it combines with B_{12} and travels down to the ileum where it reacts with a receptor in the brush border of the mucosal cells[153] in the presence of calcium ion at a pH above 6. The B_{12} is liberated on the serosal side and binds to a β-globulin in blood called transcobalamin II, which delivers the vitamin to the cells.[136] Vitamin B_{12} also circulates in the blood bound to an α-1 globulin, transcobalamin I.[127] The B_{12} bound to transcobalamin II reacts with a cell surface receptor and is internalized by endocytosis into vesicles. There the transcobalamin is digested by lysosomal proteases and B_{12} is released into the cells.[148]

This absorptive mechanism has a carrying capacity of only 1.5 to 3 μg of vitamin B_{12}.[136] Larger amounts may be absorbed by passive diffusion. Fifty to ninety percent of the stored B_{12} is in liver, which contains between 1 and 10 mg of total vitamin B_{12}. The vitamin is secreted to the extent of 0.1 to 0.2% of the body stores daily via the bile. The excretory product is mainly unchanged B_{12} which is the minute amount that escapes efficient reabsorption by the enterohepatic circulation. This very slow excretion rate probably accounts for the reason why strict vegetarians require at least 3 to 6 years to develop vitamin B_{12} deficiency.[136]

Toxicity

A few hypersensitivity reactions have been recorded for intradermal injections of vitamin B_{12}.[63] The cyano group of cyanocobalamin does not appear to be toxic even at 10,000 times the NRC requirement of 3 μg.[136] The mol wt of B_{12} is 1355 of which the cyano group represents only 26 or less than 1/50 of the total. Therefore, cyanide poisoning from overdosing with vitamin B_{12} would be extremely remote.

PANTOTHENIC ACID

Discovery and Nutritional Background

Williams and associates[154] in 1933 found that tissue extracts from 11 phyla stimulated growth of a strain of yeast called Gebrude Mayer. They called this growth factor pantothenic acid after a Greek word meaning "from everywhere". Pantothenic acid deficiency has been shown to be responsible for a type of chick dermatitis, graying of hair in rats, and hemorrhagic adrenal necrosis in the rat.[3]

Isolation, Structure, and Chemical Synthesis

Pantothenic acid was very difficult to isolate in pure form, because of its small size and water solubility. The best that could be obtained was about 90% purity. Oxidation equivalent analysis and combustion analysis data gave the formula $(C_8H_{14}O_5N)_2Ca$ for the calcium salt. It was shown to have one carboxyl, two hydroxyl, and probably a substituted amide group.[155] Hydrolysis of pantothenic acid gave β-alanine which was identified as its β-naphthalene sulfo derivative.[156] The other part of the molecule was isolated as a lactone.[157] All of this groundwork was done in Williams' laboratory. He then handed the problem over to Stiller and co-workers at Merck and Co., Inc. They were able to isolate the crystalline lactone of α,γ-dihydroxy-β,B-dimethylbutyric acid.[158] In the same year, 1940, they were successful in synthesizing the complete vitamin by a cyanohydrin reaction on α,α-dimethyl-β-hydroxypropionaldehyde and then condensing the product with β-alanine ethyl ester.[159] The lactones were resolved into their isomers by crystallization with quinine in alkaline solution. The (+) pantothenic acid, synthesized from the (−) lactone and β-alanine, was the biologically active isomer.[159] Some physical properties of this vitamin are given in Table 2.

Deficiency Syndrome

Because pantothenic acid is so generally distributed, a deficiency disease in man was difficult to demonstrate. An experimental diet deficient in pantothenate produced signs of stomach cramps, malaise, vomiting, and insomnia.[160] Another study incorporating the pantothenic acid antagonist ω-methylpantothenic acid in a deficient diet produced the same symptoms but earlier. Supplementing with pantothenic acid at the end of the study cured the symptoms.

Dietary Sources

As was mentioned, pantothenic acid was so named by Williams because it meant "from everywhere".[154] Foods rich in pantothenic acid are animal products, whole grain cereals, and legumes and, to a lesser extent, milk. However, any balanced diet should supply the minimum daily requirements, which are 2 to 3 mg/day for infants and 4 to 7 mg/day for adults. Human milk contains 2 mg/ℓ and cow's milk has 3.5 mg/ℓ.[21] Even though pantothenic acid is considered to be one of the more labile vitamins, it appears to be preserved during food processing fairly well. Stability is favored near neutrality.[22]

Structure-Activity Relationships

Pantothenic acid, pantotheine, and the co-enzyme form of the vitamin, co-enzyme A (Figure 21) are equally active in animals.[160] However, giving pantoic acid and β-alanine separately rather than linked together as the vitamin to deficient animals did not cure the deficiency disease. This meant that the amide bond joining the two halves of the vitamin is stable to hydrolysis in the gastrointestinal tract.[17]

Another combined form of pantothenic acid has been isolated from tomatoes. This is 4'-D(β-D-glucopyranosyl)-D-pantothenic acid.[160] The function of this compound is unknown at present.

Vitamin Antagonists

Bird et al.[161] cited studies with ω-methylpantothenic acid used to hasten the onset of pantothenic acid deficiency symptoms in humans described earlier. All of the other antagonists mentioned, such as pantoyltaurine, were antagonists of bacterial growth but failed to produce signs of pantothenate deficiency in experimental animals.

Mechanism of Action

Pantothenic acid functions as an integral part of co-enzyme A and acyl carrier protein. This vitamin is responsible for transfer of acyl groups in biosynthetic, degradative and oxidative metabolic pathways.

The synthesis of citric acid in the citric acid cycle takes place by the condensation of

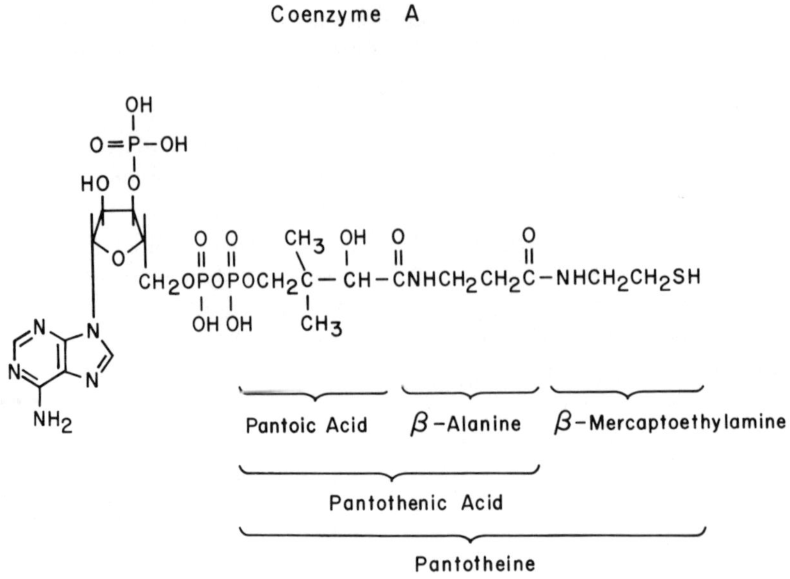

Coenzyme A

FIGURE 21. Co-enzyme A and constituent fragments.

acetyl co-enzyme A and oxaloacetate in the presence of the co-enzyme forms of the other vitamins thiamin pyrophosphate, nicotinamide adenine dinucleotide, and flavin adenine dinucleotide. These are combined in the pyruvate dehydrogenase complex within the matrix of the mitochondrion.[17] The oxidation of α-ketoglutarate to succinate in the citric acid cycle is analogous to the pyruvate to acetyl CoA conversion. Co-enzyme A is also involved in the formation of acetyl CoA units for fatty acid biosynthesis from citrate by the cytosolic enzyme ATP citrate lyase. Acetyl CoA is employed for the synthesis of acetylcholine by choline acetyl transferase in nerves.

Pantothenic acid, together with biotin, play a major role in the biosynthesis of fatty acids.[162] Co-enzyme A and apo acyl carrier protein (ACP) react to form the metabolically active ACP by the enzyme acyl carrier protein synthetase. A serine residue on the protein is phosphorylated to give the 4′-phosphopantetheine derivative of ACP and the by-product 3′,5′-adenosine diphosphate. The SH group on the phosphopantotheine residue of ACP is the acyl group acceptor during fatty acid synthesis. An acetyl group from acetyl CoA is transferred to the acceptor to form acetyl-SH-ACP. After the acetyl group is temporarily transferred to the condensing enzyme, ACP combines with a malonyl group from malonyl CoA and then adds the acetyl group from condensing enzymes back to give the 4-carbon intermediate. ACP takes the biosynthetic process to the palmitate level before starting over again. Pantothenic acid is a component of active ACP and co-enzyme A in these reactions.[162]

Oxidation of fatty acids via thioesters of co-enzyme A yields energy by their introduction into the citric acid cycle as acetyl CoA units for the ultimate generation of ATP. In the process of transferring fatty acids into and out of mitochondria, carnitine is employed as a carrier of acyl groups. Acyl transferase forms acyl carnitine on one side of the membrane from carnitine and acyl CoA and hands the acyl group back to CoA on the other side of the membrane.[17]

Co-enzyme A is involved in the biosynthesis of cholesterol by the rate determining step employing 3-hydroxy-3-methylglutaryl co-enzyme A.[17] These metabolic transformations involving pantothenic acid are presented as examples of at least seventy enzymatic reactions using coenzyme A or 4′-phosphopantetheine as prosthetic groups.

Biosynthesis

Pantothenic acid is synthesized from metabolic intermediates in green plants and micro-organisms. α-Ketoisovalerate, the immediate precursor of valine, is formed from pyruvic acid. A folate co-enzyme, N^5, N^{10}-methylene THF, is responsible for the addition of the formyl group to α-ketoisovalerate to yield ketopantoic acid which is reduced by the niacin co-enzyme, NADPH, to give pantoic acid.[106] The final step in the sequence, the addition of β-alanine, completes the biosynthesis of pantothenic acid. β-Alanine has been shown to be derived from aspartic acid by decarboxylation.[106]

Pharmacokinetics

The metabolic degradation of pantothenic acid has been studied in rat liver and kidney and in horse kidney. According to the citation,[17] co-enzyme A is dephosphorylated and then split into 4'-phosphopantetheine and adenine nucleotide.

Toxicity

No toxic reactions to pantothenic acid have been reported to date.[63] When 10 or 20 g of calcium pantothenate were taken by humans, sporadic diarrhea was recorded.[160]

BIOTIN

Discovery and Nutritional Background

The history of the discovery of biotin took many paths as did that for other vitamins. It was known as vitamin H, the curative factor for egg white injury, bios II or IIB, co-enzyme R, or Factor X.[163] Factor X, vitamin H, and the protective factor against egg white injury were isolated from liver.[5] Bios fractions were found to be essential growth factors for yeast.[3] Co-enzyme R was found to be a factor that was necessary for the respiration of legume nodule bacteria.[5] The name biotin was conferred by Kogl in 1935.[163] The investigators that were instrumental in the discovery of what proved to be this vitamin were: Parson, who described egg white injury; Gyorgy, who helped identify the factor (vitamin H) that cured egg white injury; and Miller, who studied the bios factors.[3]

Isolation, Structure, and Chemical Synthesis

In 1936, Kogl and Tonnis isolated biotin as a growth factor for yeast as its crystalline methyl ester from the yolk of duck eggs. This newly isolated substance was not identical with vitamins B_1 or C or amino acids. It was an extremely potent stimulant, being effective at a 1 to 400,000 dilution. When dried egg yolk was used as the starting material, 250 kg gave 1.1 mg of crystalline biotin with a yield of 1.4%.[5]

The structure of biotin (Figure 22) was determined, in part, by barium hydroxide removal of the carbonyl group to give the diaminocarboxylic acid.[5] This compound was shown to have two primary amino groups by the Van Slyke nitrous acid analysis.[163] Oxidation of the diaminocarboxylic acid with alkakine permanganate gave adipic acid, which identified the side chain. Biotin contains three chiral centers.[5] Two are at the junction of the rings and the third is at the site of attachment of the side chain. Synthesis of all stereoisomers and biological testing revealed that the compound in the *cis* configuration with a (+) rotation was the biologically active one. The first chemical synthesis of biotin was accomplished in 1944 by S. A. Harris and co-workers at Merck.[164] Racemic biotin was resolved by forming a salt with L (+) arginine and separating the diastereoisomers.[165] Some physical properties of biotin are given in Table 2.

Deficiency Symptoms

Biotin deficiency can be produced in animals by feeding diets containing the antagonist

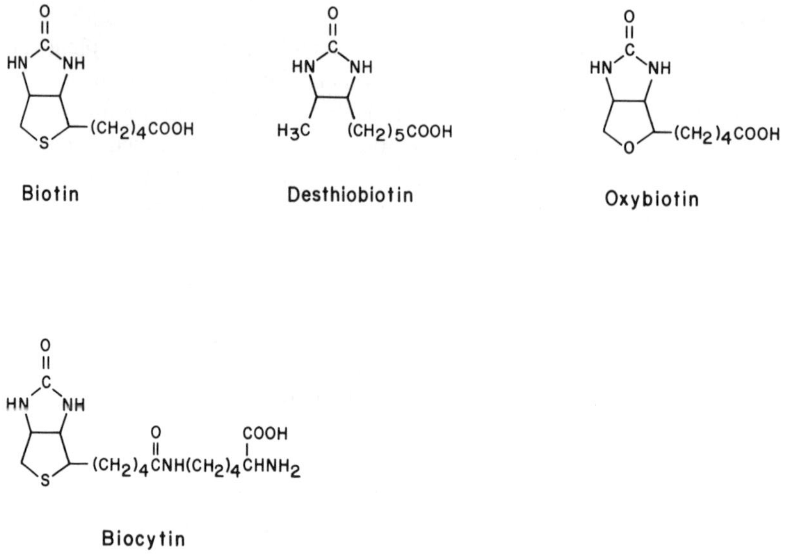

FIGURE 22.   Biotin and analogs.

avidin found in raw egg white and/or including antibiotics in the feed to decrease biotin synthesis by bacteria in the intestinal tract. Signs of deficiency are alopecia, initially about the eyes, dry and scaly skin, a spastic gait, and reproductive failure.[163,166] Biotin deficiency in man may develop on a diet containing a large number of raw eggs. One bizarre example[163] was a 66-year-old man, who consumed 1 to 4 quarts of wine daily for 6 years prior to hospital admission wherein each glass of wine contained a raw egg. Thus, even though egg yolk contained sufficient biotin to serve as a source for isolation by Kogl and Tonnis, the amount of avidin in the raw egg white was in excess of the amount needed for binding the vitamin.

Pantothenic acid and biotin appear to share certain characteristics in terms of one protecting against the severity of the deficiency of the other.[163] This will become more apparent when the metabolic role of biotin is discussed.

Dietary Sources

Good sources of biotin are liver, kidney, and yeast with lesser amounts found in nuts, cauliflower, mackerel, and sardines. Poorer sources are most cereal grains, meat, dairy products, and fruit.[21,166] The bioavailability of biotin in foods is reduced if it is bound as in wheat compared with the biotin in corn or soybeans where it is free. Biotin is synthesized by many different microorganisms. The daily requirement for this vitamin is partially met through its production by the flora of the intestinal tract. Therefore, the daily requirement for biotin in the diet is only an approximation and is based on caloric intake. The average American adult consumes between 100 and 300 μg of biotin daily.[21] Biotin is generally stable to food storage and processing.[22]

Structure-Activity Relationships

The four sets of diastereoisomers of biotin are (±)-biotin, (±)-*epi*-biotin, (+)-allobiotin, and (±)-*epi* allobiotin.[118] The only biological activity resides with (+)-biotin.

Desthiobiotin (Figure 22) has growth promoting activity for the yeast *Saccharomyces cerevisiae*, but it inhibited the use of biotin by *Lactobacillus casei*.[118] Its biological activity was attributed to its conversion to biotin. Oxybiotin, which consists of the *cis* isomer only, has biological activity attributed to the intact structure.[5] Other analogs such as the sulfoxide

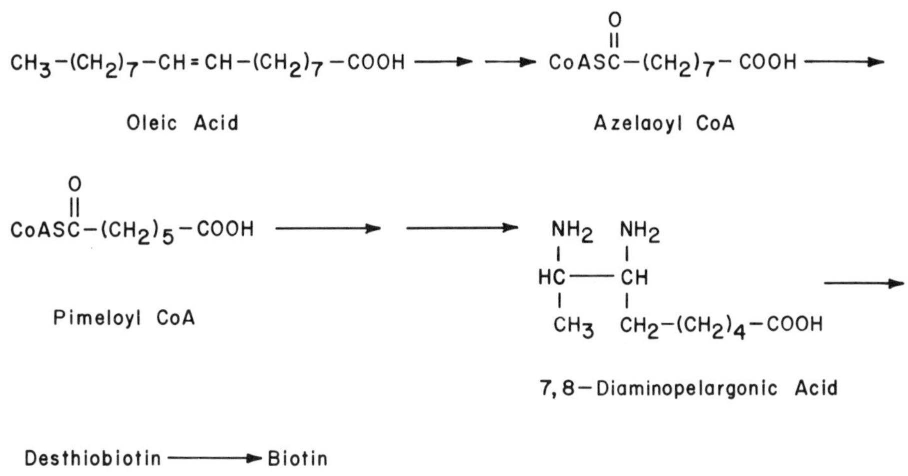

$$CH_3-(CH_2)_7-CH=CH-(CH_2)_7-COOH \longrightarrow \longrightarrow CoASC\overset{\overset{\displaystyle O}{\|}}{}-(CH_2)_7-COOH \longrightarrow$$

Oleic Acid   Azelaoyl CoA

$$CoASC\overset{\overset{\displaystyle O}{\|}}{}-(CH_2)_5-COOH \longrightarrow \longrightarrow$$

Pimeloyl CoA

7,8—Diaminopelargonic Acid

Desthiobiotin ⟶ Biotin

FIGURE 23.   Biosynthesis of biotin.

and sulfone have been synthesized. The former is biologically active, but the sulfone is a growth promoter only for yeast and not *L. casei*.[118]

One of the bound forms of biotin is biocytin (Figure 22). In yeast, biotin is combined in amide linkage with the ε-amino group of lysine. Due to its liberation of biotin, biocytin is biologically active in most systems tested. A biotin complex of very strong affinity (kdalton $= 10^{-15}$ M) is that with avidin. Avidin was mentioned as being a constituent of raw egg white and responsible for so-called egg white injury. It is a glycoprotein with a mol wt of 67,000. Four tryptophan residues compete for binding with the ureido group of biotin for reasons that are not clear. Nevertheless, avidin is a useful tool for the localization of biotin within the cell.[167]

Mechanism of Action

Biotin, in its protein bound form, is the co-enzyme responsible for carboxylation reactions in the body. It has been shown that, as in biocytin, the carboxyl group of biotin is linked with the ε-amino group of a lysine residue of the enzyme which it serves. In the reaction carried out by acetyl CoA carboxylase,[162] the initial step in fatty acid synthesis, CO_2 from bicarbonate attaches to an imino group of the biotin-containing unit called biotin carboxyl carrier protein. The reaction is driven by ATP and biotin carboxylase. In a second reaction catalyzed by transcarboxylase, acetyl CoA accepts the bound CO_2 from biotin to yield malonyl CoA and the free biotin carboxyl carrier protein. Other carboxylase enzymes for which biotin is the cofactor, are propionyl CoA carboxylase, pyruvate carboxylase, and β-methyl crotonyl CoA carboxylase.[168] Patients with a genetic lack of one or more of these enzymes have been identified. Biotin is ineffective in treating such patients, because the enzyme to which it is attached is missing or defective.

Biosynthesis

The biosynthetic pathway of biotin in microorganisms has been studied by measuring the efficiency of incorporation of carbon atoms from candidate precursors into the vitamin.[17] A proposed scheme, given in Figure 23, begins with oleic acid which is cleaved at the double bond to give azelaic acid, which is then transformed into azelaoyl coenzyme A. Beta-oxidation reduces the number of carbons by two to give pimeloyl CoA. The ethyl amino group in 7,8-diaminopelargonic acid comes from the fusion of alanine with the aid of pyridoxal phosphate. The resulting intermediate ketone is then aminated. The ureido group is completed by an energy dependent carboxylation reaction and sulfur from an unknown source is added to generate biotin.

Pharmacokinetics

Absorption of biotin occurs within the upper third to half of the intestinal tract by passive diffusion.[168] Much of the biotin is derived from bacterial synthesis in the intestinal tract. Biotin circulates in the blood stream bound to plasma proteins. Degradation of the side chain of biotin is known to take place[17] but the ring system may be excreted intact.

Toxicity

When 5 to 10 mg of biotin were given to young patients each day for the treatment of seborrheic dermatitis, no toxic reactions were encountered.[166] Although no formal toxicological studies were performed, no adverse reactions to biotin have been noted.[63]

ASCORBIC ACID

Discovery and Nutritional Background

Scurvy has been the subject of writings beginning in early Egyptian times and extending through the first part of this century. James Lind (1716 to 1794) has been credited with one of the first descriptions of scurvy, that afflicted explorers led by Jacques Cartier in 1536. With the help of friendly Indians, his men were cured by taking an extract of evergreen leaves containing vitamin C.[3] Calling British seamen "limeys" stemmed from their eating citrus fruit for the prevention of scurvy. Armies far from supply lines were also subject to this disease. Scurvy debilitated men in the Hungarian army in 1734 and in Poland in 1737. As late as 1912, the explorer Captain Robert Scott and his men died of scurvy during their expedition to the South Pole.[169] Captain James Cook during the mid to late 1700s took Lind's recommendations seriously. He demonstrated, by collecting fresh fruit and green vegetables during his voyages, that scurvy need not afflict explorers far from home. Not until ascorbic acid had been isolated and tested for the treatment of scurvy did this vitamin deficiency disease become a rare occurrence.

Isolation, Structure, and Chemical Synthesis

Szent-Györgyi in 1928 described the isolation of a carbohydrate that acted as an antioxidant. This substance which he named hexuronic acid was obtained in crystalline form from oranges, cabbages, and adrenal cortices of animals.[170] He received the Nobel Prize in physiology and medicine in 1937 for his work on actin, a muscle protein, and on vitamin C. The structure of ascorbic acid was found to be a 6-carbon enediol γ-lactone with two labile hydrogens which reacted with oxidizing agents and metal ions such as copper. It behaved as a monobasic acid.[5] Physical properties of ascorbic acid are given in Table 2.

Synthesis of ascorbic acid was accomplished by Reichstein, Grüssner and Oppenauer[171] by the addition of cyanide to xylosone. The 6-carbon cyanohydrin intermediate cyclized to formiminoascorbic acid which was hydrolyzed in dilute hydrochloric acid to ascorbic acid.

Deficiency Symptoms

Ascorbic acid deficiency occurs only in those animals that are unable to synthesize the vitamin. This includes man, nonhuman primates, guinea pigs, some fish such as the channel and blue catfish, and a few kinds of bats and birds.[32] Symptoms of the deficiency are reflected in tissues of mesenchymal origin: connective tissue, blood, bone, and cartilage.[100] The symptoms appear between 60 and 90 days after cessation of vitamin C intake. Petechiae and ecchymoses occur on the legs and buttocks, the pilosebaceous canals become hyperkeratotic, the skin becomes dry and itchy, and wounds fail to heal. Joints become painful, gums may bleed and teeth may become loose and fall out. Psychological disturbances have also been noted.

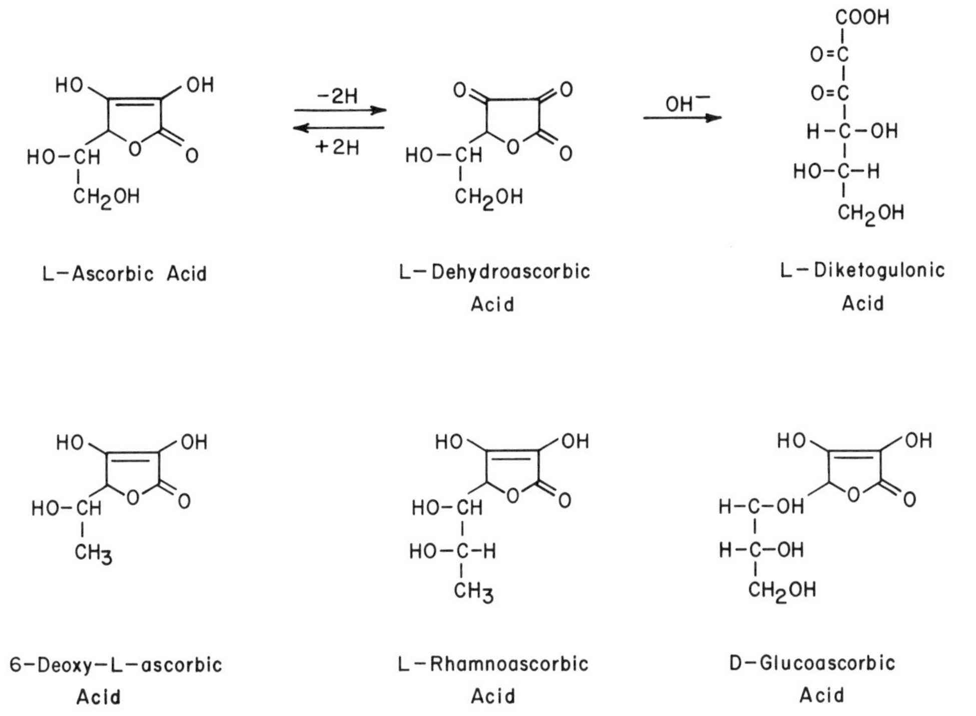

FIGURE 24. Ascorbic acid and its analogs.

Dietary Sources

Rich sources of vitamin C are green leafy vegetables, citrus fruit, sweet and hot peppers, cabbage, turnips, cauliflower, and potatoes. This vitamin is so broadly distributed that poor people are able to receive adequate dietary levels. The recommended dietary allowance of vitamin C, as given in tables by the Food and Nutrition Board, National Academy of Sciences, is 35 mg for infants, 45 mg for children 1 to 10 years of age, and 60 mg per day for adults.[21] A recent paper[172] recommends 100 mg/day for adult males to take into account incomplete absorption from the diet and individuals at the high end of the statistical requirement scale. Cooking for a long period of time and/or in a large volume of water will result in the loss of much of the ascorbic acid content. Metals such as iron or copper may hasten the destruction of this vitamin as will exposure to alkaline pHs. However, foodstuffs rich in vitamin C usually contain organic acids and natural antioxidants such as vitamin E which serve to protect this vitamin from destruction.

Structure-Activity Relationships

The biologically active form of the vitamin is L-ascorbic acid. Ascorbic acid may be reversibly oxidized to L-dehydroascorbic acid which has equivalent biological activity. Opening of the lactone ring as in L-diketogulonic acid (Figure 24) results in loss of vitamin activity.[32] A large number of structural analogs have been prepared and tested for antiscorbutic activity. 6-Deoxy-L-ascorbic acid and L-rhamnoascorbic acid were reported to have 1/3 and 1/5 of the activity of L-ascorbic acid, respectively (Figure 24).[173]

Ascorbic Acid Antagonists

Glucoascorbic acid (Figure 24) was reported to induce scurvy in rats, which normally synthesize their own ascorbic acid. However, supplementing with ascorbic acid did not reverse the symptoms produced by the antagonist. Therefore, this analog appeared to have a toxic effect of its own that was not related to the vitamin activity of ascorbic acid.[174]

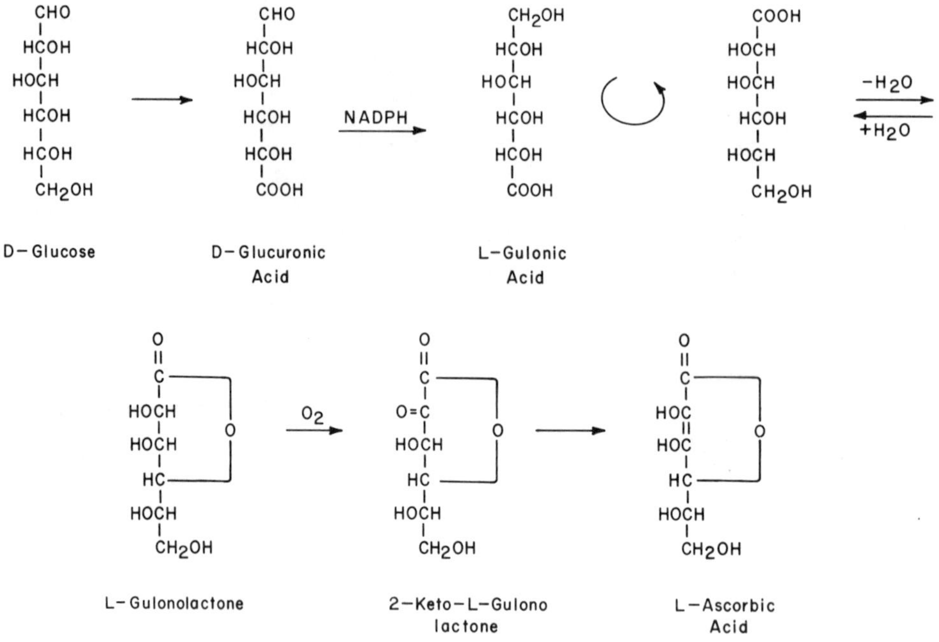

FIGURE 25.   Biosynthesis of ascorbic acid.

Mechanism of Action

It was related earlier that ascorbic acid deficiency was observed mainly in mesenchymal tissue.[100] It has been known for some time that ascorbic acid is necessary for the hydroxylation of proline to hydroxyproline and for the conversion of lysine to hydroxylysine in connective tissue. Hydroxyproline is required for the secretion of collagen and for its helical structure while hydroxylysine is necessary for crosslinkages. Vitamin C also may have an independent effect on stimulating collagen mRNA formation.[175] Ascorbic acid is involved in the hydroxylation of dopamine to norepinephrine and of tryptophan to 5-hydroxytryptophan.[17] Ascorbic acid has not been found to be responsible for maintaining the integrity of connective tissue surrounding the capillary blood vessel walls. Its role in capillary fragility is still unknown.[169] Vitamin C is required for the transport of iron from blood plasma to its storage form, ferritin, in the liver.[32] Thus, vitamin C is instrumental in the biosynthesis of collagen but its actions on other systems appear scattered compared with the well-known co-enzyme functions of the B vitamins.

Biosynthesis

Ascorbic acid is synthesized by animals and plants by two different pathways. Ascorbic acid in mammals is derived from D-glucose by the glucuronic acid pathway in the cytosol of liver.[176] D-Glucuronic acid is then enzymatically reduced by NADPH to L-gulonic acid at which point the stereochemistry of the carbohydrate chain changes from D to L and carbon 1 of D-glucose becomes carbon 6 of L-gulonic acid.[177] Gulonic acid then forms the γ-lactone and is finally oxidized by a microsomal enzyme L-galonolactone oxidase through 2-keto-L-gulonolactone to L-ascorbic acid (Figure 25). It has been shown that animals dependent on a dietary source for their ascorbic acid have a genetic lack of L-gulonolactone oxidase.

Green plants synthesize L-ascorbate-1-^{14}C from D-glucose-1-^{14}C and L-ascorbate-6-^{14}C from D-glucose-6-[14]C. The expected inversion of configuration does not occur. An epimerization at carbon 5 must take place but the nature of the inversion is unknown.[177]

Pharmacokinetics

Early reports indicated that ascorbic acid was absorbed by a passive process.[127] More recent studies demonstrated that absorption in the ileum is by active transport.[178] Ascorbate is taken up by the human ileum or placenta against a concentration gradient which is sodium-ion dependent and ouabain sensitive, indicating the participation of Na^+,K^+-ATPase.[178,179] At very high levels, ascorbate may cross the placenta by simple diffusion.

The body pool size was determined by giving radioactively labeled ascorbate to human subjects on a deficient diet and measuring urinary output at various stages of repletion.[172] In the depleted state, turnover was about 3% of the existing body pool, which under well nourished conditions was approximately 1500 mg. The first signs of scurvy appeared at a pool size of 300 to 400 mg and the last of the signs, hyperkeratosis, disappeared at a body pool size of 1000 mg of ascorbic acid. Daily turnover in the normal human was about 60 mg which gives a plasma level between 0.8 and 0.9 mg/100 mℓ.

Metabolism of ascorbic acid in rats and guinea pigs was different from man. Guinea pigs converted about 70% of their ascorbate to CO_2 and another 2%, approximately, to oxalate. The remainder was ascorbic acid and other unidentified water soluble metabolites.[180] Of the urinary metabolites in man, 20% was diketogulonic acid, less than 2% was dehydroascorbate, 44% was oxalic acid, and 20% was unchanged ascorbic acid. Virtually no CO_2 was formed in humans.[181] The halflife of ascorbate in man was 16 days while it was only 4 days in guinea pigs. This might account for the larger daily requirement for this vitamin by the guinea pig. Also, guinea pigs on a deficient diet develop scurvy in 21 days compared with 3 to 4 months in the case of humans.

Toxicity

Ascorbic acid is not as innocuous as some proponents would have the reader believe nor is it as toxic as others would propose considering the multigram quantities that are consumed. Intake of large amounts of vitamin C over an extended period of time induces enzymes to metabolize these excess amounts. Abrupt discontinuance of ascorbate supplements causes blood and tissue levels to drop below normal, resulting in the appearance of scurvy.[100]

Since oxalic acid is derived from carbons 1 and 2 of ascorbate,[181] the risk of producing kidney and bladder stones with excessive intake of this vitamin is enhanced. One individual took 4 g of ascorbic acid each day for 7 days. His 24-hr urinary oxalate excretion rose from a normal of 58 mg to 622 mg.[182] Moser and Hornig[183] found that the enzymatic formation of oxalate was saturable. Therefore, the probability of producing stones by ascorbic acid excess is unlikely except for individuals with a metabolic abnormality who synthesize large amounts of oxalate from glycine.

Ascorbic acid has been demonstrated to increase the intestinal absorption of iron.[184] This could lead to excessive iron storage and hemochromatosis with tissue damage manifested as cirrhosis, diabetes, and hyperpigmentation of the skin.[185]

Claims have been made for the protective and therapeutic effects of megadoses of ascorbate on the common cold. Some clinical studies have shown promising effects while others have been negative.[169] In light of the serious toxic effects of high vitamin C intake, the use of this agent for treatment of colds is inadvisable. In fact, overdosage by any vitamin, mineral or other so-called natural product is likely to be hazardous to a person's health.

REFERENCES

1. **Funk, C.,** Etiology of deficiency diseases — beri-beri, polyneuritis in birds, epidemic dropsy, scurvy in animals (experimental), infantile scurvy, ship beri-beri,, pellagra; *J. State Med.,* 20, 341, 1912; cited in *Chem. Astr.,* 7, 1899, 1913.

2. **Lester Smith, E.**, *Vitamin B$_{12}$*, 3rd ed., Methuen, London, 1965, 22.

3. **McCollum, E. V.**, *A History of Nutrition*, Houghton-Mifflin, Boston, 1957, 201.

4. **Cheldelin, V. H.**, New and unidentified growth factors, in *The Vitamins. Chemistry, Physiology, Pathology*, Vol. 3, Sebrell, W. H., Jr. and Harris, R. S., Eds., Academic Press, New York, 1954, 577, 596.

5. **Wagner, A. F. and Folkers, K.**, *Vitamins and Coenzymes*, Interscience, New York, 1964.

6. **Herbert, V.**, Pangamic acid (''vitamin B$_{15}$''), *Am. J. Clin. Nutr.*, 32, 1534, 1979.

7. **Anon.**, Laetrile (vitamin B$_{17}$) — a statement by the National Nutrition Consortium, *J. Am. Diet. Assn.*, 70, 354, 1977.

8. **McCollum, E. V. and Davis, M.**, Necessity of certain lipids in the diet during growth, *J. Biol. Chem.*, 15, 167, 1913.

9. **Osborne, T. B. and Mendel, L. B.**, The influence of butter-fat on growth, *J. Biol. Chem.*, 16, 423, 1913.

10. **McCollum, E. V. and Davis, M.**, Observations on the isolation of the substance in butter fat which exerts a stimulating influence on growth, *J. Biol. Chem.*, 19, 245, 1914.

11. **Steenbock, H. and Gross, E. G.**, Fat soluble vitamine II. The fat-soluble vitamine content of roots, together with some observations on their water-soluble vitamine content, *J. Biol. Chem.*, 40, 501, 1919.

12. **Palmer, L. S. and Kempster, H. L.**, Relation of plant carotenoids to growth, fecundity and reproduction of fowls, *J. Biol. Chem.*, 39, 299, 1919.

13. **Moore, T.**, The relation of carotin to vitamin A, *Lancet*, II, 380, 1929.

14. **Karrer, P., Morf, R., and Schöpp, K.**, Zur Kenntnis des Vitamins A aus Fischtranen II, *Helv. Chim. Acta*, 14, 1431, 1931.

15. **Fuson, R. C. and Christ, R. E.**, Condensation of β-cyclocitral with dimethyl acrolein, *Science*, 84, 294, 1936; as cited in *Chem. Abstr.*, 30, 8153, 1936.

16. **Kuhn, R. and Morris, C. J. O. R.**, Syntheses von vitamin A, *Ber. Dtsch. Chem. Ges.*, 70, 753, 1937.

17. **White, A., Handler, P., Smith, E. L., Hill, R. L., and Lehman, I. R.**, *Principles of Biochemistry*, 6th ed., McGraw-Hill, New York, 1978.

18. **McLaren, D. S.**, Cutaneous lesions in nutritional deficiencies, in *Dermatology in General Medicine*, Fitzpatrick, T. B., Arndt, K. A., Clark, W. H., Jr., Eisen, A. Z., Van Scott, E. J., and Vaughan, J. H., Eds., McGraw-Hill, New York, 1971, chap. 19.

19. **Maynard, L. A.** *Animal Nutrition*, McGraw-Hill, New York, 1951, 381.

20. **Watt, B. K. and Merrill, A. L.**, Handbook of the Nutritional Contents of Foods, U.S. Department of Agriculture Handbook, Dover, New York, 1975.

21. **Anon.**, *Recommended Dietary Allowances*, 9th ed., N.A.S.-N.R.C. Publ., Washington, D.C., 1980, 55.

22. **Borenstein, B.**, Effect of processing on the nutritional value of foods, in *Modern Nutrition in Health and Disease*, 6th ed., Goodhart, R. A. and Shils, M. E., Eds., Lea and Febiger, Philadelphia, 1981, 497.

23. **Bownds, M. D.**, Molecular mechanisms of visual transduction, *Trends Neurosci.*, 4, 214, 1981.

24. **Bollag, W. and Matter, A.**, From vitamin A to retinoids in experimental and clinical oncology: achievements, failures and outlook, *Ann. N.Y. Acad. Sci. U.S.A.*, 359, 9, 1981.

25. **Kligman, A. M., Fulton, J. E., and Plewig, G.**, Topical vitamin A acid in acne vulgaris, *Arch. Dermatol.*, 99, 469, 1969.

26. **Mirrer, E. and McGuire, J.**, Lamellar ichthyosis-response to retinoic acid (tretinoin), *Arch. Dermatol.*, 102, 548, 1970.

27. **Kaidbey, K. H., Petrozzi, J. W., and Kligman, A. M.**, Treatment of psoriasis with topically applied tretinoin and steroid ointment, *Arch. Dermatol.*, 111, 1001, 1975.

28. **Voorhees, J. J. and Orfanos, C. E.**, Oral retinoids. Broadspectrum dermatologic therapy for the 1980's, *Arch. Dermatol.*, 117, 418, 1981.

29. **Pochi, P.**, Oral retinoids in dermatology, *Arch. Dermatol.*, 118, 57, 1982.

30. **Meyskens, F. L., Jr.**, Modulation of abnormal growth by retinoids: a clinical perspective of the biological phenomenon, *Life Sci.*, 28, 2323, 1981.

31. **Douer, D. and Koeffler, H. P.**, Retinoic acid. Inhibition of the clonal growth of human myeloid leukemic cells, *J. Clin. Invest.*, 69, 277, 1982.

32. **Pike, R. L. and Brown, M. L.**, *Nutrition: An Integrated Approach*, 2nd ed., John Wiley & Sons, New York, 1975, 80.

33. **Hassell, J. R. and Newsome, D. A.**, Vitamin A — induced alterations in corneal and conjunctival epithelial glycoprotein biosynthesis, *Ann. N.Y. Acad. Sci. U.S.A.*, 359, 358, 1981.

34. **Shidoji, Y., Sasak, W., Silverman-Jones, C. S., and DeLuca, L. M.**, Recent studies on the involvement of retinyl phosphate as a carrier of mannose in biological membranes, *Ann. N.Y. Acad. Sci. U.S.A.*, 359, 345, 1981.

35. **Zile, M. H. and Cullum, M. E.**, The function of vitamin A: current concepts, *Proc. Soc. Exp. Biol. Med.*, 172, 139, 1983.

36. **Goodwin, T. W.**, Biosynthesis of carotenoids and plant terpenes, *Biochem. J.*, 23, 293, 1971.

37. **Rask, L., Anundi, H., Böhme, J., Erikson, U., Ronne, H., Sege, K., and Peterson, P. A.**, Structural and functional studies of vitamin A-binding proteins, *Ann. N.Y. Acad. Sci. U.S.A.*, 359, 79, 1981.

38. **Goodman, D. S.,** Retinoid-binding proteins in plasma and in cells, *Ann. N.Y. Acad. Sci. U.S.A.,* 359, 69, 1981.

39. **DeLuca, H. F., Zile, M., and Sietsema, W. K.,** The metabolism of retinoic acid to 5,6-epoxyretinoic acid, retinoyl-β-glucuronide, and other polar metabolites, *Ann. N.Y. Acad. Sci. U.S.A.,* 359, 25, 1981.

40. **Frolik, C. A.,** In vitro and in vivo metabolism of all-trans and 13-cis-retinoic acid in the hamster, *Ann. N.Y. Acad. Sci. U.S.A.,* 359, 37, 1981.

41. **Frolik, C. A., Swanson, B. N., Dort, L. L., and Sporn, M. B.,** Metabolism of 13-cis-retinoic acid: identification of 13-cis-retinoyl and 13-cis-4-oxoretinyl-β-glucuronides in the bile of vitamin A-normal rats, *Arch. Biochem. Biophys.,* 208, 344, 1981.

42. **Lotan, R.,** Effects of vitamin A and its analogs (retinoids) on normal and neoplastic cells, *Biochim. Biophys. Acta,* 605, 33, 1980.

43. **Randle, H. W., Diaz-Perez, J. L., and Winkelmann, R. K.,** Toxic doses of vitamin A for pityriasis rubra pilaris, *Arch. Dermatol.,* 116, 888, 1980.

44. **Thomas, J. R., III, Cooke, J. P., and Winkelmann, R. K.,** High-dose vitamin A therapy for Darier's disease, *Arch. Dermatol.,* 118, 891, 1982.

45. **Peto, R., Doll, R., Buckley, J. D., and Sporn, M. B.,** Can dietary beta-carotene materially reduce human cancer rates?, *Nature (London),* 290, 201, 1981.

46. **Nieman, C. and Klein Obbink, H. J.,** The biochemistry and pathology of hypervitaminosis A, *Vitam. Hormones N.Y.,* 12, 69, 1954.

47. **Muenter, M. D., Perry, H. O., and Ludwig, J.,** Chronic vitamin A intoxication in adults, *Am. J. Med.,* 50, 129, 1971.

48. **Pitha, J. and Szente, L.,** Rescue from hypervitaminosis A or potentiation of retinoid toxicity by different modes of cyclodextrin administration, *Life Sci.,* 32, 719, 1983.

49. **Lui, N. S. T. and Roels, D. A.,** Vitamin A and carotene, in *Modern Nutrition in Health and Disease,* 6th ed., Goodhart, R. A. and Shils, M. E., Eds., Lea and Febiger, Philadelphia, 1981, 142.

50. **Askew, F. A., Bourdillou, R. B., Bruce, H. M., Jenkins, R. G. C., and Webster, T. A.,** Distillation of vitamin D, *Proc. R. Soc. London Ser. B,* 107B, 1930, as cited in *Chem. Abstr.,* 24, 5802, 1930.

51. **DeLuca, H. F.,** The transformation of a vitamin into a hormone: the vitamin D story, *Harvey Lectures,* Ser. 75, Academic Press, New York, 1981, 333.

52. **Halloran, B. P. and DeLuca, H. F.,** Effect of vitamin D deficiency on skeletal development during early growth in the rat, *Arch. Biochem. Biophys.,* 209, 7, 1981.

53. **Haussler, M. R. and Cordy, P. E.,** Metabolites and analogs of vitamin D. Which for what?, *JAMA,* 247, 841, 1982.

54. **Corrandino, R. A., Ikekawa, N., and DeLuca, H. F.,** Induction of calcium-binding protein in organ-cultured chick intestine by fluoro analogs of vitamin D3, *Arch. Biochem. Biophys.,* 208, 273, 1981.

55. **Coty, W. A., McConkey, C. L., Jr., and Brown, T. A.,** A specific binding protein for 1α, 25-dihydroxyvitamin D in the chick embryo chorioallantoic membrane, *J. Biol. Chem.,* 256, 5545, 1981.

56. **Halloran, B. P. and DeLuca, H.,** Intestinal calcium transport: evidence for two distinct mechanisms of action of 1,25-dihydroxyvitamin D3, *Arch. Biochem. Biophys.,* 208, 477, 1981.

57. **Bronner, F., Lipton, J., Pansu, D., Buckley, M., Singh, R., and Miller, A., III,** Molecular and transport effects of 1,25-dihydroxyvitamin D3 in rat duodenum, *Fed. Proc. Fed. Am. Soc. Exp. Biol.,* 41, 61, 1982.

58. **Dueland, S., Pedersen, J. I., Helgerund, P., and Drevon, C. A.,** Transport of vitamin D3 from rat intestine, *J. Biol. Chem.,* 257, 146, 1982.

59. **Bruns, M. E., Vollmer, S., Wallshein, V., and Bruns, D. E.,** Vitamin D-dependent calcium-binding protein, *J. Biol. Chem.,* 256, 4649, 1981.

60. **Franceschi, R. T. and DeLuca, H. F.,** The effect of inhibitors of protein and RNA synthesis on 1α,25-dihydroxyvitamin D3-dependent calcium uptake in cultured embryonic chick duodenum, *J. Biol. Chem.,* 256, 3848, 1981.

61. **Rasmussen, H., Matsumoto, T., Fontaine, O., and Goodman, D. B. P.,** Role of changes in membrane lipid structure in the action of 1,25-dihydroxyvitamin D3, *Fed. Proc. Fed. Am. Soc. Exp. Biol.,* 41, 72, 1982.

62. **Pierides, A. M.,** Pharmacology and therapeutic use of vitamin D and its analogs, *Drugs,* 21, 241, 1981.

63. **Cumming, F., Briggs, M., and Briggs, M.,** Clinical toxicology of vitamin supplements, in *Vitamins in Human Biology and Medicine,* Briggs, M. H., Ed., CRC Press, Boca Raton, Fla., 1981, 187.

64. **Parfitt, A. M., Gallagher, J. C., Heaney, R. P., Johnston, C. C., Neer, R., and Whedon, G. D.,** Vitamin D and bone health in the elderly, *Am. J. Clin. Nutr.,* 36, 1014, 1982.

65. **Pennock, J. F., Hemming, F. W., and Kerr, J. D.,** A reassessment of tocopherol chemistry, *Biochem. Biophys. Res. Commun.,* 17, 542, 1964.

66. **Horwitt, M. K.,** Vitamin E, in *Modern Nutrition in Health and Disease,* 6th ed., Goodhart, R. A. and Shils, M. E., Eds., Lea and Febiger, Philadelphia, 1981, 180.

67. **Editors,** Vitamin E and cholestatic liver disease, *Nutr. M. D.,* 7, 3, 1981.

68. **Wasserman, R. H. and Taylor, A. N.,** Metabolic roles of fat-soluble vitamins D, E, and K, *Annu. Rev. Biochem.,* 41, 179, 1972.

69. **Century, B. and Horwitt, M. K.,** Biological availability of various forms of vitamin E with respect to different indices of deficiency, *Fed. Proc. Fed. Am. Soc. Exp. Biol.,* 24, 906, 1965.

70. **Green, J., Edwin, E. E., Diplock, A. T., and Bunyan, J.,** The effect of a water-soluble metabolite of α-tocopherol on ubiquinone in the rat, *Biochim. Biophys. Acta,* 49, 417, 1961.

71. **MacKenzie, J. B. and MacKenzie, C. G.,** The antisterility activity of α-tocohydroquinone in the female rat, *J. Nutr.,* 72, 322, 1960.

72. **Smith, L. I., Renfrow, W. B., and Opie, J. W.,** The chemistry of vitamin E. XXXVIII. α-Tocopheramine, a new vitamin E factor, *J. Am. Chem. Soc.,* 64, 1082, 1942.

73. **Schweiter, U., Tamm, R., Weiser, H., and Wiss, O.,** Zur Synthese und Vitamin-E-Wirksamkeit von Tocopheraminen und ihren N-alkyl-Derivaten, *Helv. Chim. Acta,* 49, 2297, 1966.

74. **Bieri, J. G. and Prival, E. L.,** Vitamin E activity and metabolism of N-methyltocopheramines, *Biochemistry,* 6, 2153, 1967.

75. **Scott, M. L.,** Advances in our understanding of vitamin E, *Fed. Proc. Fed. Am. Soc. Exp. Biol.,* 39, 2736, 1980.

76. **Threlfall, D. R.,** The biosynthesis of vitamin E and K and related compounds, *Vitam. Hormones N.Y.,* 29, 153, 1971.

77. **Hollander, D.,** Intestinal absorption of vitamins A, E, D and K, *J. Lab. Clin. Med.,* 97, 449, 1981.

78. **Bieri, J. G. and Farrell, P. M.,** Vitamin E, *Vitam. Hormones N.Y.,* 34, 31, 1976.

79. **Simon, E. J., Eisengart, A., Sundhein, L., and Milhorat, A. T.,** The metabolism of vitamin E. II. Purification and characterization of urinary metabolites of α-tocopherol, *J. Biol. Chem.,* 221, 807, 1956.

80. **Roberts, H. J.,** Perspective on vitamin E as therapy, *JAMA,* 246, 129, 1981.

81. **Karrer, P., Geiger, A., Legler, R., Ruegger, A., and Salomon, H.,** Über die Isolierung des α-phyllochinons (Vitamin K aus Alfalfa) sowie über dessen Entdeckungsgeschichte, *Helv. Chim. Acta,* 22, 1464, 1939.

82. **Binkley, S. B., MacCorquodale, D. W., Thayer, S. A., and Doisy, E. A.,** The isolation of vitamin K1, *J. Biol. Chem.,* 130, 219, 1939.

83. **McKee, R. W., Binkley, S. B., Thayer, S. A., MacCorquodale, D. W., and Doisy, E. A.,** The isolation of vitamin K2, *J. Biol. Chem.,* 131, 327, 1939.

84. **Binkley, S. B., MacCorquodale, D. W., Cheney, L. C., Thayer, S. A., McKee, R. W., and Doisy, E. A.,** Derivatives of vitamins K1 and K2, *J. Am. Chem. Soc.,* 61, 1612, 1939.

85. **Binkley, S. B., Cheney, L. C., Holcomb, W. F., McKee, R. W., Thayer, S. A., MacCorquodale, D. W., and Doisy, E. A.,** The constitution and synthesis of vitamin K1, *J. Am. Chem. Soc.,* 61, 2558, 1939.

86. **Fieser, L. F., Tishler, M., and Sampson, W. L.,** Vitamin K activity and structure, *J. Biol. Chem.,* 137, 659, 1941.

87. **Arora, R. B. and Mathur, C. H.,** Relationship between structure and anticoagulant activity of coumarin derivatives, *Br. J. Pharmacol.,* 20, 29, 1963.

88. **Davie, F. W. and Fujikawa, K.,** Basic mechanisms in blood coagulation, *Annu. Rev. Biochem.,* 44, 799, 1975.

89. **Suttie, J. W. and Jackson, C. M.,** Prothrombin structure, activation and biosynthesis, *Physiol. Rev.,* 57, 1, 1977.

90. **Suttie, J. W.,** The metabolic role of vitamin K, *Fed. Proc. Fed. Am. Soc. Exp. Biol.,* 39, 2730, 1980.

91. **Uotila, L. and Suttie, J. W.,** Characterization of vitamin K-dependent carboxylase from the livers of the adult ox and dicoumarol-treated calf, *Biochem. J.,* 201, 249, 1982.

92. **Dansette, P. and Azerad, R.,** A new intermediate in naphthoquinone and menaquinone biosynthesis, *Biochem. Biophys. Res. Commun.,* 40, 1090, 1970.

93. **Shearer, M. J., McBurney, A., and Barkhan, P.,** Studies on the absorption and metabolism of phylloquinone (Vitamin K) in man, *Vitam. Hormones N.Y.,* 32, 513, 1974.

94. **Funk, C.,** Substance from yeast and certain foodstuffs which prevents polyneuritis, *Br. Med. J.,* II, 787, 1912.

95. **McCollum, E. V. and Kennedy, C.,** The dietary factors operating in the production of polyneuritis, *J. Biol. Chem.,* 24, 491, 1916.

96. **Williams, R. R., Waterman, R. E., and Keresztesy, J. C.,** Larger yields of crystalline antineuritic vitamin, *J. Am. Chem. Soc.,* 56, 1187, 1934.

97. **Williams, R. R.,** Structure of vitamin B1, *J. Am. Chem. Soc.,* 58, 1063, 1936.

98. **Williams, R. R. and Cline, J. K.,** Synthesis of vitamin B1, *J. Am. Chem. Soc.,* 58, 1504, 1936.

99. **Buchman, E. R.,** Studies of crystalline vitamin B1. XIV. Sulfite cleavage. IV. The thiazole half, *J. Am. Chem. Soc.,* 58, 1803, 1936.

100. **Sanstead, H. H.,** Clinical manifestations of certain classical deficiency diseases, in *Modern Nutrition in Health and Disease,* 6th ed., Goodhart, R. S. and Shils, M. E., Eds., Lea and Febiger, Philadelphia, 1981, chap. 23.

101. **Dreyfus, P. M.,** Neurologic disease and nutrition, *Resident Staff Physician,* August 1981, p. 77.
102. **Matsuda, T. and Cooper, J. R.,** The separation and determination of thiamin and its phosphate esters in brain, *Anal. Biochem.,* 117, 203, 1981.
103. **Cerecedo, L. R.,** Thiamin antagonists, *Am. J. Clin. Nutr.,* 3, 273, 1955.
104. **Rogers, E. F.,** Thiamin antagonists, *Meth. Enzymol.,* 18, 245, 1970.
105. **Wittliff, J. L. and Airth, R. L.,** Thiaminase I, *Meth. Enzymol.,* 18, 229, 1970.
106. **Brown, G. M. and Williamson, M.,** Biosynthesis of riboflavin, folic acid, thiamin and pantothenic acid, *Adv. Enzymol. Rel. Areas Mol. Biol.,* 53, 345, 1982.
107. **White, R. H.,** Incorporation of 4-amino-5-hydroxymethylpyrimidine into thiamin by microorganisms, *Science,* 214, 797, 1981.
108. **Neal, R. A. and Sanberlick, H. E.,** Thiamin, in *Modern Nutrition in Health and Disease,* 6th ed., Goodhart, R. S. and Shils, M. E., Eds., Lea and Febiger, Philadelphia, 1981, 191.
109. **Iber, F. L., Blass, J. P., Brin, M., and Leavy, C. M.,** Thiamin in the elderly — relation to alcoholism and to neurological degenerative disease, *Am. J. Clin. Nutr.,* 36, 1067, 1982.
110. **Hauge, S. M. and Carrick, C. W.,** A differentiation between the water-soluble growth-promoting and anti-neuritic substances, *J. Biol. Chem.,* 69, 403, 1926.
111. **Salmon, W. D., Guerrant, N. B., and Hays, I. M.,** The effect of hydrogen ion concentration upon adsorption of the active factors of vitamin B complex by fuller's earth, *J. Biol. Chem.,* 80, 91, 1928.
112. **Kuhn, R., György, P., and Wagner-Jauregg, T.,** Über eine neue Klasse von Naturfarbstoffen, *Ber. Dtsch. Chem. Ges.,* 66, 317, 1933.
113. **Karrer, P., Schöpp, K., Benz, F., and Pfaehler, K.,** Synthesen von Falvinen III, *Helv. Chim. Acta,* 18, 69, 1935.
114. **Karrer, P., Schöpp, K., and Benz, F.,** Synthesen von Falvinen IV, *Helv. Chim. Acta,* 18, 426, 1935.
115. **Kuhn, R., Reinemund, K., Wegand, F., and Ströbele, R.,** Über die Synthese des Lactoflavins (Vitamin B2), *Ber. Dtsch. Chem. Ges.,* 68, 1765, 1935.
116. **Horwitt, M. K.,** Riboflavin, in *Modern Nutrition in Health and Disease,* 6th ed., Goodhart, R. S. and Shils, M. E., Eds., Lea and Febiger, Philadelphia, 1980, 197.
117. **Lambooy, J. P.,** Riboflavin antagonists, *Am. J. Clin. Nutr.,* 3, 282, 1955.
118. **Williams, R. J., Eakin, R. E., Beerstecher, E., and Shive, W.,** *The Biochemistry of B Vitamins,* Reinhold, New York, 1950, 669.
119. **Wagner-Jauregg, T.,** in *The Vitamins. Chemistry, Physiology, Pathology,* Vol. 3, Sebrell, W. H. Jr. and Harris, R. S., Eds., Academic Press, New York, 1954, 325.
120. **Al-Hassan, S. S., Kulick, R. J., Livingstone, D. B., Suckling, C. J., Wood, H. C. S., Wrigglesworth, R., and Ferone, R.,** Specific enzyme inhibitors in vitamin biosynthesis. Part 3. The synthesis and inhibitory properties of some substrates and transition state analogues of riboflavin synthase, *J. Chem. Soc. Perkin Trans.,* 1, 2645, 1980.
121. **Akiyama, T., Selhub, J., and Rosenberg, I. H.,** FMN phosphatase and FAD pyrophosphatase in rat intestinal brush borders: role in intestinal absorption of dietary riboflavin, *J. Nutr.,* 112, 263, 1982.
122. **Miller, M. S., Bruch, R. C., and White, H. B., III,** Carbohydrate compositional effects on tissue distribution of chicken riboflavin-binding protein, *Biochim. Biophys. Acta,* 715, 126, 1982.
123. **Kumosinski, T. F., Pessen, H., and Farrell, H. M., Jr.,** Structure and mechanism of action of riboflavin-binding protein: small-angle x-ray scattering, sedimentation, and circular dichroism studies on the holo- and apoproteins, *Arch. Biochem. Biophys.,* 214, 714, 1982.
124. **Christensen, S.,** The biological fate of riboflavin in mammals, *Acta Pharmacol. Toxicol.,* 32(Suppl.2), 1, 1973.
125. **Syndenstricker, V. P.,** The history of pellagra, its recognition as a disorder of nutrition and its conquest, *Am. J. Clin. Nutr.,* 6, 409, 1958.
126. **Horwitt, M. K.,** Niacin, in *Modern Nutrition in Health and Disease,* 6th ed., Goodhart, R. S. and Shils, M. E., Eds., Lea and Febiger, Philadelphia, 1980, 204.
127. **Mattews, D. M.,** Absorption of water-soluble vitamins, *Br. Med. Bull.,* 23, 258, 1967.
128. **Sauberlich, H. E. and Canham, J. E.,** Vitamin B6, in *Modern Nutrition in Health and Disease,* 6th ed., Goodhart, R. S. and Shils, M. E., Eds., Lea and Febiger, Philadelphia, 1980, 216.
129. **Umbreit, W. W.,** Vitamin B6 antagonists, *Am. J. Clin. Nutr.,* 3, 291, 1955.
130. **Makino, K. and Koike, M.,** Competitive inhibition of pyridoxal phosphate action by toxopyrimidine phosphate in the tyrosine decarboxylase system (anticoenzyme), *Enzymologia,* 17, 157, 1954; as cited in *Chem. Abstr.,* 49, 11069, 1955.
131. **Hill, R. E., Gupta, R. N., Rowell, F. J., and Spenser, I. D.,** Biosynthesis of pyridoxine, *J. Am. Chem. Soc.,* 93, 518, 1971.
132. **Middleton, H. M., III,** Characterization of pyridoxal 5'-phosphate disappearance from in vivo perfused segments of rat jejunum, *J. Nutr.,* 112, 269, 1982.

133. **Lui, A., Lumeng, L., and Li, T.-K.,** Metabolism of vitamin B6 in rat liver mitochondria, *J. Biol. Chem.,* 256, 6041, 1981.

134. **Pfiffner, J. J., Binkley, S. B., Bloom, E. S., and O'Dell, B. L.,** Isolation and characterization of vitamin Bc from liver and yeast. Occurrence of an acid-labile chick antianemia factor in liver, *J. Am. Chem. Soc.,* 69, 1476, 1947.

135. **Waller, C. W., Hutchings, B. L., Mowat, J. H., Stokstad, E. L. R., Boothe, J. H., Angier, R. B., Semb, J., SubbaRow, Y., Cosulich, D. B., Fahrenbach, M. J., Hultquist, M. E., Kuh, E., Northey, E. H., Seeger, D. R., Sickels, J. P., and Smith, J. M., Jr.,** Synthesis of pteroylglutamic acid (liver L. casei factor) and pteroic acid. I, *J. Am. Chem. Soc.,* 70, 19, 1948.

136. **Herbert, V., Colman, N., and Jacob, E.,** Folic acid and vitamin B12, in *Modern Nutrition in Health and Disease,* 6th ed., Goodhart, R. S. and Shils, M. E., Eds., Lea and Febiger, Philadelphia, 1980, 229.

137. **Herbert, V. and Das, K. C.,** The role of vitamin B12 and folic acid in hemato- and other cell-poisis, *Vitam. Hormones N.Y.,* 34, 1, 1976.

138. **Herbert, V.,** Folic acid deficiency in man, *Vitam. Hormones N.Y.,* 26, 525, 1968.

139. **Blakley, R. L.,** *The Biochemistry of Folic Acid and Related Pteridines, Front. Biol.,* Vol. 13, Neuberger, A. and Tatum, E. L., Eds., North Holland, Amsterdam, 1969, 8.

140. **Wood, H. C. S.,** Specific inhibitors of the enzymes of vitamin biosynthesis, *Chem. Ind. (London),* 150, 1981.

141. **Jukes, T. H. and Broquist, H. P.,** Sulfonamides and folic acid antagonists, in *Metabolic Inhibitors, A Comprehensive Treatise,* Vol. I, Hochster, R. M. and Quastel, J. H., Eds., Academic Press, New York, 1963, chap. 13.

142. **Stokstad, E. L. R.,** in *The Vitamins. Chemistry, Physiology, Pathology,* Vol. 3, Sebrell, W. H., Jr. and Harris, R. S., Eds., Academic Press, New York, 1954, 142.

143. **Selhub, J. and Rosenberg, I. H.,** Folate transport in isolated brush border membrane vesicles from rat intestine, *J. Biol. Chem.,* 256, 4489, 1981.

144. **Rubin, M. and Bird, H. R.,** A chick-growth factor in cow manure. V. Relation to quantity and quality of soybean-oil meal in the diet, *J. Nutr.,* 34, 233, 1947; as cited in *Chem. Abstr.,* 41, 6943, 1947.

145. **Minot, G. R. and Murphy, W. P.** Treatment of pernicious anemia by a special diet, *JAMA,* 87, 470, 1926; as cited in Ref. 2.

146. **Maugh, T. H. II,** Vitamin B12: after 25 years the first synthesis, *Science,* 179, 266, 1973.

147. **Holvey, D. N., Ed.,** *The Merck Manual of Diagnosis and Therapy,* 12 ed., Merck, Sharp and Dohme, Rahway, N.J., 1972, 258.

148. **Sennett, C., Rosenberg, L. E., and Mellman, I. S.,** Transmembrane transport of cobalamine in prokaryotic and eukaryotic cells, *Annu. Rev. Biochem.,* 50, 1053, 1981.

149. **Brumm, P. J. and Friedmann, H. C.,** Succinylactone pyrrole, a powerful inhibitor of vitamin B12 biosynthesis: effect on δ-aminolevulinic acid dehydratase, *Biochem. Biophys. Res. Commun.,* 102, 854, 1981.

150. **Katzen, H. M. and Buchanan, J. M.,** Enzymatic synthesis of the methyl group of methionine. VIII. Repression-derepression, purification and properties of 5,10-methylenetetrahydrofolate reductase from Escherichia coli, *J. Biol. Chem.,* 240, 825, 1965.

151. **Katsuhiko, F., Hagasaki, T., and Huennekens, F. M.,** Accumulation of 5-methyltetrahydrofolate in cobalamin-deficient L1210 mouse leukemia cells, *J. Biol. Chem.,* 257, 2144, 1982.

152. **Pezacka, E. and Walerych, W.,** Biosynthesis of vitamin B12. I. Role of the ribosomal proteins in vitamin B12 biosynthesis, *Biochim. Biophys. Acta,* 678, 300, 1981.

153. **Seetharam, B., Bagur, S. S., and Alpers, D. H.,** Isolation and characterization of proteolytically derived ileal receptor for intrinsic factor — cobalamine, *J. Biol. Chem.,* 257, 183, 1982.

154. **Williams, R. J., Lyman, C. M., Goodyear, G. H., Truesdail, J. H., and Holiday, D.,** "Pantothenic acid", a growth determinant of universal biological occurrence, *J. Am. Chem. Soc.,* 55, 2912, 1933.

155. **Williams, R. J., Weinstock, H. H., Jr., Rohrman, E., Truesdail, J. H., Mitchell, H. K., and Meyer, C. E.,** Pantothenic acid. III. Analysis and determination of constituent groups, *J. Am. Chem. Soc.,* 61, 454, 1939.

156. **Weinstock, H. H., Jr., Mitchell, H. K., Pratt, E. F., and Williams, R. J.,** Pantothenic acid. IV. Formation of β-alanine by cleavage, *J. Am. Chem. Soc.,* 61, 1421, 1939.

157. **Mitchell, H. K., Weinstock, H. H., Jr., Snell, E. E., Stanberry, S. R., and Williams, R. J.,** Pantothenic acid. V. Evidence for structure of non-β-alanine portion, *J. Am. Chem. Soc.,* 62, 1776, 1940.

158. **Stiller, E. T., Keresztesy, J. C., and Finkelstein, J.,** Pantothenic acid. VI. The isolation and structure of the lactone moiety, *J. Am. Chem. Soc.,* 62, 1779, 1940.

159. **Stiller, E. T., Harris, S. A., Finkelstein, J., Keresztesy, J. C., and Folkers, K.,** Pantothenic acid. VIII. The total synthesis of pure pantothenic acid, *J. Am. Chem. Soc.,* 62, 1785, 1940.

160. **Sauberlich, H. E.,** Pantothenic acid, in *Modern Nutrition in Health and Disease,* 6th ed., Goodhart, R. S. and Shils, M. E., Eds., Lea and Febiger, Philadelphia, 1980, 209.

161. **Bird, O. D., Wittle, E. L., Thompson, R. Q., and McGlohon, V. M.,** Pantothenic acid antagonists, *Am. J. Clin. Nutr.*, 3, 298, 1955.
162. **Vagelos, P. R.,** Vitamins and their carrier proteins in fatty acid synthesis, *Harvey Lect. Ser.*, 70, 21, 1976.
163. **Harris, R. S. and Györgi, P.,** Biotin, in *The Vitamins. Chemistry, Physiology, Pathology*, Vol. I, Sebrell, W. H., Jr. and Harris, R. S., Eds., Academic Press, New York, 1954, 526.
164. **Harris, S. A., Wolf, D. E., Mozingo, R., Anderson, R. C., Arth, G. E., Easton, N. R., Heyl, D., Wilson, A. N., and Folkers, K.,** Biotin II. Synthesis of biotin, *J. Am. Chem. Soc.*, 66, 1756, 1944.
165. **Wolf, D. E., Mozingo, R., Harris, S. A., Anderson, R. C., and Folkers, K.,** Biotin VI. Resolution of dl biotin, *J. Am. Chem. Soc.*, 67, 2100, 1945.
166. **Appel, J. A. and Briggs, G. M.,** Biotin, in *Modern Nutrition in Health and Disease*, 6th ed., Goodhart, R. S. and Shils, M. E., Eds., Lea and Febiger, Philadelphia, 1980, 274.
167. **Bayer, E. A. and Wilcheck, M.,** The use of the avidin-biotin complex as a tool in molecular biology, *Meth. Biochem. Anal.*, 26, 1, 1980.
168. **Roth, K. S.,** Biotin in clinical medicine. A review, *Am. J. Clin. Nutr.*, 34, 1967, 1981.
169. **Hodges, R. E.,** Ascorbic acid, in *Modern Nutrition in Health and Disease*, 6th ed., Goodhart, R. S. and Shils, M. E., Eds., Lea and Febiger, Philadelphia, 1980, 259.
170. **Szent-Györgi, A.,** Observations on the function of peroxidase systems and the chemistry of the adrenal cortex. Description of a new carbohydrate derivative, *Biochem. J.*, 22, 1387, 1928.
171. **Richstein, T., Grüssner, A., and Oppenauer, R.,** Synthese der d- und l- Ascorbinsäure (C-Vitamin), *Helv. Chim. Acta*, 16, 1019, 1933.
172. **Hornig, D.,** Requirement of vitamin C in man, *Trends Pharmacol. Sci.*, 3, 294, 1982.
173. **Smith, F.,** in *The Vitamins. Chemistry, Physiology, Pathology* Vol. 1, Sebrell, W. H., Jr. and Harris, R. S., Eds., Academic Press, New York, 1954, 180.
174. **Mapson, L. W.,** in *The Vitamins. Chemistry, Physiology, Pathology*, Vol. 1, Sebrell, W. H., Jr. and Harris, R. S., Eds., Academic Press, New York, 1954, 223.
175. **Tajima, S. and Pinell, S. R.,** Regulation of collagen synthesis by ascorbic acid. Ascorbic acid increases type I procollagen mRNA, *Biochem. Biophys. Res. Commun.*, 106, 632, 1982.
176. **Sato, P. and Udenfriend, S.,** Studies on ascorbic acid related to the genetic basis of scurvy, *Vitam. Hormones N.Y.*, 36, 33, 1978.
177. **Burns, J. J.,** Biosynthesis of L-ascorbic acid; basic defect in scurvy, *Am. J. Med.*, 26, 740, 1959.
178. **Stevenson, N.,** Active transport of L-ascorbic acid in the human ileum, *Gastroenterology*, 67, 952, 1974.
179. **Streeter, M. L. and Rosso, P.,** Transport mechanisms for ascorbic acid in the human placenta, *Am. J. Clin. Nutr.*, 34, 1706, 1981.
180. **Burns, J. J., Burch, H. B., and King, C. G.,** The metabolism of 1-C14-ascorbic acid in guinea pigs, *J. Biol. Chem.*, 191, 501, 1951.
181. **Hellman, L. and Burns, J. J.,** Metabolism of L-ascorbic acid in 1-C14 in man, *J. Biol. Chem.*, 230, 923, 1958.
182. **Briggs, M. H., Garcia-Webb, P., and Davies, P.,** Urinary oxalate and vitamin C supplements, *Lancet*, II, 201, 1973.
183. **Moser, U. and Hornig, D.,** High intakes of vitamin C: a contributor to oxalate formation in man?, *Trends Pharmacol. Sci.*, 3, 480, 1982.
184. **Pirzio-Biroli, G., Bothwell, T. H., and Finch, C. A.,** Iron absorption. II. The absorption of radioiron administered with a standard meal in man, *J. Lab. Clin. Med.*, 51, 37, 1958.
185. **Beutler, E.,** Iron, in *Modern Nutrition in Health and Disease*, 6th ed., Goodhart, R. S. and Shils, M. E., Eds., Lea and Febiger, Philadelphia, 1980, 324.
186. **Windholz, M., Ed.,** *The Merck Index*, 9th ed., Merck and Co., Rahway, N.J., 1976.
187. **Newton, D. W. and Kluza, R. B.,** pKa values of medicinal compounds in pharmacy practice, *Drug Intell. Clin. Pharm.*, 12, 546, 1978.
188. **Dean, J. A., Ed.,** *Lange's Handbook of Chemistry*, 12th ed., McGraw-Hill, New York, 1979, 5.
189. **Lepkovsky, A.,** Pathothenic acid chemistry, in *The Vitamins. Chemistry, Physiology, Pathology*, Vol. 2, Sebrell, W. H., Jr. and Harris, R. S., Eds., Academic Press, New York, 1954, 593.

INDEX

S